AF903257

Hepato-Pancreatico Biliary Imaging

Binit Sureka
Editor

Hepato-Pancreatico Biliary Imaging

Keeping it Clear and Simple

Springer

Editor
Binit Sureka
Department of Diagnostic & Interventional Radiology
All India Institute of Medical Sciences
Jodhpur, Rajasthan, India

ISBN 978-981-95-1698-8 ISBN 978-981-95-1699-5 (eBook)
https://doi.org/10.1007/978-981-95-1699-5

© The Editor(s) (if applicable) and The Author(s), under exclusive license to Springer Nature Singapore Pte Ltd. 2025, corrected publication 2026

This work is subject to copyright. All rights are solely and exclusively licensed by the Publisher, whether the whole or part of the material is concerned, specifically the rights of translation, reprinting, reuse of illustrations, recitation, broadcasting, reproduction on microfilms or in any other physical way, and transmission or information storage and retrieval, electronic adaptation, computer software, or by similar or dissimilar methodology now known or hereafter developed.
The use of general descriptive names, registered names, trademarks, service marks, etc. in this publication does not imply, even in the absence of a specific statement, that such names are exempt from the relevant protective laws and regulations and therefore free for general use.
The publisher, the authors and the editors are safe to assume that the advice and information in this book are believed to be true and accurate at the date of publication. Neither the publisher nor the authors or the editors give a warranty, expressed or implied, with respect to the material contained herein or for any errors or omissions that may have been made. The publisher remains neutral with regard to jurisdictional claims in published maps and institutional affiliations.

This Springer imprint is published by the registered company Springer Nature Singapore Pte Ltd.
The registered company address is: 152 Beach Road, #21-01/04 Gateway East, Singapore 189721, Singapore

If disposing of this product, please recycle the paper.

Foreword

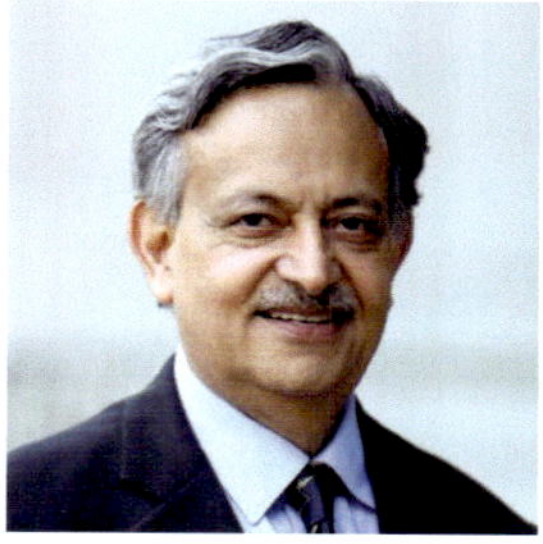

High-quality imaging and its proper interpretation is the corner stone of precise clinical diagnosis. Computed Tomography (CT) and Magnetic resonance Imaging (MRI) are contributing immensely in the diagnosis and follow-up of hepatobiliary and pancreatic diseases. The most appropriate investigation for each pathology or organ to be examined must be selected by the clinicians and the advantages and disadvantages of each investigation appreciated by the radiologist in order to provide holistic cost-effective management.

MRI of the abdomen especially in keeping focus on liver, biliary, and pancreatic tumors plays a vital role in imaging, and radiologists require certain level of advanced training in interpreting these pathologies as there is limited exposure in MRI of the abdomen during residency training.

This book compiled by Prof. Binit Sureka contains 21 chapters which are highly relevant to the abdominal radiologists, interventional radiologists, radiology residents, and also to the hepatologists and transplant surgeons. Important day-to-day challenges in reporting liver vascular anatomical variations, common and uncommon liver, biliary, and pancreatic pathologies, and basics on hardware in interventional radiology are covered in detail by distinguished national and international experts.

I had the pleasure of having Prof. Sureka at the Institute of Liver and Biliary Sciences (ILBS, New Delhi). While gaining expertise in hepatopancreatobiliary diseases, he also contributed immensely to the growth of the radiology services at ILBS. The selection of the topics for the book reveals his deep understanding on the subject. There is no doubt that the book will be a valuable addition to possess by the clinicians dealing with hepato-pancreatico biliary pathologies and to all the radiologists who want to make career in abdominal imaging.

Director, Institute of Liver & Biliary Sciences
New Delhi, India

Shiv Kumar Sarin, DM

Foreword

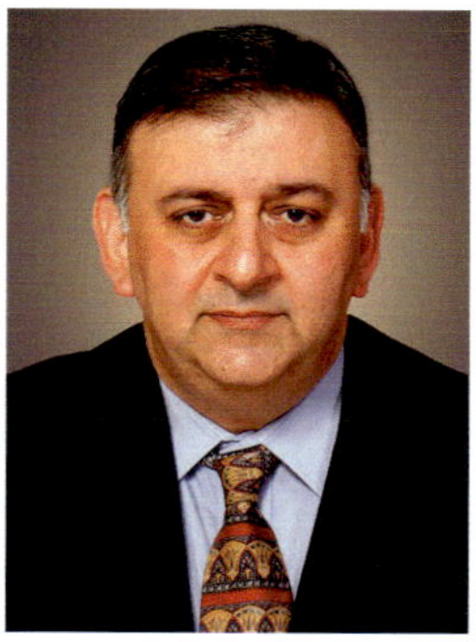

It is both a privilege and a pleasure to write the foreword to this remarkable work. This book was conceptualized in 2021 but got delayed due to the COVID pandemic.

Dr. Sureka has a brilliant and exceptional academic record. I am deeply impressed by the academic deeds and contributions made by Dr. Binit. Having had the opportunity to watch the author grow through his medical journey as a faculty, I have been consistently impressed by his keen interest in abdominal radiology. This book is a testament to those qualities.

This well-written educational book entitled *Hepato-Pancreatico Biliary Imaging* is not just a book for abdominal radiologists, it is a book for general radiologists, surgeons, and students of radiology and surgery, anyone interested in the imaging of the liver, bile ducts, and pancreas.

I commend the author for undertaking this endeavor and for contributing meaningfully to the growing dialogue between the radiologists and the surgeons. I am confident that readers will find this work engaging and enlightening.

Vice Chancellor
Atal Bihari Vajpayee
Medical University
Lucknow, Uttar Pradesh, India

Sanjeev Misra, MS, MCh, FAMS, DSc.

Foreword

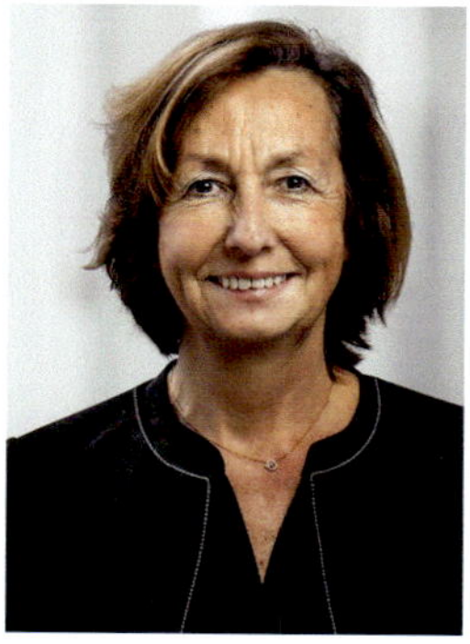

This well-written educational book entitled *Hepato-Pancreatico Biliary Imaging* published by Springer consists of 21 chapters on medical imaging of the liver, bile ducts, and pancreas, written by internationally renowned experts in their field. There is a clear logic to organizing a book on these three organs, not only because of their anatomy and interconnection but also because identical processes frequently affect the liver, bile ducts, and pancreas, such as inflammation, fibrosis, tumors, and trauma.

This book also covers the anatomy of the liver, bile ducts, and pancreas, as well as the anatomical variations that all radiologists need to know, as some of them have significant consequences. Finally, it addresses important topics for improving patient care: the role of PET-CT, surgical techniques, and interventional radiology.

The text is well illustrated with numerous tables and figures that aid understanding and memorization.

Dr. Binit Sureka not only did a remarkable job coordinating this book but also contributed to the writing of three chapters. It is a useful textbook for radiologists in training and radiologists interested in subspecializing in abdominal radiology.

Department of Radiology
Beaujon Hospital, Université, Paris Cité
Paris, France

Valérie Vilgrain

Foreword

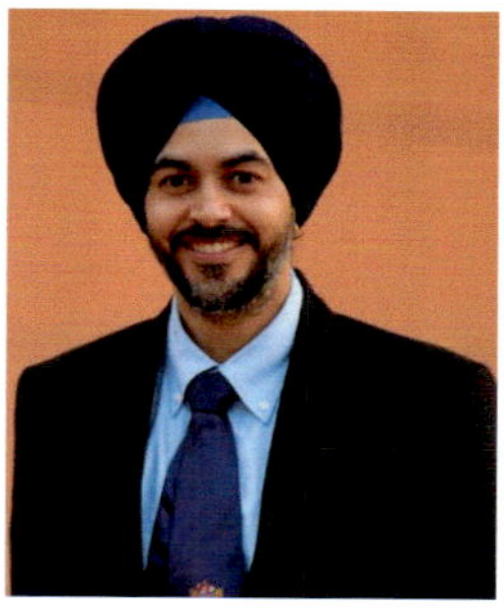

It is my privilege to write a foreword for this book.

The liver and biliary system present some of the most complex and diagnostically challenging regions in medical imaging. Hepatobiliary imaging has evolved into a critical subspecialty within radiology, integrating advances in cross-sectional imaging, contrast-enhanced techniques, functional studies, and image-guided interventions to aid in the diagnosis and management of a wide spectrum of hepatic and biliary diseases.

This book arrives at a time when the demand for precision in hepatobiliary diagnosis has never been greater. From the early detection of hepatic malignancies and evaluation of diffuse liver disease to the intricate anatomy of the biliary tree in post-surgical patients, high-quality imaging plays a central role in guiding clinical care.

The authors have brought together a wealth of knowledge and experience to craft a resource that is both comprehensive and accessible. Their focus on clinical relevance, imaging-pathologic correlation, and practical decision-making will serve learners and practitioners alike—radiologists, hepatologists, surgeons, and trainees—who are engaged in the care of patients with liver and biliary disorders.

The sections on interventional radiology cover all the important aspects involved in planning and performing a minimally invasive image-guided procedure in this region and would be of immense value to both practicing and trainee interventional radiologists.

This text not only reflects the current state of the art in hepatobiliary imaging but also highlights the importance of collaboration across specialties. It is a valuable contribution to the field and an essential reference for anyone seeking to deepen their expertise in this rapidly advancing area.

I congratulate the editors and authors for this effort of theirs and wish them well for their future academic endeavors.

Pushpinder S. Khera, MD, FRCR
Professor & Head, Department of Diagnostic and Interventional Radiology, All India Institute of Medical Sciences
Jodhpur, Rajasthan, India

Preface

Cross-sectional imaging has made a significant impact in the field of modern medicine and diagnostic radiology, offering unprecedented clarity and depth in visualizing anatomical structures and pathological processes. The new generation CT scanners and advanced MRI sequences help the radiologists provide more accurate anatomical details and diagnoses and guide minimally invasive interventions contributing to better patient care.

This book was conceived in 2021 but got slightly delayed due to COVID pandemic. From my experience as a teacher, I find many radiologists are unable to answer many key questions asked by the surgeons and hepatologists. This book is a comprehensive guide to the principles and applications of cross-sectional imaging. The chapters in the book will help in bridging the gap between theoretical understanding and support clinical decision-making by providing detailed explanations, high-quality images, and practical insights drawn from real-world case scenarios. Each chapter is relevant for the radiologists in writing relevant findings in terms of "what the clinician wants."

As imaging continues to play an ever-growing role in modern medicine, proficiency in cross-sectional modalities is no longer optional—it is foundational. We hope this book will serve not only as a learning tool but also as a long-term reference for those committed to excellence in abdominal radiology.

I extend my gratitude to all the contributors, mentors, and colleagues who have supported this project, and most importantly, to the readers who continually push the boundaries of learning and practicing medicine.

Additional Professor, Department of
Diagnostic & Interventional Radiology
All India Institute of Medical Sciences
Jodhpur, Rajasthan, India

Binit Sureka, MD, MBA
DNB, FICR, FESGAR

Acknowledgements

This book would not have been possible without the guidance, support, and blessings of the stalwarts in the field of Hepatology, Abdominal radiology, GI surgery, and Oncosurgery.

I am extremely thankful to

Prof. SK Sarin, Director, Institute of Liver & Biliary Sciences, New Delhi
Prof. Sanjeev Misra, Vice Chancellor, Atal Bihari Vajpayee Medical University, UP and Founder Director AIIMS Jodhpur
Prof. Roberto Pozzi Mucelli, University of Verona, Italy
Prof. Riccardo Manfredi, University of Rome, Italy
Prof. Giulia Zamboni, University of Verona, Italy
Prof. Mirko D'Onofrio, University of Verona, Italy
Prof. Jeong Min Lee, Seoul National University Hospital, South Korea
Prof. Jae Young Lee, Seoul National University Hospital, South Korea
Prof. Valérie Vilgrain, Beaujon Hospital, Clichy, France
Prof. Maxime Ronot, Beaujon Hospital, Clichy, France

I wish to express my sincere thanks to my colleagues Dr. Pushpinder Singh Khera, Dr. Pawan Garg, Dr. Taruna Yadav, Dr. Sarbesh Tiwari, Dr. Rengarajan, Dr. Vaibhav Varshney, Dr. Subhash Soni, Dr. Ashish Agarwal, Dr. Chhagan Lal Birda. My earnest thanks to all the faculty members in the Institute and my teachers at PGIMER Chandigarh (Dr. N. Khandelwal, Dr. Mandeep Kang, Dr. Naveen Kalra, Dr. Anupam Lal) who have constantly motivated me to grow in my speciality.

I would like to express my deepest gratitude to my parents, Smt. Sulochana Sureka and Shree Jagdish Prasad Sureka, thank you for instilling in me the value of hard work and the courage to follow my passion.

The list would be incomplete without mentioning name of my wife, Dr. Aliza, and son, Viraaj, who have been supporting me constantly in my journey.

Contents

1 Anatomic Variations in the Biliary and Vascular Anatomy of the Liver

Binit Sureka and Siddhi Chawla

Table 1.1 Imaging modalities for the biliary tree

Modality	Advantages	Disadvantages
Magnetic resonance cholangiopancreatography (MRCP)	Non-invasive, anatomy well-delineated	Therapeutic procedures cannot be performed
Endoscopic retrograde cholangiopancreatography (ERCP)	Accurate	Invasive procedure
Intraoperative cholangiography	Highly Accurate	Used by surgeons while performing complex surgeries; not for routine use for diagnostic purpose

1.1 Biliary Tree

1.1.1 Imaging Protocol

There are various techniques available for the visualization of the biliary tree as mentioned in Table 1.1 [1].

1.2 Embryology

Intrahepatic bile ducts are formed from the bipotent progenitor cells and the ductal plate. Bile ducts are formed after remodeling which typically begins in the 12th week of gestation and is completed by the postnatal period [2]. Due to this process of development, the variations in the biliary tract are associated with variations in the portal vein.

1.3 Normal Anatomy

1.3.1 Intrahepatic Bile Ducts

The normal intrahepatic biliary anatomy consists of right and left hepatic ducts and their branches (Fig. 1.1). The right hepatic duct has two major branches—the right posterior duct and the right anterior duct [3]. The right posterior duct unites with the anterior sectoral duct medially to form the right hepatic duct. The left hepatic duct is formed by tributaries draining segments II-IV of the liver [1].

B. Sureka (✉) · S. Chawla
Department of Diagnostic & Interventional Radiology, AIIMS Jodhpur, Jodhpur, Rajasthan, India

© The Author(s), under exclusive license to Springer Nature Singapore Pte Ltd. 2025

B. Sureka (ed.), *Hepato-Pancreatico Biliary Imaging*, https://doi.org/10.1007/978-981-95-1699-5_1

1.3.2 Extrahepatic Bile Ducts

In almost 58% of the population, normal biliary anatomy is seen (Fig. 1.1) [6]. The right hepatic duct (RHD) and left hepatic duct (LHD) join to form the common hepatic duct (CHD). The bile duct draining the caudate lobe can join the origin of either LHD or RHD [3, 4]. The cystic duct joins the CHD and usually measures 2—4 cm in length and 1—5 mm in diameter.

1.4 Common and Uncommon Anatomic Variations

The drainage of the right posterior sectoral duct into the left hepatic duct is the most frequently encountered anatomic variation. Other variations are the right posterior sectoral duct draining into the CHD or the cystic duct and trifurcation anomaly (Fig. 1.2). Similarly, variations are encountered in the left hepatic duct—tri-confluence of segmental ducts, common trunk of segment III-IV duct, etc. [4, 5].

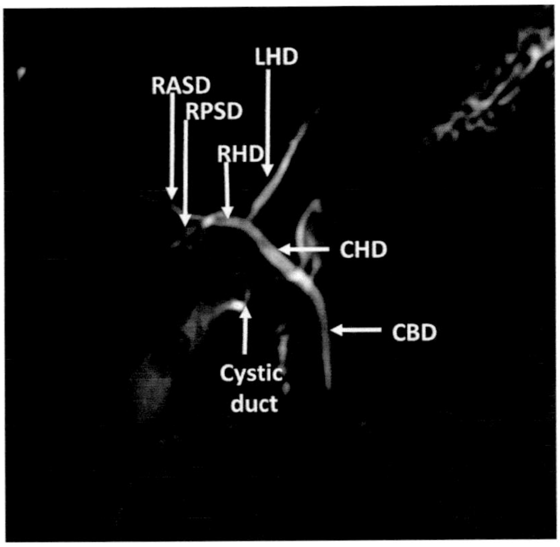

Fig. 1.1 Normal anatomy of the intra- and extrahepatic biliary ducts on MRCP

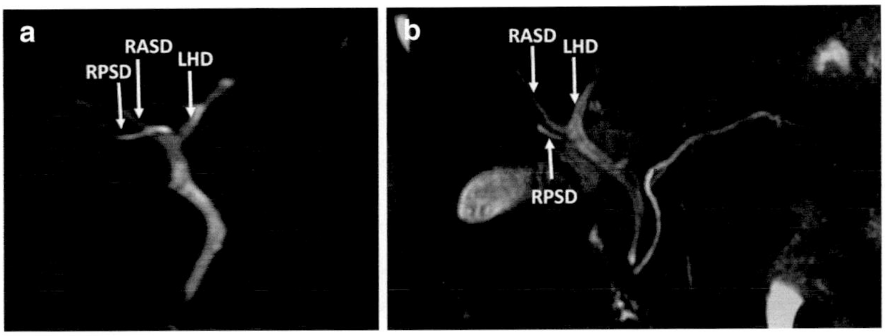

Fig. 1.2 MRCP images showing anatomical variations: (**a**) trifurcation anomaly and (**b**) aberrant drainage of RPSD into the CHD

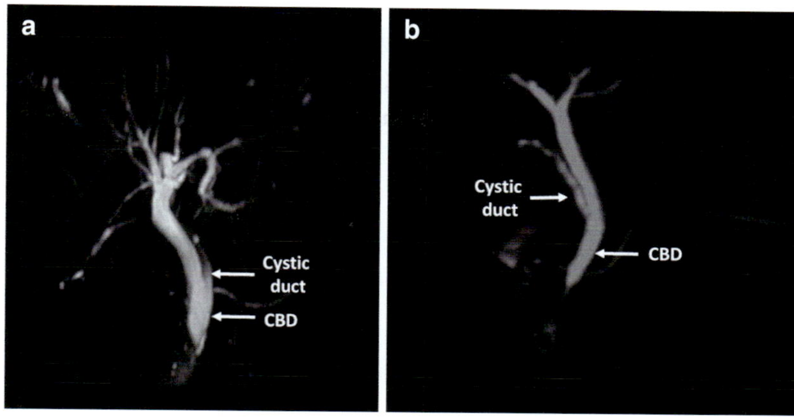

Fig. 1.3 MRCP images showing (**a**) medial insertion of cystic duct into CBD and (**b**) low insertion of cystic duct

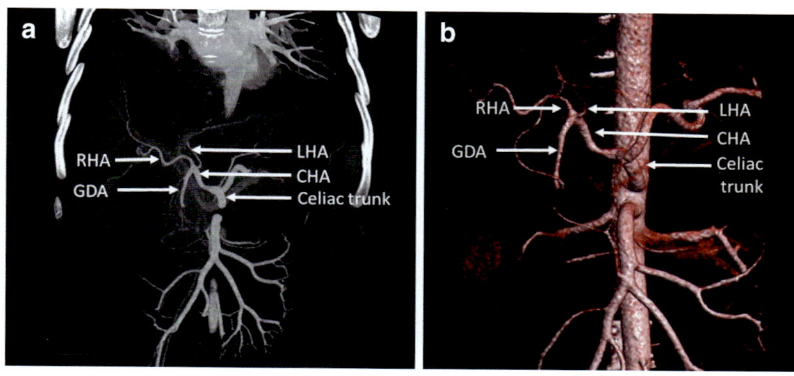

Fig. 1.4 (**a**) Coronal MIP and VRT. (**b**) Images show the normal arterial anatomy of CHA, RHA, and LHA

1.5 Aberrant and Accessory Bile Ducts

An aberrant bile duct is defined as any duct draining a certain segment of liver but has an anomalous confluence pattern. The cystohepatic duct is an aberrant duct which courses through the gallbladder fossa and drains into the cystic duct or into the right hepatic duct. The cholecystohepatic duct drains directly into the gallbladder. An accessory bile duct on the other hand is an additional bile duct draining a particular segment of the liver. Ducts of Luschka are blind ending ducts ~1–2 mm in diameter usually seen in the gallbladder fossa draining into the right hepatic duct [6].

1.6 Cystic Duct Variations

Parallel course of cystic duct, medial insertion of cystic duct, low or high insertion, and spiral course are a few anatomic variations encountered in cystic duct insertion (Fig. 1.3). If the length of the cystic duct is less than 5 mm, it is labeled as a short cystic duct, while if its diameter is > 5mm, it is labeled as a cystic duct hypertrophy [5].

1.7 Vascular Anatomy and Variations

1.7.1 Hepatic Artery

1.7.1.1 Normal Anatomy

The celiac axis arises from the aorta gives rise to the left gastric artery (LGA), the splenic artery, and the common hepatic artery (CHA). CHA divides into the proper hepatic artery (PHA) and the gastroduodenal artery (GDA). PHA divides into the left and right hepatic artery (Fig. 1.4). The middle hepatic artery (MHA) is the artery which supplies segment IV and can arise from either LHA or RHA [7].

Table 1.2 Hepatic arterial variants according to Michel's classification [7]

Type	Description
I	Right and left hepatic artery (RHA, LHA), middle hepatic artery origin from CHA
II	Replaced LHA from the left gastric artery (LGA)
III	Replaced RHA from the superior mesenteric artery (SMA)
IV	Replaced RHA and LHA
V	Accessory LHA from the LGA
VI	Accessory RHA
VII	Accessory both RHA and LHA
VIII	Replaced RHA and accessory LHA or replaced LHA and accessory RHA
IX	Entire hepatic trunk origin from SMA
X	Entire hepatic trunk origin from LGA

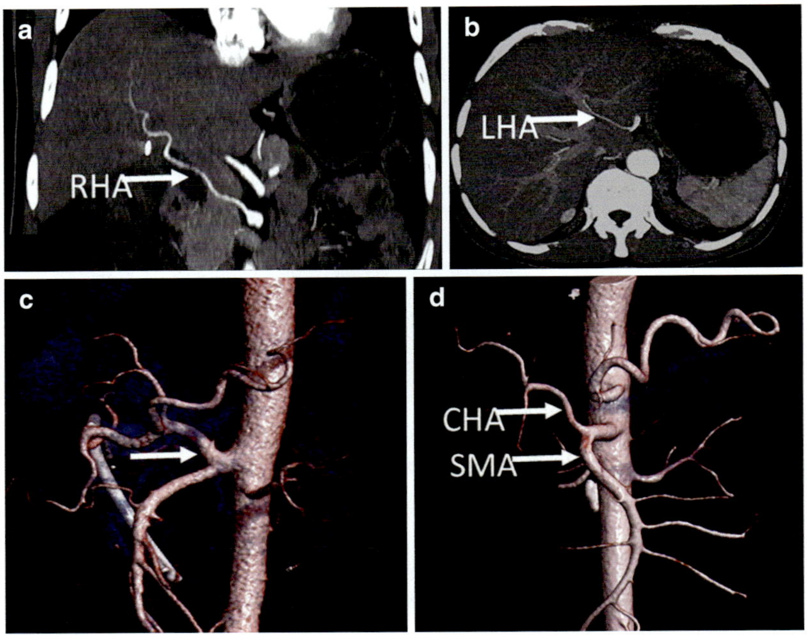

Fig. 1.5 Axial and coronal MIP and VRT images showing anatomical variations in hepatic artery: (**a**) replaced RHA from SMA, (**b**) replaced LHA from LGA, (**c**) common origin of celiac trunk and SMA, and (**d**) common origin of CHA and SMA

1.8 Common Anatomical Variations

Table 1.2 shows hepatic arterial variations defined by Michel et al [7]. The relevant anatomic variations from the surgeon's perspective are the replaced origin of the right hepatic artery from the superior mesenteric artery (SMA), the replaced left hepatic artery from the left gastric artery, the common origin of the celiac trunk and SMA, and the single trunk of the common hepatic artery and SMA (Fig. 1.5).

1.9 Hepatic Vein

1.9.1 Embryology

At around the fourth week of embryonic development, the ventral endodermal wall of the foregut begins to develop the liver bud which eventually forms the entire liver secondary to complex remodeling [8]. Between the 4th and 6th weeks, the cranial portions of the vitelline veins and umbilical veins are interrupted which form the hepatic sinusoids. The cranial part of the left vitelline vein atrophies and disappears by the fifth

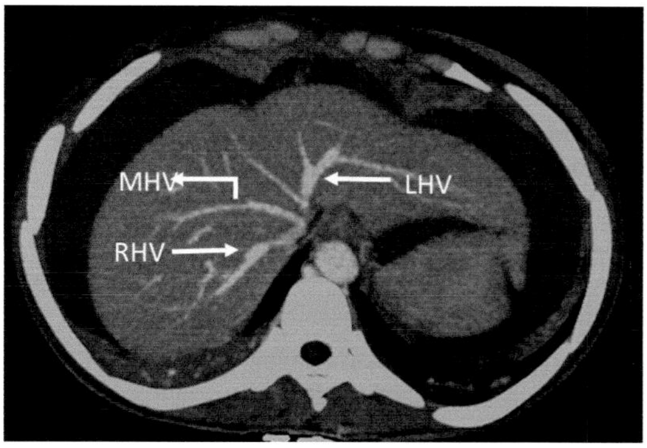

Fig. 1.6 Axial MIP images showing normal anatomy of hepatic veins draining into the inferior vena cava

week of development. The proximal right vitelline vein after fusion with the primary hepatic vein forms the three major hepatic veins [9].

1.10 Normal Anatomy

The hepatic veins are usually three in number (Fig. 1.6). About 75% of the blood supply to the liver is from the portal vein, and the remaining 25% is from the hepatic artery. The outflow from the liver is only through the hepatic veins [8]. Small accessory unnamed veins also can be present which drain directly into the inferior vena cava (IVC). The middle hepatic vein (MHV) and the left hepatic vein (LHV) have a common trunk in 65–85% of patients [10]. The right hepatic vein (RHV) drains into the IVC separately.

1.11 Anatomic Variations

The most common variations in hepatic veins are single RHV, early branching of RHV, and accessory inferior RHV (venous tributary > 3mm in caliber draining into IVC) [8, 10, 11].

1.12 Portal Vein

1.12.1 Embryology

Development of the portal vein (PV) occurs between the 4th and 10th weeks. Umbilical veins, vitelline veins, and cardinal veins are three paired venous systems present in the fetus. At around the second month of gestation, there is selective involution of the vitelline veins which results in the formation of PV. The stem of PV and the left branch of PV are formed by the left vitelline vein, while the right branch of the portal vein is formed by the right vitelline vein. Any alteration in this process can result in variations in PV [12, 13].

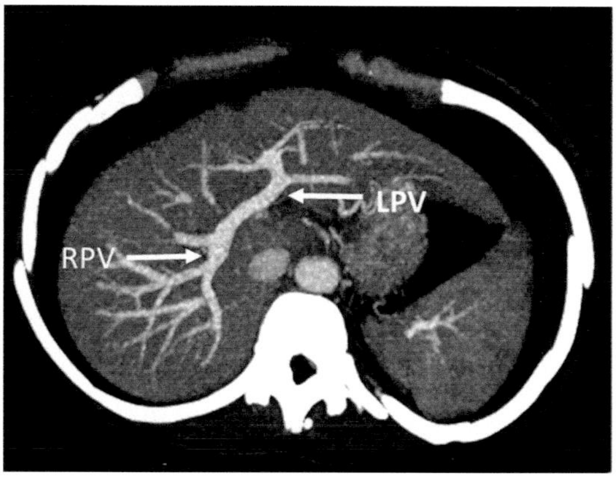

Fig. 1.7 Axial MIP images showing normal anatomy of intrahepatic branches of the main portal vein

1.13 Normal Anatomy

The PV is formed by the union of the superior mesenteric vein and the splenic vein. At the hilum, the main portal vein (MPV) divides into the right portal vein (RPV) and the left portal vein (LPV) (Fig. 1.7). The RPV divides into the right anterior portal vein (RAPV) and the right posterior portal vein (RPPV) branches. The LPV in the proximal part courses horizontally to the left and in the distal part turns medially toward the ligamentum teres. Normal portal blood flow in humans is about 1000–1200 ml/min [12, 14].

1.14 Anatomic Variations

Normal anatomy of PV and its branches is seen in only 65% of the cases. Anatomic variations in the portal vein are trifurcation (Fig. 1.8), RPPV originating as a first branch of MPV,

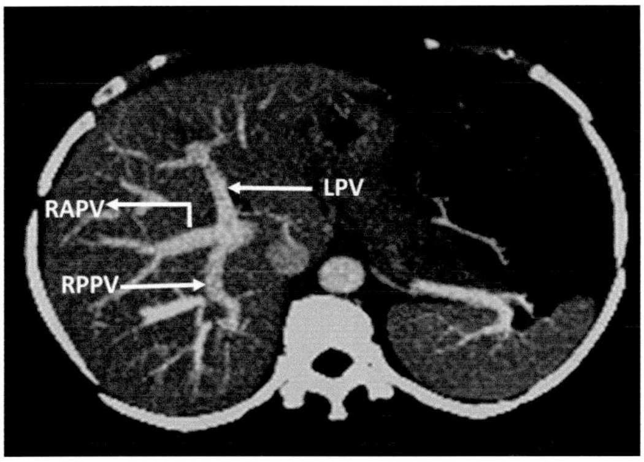

Fig. 1.8 Axial MIP images showing trifurcation of the main portal vein into LPV, RPPV, and RAPV

absence of PV bifurcation, total ramification, etc. Separate origins of segmental branches from RPV can also be seen. Dual supply of segment VIII from both right and left PV branches or only from the left portal vein can also be seen [14].

1.15 Conclusion

In the era of an increasing trend toward liver transplant, selective lobectomies, and super-selective hepatic lobe–specific interventional procedures to treat various liver lesions, preoperative assessment is essential. Especially in cases of liver transplant, both liver donors and liver recipients need meticulous preoperative assessment to avoid dreadful complications like hepatic necrosis or bile leakage, which are invariably responsible for poor postoperative outcomes. MDCT with its various post-processing tools depicting the vascular structures and MRI with MRCP do an excellent depiction of biliary anatomy, making them the most accurate imaging modalities to delineate anatomy preoperatively. It helps the surgeon or interventionist to form a roadmap before they operate, and hence, management of any anatomical variants can be planned beforehand, drastically improving the post-procedural patient outcome and thus making accurate identification of anatomical variants quintessential.

References

1. Sureka B, Bansal K, Patidar Y, Arora A. Magnetic resonance cholangiographic evaluation of intrahepatic and extrahepatic bile duct variations. Indian J Radiol Imaging. 2016;26:22–32.
2. Sureka B, Rastogi A, Bihari C, Bharathy KGS, Sood V, Alam S. Imaging in ductal plate malformations. Indian J Radiol Imaging. 2017;27(1):6–12. https://doi.org/10.4103/0971-3026.202966.
3. Mortelé KJ, Ros PR. Anatomic variants of the biliary tree: MR cholangiographic findings and clinical applications. AJR Am J Roentgenol. 2001;177:389–94.
4. Choi JW, Kim TK, Kim KW, Kim AY, Kim PN, Ha HK, et al. Anatomic variation in intrahepatic bile ducts: an analysis of intraoperative cholangiograms in 300 consecutive donors for living donor liver transplantation. Korean J Radiol. 2003;4:85–90.
5. Maheshwari P. Cystic malformation of cystic duct: 10 cases and review of literature. World J Radiol. 2012;4:413–7.
6. Minutoli F, Naso S, Visalli C, Iannelli D, Silipigni S, Pitrone A, et al. A new variant of cholecystohepatic duct: MR cholangiography demonstration. SurgRadiolAnat. 2014; [Epub ahead of print]
7. Sureka B, Mittal MK, Mittal A, Sinha M, Bhambri NK, Thukral BB. Variations of celiac axis, common hepatic artery and its branches in 600 patients. Indian J Radiol Imaging. 2013;23:223–33.
8. Sureka B, Sharma N, Khera PS, Garg PK, Yadav T. Hepatic vein variations in 500 patients: surgical and radiological significance. Br J Radiol. 2019;92(1102):20190487. https://doi.org/10.1259/bjr.20190487.
9. Yagel S, Kivilevitch Z, Cohen SM, Valsky DV, Messing B, Shen O, et al. The fetal venous system, Part I: Normal embryology, anatomy, hemodynamics, ultrasound evaluation and Doppler investigation. Ultrasound Obstet Gynecol. 2010;35:n/a–50.
10. Soyer P, Bluemke DA, Choti MA, Fishman EK. Variations in the intrahepatic portions of the hepatic and portal veins: findings on helical CT scans during arterial portography. AJR Am J Roentgenol. 1995;164:103–8.
11. Mišič J, Popović P, Hribernik M, Starc A, Dahmane R. Morphological characteristics and frequency of accessory right hepatic veins – evaluation with Computed Tomography. ActaClin Croat. 2018;57:71–81.
12. Sureka B, Patidar Y, Bansal K, Rajesh S, Agrawal N, Arora A. Portal vein variations in 1000 patients: surgical and radiological importance. Br J Radiol. 2015;88:20150326.
13. Walsh G, Williams MP. Congenital anomalies of the portal venous system: CT appearances with embryological considerations. Clin Radiol. 1995;50:174–6.
14. Covey AM, Brody LA, Getrajdman GI, Sofocleous CT, Brown KT. Incidence, patterns, and clinical relevance of variant portal vein anatomy. AJR Am J Roentgenol. 2004;183:1055–64.

2 Normal Anatomy and Anatomic Variations of the Pancreas

Satya Jha and Binit Sureka

2.1 Introduction

The pancreas lies in contact with the peritoneal ligament, which serves as a potential space for the spread of pancreatic disease. Understanding embryology can help one understand these complex anatomic relations [1]. Moreover, understanding the anatomy gives us insight into why certain anatomical variations occur and what associations can be expected with them.

We can classify significant anatomical variations as variations of the pancreatic duct and those of the pancreatic head, uncinate process, body, and tail. The pancreatic head and neck variations can be either in the form of fusion anomalies, like pancreatic divisum, or pancreatic contour variations involving the head, body, or tail [2].

It is essential to identify these variations as they give a pseudo-mass appearance. The objective is to make its readers familiar with these variations, also known as pancreatic pseudo-mass, which can otherwise be mistaken for a lesion [3, 4].

S. Jha · B. Sureka (✉)
Department of Diagnostic & Interventional Radiology, AIIMS Jodhpur, Jodhpur, Rajasthan, India

2.2 Embryology, Development, and Anatomy

The development of the pancreas occurs during the fourth week of gestation, from the ventral and dorsal pancreatic buds at the primitive foregut-midgut junction. The development of the primitive gut tube occurs between the 3rd and 4th weeks. It further divides into foregut, midgut, and hindgut [5]. Hepatic diverticulum, which arises from the primitive foregut, gives rise to a cranial and a caudal bud. Its cranial bud becomes the liver and the extrahepatic biliary tree. The caudal bud develops into the gall bladder; the cystic duct appears, as well as the ventral pancreas through further complex budding [6, 7]. Another diverticulum arises cranial and dorsal to the hepatic diverticulum and grows into the dorsal mesogastrium. This gives rise to the dorsal portion of the pancreas and its ducts. The dorsal mesogastrium gives rise to the gastrophrenic ligament, the gastrosplenic and splenorenal ligaments, and the lesser and greater omenta. Usually, the ventral pancreatic bud fuses alongside the dorsal bud. The dorsal pancreatic bud forms the upper/anterior head, body, and tail of the pancreas. The ventral bud forms the inferior/posterior head and uncinate process. The dorsal and ventral pancreatic buds give rise to their own ductal systems that fuse with each other and duodenum, hence giving rise to a new duct that joins the distal part of the dorsal pancreatic duct with the duct of the ventral pancreas, thus forming the main

© The Author(s), under exclusive license to Springer Nature Singapore Pte Ltd. 2025

B. Sureka (ed.), *Hepato-Pancreatico Biliary Imaging*, https://doi.org/10.1007/978-981-95-1699-5_2

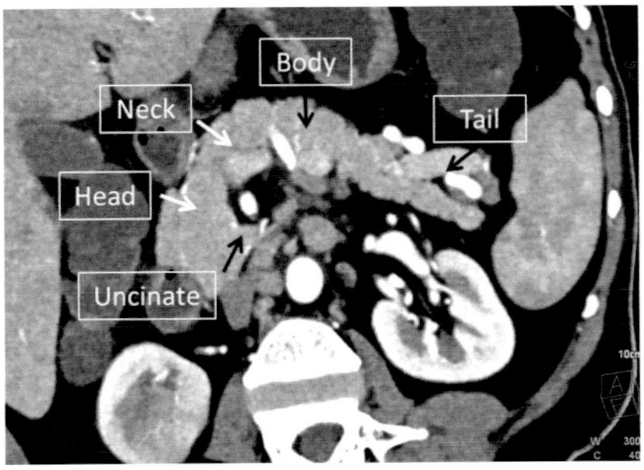

Fig. 2.1 Oblique reformatted CT image showing cross-sectional anatomy of the pancreas

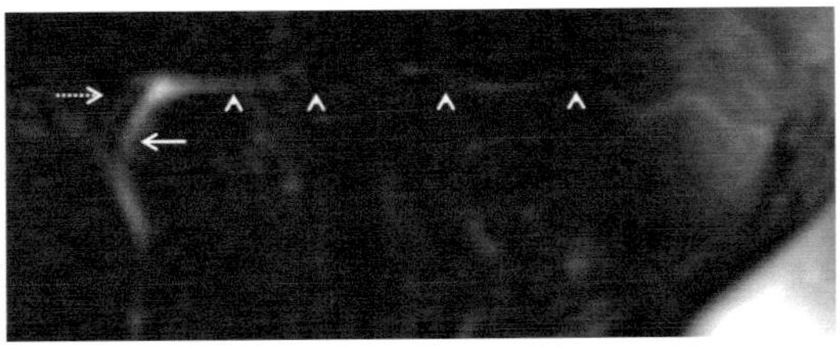

Fig. 2.2 Axial MRCP image showing the main pancreatic duct (arrowheads) with a bifid configuration showing the ventral duct of Wirsung (arrow) and the dorsal duct of Santorini (dashed arrow)

pancreatic duct, or the duct of Wirsung that drains into major duodenal papilla. The remnant of the dorsal duct forms the accessory pancreatic duct of Santorini that empties into the minor duodenal papilla. Due to this complex process of pancreatic development and fusion, any change from usual in the development course can lead to an armamentarium of anatomic variants [3, 7].

2.3 Segmental/Cross-Sectional Anatomy of Pancreas

The normal pancreas can have a smooth as well as a coarsely lobulated contour and is located in the anterior pararenal space of the retroperitoneum. It is divided into four parts, i.e., head, neck, body, and tail (Fig. 2.1). It usually measures 15–20 cm in length. Measurements in axial dimension on average are 23 mm, 19 mm, 20 mm, and 15 mm in the head, neck, body, and tail of the pancreas, respectively. The pancreatic head is nested within the C loop of the duodenum. The uncinate process is a triangle-shaped, caudal extension of the pancreatic head.

The pancreatic neck lies to the left of the head and is seen as a constricted part. The superior mesenteric vein acts as a landmark to delineate the head from the neck of the pancreas, as the head lies to its right, while the SMV lies ventral to it. The delineation between the pancreatic body and tail is done by dividing the distance between the neck and pancreatic tail into equal halves [4, 8].

2.4 Pancreatic Ducts

The most common normally encountered downstream ductal configuration is a bifid configuration with patent ducts of Wirsung (ventral duct) and Santorini (dorsal duct) (Fig. 2.2). Other common configurations that can be seen are those of either a dominant or a rudimentary duct of Santorini. Approximately 20–30 side branches enter the main pancreatic duct at right angles.

2.5 Anatomy of the Pancreaticobiliary Junction

In the most frequently seen pattern, the duct of Wirsung joins with the common bile duct (CBD) and then together drains into the duodenum at an opening called the major papilla.

Smooth muscles encircle this distal-most portion of the common bile duct and duct of Wirsung, called the sphincter choledochus and sphincter pancreaticus, respectively, together forming the Sphincter of Oddi, which is approximately 10–15 mm in length. In about 40% of cases, a dilated channel called the ampulla is formed by joining the duct of Wirsung and the CBD at the major papilla.

2.6 Retroportal Lamina

Retroportal lamina or right right-portal lamina, also known as right retropancreatic lamina, is a connective tissue containing lymphatics, neural

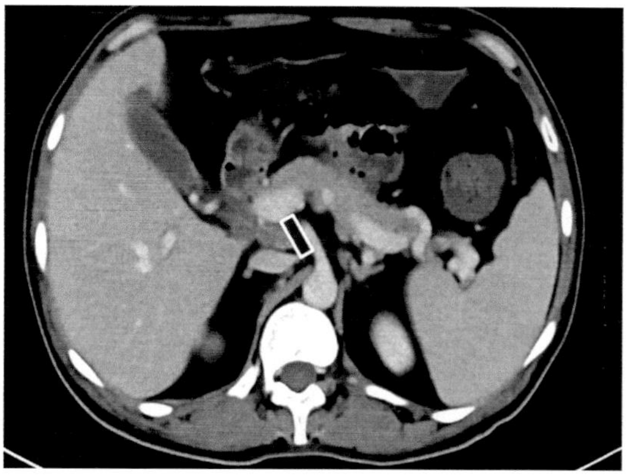

Fig. 2.3 Axial contrast CT image showing retroportal lamina (box)

elements, and a part of the posterior pancreaticoduodenal artery. It lies between the uncinate process of the pancreas and the superior mesenteric artery. It plays an important role in decision-making regarding the prediction of healthy margins while planning surgical resection (Fig. 2.3) [9]. The aberrant right hepatic artery, when arising from the superior mesenteric artery, passes through the retroportal lamina; hence, it is important to communicate this to the surgeons.

2.7 Pancreatic Divisum

It is the most common pancreatic ductal anatomic variation [10]. It is divided into three subtypes:

- *Type 1 (classic)*: Most common type: No connection between the main and minor pancreatic duct (Fig. 2.4).
- *Type 2*: Major pancreatic duct or ventral duct is absent, and the entire pancreatic tissue is drained by the minor/dorsal duct.
- *Type 3*: A thin filamentous connection between dorsal and ventral ducts; it is the least common type (Fig. 2.5).

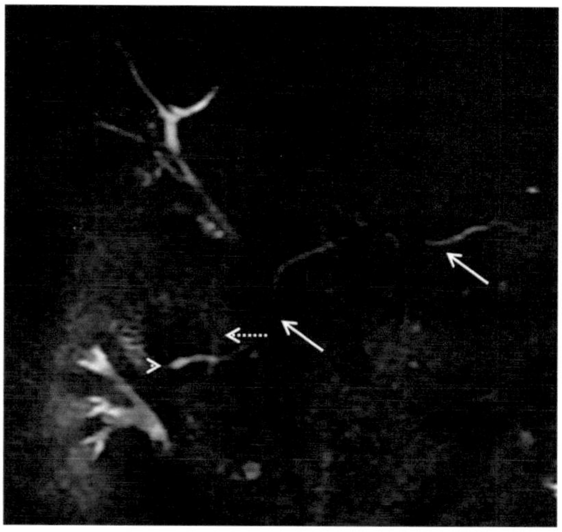

Fig. 2.4 MRCP showing the dominant dorsal pancreatic duct (arrows) anterior to the bile duct (dashed arrow) draining into the minor papilla in a case of type 2 pancreas divisum. Incidental note is made of Santorinocele (arrowhead)

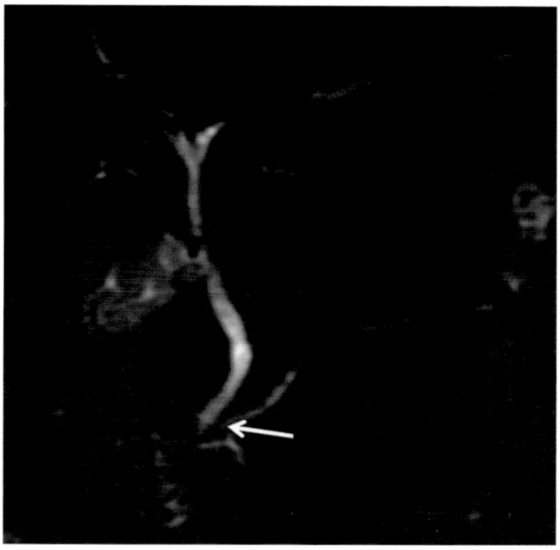

Fig. 2.5 MRCP image showing thin filamentous (arrow) connection between the dorsal and ventral ducts in a case of type 3 pancreas divisum

2.8 Reverse Pancreas Divisum

Reverse pancreas divisum is the term used for an anomaly where the main pancreatic duct fuses with the ventral duct. In such cases, a small dorsal duct may be seen as a remnant that does not communicate with the main duct. This is contrary to the commonly described pancreatic divisum, where the main pancreatic duct fuses with the dorsal duct and opens at the minor papilla, showing no communication with the ventral duct [11].

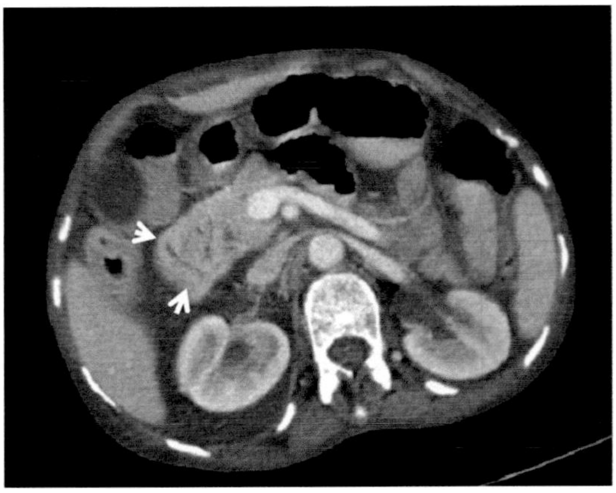

Fig. 2.6 Axial contrast CT showing a ring of pancreatic tissue (arrowheads) encircling the second part of the duodenum in a case of complete annular pancreas

2.9 Annular Pancreas

Sometimes, the ventral pancreatic bud, instead of rotating clockwise with the duodenum, persists along the lateral wall of the duodenal C loop. This persistent pancreatic tissue fuses with the pancreatic head and encircles the duodenum, giving rise to an annular pancreas. It can be of two types—complete or incomplete.

Complete annular pancreas leads to presentation with bilious vomiting in the neonatal period due to obstruction of the duodenal lumen. There are often no symptoms throughout life, and they may be detected incidentally on imaging for a different indication. Presentation in adulthood with episodes of pancreatitis or gastric outlet obstruction is also seen.

Visualization of the pancreatic duct encircling the duodenum on magnetic resonance cholangiopancreatography (MRCP) or endoscopic retrograde cholangiopancreatography (ERCP) is diagnostic of this entity. Secretin MRCP is better than routine MRCP for the demonstration of ductal anatomy. CT shows a ring of pancreatic parenchyma encircling the second part of the duodenum (Fig. 2.6).

Sometimes, only a thin rim of pancreatic parenchyma extends anterolateral or posterolateral to the duodenum, and this is known as an incomplete annular pancreas. This gives a "crocodile jaw" configuration. Rarely, in these cases, a thin rim of pancreatic parenchyma is embedded within the duodenal wall (Fig. 2.7).

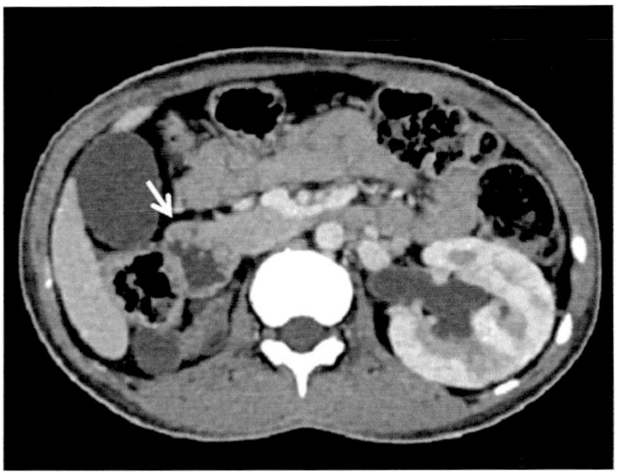

Fig. 2.7 Axial contrast CT showing rim of pancreatic tissue (arrow) anterolateral to the duodenum in a case of incomplete annular pancreas

Annular pancreas may be frequently associated with duodenal stenosis, duodenal atresia, and Down syndrome.

2.10 Portal Annular Pancreas

Portal annular pancreas [12], also known as circumportal pancreas, is an extremely rare pancreatic anomaly. It results from a bizarre fusion of the main pancreatic body to the uncinate process occurring on the left of the portal vein-superior mesenteric vein junction, leading to encasement of the vessels within pancreatic tissue.

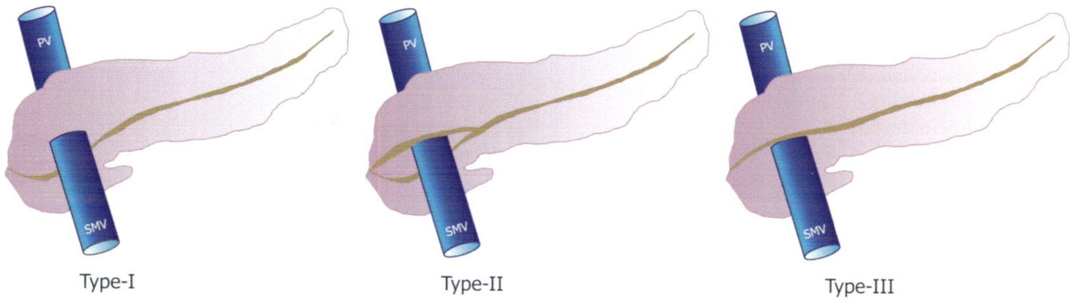

Fig. 2.8 Line diagram showing various types of the circumportal pancreas

It is subgrouped into three types: I, II, and III. In type I, the ventral bud of the pancreas fuses with the dorsal bud posterior to the portal vein so that the pancreatic duct courses posterior to the portal vein (retroportal pancreatic duct). Type II is associated with pancreas divisum. In type III, the uncinate process alone is involved, and the pancreatic duct courses anterior to the portal vein (anteportal pancreatic duct) (Fig. 2.8).

2.11 Ectopic Pancreas

Ectopic pancreas is the presence of pancreatic tissue located at a site other than the pancreas. The most common site is the submucosa of the stomach or proximal small bowel. It can however be found at any part of the bowel and has been notably associated with Meckel's diverticulum. It is usually small in size (a few mm to cm) and is detected incidentally on gastroscopy or sometimes on barium meal as a smooth broad-based lesion with central umbilication. On cross-sectional imaging, ectopic pancreatic tissue has attenuation and enhancement similar to the pancreas [13].

2.12 Dorsal Pancreatic Agenesis

Pancreatic agenesis results from the nondevelopment of either dorsal or ventral pancreatic buds, or both (i.e., complete agenesis), the latter being incompatible with life. Partial agenesis of the dorsal bud leading to dorsal pancreatic agenesis is more common than ventral pancreatic agenesis. *Dependent stomach sign* and *dependent intestine sign* are described in dorsal pancreatic agenesis in which the stomach and intestines lie in the pancreatic bed anterior to the splenic vein (Fig. 2.9). The term pseudo-agenesis is used when there is atrophy secondary to chronic pancreatitis [13].

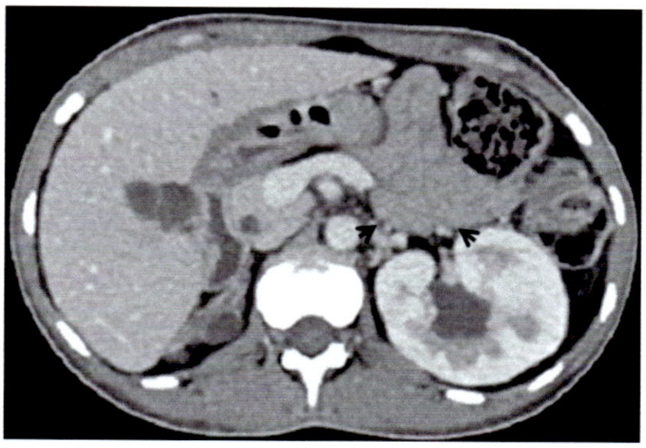

Fig. 2.9 Axial CT image showing the *dependent intestine sign* in the pancreatic bed in a case of dorsal pancreatic agenesis

2.13 Accessory Pancreatic Lobe

Another rare anomaly is an accessory pancreatic lobe. It is connected to the main pancreatic parenchyma via an accessory duct. It has an association with gastric duplication cyst, wherein the aberrant duct communicates with the main pancreatic duct as well as the cyst [13].

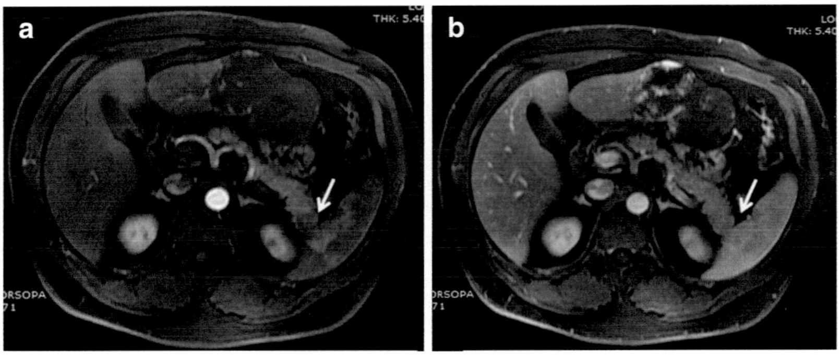

Fig. 2.10 Contrast-enhanced MR images: (**a**) arterial phase and (**b**) venous phase showing nodular lesion in the tail of the pancreas with enhancement characteristics similar to splenic parenchyma in a case of intrapancreatic accessory spleen

2.14 Variations of Pancreatic Contours

These contour variations occur because of the presence of fetal lobulations, which are nothing but protrusions from the head and neck of the pancreas. This protrusion should be more than 1cm beyond the anterior superior pancreaticoduodenal artery or gastroduodenal artery [2]. These protrusions are of three types and are found in approximately 30% population: type I being the anterior protrusion; type II, i.e., posterior protrusion; and type III (horizontal) protrusion. From the pancreatic neck and body, an anterior or posterior projection may be seen [2]. The tail of the pancreas may be lobulated, globular, tapering, or bifid in appearance [14].

2.15 Tuber Omentale

Sometimes, the pancreatic body may appear prominent along its anterior surface, which is seen in contact with the lesser omentum. This appearance is called the omental tuberosity or tuber omentale. It should be differentiated from a mass or lymph node on a cross-sectional image [15].

2.16 Pancreatic Cleft

When there is invagination of peripancreatic fat into the pancreas, it gives rise to a cleft-like appearance. This can mimic a fractured pancreas, especially if the patient has a history of trauma. In the pancreatic cleft, the surrounding fat does not show haziness or stranding.

2.17 Intrapancreatic Accessory Spleen

Intrapancreatic accessory spleen (IPAS) is a rare entity. The most common location is in the pancreatic tail. Since normal attenuation of the spleen is higher than the normal pancreatic parenchyma density and so is the post-contrast enhancement, an intrapancreatic splenic tissue may simulate a hypervascular mass on CT or MRI. An IPAS has similar attenuation values and enhancement characteristics to those of the normal spleen (Fig. 2.10) [16].

2.18 Anomalous Pancreatobiliary Junction

It describes an abnormal fusion of the common bile duct and pancreatic duct outside the sphincter of Oddi, resulting in the formation of a long common channel of more than 15 mm (Fig. 2.11). As it is located outside the sphincter of Oddi, there may be reflux of pancreatic secretions into the biliary system, leading to the formation of a choledochal cyst, or reflux into the pancreatic duct, leading to recurrent episodes of acute pancreatitis [13].

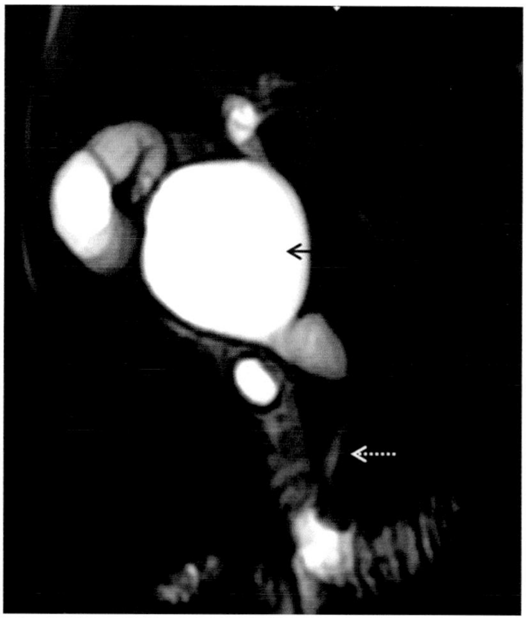

Fig. 2.11 MRCP image showing an anomalous long common channel (dashed arrow) in a case of choledochal cyst (arrow)

References

1. Pancreas: Peritoneal Reflections, Ligamentous Connections, and Pathways of Disease Spread | RadioGraphics [Internet]. [cited 2021 Jun 13]. Available from: https://pubs.rsna.org/doi/full/10.1148/rg.e34
2. Ross BA, Jeffrey RB, Mindelzun RE. Normal variations in the lateral contour of the head and neck of the pancreas mimicking neoplasm: evaluation with dual-phase helical CT. Am J Roentgenol. 1996;166(4):799–801.
3. Borghei P, Sokhandon F, Shirkhoda A, Morgan DE. Anomalies, anatomic variants, and sources of diagnostic pitfalls in pancreatic imaging. Radiology. 2013;266(1):28–36.
4. Mortelé KJ, Rocha TC, Streeter JL, Taylor AJ. Multimodality imaging of pancreatic and biliary congenital anomalies. RadioGraphics. 2006;26(3):715–31.
5. Hurtado CW, Waasdorp C, Sferra T, Polk B. Embryology and anatomy of the gastrointestinal tract:14.
6. Ando H. Embryology of the biliary tract. Dig Surg. 2010;27(2):87–9.
7. Tadokoro H, Takase M, Nobukawa B. Development and congenital anomalies of the pancreas. Anat Res Int. 2011;14(2011):1–7.
8. Raichholz G, Giménez S, Dumoulin S, Sañudo JL. Segmental anatomy of the pancreas and its developmental variants. 2016;5:10.
9. Bouassida M, Mighri MM, Chtourou MF, Sassi S, Touinsi H, Hajji H, et al. Retroportal lamina or mesopancreas? Lessons learned by anatomical and histological study of thirty three cadaveric dissections. Int J Surg. 2013;11(9):834–6.
10. Dimitriou I, Katsourakis A, Nikolaidou E, Noussios G. The main anatomical variations of the pancreatic duct system: review of the literature and its importance in surgical practice. J Clin Med Res. 2018;10(5):370–5.
11. Soulen MC, Zerhouni EA, Fishman EK, Gayler BW, Milligan F, Siegelman SS. Enlargement of the pancreatic head in patients with pancreas divisum. Clin Imaging. 1989;13(1):51–7.
12. John R, Simon B, Eapen A, Putta T, Joseph P, Raju RS, et al. Portal annular pancreas: an underrecognized variant, prevalence, and clinical relevance. Trop Gastroenterol. 2020;40(4):132–6.
13. Türkvatan A, Erden A, Türkoğlu MA, Yener Ö. Congenital variants and anomalies of the pancreas and pancreatic duct: imaging by magnetic resonance cholangiopancreaticography and multidetector computed tomography. Korean J Radiol. 2013;14(6):905.
14. Omeri AK, Matsumoto S, Kiyonaga M, Takaji R, Yamada Y, Kosen K, et al. Contour variations of the body and tail of the pancreas: evaluation with MDCT. Jpn J Radiol. 2017;35(6):310–8.
15. Mortelé KJ. Mimics, miscalls, and misses in pancreatic disease. 8.
16. Kim SH, Lee JM, Han JK, Lee JY, Kim KW, Cho KC, Choi BI. Intrapancreatic accessory spleen: findings on MR Imaging, CT, US and scintigraphy, and the pathologic analysis. Korean J Radiol. 2008;9(2):162–74.

3 Imaging in Hepatic Infections

Reettika Chanda, Kirthi Sathyakumar,
and Anu Eapen

3.1 Introduction

A wide range of bacterial, parasitic, fungal, and viral infections can affect the liver, causing a spectrum of pyogenic and non-pyogenic abscesses, focal parenchymal lesions, cholangitis, hepatitis, and granulomatous diseases [1–3].

Imaging plays a crucial role in the identification, diagnosis, and management of hepatobiliary infections.

3.2 Imaging Modalities

3.2.1 Plain Radiographs

Although radiographs are not primarily used in the diagnosis of hepatobiliary infections, a focal bulge in liver contour, air in the liver, pneumobilia, and portal venous air on abdominal X-rays provide clues toward the presence of hepatobiliary infections.

3.2.2 Ultrasound

Ultrasound is often used as the initial modality to identify and characterize liver abscesses and hydatid cysts and to assess biliary involvement [2, 4].

R. Chanda · K. Sathyakumar · A. Eapen (✉)
Christian Medical College, Vellore, India

3.2.3 Computed Tomography (CT)

CT helps in assessing the extent of liver involvement, identifying complications as well as in evaluating a local or remote source of spread [1, 2, 4].

3.2.4 Magnetic Resonance Imaging (MRI)

Specific signal characteristics, appearance, and enhancement pattern on MRI aid in differentiating liver infections from other conditions such as neoplasm [1, 2].

3.3 Bacterial Infections

3.3.1 Pyogenic Liver Abscess

Causative Organism(s): Most liver abscesses have polymicrobial growth. Among individual bacteria, *Klebsiella pneumoniae* is the most common cause of solitary abscesses, while *Escherichia coli* is most frequently identified from cholangitic abscesses [5, 6].

3.3.1.1 Mode of Transmission

While ascending cholangitis from infections of the biliary tree is the most well-known mechanism through which hepatic infections occur,

© The Author(s), under exclusive license to Springer Nature Singapore Pte Ltd. 2025
B. Sureka (ed.), *Hepato-Pancreatico Biliary Imaging*, https://doi.org/10.1007/978-981-95-1699-5_3

other routes include portal phlebitis due to gastrointestinal infections, hematogenous dissemination of systemic infections through the hepatic artery, direct extension from a local source, and traumatic inoculation of the pathogen [5–7]. The cause of liver abscess cannot be determined in about 20% [4, 6].

3.3.1.2 Imaging

Pyogenic abscesses less than 2 cm are called microabscesses, while those larger than 2 cm are termed macroabscesses (Fig. 3.1) [1]. While pyogenic liver abscesses are often solitary, liver involvement in disseminated infections and sepsis can lead to the formation of multiple abscesses. Clusters of microabscesses are common with ascending cholangitis; coliforms and enteric bacteria are the likely cause (Figs. 3.2 and 3.3) [5, 7].

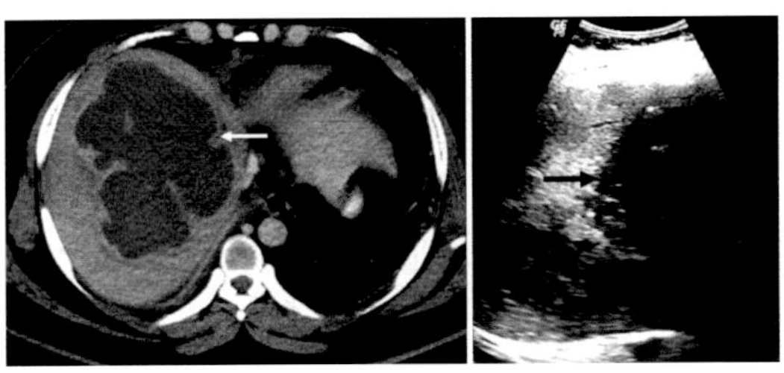

Fig. 3.1 Liver abscess. Contrast-enhanced CT shows a large, coalesced macroabscess in the liver (arrow)

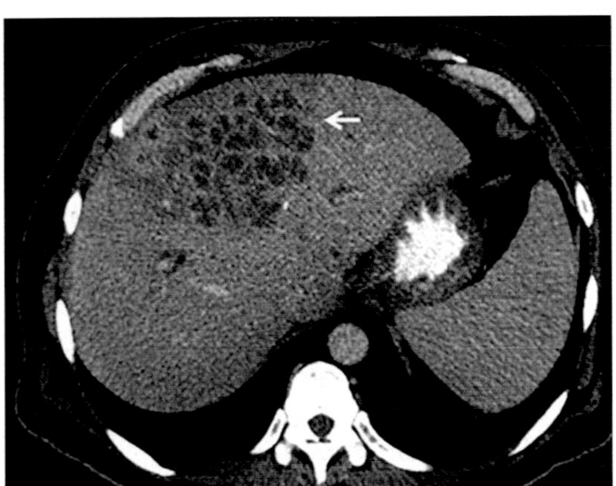

Fig. 3.2 Cluster sign. Contrast-enhanced CT of the liver shows a cluster of multiple small abscesses in the central liver, the so-called cluster sign (arrow), described with pyogenic liver abscess

Ultrasound appearance of liver abscess is determined by its size and stage of liquefaction. Early in the disease, they either appear as round, solid hypoechoic lesions or an ill-defined area of altered hepatic parenchyma. Debris and anechoic liquefied components can be seen gradually [1, 2]. Gas within the abscess appears as high-intensity echoes with dirty acoustic shadowing [8].

On CT, abscesses are hypodense with faint wall enhancement. The double target sign is used to describe the enhancing wall surrounded by a hypodense halo due to perilesional edema [1–3, 9]. Gas within an abscess, though uncommon, is highly specific for a pyogenic cause, *Klebsiella* being the most common (Fig. 3.4). Widely scattered microabscesses occur with staphylococcal infections and in septicemia.

On MRI, a pyogenic abscess is hypointense on T1w and hyperintense on T2w. Perilesional edema appears as confluent T2w hyperintensity in the adjacent parenchyma [1–3]. The wall shows early and persistent enhancement post-contrast. Multiple fine interrupted septa within an abscess form the "turquoise sign," a feature commonly associated with *K. pneumoniae* [3, 10].

3.3.1.3 Complications

Rupture of a liver abscess into the peritoneal or pleural cavity is a dreaded complication. Disseminated pyogenic infection and sepsis may also occur with untreated abscesses [2–4].

3.3.1.4 Management

Image-guided (USG/CT) catheter drainage acts as an accompaniment to medical management for large liver abscesses [2, 11–13]. For smaller abscesses, where catheter placement may not be possible, fine needle aspiration can be done for diagnostic as well as therapeutic purposes. Surgical drainage requires consideration when there are multiple pyogenic abscesses, loculated abscess, underlying disease requiring surgery, inadequate response to treatment, failed percutaneous drainage, and in cases complicated by perforation or fistula formation [2, 11–14].

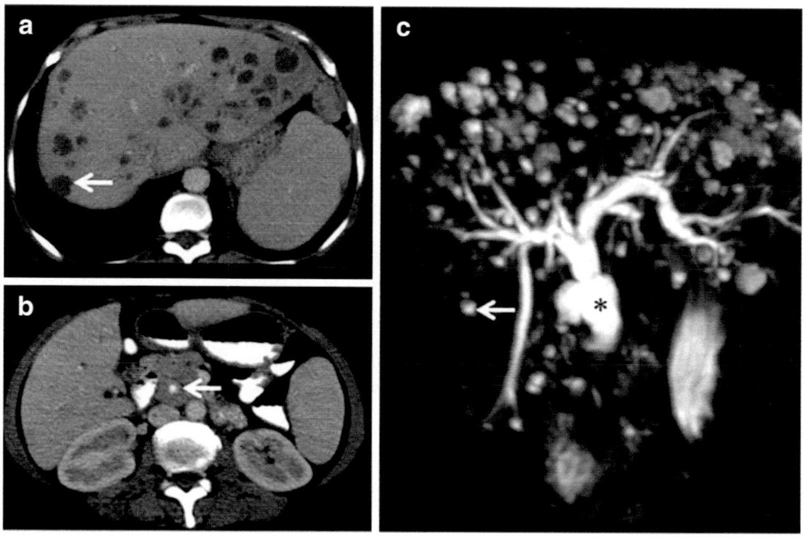

Fig. 3.3 Cholangitic abscesses. Contrast-enhanced CT of the liver shows multiple small, scattered liver abscesses (arrow in **a**), a calculus in the distal CBD (arrow in **b**). On MRCP, the biliary tree is dilated (*), and the liver lesions appear round and hyperintense (arrow in **c**)

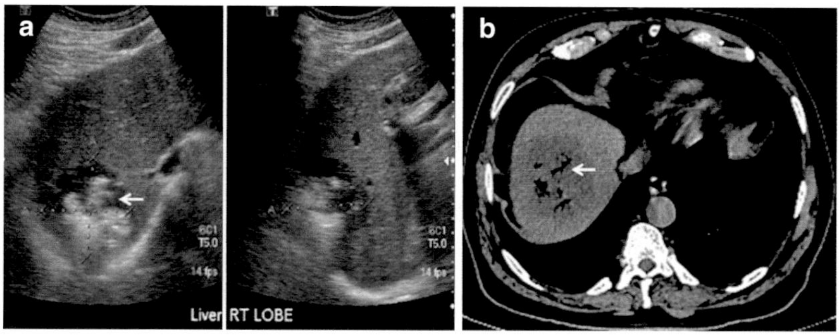

Fig. 3.4 Pyogenic liver abscess. Ultrasound (**a**) and noncontrast CT (**b**) images show air within a large abscess in the right lobe of the liver, confirming the pyogenic origin of the abscess (arrows)

3.4 Parasitic Infections

3.4.1 Liver Parenchymal Infections

3.4.1.1 Amebic Liver Abscess

Causative Organism

Entamoeba histolytica is a protozoan endemic to Southeast Asia, Africa, and Central and South America.

Mode of Transmission

The liver is the most common site of extraintestinal involvement in amebiasis. The organism gains entry into the liver from the colon via the portal venous circulation [2, 15].

Pathology

Amebic liver abscesses have a shaggy wall with chocolate-colored content within, formed due to hemorrhage within the abscess.

Imaging

Amebic liver abscess is often solitary and commonly affects the right lobe of the liver in a subcapsular location [1, 2]. Cysts are unilocular; a few septa may be present. The size of the cysts is variable.

On ultrasound, the abscess appears as a thin-walled, well-defined, round, homogeneous, hypoechoic lesion with low-level internal echoes and posterior acoustic enhancement (Fig. 3.5) [1–4].

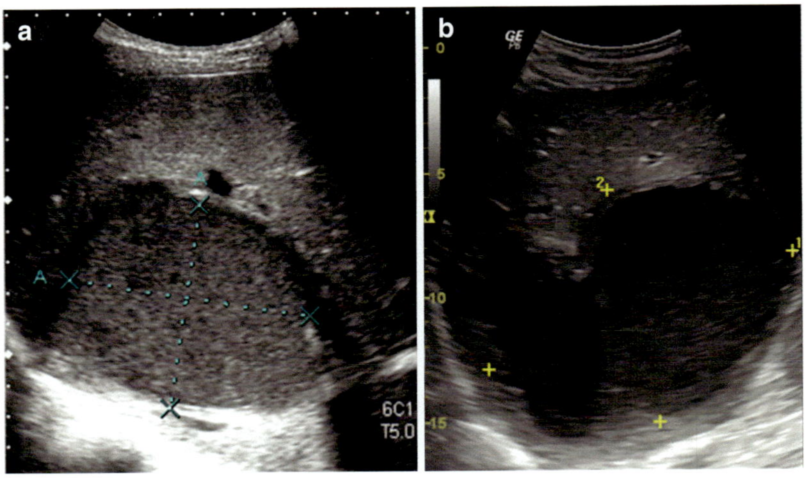

Fig. 3.5 (**a** and **b**) Amoebic liver abscess. Ultrasound images of the liver abscess show a large solitary lesion located in the right lobe of the liver in a peripheral subcapsular location with low-level internal echoes

On CT, similar to a pyogenic abscess, the wall of an amebic abscess may also show a double-enhancing rim or a target appearance (Fig. 3.6). Presence of intralesional air is unusual.

MRI features of intralesional T1w hypointensity and T2w hyperintensity with perilesional edema are indistinguishable from a pyogenic abscess. Table 3.1 enlists common differences between pyogenic and amoebic liver abscesses [2, 3].

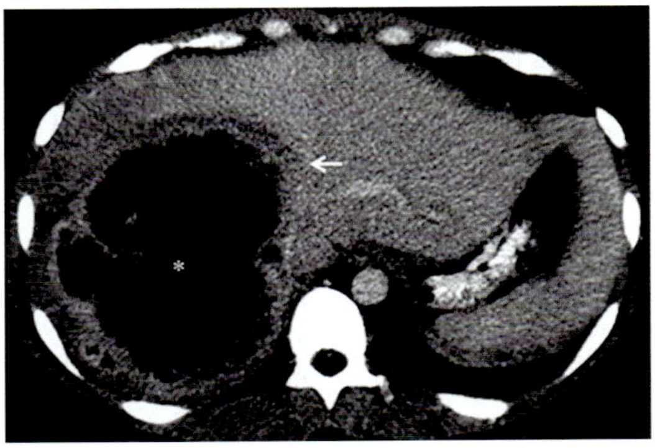

Fig. 3.6 Amoebic liver abscess. Contrast-enhanced CT of the liver shows a fluid attenuation lesion (*) with a thick enhancing wall (arrow) which shows double rim or target appearance and a peripheral zone of edema in the surrounding liver parenchyma

Complications

Extrahepatic extension through capsular or diaphragmatic rupture is common and a hallmark of this disease [3, 16].

Management

Treatment with oral metronidazole suffices in most patients with amebic liver abscess. Image-guided percutaneous drainage is reserved for large abscesses, those in whom metronidazole therapy fails, in suspected superadded bacterial infections, in impending rupture, or in pregnancy (Fig. 3.7) [4, 11, 12, 17–19].

3.4.1.2 Hydatid Liver

Causative Organism(s)

Echinococcus granulosus—most common; *Echinococcus alveolaris/multilocularis*—rare

Table 3.1 Common differences between amebic and pyogenic liver abscesses (Ref. [1])

Characteristic	Amoebic liver abscess	Pyogenic liver abscess
Age	Relatively younger	Middle aged
Symptoms	Acute illness	Acute illness/ clinically occult
Number	Single	Single/multiple
Location	Right lobe, close to the capsule	Single lesion—right lobe Multiple lesions—cluster sign
Intralesional air	Absent	Present in gas-forming organism infection

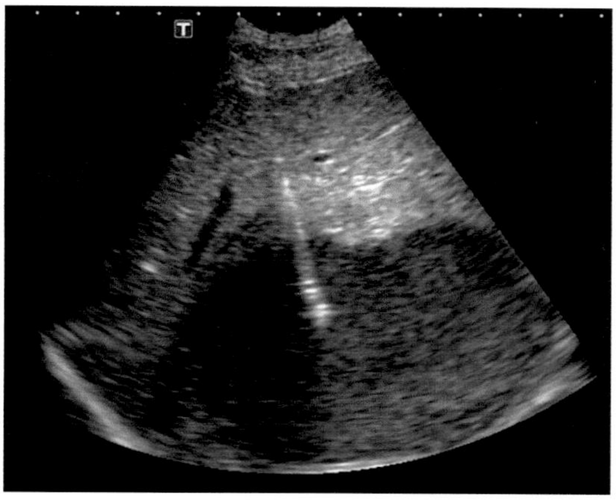

Fig. 3.7 Ultrasound-guided drainage of liver abscess. Ultrasound shows an aspiration needle within a large abscess in the right lobe of the liver

Mode of transmission: feco-oral route
Definitive hosts: dogs, cats, and other carnivores.
Intermediate host: cattle, sheep, and goats
Accidental host: humans

Pathology

The parasite resides in the gut of the definitive host and is shed in its feces. Ruminants grazing on this contaminated soil act as intermediate hosts and ingest the ova, which penetrate the gut wall and enter the liver through the portal venous circulation. The parasite can enter into systemic circulation through the liver and colonize other organs such as the lungs, brain, etc. In the infected organ, the liver being the most common, the ovum develops into a cyst gradually increasing in size. The parasitic cycle is completed when the definitive host feeds on the intermediate host.

There are three layers in a mature hydatid cyst. The innermost layer is the endocyst or germinal layer that is one cell layer thick and contains live tissue surrounding a central fluid-filled hydatid cavity. The intermediate layer is an acellular layer secreted by the germinal membrane and is called the ectocyst. It is a laminated layer that is 1–2 mm thick. The outermost layer or the pericyst is a thick fibrous capsule formed as a result of the host response to the hydatid [1, 2, 24, 25].

Imaging

The spectrum of imaging appearances in hydatid cysts of the liver and the World Health Organization classification are described in Table 3.2.

Ultrasound

A simple hydatid cyst is anechoic on ultrasound (Fig. 3.8a). The cyst wall is seen as a "trilaminar layer" or double echogenic line with a hypoechoic layer in between, on high-frequency ultrasound (Fig. 3.9).

Mobile hydatid sand appears as tiny low-level internal echoes known as snowflake or snowstorm sign.

A "spoke-wheel pattern" is formed by multiple daughter cysts within the mother cyst (Fig. 3.10).

The endocyst appears as a floating, undulating membrane as it matures and starts separating from the ectocyst, forming the "water lily sign" on complete separation. At a later transitional stage, daughter cysts are seen within a solid matrix (Fig. 3.11).

The wall begins to calcify on further maturation, gradually progressing toward the center of the cyst [3, 20–24, 26].

On CT, simple cysts are round, with homogeneous fluid density and well-defined walls. Daughter cysts appear as multiple small, round, simple cysts within a larger mother cyst containing fluid of higher density, forming a "rosette-like" pattern. Detached, floating membranes of the endocyst appear as thin, wavy structures within the cysts. Hydatid calcification occurs as the cyst matures (Fig. 3.12) [3, 24].

Magnetic Resonance Imaging

The trilaminar wall of the hydatid cyst can be seen on high resolution T2-weighted sequence. Simple cysts are well defined, round, T1w hypointense, and T2w hyperintense (Fig. 3.8b). The appearance of the detached floating endocyst membrane is described as "serpent sign" or "snake sign" [27, 28].

Table 3.2 Types of hydatid cyst (Refs. [3, 21])

Who Classification	CL	CE 1	CE 2	CE 3A	CE 3B	CE 4	CE 5
Gharbi classification		I	III	II	III	IV	V
Activity	Active	Active	Active	Transitional	Transitional	Inactive	Inactive
Description	Simple unilocular cyst with imperceptible wall	CL with the wall	Multiple daughter cysts	Detached membranes	Daughter cysts within a solid matrix	Heterogeneous cyst contents, absent daughter cysts	Solid cyst with thick wall calcification and variable intralesional calcification
US feature	Anechoic	Double line sign, trilaminar sign	Spoke-wheel pattern	Water lily sign	Cysts embedded in an echogenic matrix	Ball of wool sign	Thick calcified wall with dense posterior acoustic corridor
US appearance		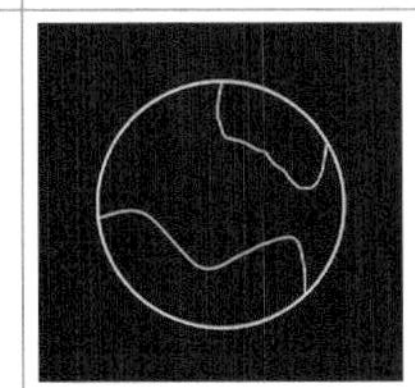	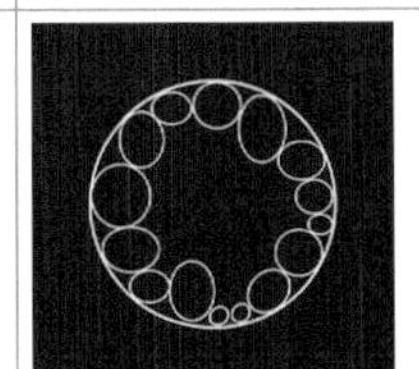	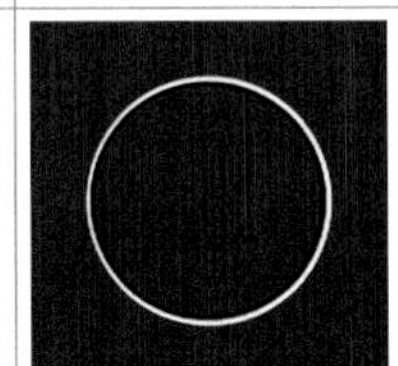	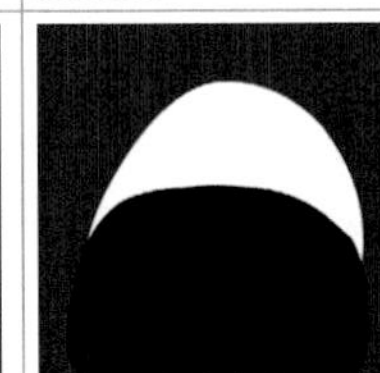	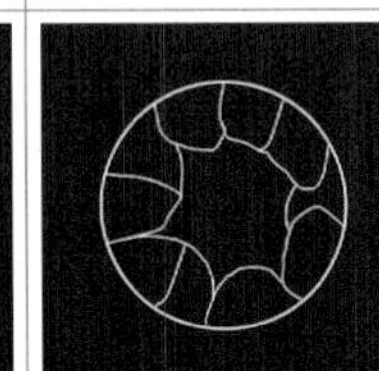	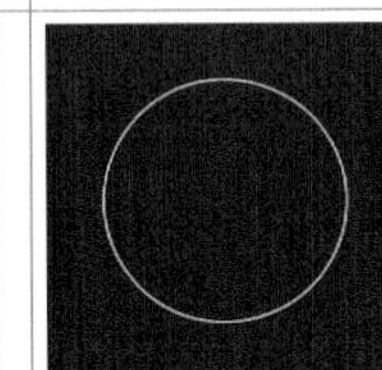
CT feature	Homogeneous hypodense	Thin, perceptible wall	Rosette pattern	Thin hypodense wavy structures		Central solid non-enhancing areas	Dense wall calcification
MRI feature	T1 hypointense and T2 hyperintense	Trilaminar sign	Multiple cysts within a larger cyst	Snake sign		Calcification	T1 hyperintense and T2 hypointense
PAIR feasibility	Yes	Yes	No	Yes	No	No	No

CL cystic lesion, *CE* cystic echinococcosis

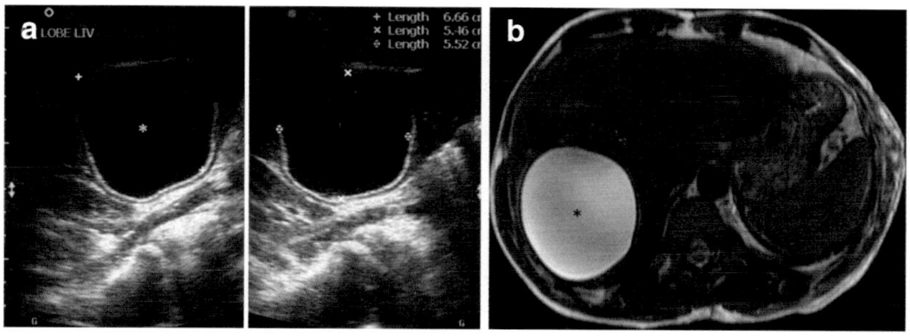

Fig. 3.8 Hydatid cyst liver, WHO grade CE 1. Unilocular hepatic hydatid cyst seen as a well-defined anechoic lesion with posterior acoustic enhancement on ultrasound (white asterisk in **a**) and a homogeneously T2w hyperintense lesion with a hypointense rim on MRI (black asterisk in **b**)

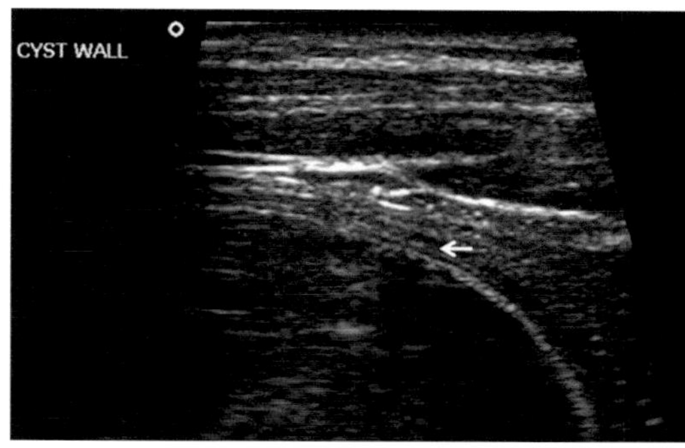

Fig. 3.9 Hydatid cyst liver. Ultrasound shows the laminar wall or trilaminar membrane of a hydatid cyst on high-frequency ultrasound with double echogenic layers and an intervening hypoechoic layer (arrow)

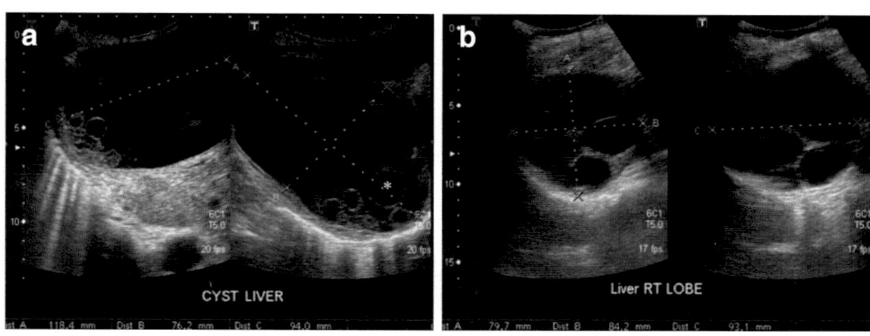

Fig. 3.10 Hydatid cyst liver, WHO grade CE 2. Ultrasound images show multiple daughter cysts within a large anechoic cyst (**a**). Spoke wheel pattern formed by the daughter cysts filling in the mother cyst (**b**)

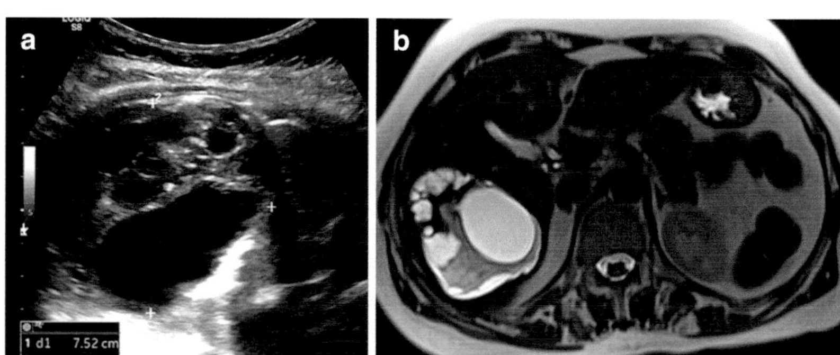

Fig. 3.11 Hydatid cyst liver, WHO grade CE 3b. Ultrasound (**a**) and T2-weighted MRI (**b**) images show a hydatid cyst with multiple daughter cysts within a partly solid matrix, representing the transitional stage

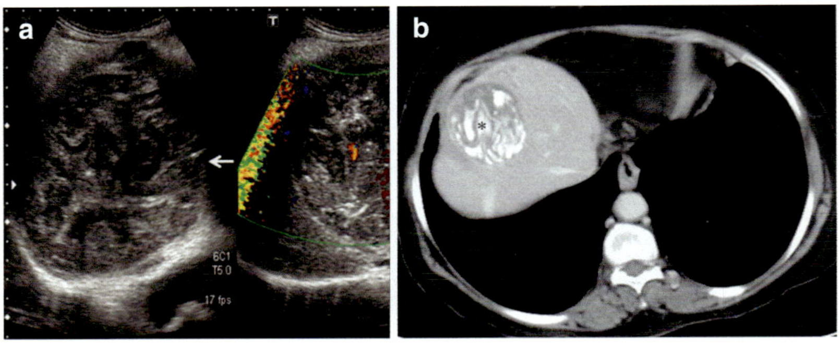

Fig. 3.12 Hydatid cyst liver, WHO grade CE 4. Ultrasound (**a**) and CT (**b**) images show a well-defined lesion in the liver with a heterogeneous solid component intermixed with calcification

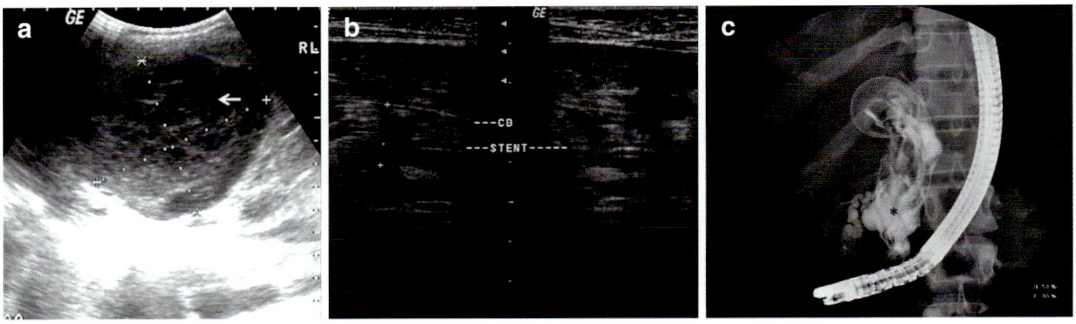

Fig. 3.13 Biliary rupture of hydatid cyst. Ultrasound of the liver shows a complex cyst with collapsed membranes and heterogeneous content with absent daughter cysts (**a**). Dilated CBD with stent in situ and extension of membranes seen as linear echogenic material within CBD (**b**). ERCP image shows the ruptured membranes appearing as filling defects within a dilated CBD (**c**)

Complications of Liver Hydatid

Disintegration of the hydatid membrane with time or due to the rise in intra-cystic pressure can lead to the following forms of rupture [24, 27]:

(i) Contained rupture—only the endocyst ruptures, while the ectocyst and pericyst remain intact.
(ii) Communicating rupture—cyst ruptures into the biliary system (Fig. 3.13).
(iii) Direct rupture—all three layers tear with spillage into the peritoneal and pleural cavities and adjacent organs (Fig. 3.14).

Hepatic Hydatid Mimics [3]

Mucinous Cystic Neoplasm (MCN): These are uniloculated or multiloculated cystic lesions with enhancing internal septations on CT, unlike hydatid contents which do not enhance (Fig. 3.15) [3]. Intralesional solid enhancing areas are present in invasive MCN (Fig. 3.16).

Liver Abscess: Cyst wall is trilaminar and can have focal calcifications in hydatid.

Radiological Management

Image-guided PAIR (percutaneous puncture, aspiration, injection, and re-aspiration) procedure can be done for CE 1 and CE 3A (WHO grading of cystic echinococcosis (CE) of the liver of size more than 5 cm) (Fig. 3.17).

The procedure involves USG-guided or occasionally CT-guided puncture of the cyst, aspiration of cyst contents, followed by injection of scolicidal agent, and then re-aspiration of cyst contents after a 15-min wait. Traditionally, absolute alcohol has been used as a scolicidal agent. Other substances like chlorhexidine, betadine, hypertonic saline, formalin, and hydrogen peroxide have also shown promising results [21, 29–31].

Cyst fluid obtained with the initial aspiration is assessed for scolices and the presence of bilirubin. Bilirubin in hydatid fluid is confirmatory for

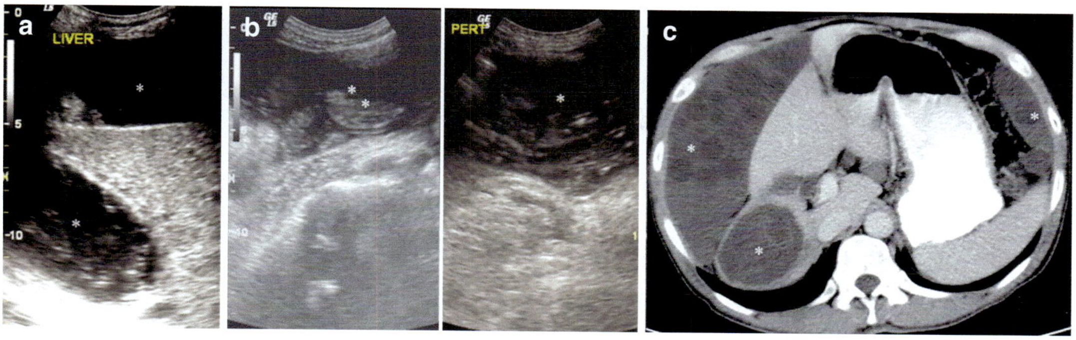

Fig. 3.14 Peritoneal hydatidosis. Ultrasound images show cystic lesions with internal echogenic content in the perihepatic spaces and in the pelvis (asterisk in **a**, **b**). (**c**) On CT, peritoneal complex cystic lesions show the presence of multiple internal smaller cysts or daughter cysts

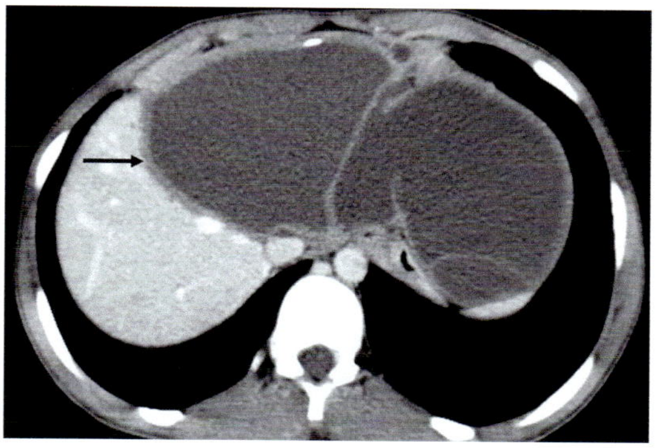

Fig. 3.15 Mucinous cystic neoplasm. Contrast-enhanced CT image shows a large multiloculated cystic lesion in the left lobe of the liver with internal septations, confirmed histologically to be a mucinous cystic neoplasm

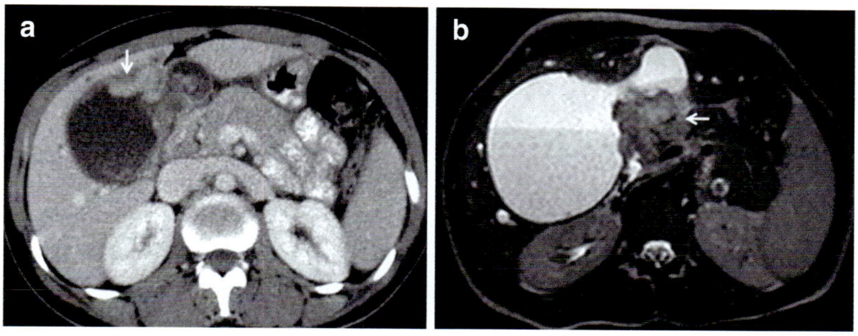

Fig. 3.16 Invasive mucinous cystic neoplasm. Contrast-enhanced CT of the liver shows a cystic lesion in the liver with intralesional solid, nodular enhancing areas (arrow in **a**). The solid component is of intermediate signal intensity on T2-weighted MRI (**b**). Lesion was confirmed on histology to be an invasive mucinous cystic neoplasm of the liver

biliary communication. Injection of scolicidal agent is contraindicated in these cysts.

Echinococcus multilocularis

This is a rare form of hydatid infection, also known as alveolar echinococcosis. The disease has a slow-growing course and an infiltrative pattern of involvement, often mimicking malignancies. The liver is the most commonly affected organ [32, 33].

3.4.1.3 Imaging

On Ultrasound there are single or multiple echogenic lesions with irregular necrotic areas within and microcalcification demonstrating a “hail-

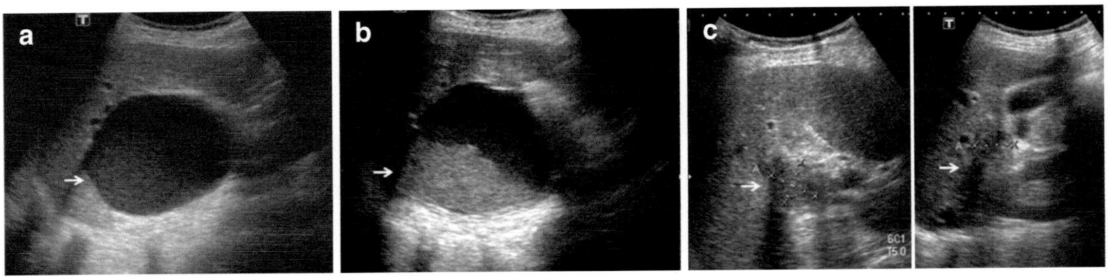

Fig. 3.17 PAIR procedure. Pre-procedure ultrasound appearance of a hepatic hydatid cyst containing low-level internal echoes (**a**). One week after PAIR, there is a mild reduction in the size of the cyst with an increase in non-enhancing debris within (**b**). Four months after the procedure, the cyst has shrunk, and fluid within it has disappeared (**c**)

storm," "vesicular," and "alveolar" patterns on ultrasound. Infiltration of the liver hilum can mimic the appearance of a tumor. Dead cysts have a heterogeneous, solid, tumor-like appearance resembling a "ball of wool" with wall calcification [32, 34].

On CT, hepatic lesions appear as multiple hypodense masses with a variable solid component. Punctate or amorphous patterns of intralesional as well as peripheral calcification are common. Larger lesions resemble "geographic maps."

CT is an important tool for the assessment of biliary and vascular infiltration as well as for detecting direct infiltration of surrounding structures and distant spread [32, 34–36].

On MRI, infiltrative, necrotic liver lesions have irregular margins with variable, heterogeneous signal intensity of the internal contents on T1w and T2w images. An important feature that helps differentiate hepatic tumors is the absence of post-contrast enhancement in these lesions [32, 34–38].

Management

There is no parasiticidal drug available for the treatment of *E. alveolaris*. Radical surgery is the treatment of choice for resectable lesions, while liver transplant is considered a last resort measure in the treatment of intractable, symptomatic biliary disease.

The role of image-guided procedures ranges from specimen collection for diagnosis, percutaneous liver abscess drainage, to symptomatic relief by percutaneous stenting of biliary and vascular obstructions [32, 38, 39].

3.4.2 Hepatic Vascular Infections

3.4.2.1 Schistosomiasis

Causative Organism: Of the five species of trematode blood flukes infecting humans, *Schistosoma mansoni* and *Schistosoma japonicum* are the most common that affect the liver [1, 2, 40].

Mode of Transmission and Pathology

The parasite enters the bloodstream by penetrating the skin and migrates to the mesenteric veins where it lays eggs. These eggs are carried to the hepatic venules through the portal circulation where they form granulomas. *S. mansoni* eggs, due to their size, lodge in the larger portal veins at the hilum, while *S. japonicum* eggs, being smaller in size, reach up to the peripheral branches. Schistosomiasis is a presinusoidal cause of portal hypertension.

Imaging

Ultrasound

Periportal fibrosis appears as thick, hyperechoic bands along the portal vein and its branches on ultrasound. Central anechoic blood in the portal vein surrounded by hyperechoic wall fibrosis forms a bull's eye appearance around the hilum in *S. mansoni* infection. A mosaic pattern of polygonal hyperechoic septa or a "fish scale

Table 3.3 Phases of *Fasciola hepatica* infection in the definitive host (Refs. [3, 4])

	Hepatic phase	Biliary phase
Mechanism	Digests hepatocytes	Enters the biliary ducts
Pathology	Small necrotic cavities/abscess	Migrate to the central & extrahepatic biliary ducts
Imaging	Ill-defined linear or patchy subcapsular nodules on CT, extending toward the hilum	Filling defects in the bile duct Duct wall thickening and dilatation

appearance" located peripherally in the liver can be seen with *S. japonicum* infection [1–4].

CT and MRI

On CT, calcified septa perpendicular to the liver capsule, forming a "turtle-back" or "tortoise shell" appearance, are classically seen with *S. japonicum* infection. Periportal hypodense fibrous bands diffusely scattered throughout the liver are a common finding. These septa are T1w iso-to-hypointense and T2w hyperintense and demonstrate marked delayed contrast enhancement. Features of chronic liver disease and portal hypertension are often present along with an increased risk for the development of hepatocellular carcinoma [1–4, 41].

Management

Diagnosis is made by serology and by the visualization of live eggs in stool. Anthelmintic drugs like praziquantel are used as the first line of treatment.

3.4.3 Billiary Infections

3.4.3.1 *Fasciola hepatica*

Causative Organism

The trematode *Fasciola hepatica* is a fluke responsible for hepatobiliary fascioliasis.

Mode of Transmission

Ingestion of freshwater plants contaminated with the metacercaria stage of the parasite

Pathology

Infection in the definitive host is divided into two phases: The first is the hepatic or parenchymal phase, and the second is the biliary phase. In the first phase, the ingested juvenile larvae penetrate the intestinal wall, migrate through the peritoneal cavity, breach the liver capsule, and enter the liver parenchyma. This causes mechanical destruction and inflammation of the hepatic parenchyma along the tracks of the migrating larva. In the biliary phase, the larvae enter the biliary radicles where they mature into adults and lay eggs (Table 3.3) [3, 4, 42, 43].

Imaging

Ultrasound

Ultrasound in the parenchymal phase of infection shows clusters of multiple ill-defined hypoechoic nodules in a subcapsular location. In the biliary phase, mild intrahepatic biliary ductal dilatation, gallbladder, and common biliary duct wall thickening due to inflammation are common. Live parasites may appear as 5–25-mm-long, mobile, curvilinear snail-like or leaf-like internal echoes within the gallbladder or common bile duct [3, 4, 42].

CT

On CT, linear hypodense subcapsular tracts are seen along with multiple small, confluent nodules of 2–3 cm size converging from the subcapsular region toward the hilum along the portal triads (Fig. 3.18a, b). Perihepatic fluid and reactive periportal lymph nodes are ancillary findings. A rare complication is the presence of subhepatic hematoma, which could be life-threatening if ruptured [4, 32, 42].

MRI Features

There are five distinct patterns of fascioliasis described on MRI:

(i) Capsular inflammation or perihepatitis
(ii) Ill-defined linear periportal tracts in a subcapsular location

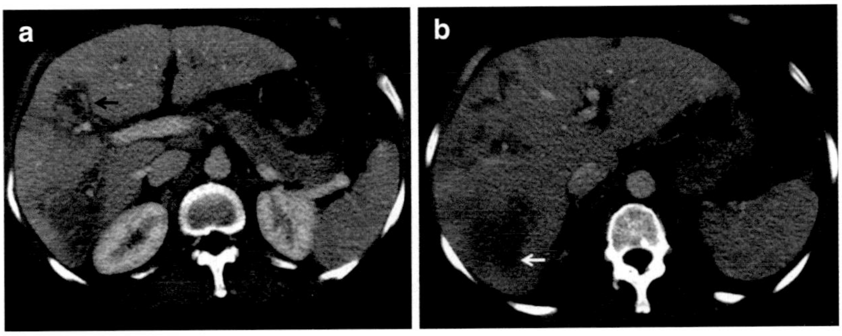

Fig. 3.18 *Fasciola hepatica* infection. Contrast-enhanced CT of the liver shows serpentine (black arrow in **a**) and hypodense foci (white arrow in **b**), extending from periphery to center (tunnel and cave sign)

(iii) Geographic borders of segmental hepatic inflammation
(iv) Rim-enhancing abscesses
(v) Post-inflammatory focal fibrosis

Active parenchymal inflammation, subcapsular tracts, and abscesses are hypointense on T1w and hyperintense on T2w and may show diffusion restriction. Late fibrosis appears hypointense on both T1- and T2-weighted images. On MR cholangiography, the parasites in the distal bile duct or gallbladder may appear as ill-defined, elongated, hypointense filling defects [3, 4, 43].

3.4.3.2 Ascariasis

Causative Organism: Ascaris lumbricoides, also known as roundworm

Mode of Transmission

On ingestion of food or water contaminated with ascaris eggs, the eggs reach the jejunum and hatch into larvae, which subsequently develop into adult worms. These worms can migrate into the biliary tree through the ampulla of Vater and cause mechanical obstruction [4].

Imaging

Ultrasound

The following signs have been described in biliary ascariasis on sonography [44–47]:

Inner-tube sign: The adult worm can be directly visualized as a long tubular echogenic structure inside a dilated biliary tree with a central hypoechoic line representing its gastrointestinal tract.

Strip sign: Thin tubular structure without an inner tube.

Spaghetti sign: Formed by the overlap of multiple worms in the common bile duct.

Occasionally, an adult worm can migrate to the liver parenchyma, where superinfection following its death can lead to the formation of a hepatic abscess.

ERCP, CT, and MRI

On ERCP, CT, and MRI, the adult worm can appear as a filling defect within a dilated bile duct. The worm may swallow contrast in the biliary tree which then outlines its gut (Fig. 3.19) [4, 45, 48, 49].

3.4.3.3 Clonorchiasis

Causative Organism: *Clonorchis sinensis*

Mode of Transmission

Ingestion of infected raw fish and snails, which are intermediate hosts. Humans, dogs, and cats are definitive hosts.

Pathology

On ingestion, action by gastric acids releases the eggs. Larvae travel through the ampulla of Vater to the second-order and smaller biliary ducts, where they reside until maturity. The adult worms migrate to the larger hepatic and biliary ducts to lay eggs. The presence of these flukes in the biliary system elicits an inflammatory response with subsequent development of adenomatous hyper-

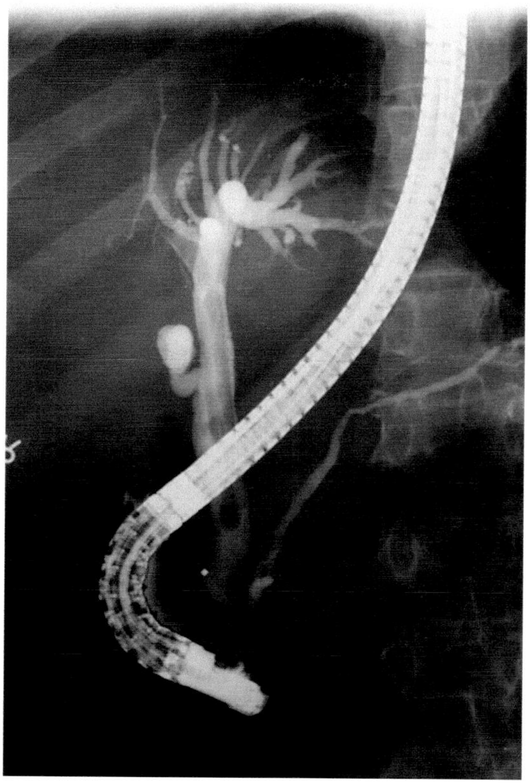

Fig. 3.19 Ascariasis. ERCP shows a linear, elongated filling defect in the CBD which has a central linear density within it, representing the gut outlined by contrast ingested by a roundworm

plasia, duct wall thickening, periductal fibrosis, and strictures.

Imaging

Peripheral mild diffuse intrahepatic biliary radicle dilatation with wall thickening, focal strictures, and sparing of the extrahepatic bile ducts is a classic feature of clonorchiasis, seen on ultrasound, CT, and MRI. Adult flukes may appear as crescent- or stilleto-shaped echogenic structures within the bile ducts on ultrasound and as small crescentic or ellipsoid filling defects on MRI. Peribiliary inflammation occurs as enhanced biliary walls on CT and MRI. Superadded infection can lead to the formation of hepatic abscesses [4, 50–53].

3.5 Hepatobiliary Tuberculosis

3.5.1 Introduction

Abdominal tuberculosis comprises 3.5% of extrapulmonary TB; isolated hepatic involvement occuring in less than 1% of cases [54]. It is usually a part of disseminated infection associated with miliary tuberculosis or secondary to tuberculosis of the lungs or gastrointestinal tract. Hematogenous dissemination via the hepatic artery predisposes to a military pattern of disease, while infection via the portal vein causes focal liver TB. Lymphatic spread is a less common pathway [55]. Concomitant splenic involvement and HIV infection are common in these patients.

Clinical Features: Patients may present with right upper quadrant pain, jaundice, and hepatosplenomegaly with other systemic symptoms such as fever, anorexia, malaise, and weight loss [55].

Imaging The imaging patterns include miliary TB, macronodular TB, serohepatic TB, and tubercular cholangitis [56].

(a) *Miliary tuberculosis*: It is the most common pattern resulting from hematogenous spread, forming multiple granulomas. It manifests as multiple random lesions measuring 0.5–2 cm in the liver parenchyma. These lesions are hypoechoic-isoechoic on sonography and appear cystic or nodular on CT and MRI. Peripheral rim enhancement indicative of microabscesses can be seen. Calcification is seen in chronic or healing stages. The other diagnostic considerations would include opportunistic fungal infections, *Pneumocystis jiroveci* infection, sarcoidosis, metastases, and lymphoma [54, 56].
(b) *Macronodular tuberculosis*: These lesions are more than 2 cm in size, manifesting either as solitary or multiple hepatic masses. Sonographic appearance is nonspecific, rang-

ing from purely hypoechoic or hyperechoic to mixed echogenicity lesions. On CT, noncaseating granulomas appear as hypodense lesions with variable rim enhancement (Fig. 3.20a). Caseating granulomas result in tubercular abscesses with central or multifocal liquefaction. Depending on the pattern of liquefaction, they can appear "honeycomb" like with multiple septations or as a cluster of conglomerating lesions. On MRI, the lesions are T1w hypointense with a hypointense rim and iso-to-hyperintense on T2w with a less hyperintense rim. Alternatively, the T2w signal may be hypointense in a caseating granuloma without liquefaction. Post-contrast rim/septal enhancement and restricted diffusion are other features. Large abscesses may rupture, forming perihepatic and peritoneal collections [54, 56].

(c) *Serohepatic tuberculosis*: This rare presentation results from tuberculous involvement of the subserosal plane and Glisson capsule. Peripheral coalescing lesions causing thickening of the liver capsule and subcapsular plane have been described as "frosted liver/sugar-coating" appearance [56].

(d) *Tubercular cholangitis*: Biliary involvement can be secondary to hematogenous spread, ascending infection from the bowel, or contiguous spread from hepatic lesions. Both the large and small calibre ducts can be involved, forming biliary strictures with bile duct wall thickening and dilatations (Fig. 3.20b). The strictures are multifocal and associated with segmental parenchymal atrophy. Miliary calcifications along the bile ducts are a characteristic finding. MRCP clearly depicts the multifocal strictures noninvasively, while ERCP is preferred for tissue sampling and placement of biliary stents. Imaging differential diagnoses in these cases include sclerosing cholangitis and cholangiocarcinoma [54, 56].

Concurrent splenic, lymph nodal, and pulmonary involvement helps in narrowing the differential diagnosis. Portal hypertension is an uncommon complication. Healing phase or scarring of multiple tubercles can result in tuberculous pseudocirrhosis [55].

Diagnosis and Treatment: A total of 75% of patients may show abnormality on the chest radiograph. Deranged liver function tests can be seen in 30–80% of cases. As the imaging patterns vary, histopathological/microbiological confirmation is usually required. Hepatobiliary TB is treated with the same regimen as any other extrapulmonary lesion using quadruple therapy with antituberculous drugs, and the prognosis is good [55].

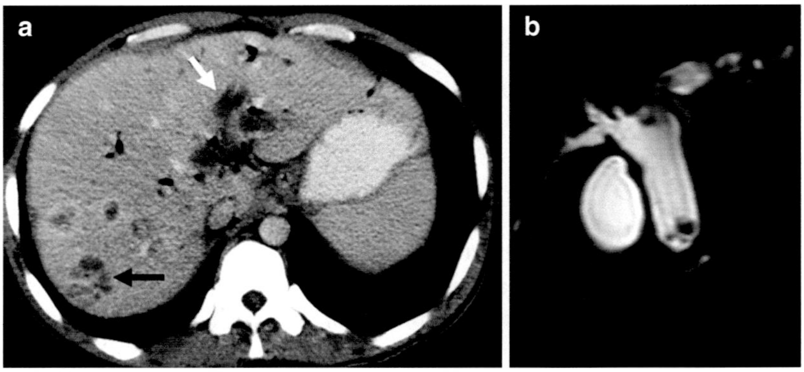

Fig. 3.20 Hepatic and biliary tuberculosis. Contrast-enhanced CT of the liver shows multiple ill-defined hypodense lesions with variable rim enhancement (black arrow in **a**) and intrahepatic biliary dilatation in the left lobe (white arrow in **b**). The MRCP image shows a dilated CBD due to a tuberculous stricture of the lower CBD. TB of the liver was confirmed on histology

3.6 Fungal Infections

Fungal infections of the liver occur typically in immunocompromised individuals or those with hematological malignancies, most commonly leukaemia [1, 57]. Infection reaches the liver via the portal venous system. The most common organism is *Candida albicans*. Some of the other less common organisms implicated are *C. neoformans* and *H. capsulatum* [58].

Imaging

Fungal infections, typically hepatic candidiasis, most commonly present as hepatic microabscesses usually less than 10 mm [2, 58].

There are four ultrasound patterns described in hepatic candidiasis.

The "bull's-eye" appearance, seen in patients with active infection and normal white cell count, comprises a central echogenic focus with a peripheral hypoechoic rim. The "wheel-within-a wheel" appearance describes a central hypoechoic area surrounded by an echogenic zone of inflammatory cells and a peripheral hypoechoic rim of fibrosis. The other patterns are a uniformly hypoechoic nodule, which is the most common appearance, and a lesion with varying echogenicity, seen in later stages of the infection (Figs. 3.21 and 3.22a) [1, 2].

On CT, microabscesses are seen as multiple, discrete, round, low attenuation lesions which usually enhance centrally (Fig. 3.22b). Peripheral enhancement may also be seen in some lesions [1, 57].

On MRI, these lesions are mildly hypointense on T1-weighted images, markedly hyperintense on T2-weighted images with a peripheral dark ring on all sequences.

Treatment is with appropriate antifungal therapy.

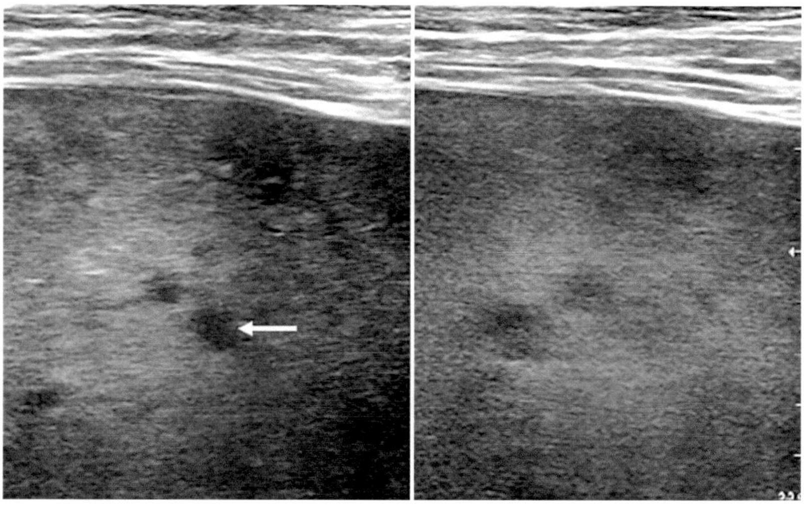

Fig. 3.21 *Candida* infection of the liver. Ultrasound images of the liver in a 52-year-old male with acute myeloid leukemia, on chemotherapy and febrile neutropenia with *Candida* microabscesses seen as ill-defined hypoechoic lesions in the liver

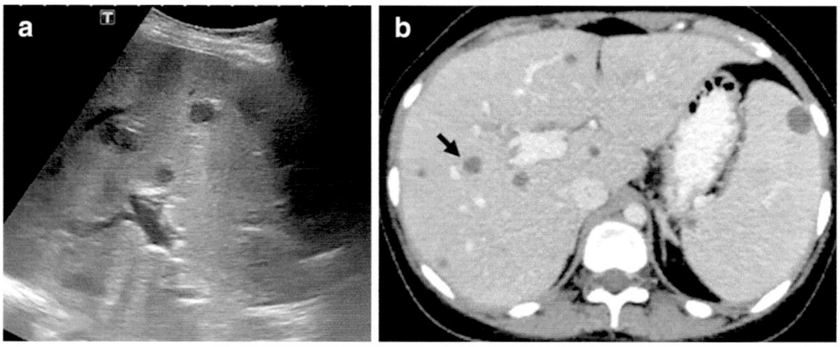

Fig. 3.22 *Candida* infection of the liver. Ultrasound shows multiple well-defined, hypoechoic lesions in a 19-year-old lady with acute leukemia and sepsis from *Candida* (**a**). CT images show discrete low attenuation lesions (**b**). *Candida* was confirmed on liver biopsy

3.7 Viral Hepatitis

Etiopathogenesis
Acute viral hepatitis is caused by the hepatitis viruses A, B, C, D (HBV-associated delta agent), and E. Histological features of acute viral hepatitis include necrosis of random isolated cells or clusters of cells, diffuse liver cell injury, reactive Kupfer cell changes, and regeneration of hepatocytes during recovery. In severe acute hepatitis, bridging necrosis involving portal tracts or central veins may be seen [1]. Persistence of inflammation and necrosis for at least 6 months is seen in chronic hepatitis. In mild chronic hepatitis, inflammation is confined to portal tracts; however, with more severe disease, piecemeal necrosis extends from portal tracts to liver parenchyma with hepatocyte necrosis. This further leads to fibrous septae formation, hepatocyte regeneration, and cirrhosis [1].

Imaging
The imaging appearances in acute hepatitis are nonspecific.

Ultrasound shows hepatomegaly with diffuse decrease in parenchymal echogenicity causing portal vein radicles to appear relatively hyperechoic, the so-called "starry night" appearance [1, 2].

On CT, hepatomegaly with heterogeneous parenchymal enhancement, well-defined areas of low attenuation, and hypoattenuation around portal radicles representing edema, may be seen.

On MRI, there are nonspecific findings such as hepatomegaly and periportal T2w hyperintense areas, representing edema. Other findings include GB wall edema and ascites [1, 59].

3.8 Melioidosis

Melioidosis is caused by a gram-negative bacterium, *Burkholderia pseudomallei*, found in soil and surface water. It is endemic in Southeast Asia and northern Australia [60].

Route of Transmission: The organism infects humans usually via percutaneous inoculation. Other routes of transmission are via inhalation and ingestion. There is a higher risk of infection among diabetics. Clinical presentation is often varied, ranging from subclinical infection to fulminating illness and septic shock [60].

Imaging
Melioidosis can affect several organs, the most common being the lungs, skin and subcutaneous tissues, liver, and spleen. The second most common solid organ affected is the liver. On imaging, lesions appear as multiple discrete lesions which are clustered or coalesce into multiple small abscesses. A typical "honeycomb" appearance on CT due to rim enhancement of these lesions may be seen [60, 61]. This is usually accompanied by lesions in other organs such as the spleen. Imaging findings are often nonspecific, but the pattern of distribution in multiple organs should arouse suspicion of melioidosis (Fig. 3.23) [60].

Treatment includes drainage of large abscesses and appropriate antibiotic therapy [60, 61].

Imaging has a significant role to play in the evaluation of hepatic infections. Several infections have classic imaging appearances, while others have nonspecific findings. Early diagnosis facilitates early medical and other therapeutic interventions.

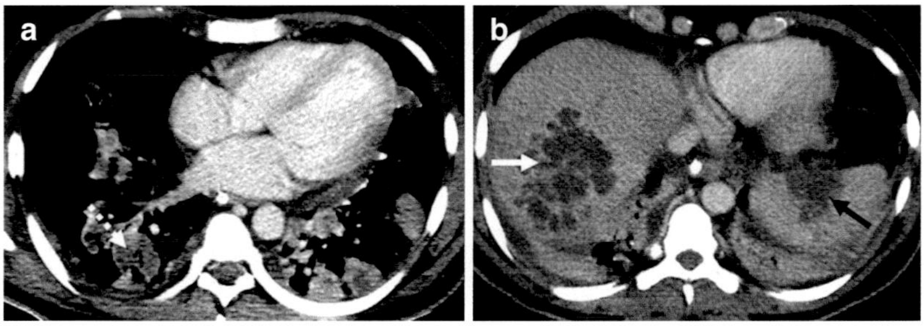

Fig. 3.23 Melioidosis. (**a** and **b**) CT images show multiple clustered, coalescing small abscesses with a honeycomb appearance in the liver (white arrow) with a splenic abscess (black arrow) and multiple lower lobe of lung consolidations with areas of breakdown (dashed white arrow)

Acknowledgements All images in the chapter are courtesy of the Department of Radiodiagnosis, Christian Medical College, Vellore, Tamil Nadu, India.

References

1. Mortelé KJ, Segatto E, Ros PR. The infected liver: radiologic-pathologic correlation. RadioGraphics. 2004;24(4):937–55.
2. Doyle DJ, Hanbidge AE, O'Malley ME. Imaging of hepatic infections. Clin Radiol. 2006;61(9):737–48.
3. Bächler P, Baladron MJ, Menias C, Beddings I, Loch R, Zalaquett E, et al. Multimodality imaging of liver infections: differential diagnosis and potential pitfalls. RadioGraphics. 2016;36(4):1001–23.
4. Malekzadeh S, Widmer L, Salahshour F, Egger B, Ronot M, Thoeny HC. Typical imaging finding of hepatic infections: a pictorial essay. Abdom Radiol N Y. 2021;46(2):544–61.
5. Chou FF, Sheen-Chen SM, Chen YS, Chen MC. Single and multiple pyogenic liver abscesses: clinical course, etiology, and results of treatment. World J Surg. 1997;21(4):384–8. discussion 388–389
6. Seeto RK, Rockey DC. Pyogenic liver abscess changes in etiology, management, and outcome. Medicine (Baltimore). 1996;75(2):99–113.
7. Shi S, Zhai Z, Zheng S. Pyogenic liver abscess of biliary origin: the existing problems and their strategies. Semin Liver Dis. 2018;38(03):270–83.
8. Subramanyam BR, Balthazar EJ, Raghavendra BN, Horii SC, Hilton S, Naidich DP. Ultrasound analysis of solid-appearing abscesses. Radiology. 1983;146(2):487–91.
9. Knochel JQ, Koehler PR, Lee TG, Welch DM. Diagnosis of abdominal abscesses with computed tomography, ultrasound, and 111In leukocyte scans. Radiology. 1980;137(2):425–32.
10. Kim S-B, Je B-K, Lee KY, Lee SH, Chung H-H, Cha SH. Computed tomographic differences of pyogenic liver abscesses caused by Klebsiella pneumoniae and non-Klebsiella pneumoniae. J Comput Assist Tomogr. 2007;31(1):59–65.
11. Surya M, Bhoil R, Sharma YP. Study of ultrasound-guided needle aspiration and catheter drainage in the management of liver abscesses. J Ultrasound. 2020;23(4):553–62.
12. Rajak CL, Gupta S, Jain S, Chawla Y, Gulati M, Suri S. Percutaneous treatment of liver abscesses: needle aspiration versus catheter drainage. AJR Am J Roentgenol. 1998;170(4):1035–9.
13. Heneghan HM, Healy NA, Martin ST, Ryan RS, Nolan N, Traynor O, et al. Modern management of pyogenic hepatic abscess: a case series and review of the literature. BMC Res Notes. 2011;4:80.
14. vanSonnenberg E, Ferrucci JT, Mueller PR, Wittenberg J, Simeone JF. Percutaneous drainage of abscesses and fluid collections: technique, results, and applications. Radiology. 1982;142(1):1–10.
15. Haque R, Huston CD, Hughes M, Houpt E, Petri WA. Amebiasis. N Engl J Med. 2003;348(16):1565–73.
16. Radin DR, Ralls PW, Colletti PM, Halls JM. CT of amebic liver abscess. AJR Am J Roentgenol. 1988;150(6):1297–301.
17. Mondal A, Lahiri A, Ray P, Bhattacharjee A. Effective treatment options in amoebic liver abscess in a tertiary care setting in West Bengal: an observational study, India. Int Surg J. 2018;5(11):3666–71.
18. Ghosh JK, Goyal SK, Behera MK, Tripathi MK, Dixit VK, Jain AK, et al. Efficacy of aspiration in amebic liver abscess. Trop Gastroenterol. 2016;36(4):251–5.
19. Tandon A, Jain AK, Dixit VK, Agarwal AK, Gupta JP. Needle aspiration in large amoebic liver abscess. Trop Gastroenterol Off J Dig Dis Found. 1997;18(1):19–21.
20. Gharbi HA, Hassine W, Brauner MW, Dupuch K. Ultrasound examination of the hydatic liver. Radiology. 1981;139(2):459–63.
21. WHO Informal Working Group. International classification of ultrasound images in cystic echinococcosis for application in clinical and field epidemiological settings. Acta Trop. 2003;85(2):253–61.
22. Turgut AT, Akhan O, Bhatt S, Dogra VS. Sonographic spectrum of hydatid disease. Ultrasound Q. 2008;24(1):17–29.
23. Pendse HA, Nawale AJ, Deshpande SS, Merchant SA. Radiologic features of hydatid disease: the importance of sonography. J Ultrasound Med Off J Am Inst Ultrasound Med. 2015;34(5):895–905.
24. Pedrosa I, Saíz A, Arrazola J, Ferreirós J, Pedrosa CS. Hydatid disease: radiologic and pathologic features and complications. RadioGraphics. 2000;20(3):795–817.
25. Lewall DB. Hydatid disease: biology, pathology, imaging and classification. Clin Radiol. 1998;53(12):863–74.
26. Lewall DB, McCorkell SJ. Hepatic echinococcal cysts: sonographic appearance and classification. Radiology. 1985;155(3):773–5.
27. Mehta P, Prakash M, Khandelwal N. Radiological manifestations of hydatid disease and its complications. Trop Parasitol. 2016;6(2):103–12.
28. Polat P, Kantarci M, Alper F, Suma S, Koruyucu MB, Okur A. Hydatid disease from head to toe. RadioGraphics. 2003;23(2):475–94.
29. Ustünsöz B, Akhan O, Kamiloğlu MA, Somuncu I, Uğurel MS, Cetiner S. Percutaneous treatment of hydatid cysts of the liver: long-term results. AJR Am J Roentgenol. 1999;172(1):91–6.
30. Kabaalioğlu A, Ceken K, Alimoglu E, Apaydin A. Percutaneous imaging-guided treatment of hydatid liver cysts: do long-term results make it a first choice? Eur J Radiol. 2006;59(1):65–73.
31. Brunetti E, Troia G, Garlaschelli AL, Gulizia R, Filice C. Twenty years of percutaneous treatments for cystic echinococcosis: a preliminary assessment of their use and safety. Parassitologia. 2004;46(4):367–70.

32. Bulakçı M, Kartal MG, Yılmaz S, Yılmaz E, Yılmaz R, Şahin D, et al. Multimodality imaging in diagnosis and management of alveolar echinococcosis: an update. Diagn Interv Radiol. 2016;22(3):247–56.
33. Bv C, O A, R H, B Z, W V, W J, et al. Echinococcosis of the liver. Abdom Imaging [Internet]. 2008;33(2) Available from: https://pubmed.ncbi.nlm.nih.gov/17912581/
34. Alveolar Echinococcosis: Spectrum of Findings at Cross-sectional Imaging | RadioGraphics [Internet]. [cited 2022 Jan 25]. Available from: https://pubs.rsna.org/doi/10.1148/rg.327125708?url_ver=Z39.88-2003&rfr_id=ori:rid:crossref.org&rfr_dat=cr_pub%20%200pubmed
35. Chouhan MD, Wiley E, Chiodini PL, Amin Z. Hepatic alveolar hydatid disease (Echinococcus multilocularis), a mimic of liver malignancy: a review for the radiologist in non-endemic areas. Clin Radiol. 2019;74(4):247–56.
36. S B-H, E D, O B, B B, S K, Jp M, et al. Imaging aspects and non-surgical interventional treatment in human alveolar echinococcosis. Parasitol Int [Internet]. 2006;55 Suppl. Available from: https://pubmed.ncbi.nlm.nih.gov/16403670/
37. Alveolar echinococcosis: MR findings in the liver – PubMed [Internet]. [cited 2022 Jan 25]. Available from: https://pubmed.ncbi.nlm.nih.gov/12750459/
38. Liu W, Delabrousse É, Blagosklonov O, Wang J, Zeng H, Jiang Y, et al. Innovation in hepatic alveolar echinococcosis imaging: best use of old tools, and necessary evaluation of new ones. Parasite [Internet]. 2014:21. Available from: https://www.ncbi.nlm.nih.gov/pmc/articles/PMC4273719/
39. M K, O A, Mt G, Bk K, H Y, G K, et al. Complete resolution of an alveolar echinococcosis liver lesion following percutaneous treatment. Cardiovasc Intervent Radiol [Internet]. 2006;29(3) Available from: https://pubmed.ncbi.nlm.nih.gov/16228851/
40. Bica I, Hamer DH, Stadecker MJ. Hepatic schistosomiasis. Infect Dis Clin North Am. 2000;14(3):583–604. viii
41. Lee D, Shaffer K. Concentric rings: updated CT appearance of hepatic schistosomiasis mansoni. Radiol Case Rep. 2015;1(4):134–9.
42. Kabaalioglu A, Ceken K, Alimoglu E, Saba R, Cubuk M, Arslan G, et al. Hepatobiliary fascioliasis: sonographic and CT findings in 87 patients during the initial phase and long-term follow-up. Am J Roentgenol. 2007;189(4):824–8.
43. Radiological Imaging Features of Fasciola hepatica Infection – A Pictorial Review [Internet]. [cited 2022 Jan 20]. Available from: https://www.ncbi.nlm.nih.gov/pmc/articles/PMC3279695/
44. Sultan Khuroo M, Ali Zargar S, Nabi Yattoo G, Yousuf Dar M, Javid G, Ahmad Khan B, et al. Sonographic findings in gallbladder ascariasis. J Clin Ultrasound. 1992;20(9):587–91.
45. Das C, Kumar J, Debnath J, Chaudhry A. Imaging of ascariasis. Australas Radiol. 2007;51(6):500–6.
46. Schulman A, Loxton A, Heydenrych J, Abdurahman K. Sonographic diagnosis of biliary ascariasis. 1982;7
47. Lynser D, Handique A, Daniala C, Phukan P, Marbaniang E. Sonographic images of hepato-pancreatico-biliary and intestinal ascariasis: a pictorial review. Insights Imaging. 2015;6(6):641–6.
48. Adaletli I, Selçuk D, Gülşen M, Savaş C, Korman U. MRCP findings of biliary ascariasis before and after medical treatment. Turk J Gastroenterol Off J Turk Soc Gastroenterol. 2005;16(2):98–101.
49. Hwang CM, Kim TK, Ha HK, Kim PN, Lee M-G. Biliary ascariasis: MR cholangiography findings in two cases. Korean J Radiol. 2001;2(3):175–8.
50. Choi D, Hong S-T. Imaging diagnosis of clonorchiasis. Korean J Parasitol. 2007;45(2):77–85.
51. Jang Y-J, Byun JH, Yoon SE, Yu E. Hepatic parasitic abscess caused by clonorchiasis: unusual CT findings of clonorchiasis. Korean J Radiol. 2007;8(1):70–3.
52. Lim JH. Radiologic findings of clonorchiasis. 1990;8.
53. Characteristic imaging features of clonorchiasis [Internet]. HKMJ. 2018 [cited 2022 Jan 20]. Available from: https://www.hkmj.org/abstracts/v24n2/206.e3.htm
54. Karaosmanoglu AD, Onur MR, Sahani DV, Tabari A, Karcaaltincaba M. Hepatobiliary tuberculosis: imaging findings. Am J Roentgenol. 2016;207(4):694–704.
55. Chaudhary P. Hepatobiliary tuberculosis. Ann Gastroenterol. 2014;27(3):207–11.
56. Kakkar C, Polnaya AM, Koteshwara P, Smiti S, Rajagopal KV, Arora A. Hepatic tuberculosis: a multimodality imaging review. Insights Imaging. 2015;6(6):647–58. https://doi.org/10.1007/s13244-015-0440-y.
57. Karaosmanoglu AD, Uysal A, Karcaaltincaba M, Akata D, Ozmen MN, Kraeft J, Hahn PF. Non-neoplastic hepatopancreatobiliary lesions simulating malignancy: can we differentiate? Insights Imaging. 2020;11(1):21.
58. Orlowski HLP, McWilliams S, Mellnick VM, Bhalla S, Lubner MG, Pickhardt PJ, Menias CO. Imaging spectrum of invasive fungal and fungal-like infections. Radiographics. 2017;37(4):1119–34.
59. Malekzadeh S, Widmer L, Salahshour F, Egger B, Ronot M, Thoeny HC. Typical imaging finding of hepatic infections: a pictorial essay. Abdom Radiol (NY). 2021;46(2):544–61.
60. Alsaif HS, Venkatesh SK. Melioidosis: spectrum of radiological manifestations. Saudi J Med Med Sci. 2016;4(2):74–8. https://doi.org/10.4103/1658-631X.178286.
61. Martin PF, Teh CS, Casupang MA. Melioidosis: a rare cause of liver abscess. Case Rep Hepatol. 2016;2016:5910375. https://doi.org/10.1155/2016/5910375.

4 Approach to Benign Liver Tumours

Pratyaksha Rana, Pavithra Subramanian, and Naveen Kalra

4.1 Introduction

Benign liver tumours are commonly encountered in day-to-day clinical practice. Most cases are asymptomatic and often incidentally detected. Although some have typical imaging appearances posing no diagnostic difficulty, atypical appearances and uncommon benign tumours can be of diagnostic challenge. Furthermore, there is significant overlap in imaging features of various benign and malignant liver tumours. Imaging plays a crucial role in the detection and characterisation of focal liver lesions. Moreover, imaging has a vital role in the detection of complications and in the surveillance of some benign liver tumours. Hence, it is very important for radiologists to be aware of the typical and atypical imaging features of both common and uncommon benign liver tumours.

This chapter addresses the imaging features of benign liver tumours. At the end, important differential diagnoses on imaging are briefly discussed.

P. Rana · P. Subramanian · N. Kalra (✉)
Department of Radiodiagnosis and Imaging, PGIMER, Chandigarh, India

4.2 Classification of Benign Liver Tumours

Classification of benign liver tumours is according to their cell of origin [1, 2]. These include tumours of hepatocellular, mesenchymal and cholangiocellular origin (Table 4.1). The tumours of hepatocellular origin include hepatic adenoma, focal nodular hyperplasia, hepatocellular nodules in cirrhosis and nodular regenerative hyperplasia. Biliary cystadenoma and bile duct adenoma are a spectrum of benign tumours of cholangiocellular origin. Hepatic cysts (including simple cyst, polycystic liver disease, foregut cyst, peribiliary cyst and biliary hamartomas) are developmental lesions rather than true neoplasms [1]. The mesenchymal benign tumours include haemangioma, angiomyolipoma, lipoma, paraganglioma, lymphangioma, leiomyoma, fibroma and inflammatory pseudotumour. Mesenchymal hamartoma and infantile haemangioma (previously called infantile haemangioendothelioma) are benign liver tumours of mesenchymal origin found predominantly in the pediatric population. Peliosis hepatis is a rare benign disorder characterised by multiple blood-filled lacunar spaces within the liver [3]. Apart from these, heterotopic tissues (adrenal and pancreatic) can be found within the liver parenchyma, giving rise to adrenal rest tumour and pancreatic heterotopia which are extremely rare [2]. Overall, hepatic haemangioma is the

© The Author(s), under exclusive license to Springer Nature Singapore Pte Ltd. 2025

B. Sureka (ed.), *Hepato-Pancreatico Biliary Imaging*, https://doi.org/10.1007/978-981-95-1699-5_4

Table 4.1 Classification of benign liver tumours

	Cell of origin	Tumours
A	Tumour-like conditions	Hepatic cyst Polycystic liver disease Ciliated hepatic foregut cyst Peribiliary cyst Biliary hamartomas Peliosis hepatis
B	Hepatocellular origin	Hepatic adenoma Focal nodular hyperplasia (FNH) Nodular regenerative hyperplasia (NRH) Hepatocellular nodules in cirrhosis
C	Mesenchymal origin	Haemangioma Mesenchymal hamartoma Infantile haemangioma Angiomyolipoma/lipoma/myelolipoma Inflammatory pseudotumour Paraganglioma Leiomyoma Fibroma Lymphangioma
D	Cholangiocellular origin	Hepatic cysts (simple cysts, polycystic disease) Bile duct adenoma Biliary cystadenoma
E	Heterotopic origin	Adrenal rest Pancreatic rest

most common benign liver tumour which has a fairly characteristic imaging appearance in most of the cases [4].

4.3 Role of Imaging and Diagnostic Approach

Accurate diagnosis of a benign liver tumour is crucial to avoid unnecessary interventions and surgeries, for timely treatment of premalignant conditions and appropriate surveillance. A combination of imaging techniques along with clinical information is often needed for arriving at a diagnosis [5]. A comprehensive evaluation of comorbidities and biochemical analysis is sometimes needed. Lesions with typical imaging features require no further diagnostic work-up or only a short-term follow-up. For indeterminate lesions, multiple cross-sectional imaging techniques can be employed which can suggest the diagnosis; however, if, still, the diagnosis dilemma persists, histological diagnosis is needed. The approach has to be individualised on a case-by-case basis (Fig. 4.1).

4.3.1 Ultrasound (US)

Abdominal US is the first-line imaging modality for the evaluation of liver diseases. It possesses the advantage of being radiation-free, easily accessible, cost-effective and non-invasive with inherent soft tissue contrast. Both grayscale and Doppler US (colour and spectral Doppler) are useful for the identification and characterisation of liver lesions. Internal features (solid versus cystic lesions, vascularity pattern), capsule and relationship to surrounding structures can be demonstrated [7]. However, it is a subjective and operator-dependent modality. Moreover, most of the benign liver tumours have a wide range of sonographic appearances, and there is significant overlap between various lesions on US. Hence, cross-sectional imaging is usually needed for further characterisation.

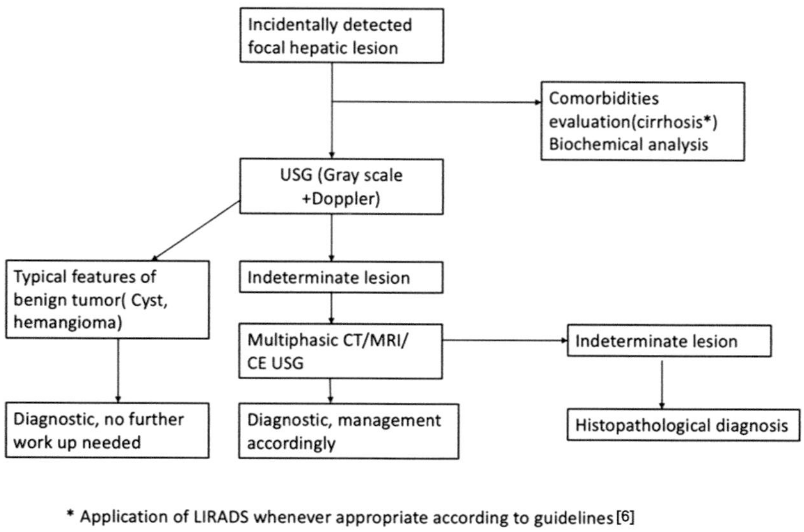

Fig. 4.1 Imaging approach to benign liver tumours

4.3.2 Contrast-Enhanced Ultrasound (CEUS)

There is a growing role of contrast-enhanced US for characterisation and evaluation of focal liver lesions [8–10]. Apart from the morphological assessment, the microcirculation and vascular enhancement pattern of the lesion are demonstrated on administration of intravenous US contrast agent. In addition to the advantages of grayscale ultrasound, it is particularly useful in patients with deranged renal function in whom contrast-enhanced cross-sectional imaging cannot be performed. It can also be used for long-term surveillance of certain liver lesions, being a radiation-free modality. SonoVue (sulfur hexafluoride in phospholipid shell) is a second-generation US contrast agent which has purely intravascular distribution and is widely available [11]. Due to the dual vascular supply of the liver, multiple enhancement phases are obtained for up to 5 min after contrast administration to study the continuous intralesional haemodynamic changes [12]. With the use of a US contrast agent, diagnostic accuracy is significantly increased for the identification as well as characterisation of the liver lesions compared to grayscale US [13].

4.3.3 Computed Tomography (CT)

Multidetector CT remains the most frequently used imaging technique for evaluation of liver lesions [14]. Apart from being objective in nature, it is more accurate and delineates the morphology, vascularity and relationship of the lesion with adjacent structures. With recent advances, substantial anatomical coverage can be achieved in a short scan time along with multiplanar and volumetric reconstructions. A multiphasic acquisition is needed to provide detailed morphological and haemodynamic information. A non-contrast-enhanced phase is added to detect calcification, fat, necrosis and intralesional haemorrhage. In the presence of dual energy CT, a virtual non-contrast image can be generated, with which the non-contrast enhanced phase can be omitted [15]. After contrast administration (non-ionic extracellular contrast agents), multiple post-contrast phases are obtained depending on the diagnostic task. An early arterial phase (10–20 s, after contrast administration) is acquired for the generation of an arterial vascular road map to see the arterial supply of the lesion and to plan intervention. A late arterial phase (25–30 s, after contrast administration) demonstrates the hypervascular lesions in the background of hypoattenuating liver parenchyma. Portal venous (60–70 s, after contrast administration) and delayed (2–3 min, after contrast administration) phases are obtained to study the intralesional haemodynamics and the lesion attenuation in relation to the adjacent liver parenchyma [16].

4.3.4 Magnetic Resonance Imaging (MRI)

MRI is a comprehensive imaging modality for morphological and functional characterisation of liver lesions [17]. Use of higher magnetic field strength (1.5–3 Tesla), dedicated phased array body coil and technical advancements in imaging sequences, including respiratory-triggered 3D data acquisition, have further expanded its role [18]. The standard MRI sequences for evaluation of the liver lesions include a pre-contrast T2-weighted (T2-W) sequence (single-shot fast-spin echo sequence, balanced steady-state free precession sequence), T1-weighted sequence (T1-W), chemical shift imaging and multiphasic dynamic 3D-spoiled gradient echo sequence performed till 3–4 min after contrast administration [19]. In addition, diffusion-weighted imaging and MRCP can be added depending on the clinical scenario. Non-specific gadolinium-based extracellular MRI contrast agents are commonly employed for post-contrast imaging, which follow the same haemodynamic principle as iodinated CT contrast. Hepatocyte-specific contrast agents (gadoxetic acid disodium, gadobenate diglumine) are partially excreted by the biliary system. This allows the combination of multiple contrast phases of extracellular non-specific agents along with a hepatocyte-specific excretory phase to the contrast-enhanced liver imaging protocol [20]. Use of these agents has been found to be better for liver lesion evaluation, especially differentiating hepatic adenoma versus focal nodular hyperplasia, which remains a diagnostic challenge [21]. Superparamagnetic iron oxide particles (SPIOs) are taken up by reticuloendothelial cells of the liver (Kupffer cells) which are present in variable amounts in various liver lesions. This property can be used for lesion detection and characterisation using T2* gradient echo sequences [22].

4.3.5 Nuclear Medicine

Due to widespread advances in cross-sectional imaging modalities, there has been a declining role of conventional scintigraphy techniques in the characterisation of liver lesions. FDG-PET/CT also has a limited role in the evaluation of benign liver tumours.

Despite technical advances and a multitude of imaging modalities available, histopathological confirmation of diagnosis may also be required.

4.4 Benign Tumour-Like Conditions

4.4.1 Hepatic Cysts

Hepatic cysts are developmental lesions rather than true tumours. There is a slight predominance of females [2]. They vary in size and number.

4.4.1.1 Pathology

Hepatic cysts are thought to be of biliary tract origin arising due to deranged development of bile ducts. The wall of the cyst is lined by cuboidal biliary epithelium; however, they do not communicate with the biliary tree [23].

4.4.1.2 Clinical Features

Most of the hepatic cysts are incidentally discovered at routine imaging. However, large cysts can cause compression of adjacent structures leading to symptoms.

4.4.1.3 Imaging Features

US

On grayscale US, they are round to oval anechoic lesions with a thin imperceptible wall (Fig. 4.2a). Posterior wall enhancement is seen with increased through-transmission. In case of complication (mostly due to haemorrhage or infection), internal

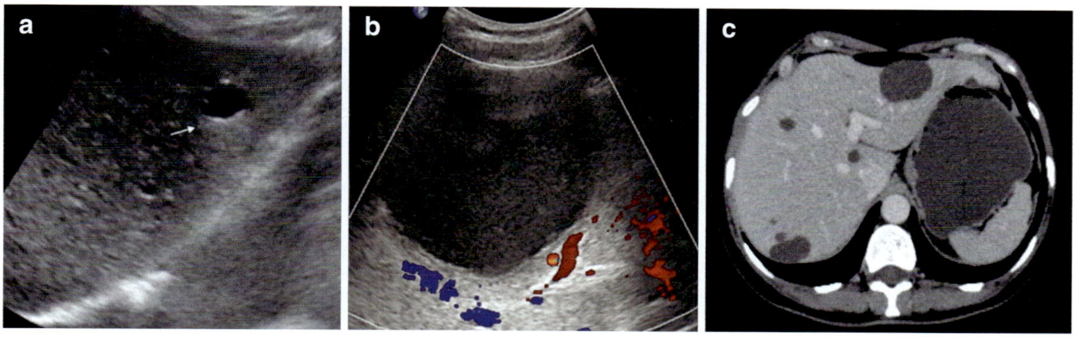

Fig. 4.2 Hepatic cysts. Grayscale US image (**a**) shows an oval, anechoic lesion with a thin imperceptible wall and posterior acoustic enhancement (arrow), characteristic of a simple hepatic cyst. Colour Doppler US image (**b**) shows a unilocular hepatic cyst with fine echoes within and no internal vascularity, suggesting a complicated cyst. Post contrast CT (venous phase), axial image (**c**) shows multiple small non-enhancing hypodense homogenous lesions scattered in both lobes consistent with simple hepatic cysts

debris, thick septation or nodularity can be noted (Fig. 4.2b) [23].

CT

Simple hepatic cysts are typically well demarcated with a homogenous appearance. The attenuation varies from 10–15 HU (Fig. 4.2c). Characteristically, contrast enhancement is absent except in cases of complication [24].

MRI

Hepatic cysts typically have a fluid signal intensity, appearing homogenously hyperintense on T2-W and hypointense on T1-W images. No diffusion restriction or post-contrast enhancement is seen (Fig. 4.3). In case of intracystic haemorrhage, high signal intensity on T1-W images can be seen.

4.4.2 Polycystic Liver Disease

Polycystic liver disease is a rare autosomal-dominant fibropolycystic disease manifesting with multiple simple hepatic cysts. Around 50% have associated autosomal-dominant polycystic kidney disease [25].

4.4.2.1 Pathology

Polycystic liver disease arises due to ductal plate malformation affecting small intrahepatic biliary ducts. It can be associated with other disorders characterised by ductal plate malformation such as Caroli's disease and biliary hamartomas. Histologically, it contains two types of cysts: simple hepatic cysts (lined by cuboidal biliary epithelium) and peribiliary cysts (dilated peribiliary glands) [25].

4.4.2.2 Clinical Features

There is an increase in the number and size of cysts after puberty, with symptoms appearing as the disease progresses. Common complications include rupture, haemorrhage and super-added infection [25].

4.4.2.3 Imaging Features

Imaging appearance is typically similar to hepatic cysts ranging in size from a few millimetres to 80mm. Complications are better depicted on MRI/CT as compared to US (Fig. 4.4) [26].

4.4.3 Ciliated Hepatic Foregut Cyst

Ciliated hepatic foregut duplication cyst is a rare congenital lesion. They are mostly benign; however, rare cases of malignant transformation to squamous cell carcinoma have been reported [27].

4.4.3.1 Pathology

Ciliated hepatic foregut cysts are thought to arise from the embryonic foregut with histology

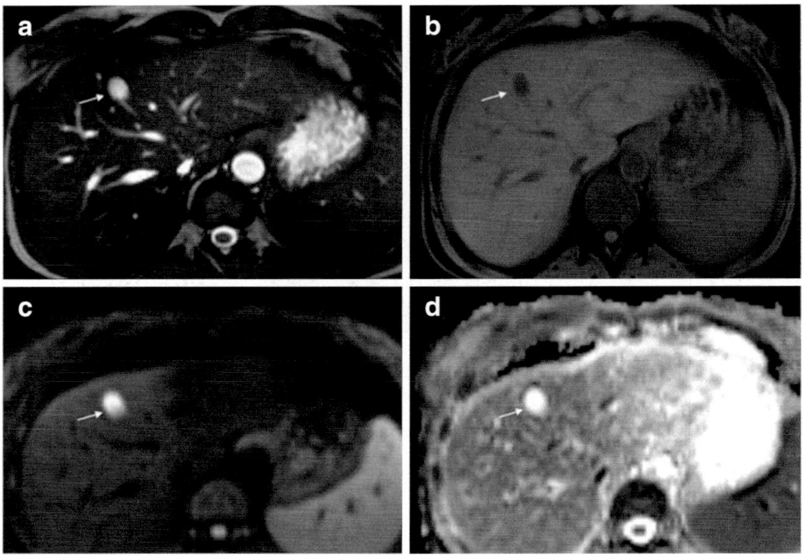

Fig. 4.3 Hepatic cyst on MRI. Axial T2-W (**a**) and T1-W (**b**) MRI images depict a circumscribed homogenous T2-W hyperintense and T1-W hypointense lesion (arrow), with fluid signal intensity. There is no diffusion restriction (DWI-b800, (**c**) with T2 shine-through on the corresponding ADC map (**d**)

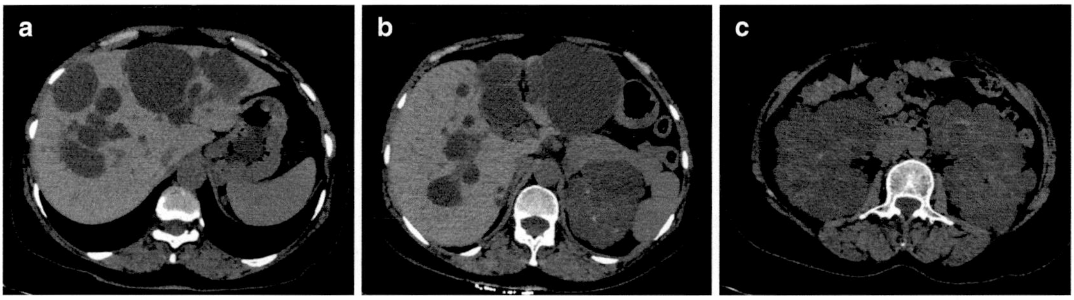

Fig. 4.4 Polycystic liver disease in a patient with autosomal dominant polycystic kidney disease (ADPKD). Axial CT images show multiple cysts of varying sizes in both lobes of the liver (**a** and **b**). Bilateral kidneys are enlarged and show numerous cysts, some of which show haemorrhagic changes (**c**)

similar to bronchogenic and oesophageal duplication cysts and are lined by pseudostratified columnar epithelium.

4.4.3.2 Clinical Features

The vast majority of patients are asymptomatic, discovered incidentally during imaging for other causes. However, portal hypertension or jaundice can occur rarely due to mass effect from the lesion [28].

4.4.3.3 Imaging Features

A ciliated hepatic foregut duplication cyst is typically a solitary lesion, measuring <3 cm, and is most commonly located in the subcapsular location. On US, they appear as anechoic or hypoechoic depending on the internal content. CT/MRI appearance also varies depending on the cyst content, whether it is serous or mucinous. Diffusion restriction or post-contrast enhancement is typically absent. In cases of cysts larger than 4 cm, with a solid enhancing component and thick irregular septations, malignant transformation should be ruled out [25, 29].

4.4.4 Peribiliary Cyst

Peribiliary cysts are a rare benign disorder, occurring in patients with cirrhosis, especially in the setting of portal hypertension. These represent cystic dilatation of the peribiliary

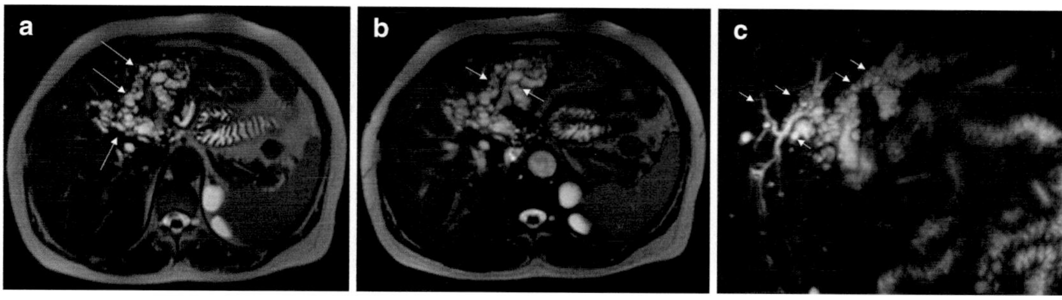

Fig. 4.5 Peribiliary cysts. Axial T2-weighted MRI image shows multiple cystic lesions of varying sizes in the left lobe of the liver (**a**), which are seen along the portal tracts, on either side of the portal vein branches (**b**). The peribiliary distribution of these lesions is better appreciated on the coronal MRCP image (**c**)

glands in the bile duct wall. They vary in size and number and are often detected incidentally. On US, well-marginated homogenous anechoic cysts are seen along the portal tracts, along both sides of the portal vein branches. This is in contrast to biliary radical dilatation, which is seen on one side. Moreover, the presence of thin septa within can help differentiate them from biliary radicle dilatation. On CT/MRI, hilar distribution is better appreciated with simple fluid attenuation/signal intensity (Fig. 4.5) [30, 31].

4.4.5 Biliary Hamartomas (von Meyenburg Complex)

Biliary hamartomas, also known as von Meyenberg complexes, are congenital cystic hamartomatous lesions, originating from embryonic bile ducts that fail to involute. They are more common in females as compared to males [25].

4.4.5.1 Pathology

Biliary hamartomas occur due to ductal plate malformation with deficient remodelling of the primitive ductal plate. They consist of dilated small bile ducts surrounded by fibrous stroma and do not communicate with the biliary tree [2].

4.4.5.2 Clinical Features

Biliary hamartomas are less commonly detected on imaging due to their small size. They are asymptomatic, requiring no treatment.

4.4.5.3 Imaging Features

US

On US, multiple, small (<15 mm), round or irregular scattered cysts are seen diffusely distributed in the liver parenchyma, with a predilection for the subcapsular region. Due to the small size, they can appear as anechoic, hypoechoic or hyperechoic, with closely placed lesions demonstrating reverberation artefacts [32].

CT

CT features of biliary hamartomas are similar to small simple cyst, showing no post-contrast enhancement.

MRI

Markedly T2-W hyperintense/T1-W hypointense small cysts are seen diffusely scattered in both lobes of the liver, with occasional rim enhancement due to adjacent compressed liver parenchyma (Fig. 4.6). In a subset of cysts, a small mural nodule composed of fibrocollagenous tissue can be seen showing post-contrast enhancement and T2-W intermediate signal intensity [33].

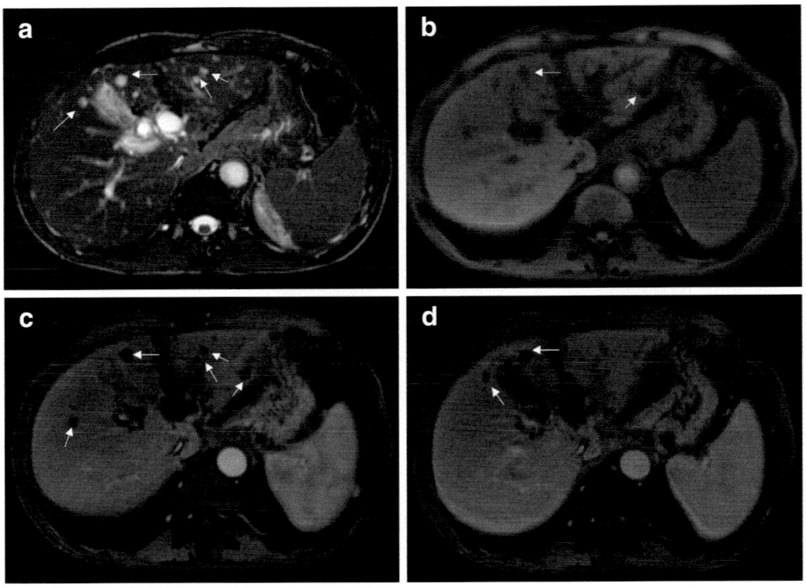

Fig. 4.6 Biliary hamartomas. (**a**) Axial T2-weighted MRI image shows small hyperintense cysts in both lobes of the liver (arrows). These appear hypointense on T1-weighted image (**b**) and show subtle rim enhancement in the arterial phase (**c**) with no washout in the delayed phase (**d**)

4.4.6 Peliosis Hepatis

Peliosis hepatis is a rare benign vascular disorder characterised by sinusoidal dilatation and multiple blood-filled lacunar spaces within the liver parenchyma. There may be involvement of other organs also such as the spleen and bone marrow [3].

4.4.6.1 Pathology

The exact etiopathogenesis of peliosis hepatis remains unclear. Several causes attributable to the development of this vascular condition include drugs (anabolic steroids, tamoxifen, oral contraceptive pills, azathioprine), toxins (polyvinyl chloride, arsenic) and chronic wasting diseases (tuberculosis, leprosy, acquired immune deficiency disorder(AIDS) and various malignancies, particularly hepatocellular cancer). The proposed primary event could be obstruction of hepatic outflow at the sinusoidal level with subsequent venous dilatation and cavity formation secondary to hepatocellular necrosis. The dilated sinusoids contain red blood cells and are bound by cords of liver cells [34].

4.4.6.2 Clinical Features

Hepatomegaly, ascites, portal hypertension and hepatic failure are common clinical presentations. However, symptoms are often absent or nonspecific. Rupture and intraperitoneal haemorrhage are potential complications [35].

4.4.6.3 Imaging Features

US

The US appearance of peliosis hepatis is variable depending on the echogenicity of the background liver parenchyma. The lesions appear as hypoechoic in the background of hepatic steatosis, hyperechoic in normal liver and heterogenous in cases of haemorrhage. On colour Doppler, perinodular and intranodular vascularity can be seen [3].

CT

The CT appearance depends on the presence of haemorrhage and thrombosis and the size of the lesion. They usually appear as multiple areas of low attenuation with interspersed high-density areas corresponding to haemorrhage. Calcification may be present. On post-contrast administration, early globular enhancement followed by progressive centrifugal enhancement is seen. In the delayed phase, diffuse homogenous enhancement is seen due to contrast pooling in the sinusoidal cavities [36].

MRI

There is a variable appearance of peliosis hepatis on MRI which is largely dependent on age and status of the blood component. On T2-W images, the lesion is usually heterogenously hyperintense, while on T1-W images, it can appear hypointense to hyperintense. A similar enhancement pattern is seen after contrast administration as on CT [37].

4.5 Benign Liver Tumours of Hepatocellular Origin

4.5.1 Hepatic Adenoma/Hepatocellular Adenoma

Hepatic adenomas are benign liver tumours of hepatocellular origin which are a heterogenous group of tumours with specific genetic and pathological abnormalities [38, 39]. They are more common in young women (90%) with predisposing factors including oral contraceptive intake, anabolic steroid use and glycogen storage disorders. A total of 80% are solitary with multiple adenomas encountered in patients with adenomatosis, glycogen storage disorders (Type 1A) and von-Gierke's disease [40]. Complications include risk of spontaneous haemorrhage and degeneration into hepatocellular carcinoma which depends on the subtype of hepatic adenomas [41, 42].

4.5.1.1 Pathology

Hepatic adenomas arise from the differentiated hepatocytes which are larger than normal hepatocytes and are arranged in cords. They typically lack bile ducts or portal triads, which is a key distinguishing feature between focal nodular hyperplasia and adenoma on histology [43].

Currently, hepatic adenomas are classified into three subtypes with each having distinct pathological and genetic alteration (genotype-phenotype classification)—inflammatory hepatocellular adenoma, hepatocyte nuclear factor 1α-mutated hepatocellular adenoma (HNF-1α) and beta-catenin-mutated hepatocellular adenoma. Few hepatic adenomas (around 10%) are without any specific genetic and pathological alterations and are labelled as unclassified hepatic adenomas. Each subtype has distinct histopathological and imaging features, although considerable overlap does exist [44]. It is important to subtype the hepatocellular adenomas due to different management strategies.

4.5.1.2 Inflammatory Hepatocellular Adenomas

Inflammatory hepatocellular adenomas are the most common subtype accounting for 40–50% of all adenomas. They typically occur in young females, on oral contraceptives and in obese patients [44]. The proposed pathogeneses are mutations in the interleukin-6 signal transducer gene (IL6ST) and overexpression of wild-type glycoprotein 130, which leads to activation of the JAK-STAT (Janus kinase-signal transducer and activator of transcription) pathway [45, 46]. Inflammatory adenomas have intense polymorphous inflammatory infiltrates, dilatation of sinusoids, haemorrhage and thick-walled arteries [47]. Of all the subtypes, the inflammatory subtype has the highest chances of bleeding which can occur in 30% of the cases. About 10% show an increased risk of malignancy transformation [38, 39].

4.5.1.3 HNF-1α-Mutated Hepatocellular Adenoma

HNF-1α-mutated hepatocellular adenomas are the second most common subtype which account for 30–35% of all cases. They occur exclusively in young women with a history of oral contraceptive pill intake. They are multiple in 50% of cases [44]. It occurs due to inactivating mutations of the HNF-1α gene, which is a tumour suppressor gene located at chromosome 12 [48]. There is impairment of fatty acid metabolism in the liver with intracellular fat deposition, with characteristic intratumoural lipid accumulation within the hepatocytes and lack of liver fatty acid–binding protein at immunochemical analysis [49]. Macroscopic fat is demonstrated in about 7% of cases, while microscopic fat is seen in 35–77% of cases [44]. They are the least aggressive type with minimal risk of bleeding and no risk for degeneration into malignancy.

4.5.1.4 Beta-Catenin-Mutated Hepatocellular Adenoma

Beta-catenin-mutated hepatocellular adenoma constitutes 10–15% of all cases of hepatocellular adenoma. They occur more commonly in men, with risk factors including anabolic steroids, glycogen storage disorder and familial adenomatosis polyposis [44]. Proposed etiopathogenesis includes activating mutations in the beta-catenin protein, an important regulator of the Wnt/beta-catenin pathway, which results in uncontrolled proliferation of hepatocytes [50]. Histologically, they are characterised by cellular proliferation with a higher nuclear-cytoplasmic ratio and nuclear atypia and are sometimes difficult to differentiate from well-differentiated hepatocellular carcinoma [51]. Overall, they carry the worst prognosis of all the hepatic adenomas, with the highest risk of malignant transformation [44].

4.5.1.5 Clinical Features

Most hepatic adenomas are asymptomatic and incidentally detected. Some may present with right upper quadrant pain and fullness. Acute abdomen with hypotensive emergency can occur in cases of spontaneous rupture. Patients with inflammatory hepatic adenoma can present with signs of systemic illness along with elevated inflammatory markers including leucocytosis, elevated C-reactive protein and serum amyloid-A [52].

4.5.1.6 Imaging

US

Hepatic adenomas are generally circumscribed lesions with heterogenous echopattern depending on the degree of haemorrhage, necrosis, fat, fibrosis and liquefaction. A hypoechoic peripheral rim may be present in some cases. On colour Doppler, internal vascularity is present with a few intralesional arteries. On CE-USG, they are hyper-enhancing in the arterial phase, with a centripetal pattern of enhancement and diffuse sustained enhancement in the venous and delayed phases. However, about 30% of adenomas can show weak washout in the delayed phase [53].

CT

In the non-contrast phase, the hepatic adenomas are of heterogenous attenuation with areas of high density corresponding to bleeding and low density corresponding to intralesional fat. After contrast administration, moderate and rapid enhancement is seen in the arterial phase, typically showing washout and becoming isodense to the adjacent liver parenchyma in the venous and delayed phases (Fig. 4.7). A hyperdense rim may be seen in some cases in the delayed phase [54, 55].

MRI

MRI is the imaging modality of choice for subtype characterisation of hepatocellular adenomas. Most are typically of high or equal signal intensity on T1-W and T2-W images, with intense arterial enhancement, becoming isointense in the venous phase on post-contrast sequences (Fig. 4.8). They may show restricted diffusion. There is a lack of uptake of hepatocyte-specific MRI contrast agents. While adenomas with microscopic fat show a characteristic signal drop on opposed-phase images, lipid-poor adenomas retain the signal intensity with no signal drop. Certain MRI features have been described, suggesting a particular subtype of hepatic adenoma, although histopathological and immunohistochemical analysis is often needed for

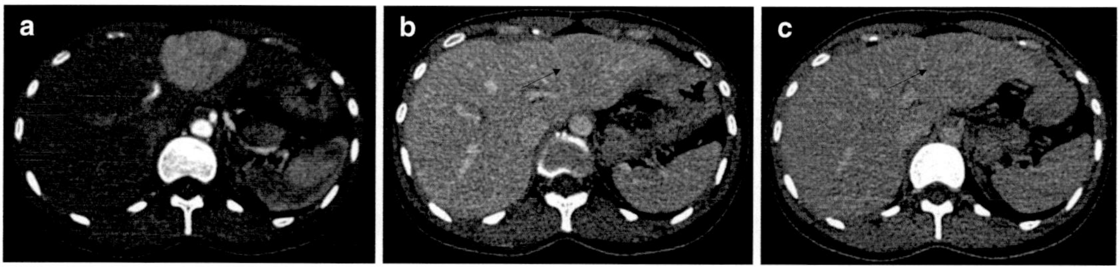

Fig. 4.7 Hepatic adenoma on CT. Axial images of a dynamic contrast CT show a lesion in segment IV (arrow), which is hyperenhancing on the arterial phase (**a**), and becomes isodense to the liver parenchyma in the venous (**b**) and delayed (**c**) phases

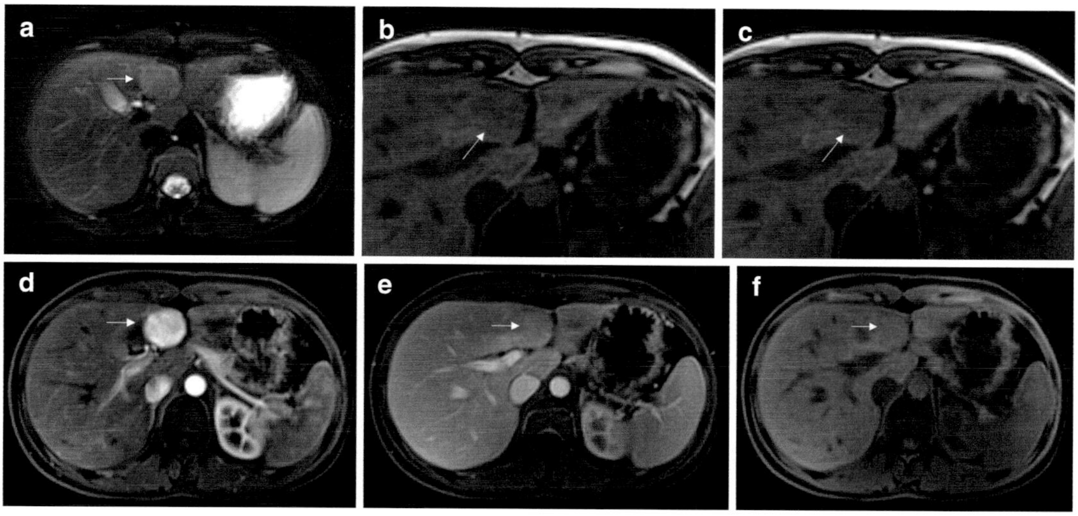

Fig. 4.8 Hepatic adenoma on MRI. Contrast-enhanced MRI shows a circumscribed lesion in segment IV of the liver (arrow), which is mildly hyperintense on T2-W sequence (**a**). On T1-W in-phase (**b**) and opposed-phase (**c**) sequences, there is a mild drop in signal intensity in the opposed phase indicating microscopic fat (arrows). The lesion is hyperenhancing in the arterial phase (**d**) and is isointense to the liver parenchyma in the venous (**e**) and delayed (**f**) phases

Table 4.2 MRI features of different subtypes of hepatic adenoma

Subtype of hepatocellular adenoma	T2-W sequence	T1-W sequence	Chemical shift imaging	Post-contrast T1-W sequence
Inflammatory hepatocellular adenoma	Diffusely hyperintense with higher signal intensity along the periphery	Isointense-mildly hyperintense	Minimal or no signal drop	Intense enhancement in the arterial phase, with persistent enhancement in the venous and delayed phases
HNF-1**α**-mutated hepatocellular adenoma	Isointense-hyperintense	Isointense-hyperintense	Diffuse signal drop on opposed-phase images	Moderate arterial enhancement, with no persistence enhancement in the venous and delayed phases
Beta-catenin-mutated hepatocellular adenoma	Homogenous/heterogenous hyperintense	Homogenous/heterogenous hyperintense	No drop in signal	Strong arterial enhancement that can or may not persist in the venous and delayed phases

complete characterisation and diagnosis of different subtypes of hepatic adenoma**.** The MRI appearances of different subtypes of hepatic adenomas are summarised in Table 4.2 [40, 44, 56–59].

4.5.2 Focal Nodular Hyperplasia

Focal nodular hyperplasia (FNH) is the most common benign liver tumour of hepatocellular origin and, overall, the second most common benign liver tumour after haemangioma [60]. It is considered a regenerative hyperplastic lesion rather than a true neoplastic lesion. They can occur in patients of all age groups and genders, although they are much more common in young women. They are solitary in 80% of cases and multiple in 20% of cases [61].

4.5.2.1 Pathology

An underlying vascular malformation or vascular injury is the proposed etiological factor for the development of FNH, leading to hepatocyte proliferation secondary to increased arterial flow. The lesion is composed of hepatocytes, fibrous tissue and a variable amount of Kupffer cells and bile ductules, which do not show communication with the adjacent biliary tree. One or more central scars containing malformed vascular structures are present in most of the cases [62]. FNHs are classified into classical (80%) and non-classical types (which comprise 20% of all cases). The classical FNH is characterised by the presence of an abnormal nodular architecture, malformed vessels and cholangiolar proliferation. The non-classical type is further divided into three subtypes: a) telangiectatic FNH (dilated sinusoids with hypertrophied arteries), b) FNH with cytological atypia and c) mixed hyperplastic and adenomatous FNH (resembles adenoma). Bile duct proliferation is present in all types of FNH; however, atypical FNH has certain features corresponding to its nomenclature [61, 63].

4.5.2.2 Clinical Features

Like hepatic adenoma, most patients with FNH are asymptomatic, and the lesion is incidentally detected. Larger lesions can cause vague abdominal symptoms due to mass effect.

4.5.2.3 Imaging

US

FNHs have a nonspecific appearance and are usually seen as isoechoic homogenous lesions, with surrounding mass effect. The grayscale US findings can be subtle, even in larger lesions. Some lesions can have a hypoechoic halo around the lesion due to compressed adjacent liver parenchyma. On colour Doppler, a central vessel may be present within a solid mass, radiating from the central scar into the surrounding lesion [64, 65]. On CE-US, it is hyperenhancing in the arterial phase, with a spoke-wheel or centrifugal filling pattern, showing sustained enhancement on venous and delayed phase images [66].

CT

FNHs are often not visualised on non-contrast CT as they are isodense to slightly hypodense to the adjacent liver parenchyma. On contrast adminis-

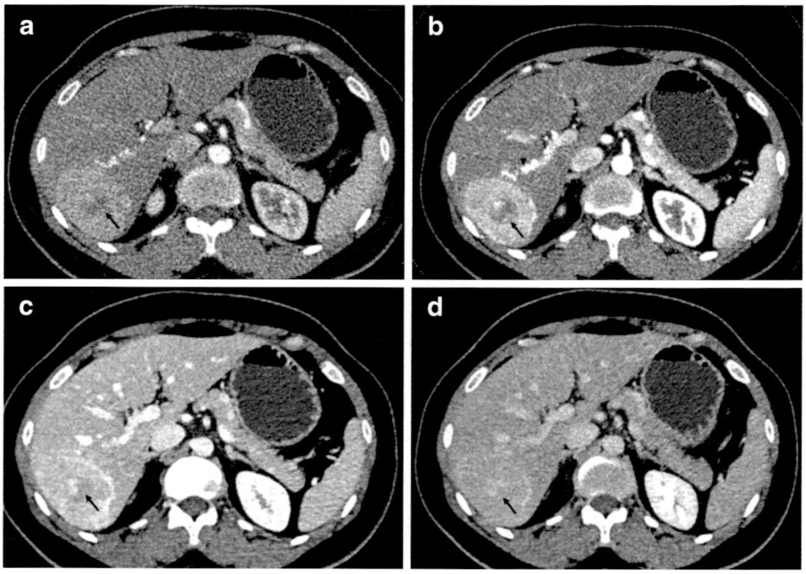

Fig. 4.9 Focal nodular hyperplasia (FNH) on CT. Axial sections of dynamic-contrast CT depicting a circumscribed homogenous arterial-enhancing lesion in segment VII (**a** and **b**), showing washout in venous (**c**) and delayed (**d**) phase images with a central scar (arrow). The central scar is hypoattenuating in the early arterial phase, with delayed enhancement in later phases, characteristic of FNH. Note the tortuous feeding vessels (arrowhead), commonly seen in FNH

tration, they are lobulated homogenously enhancing lesions in the arterial phase with some washout in the venous phase, becoming isoattenuating on delayed phase. Large feeding arteries and draining veins may be seen. They always drain into the hepatic veins. Portal venous supply is absent. A central scar is present in about 60% of cases on CT. The scar is hypoattenuating in the early arterial phase with fill-in on later phases showing delayed enhancement (Fig. 4.9) [67, 68].

MRI

FNHs are isointense to hypointense on T1-W images and isointense to mildly hyperintense on T2-W images. The scar is seen in 78% of cases and appears hyperintense on T2-W images. The imaging characteristics on post-contrast MRI sequences are similar to those of CT. There is persistent and delayed enhancement of the central scar (Fig. 4.10) [69]. Although FNH is the most common tumour with a central scar, it can be seen in some other liver lesions as well (Table 4.3). With hepatocyte-specific contrast agents, there is prolonged and excessive uptake of contrast by the tumour, with the absence of secretion within the biliary system [21]. Moreover, due to the presence of Kupffer cells, there is uptake of SPIO contrast agent within the lesion, manifesting as signal drop on T2-W GRE sequences [70].

The non-classical FNH can have different and variable imaging appearances ranging from less intense enhancement, atypical appearance of central scar, higher signal intensity on T2-W images and pseudocapsular enhancement on delayed phases. In such cases, hepatocyte-specific agents can be of help, where there is uptake of contrast by the lesion [62].

Since FNH has a benign clinical course, while hepatic adenomas have more chances of complications, differentiation is important. A more homogenous appearance, a central scar and persistent uptake with hepatocyte-specific contrast agents on MRI are more suggestive of FNH, while T1-W heterogenicity and absent or minimal uptake of hepatocyte-specific contrast agents are more suggestive of hepatic adenoma [1, 2].

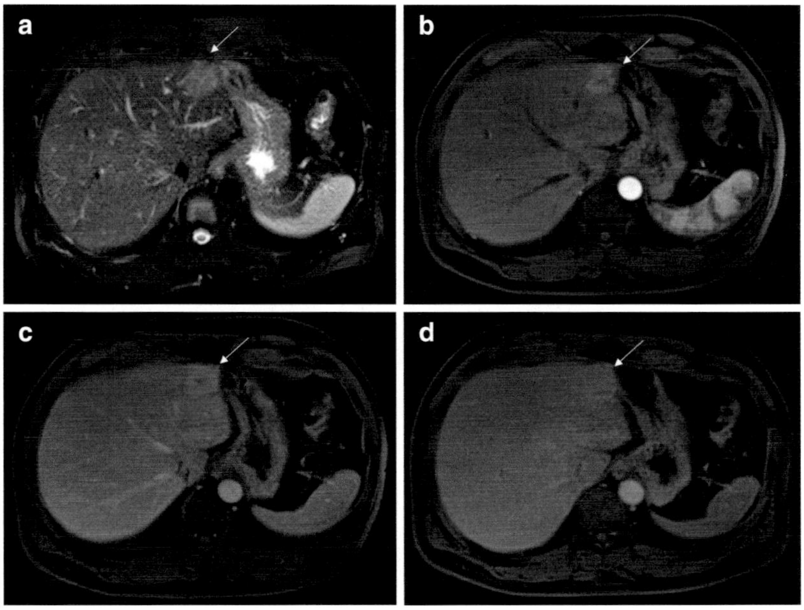

Fig. 4.10 FNH on dynamic contrast-enhanced MRI. Axial T2-weighted image (**a**) shows a well-defined, mildly hyperintense lesion in segment II (arrow). The lesion shows homogenous enhancement in the arterial phase (**b**) with a non-enhancing central scar. The lesion shows mild washout in the venous phase (**c**) and is almost isointense in the delayed phase, with delayed enhancement of the central scar (**d**)

Table 4.3 Focal hepatic lesions with central scar [62]

Lesion	Imaging feature of the scar
Focal nodular hyperplasia	Usually <2 cm, T2-W hyperintense with delayed enhancement. Calcification is rare
Fibrolamellar hepatocellular carcinoma	Larger, T2-W hypointense with no enhancement. Calcification is common
Haemangioma	Larger and brighter on T2-W images

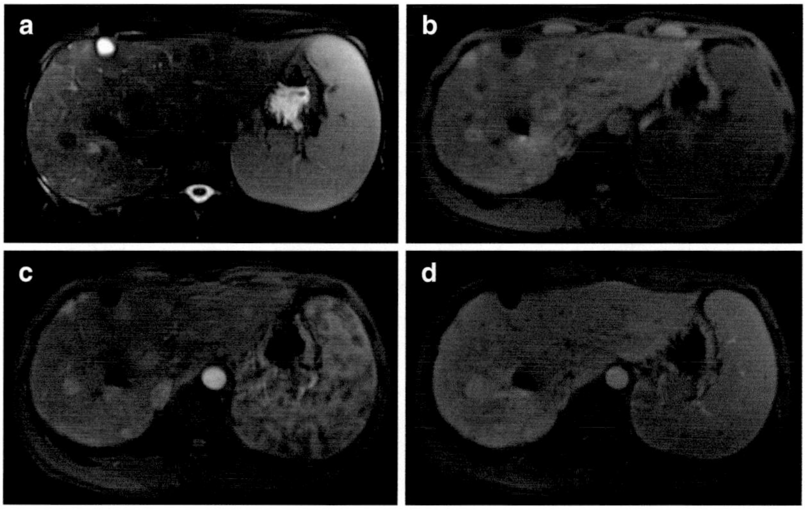

Fig. 4.11 Regenerative nodules on MRI. Multiple well-defined, hypointense nodules are seen on the T2-weighted image (**a**), which are iso- to slightly hyperintense on the T1-weighted image (**b**). These nodules show no enhancement in the arterial phase (**c**) and show mild homogenous enhancement in the delayed phase (**d**). Note is made of an incidental liver cyst in segment VIII

4.5.3 Nodular Regenerative Hyperplasia (NRH)

NRH is a hepatocyte proliferative disorder characterised by multiple nodules within the liver in the absence of fibrosis. It is a rare disease, occurring usually in adults or children with portal hypertension with no gender predilection [71].

4.5.3.1 Pathology

Although exact etiopathogenesis remains unclear, an association with various myeloproliferative disorders, collagen vascular diseases and chemotherapeutic drugs has been found [72].

4.5.3.2 Imaging

US

The US appearance can vary from being normal to multiple hypoechoic to isoechoic nodules showing internal vascularity on colour Doppler.

CT

Multiple hepatic nodules of varying sizes can be seen on CT which show homogenous arterial phase enhancement, becoming isodense on venous and delayed phase images. The nodules with central haemorrhage can have heterogenous attenuation. However, the liver can appear normal in cases of very small nodules [1].

MRI

The nodules in NRH are typically isointense on T1-W and T2-W images, with foci of T1-W hyperintensity showing homogenous arterial post-contrast enhancement. However, imaging appearances may be variable. There is diffuse uptake of hepatocyte-specific and SPIO MRI contrast agents [73].

4.5.4 Hepatocellular Nodules in Cirrhosis

The nodules encountered in cirrhosis are classified as regenerative nodules, dysplastic nodules (low grade and high grade) and malignant nodules (hepatocellular carcinoma). These may pose a diagnostic dilemma. In current clinical practice, in the presence of cirrhosis in an appropriate clinical setting, the LIRADS lexicon is applied for describing the lesions. The regenerative nodules show isointense signal intensity on T1-W and T2-W images with foci of dysplasia manifesting as high signal intensity on T2-W images. Some of the regenerative nodules show high T1 signal intensity due to the presence of metal-binding proteins, proteins or lipids (Fig. 4.11). The dysplastic nodules can have arterial phase enhancement on both CT and MRI [1, 6, 74].

4.6 Benign Liver Tumours of Mesenchymal Origin

4.6.1 Haemangioma

Liver haemangiomas are the most common benign liver tumours with a prevalence of 1–20% in the general population [75]. They occur in any age group with female predominance. Multiple haemangiomas are encountered in 10% of all cases and are associated with syndromes like Klippel-Trenaunay syndrome, Osler-Rendu-Weber disease and von Hippel-Landau syndrome [1].

4.6.1.1 Pathology

Pathologically, haemangiomas are characterised by endothelial-lined large, blood-filled vascular channels separated by fibrous septa. Depending on the size of the vascular channels, haemangiomas can be classified as cavernous or capillary type. Multiple large vascular spaces with varying degrees of haemorrhage, thrombosis and fibrosis can be seen [76].

4.6.1.2 Clinical Features

Most of the liver haemangiomas are asymptomatic and uncommonly present with abdominal pain. Rare, but clinically significant complications include spontaneous haemorrhage (intratumoural and peritoneal) and Kasabach-Merrit syndrome (consumption coagulopathy) [77].

4.6.1.3 Imaging Features

US

The classical haemangiomas are typically small in size (<3 cm), circumscribed, homogenous, hyperechoic lesions with posterior acoustic enhancement (Fig. 4.12a). Some appear as relatively hypoechoic to isoechoic lesions with an echogenic rim. In the presence of background diffuse liver disease, including hepatic steatosis and fibrosis, the echo pattern of haemangioma can be variable [78, 79]. On CE-US, a centripetal pattern of enhancement is seen with peripheral discontinuous nodular enhancement in the arterial phase,

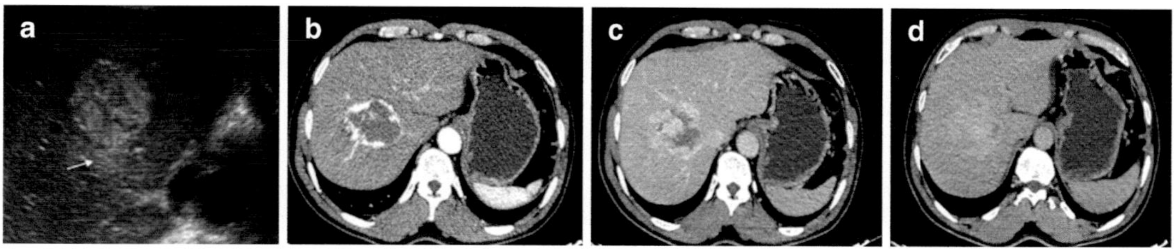

Fig. 4.12 Hepatic haemangioma. (**a**) On US, there is a circumscribed hyperechoic liver lesion with posterior acoustic enhancement (arrow). Axial section of dynamic contrast CT depicts a circumscribed lesion in segment VIII, showing peripheral nodular discontinuous enhancement in the arterial phase (**b**), with progressive, centripetal filling in the venous (**c**) and delayed (**d**) phases. The attenuation of the lesion is almost the same as that of the aorta in all phases of dynamic CT, characteristic of haemangioma

with progressive enhancement in the venous and delayed phases, filling the lesion partially or completely [12].

CT

Haemangiomas appear as hypoattenuating lesions on the non-contrast phase. After contrast administration, they show early, peripheral, nodular and discontinuous enhancement, with attenuation of the enhancing nodules equivalent to that of the aorta (Fig. 4.12b). In the venous and delayed phases, there is gradual, progressive, centripetal filling, with persistent homogenous enhancement on delayed phase images (Fig. 4.12c, d). This enhancement pattern is specific to haemangioma and differentiates it from vascular metastasis which usually have a complete rim of arterial enhancement [80, 81].

MRI

On MRI, haemangiomas are typically well circumscribed with homogenous high signal intensity on T2-W images and low signal intensity on T1-W images. No diffusion restriction is seen, and lesions retain high signal intensity on DWI and ADC maps. The imaging features on dynamic post-contrast-T1-W images are similar to those of CT. The reported sensitivity and specificity to diagnose classical haemangiomas with dynamic contrast-enhanced MRI and T2-W images are 98% with an accuracy of 99% (Fig. 4.13) [82–84].

4.6.1.4 Common Atypical Haemangiomas

Large/Giant Haemangioma

The definition of large/giant haemangioma is variably described in the literature. Some authors use a cut-off of 4 cm in diameter, while some define it as being greater than 6 cm or 12 cm in diameter [83]. Due to the larger size, the lesions undergo changes such as necrosis, haemorrhage, fibrosis and thrombosis, which are responsible for their heterogenous imaging appearance. They are of heterogenous echotexture on US. On non-contrast CT, the lesions with haemorrhage can be of higher attenuation. The MRI findings include a sharply marginated high signal intensity lesion on T2-W and low signal intensity lesion on T1-W images, with central T2-W higher signal intensity cleft-like areas and a few internal T2-W hypointense septa. On post-contrast CT/MRI sequences, there is non-uniform enhancement with non-

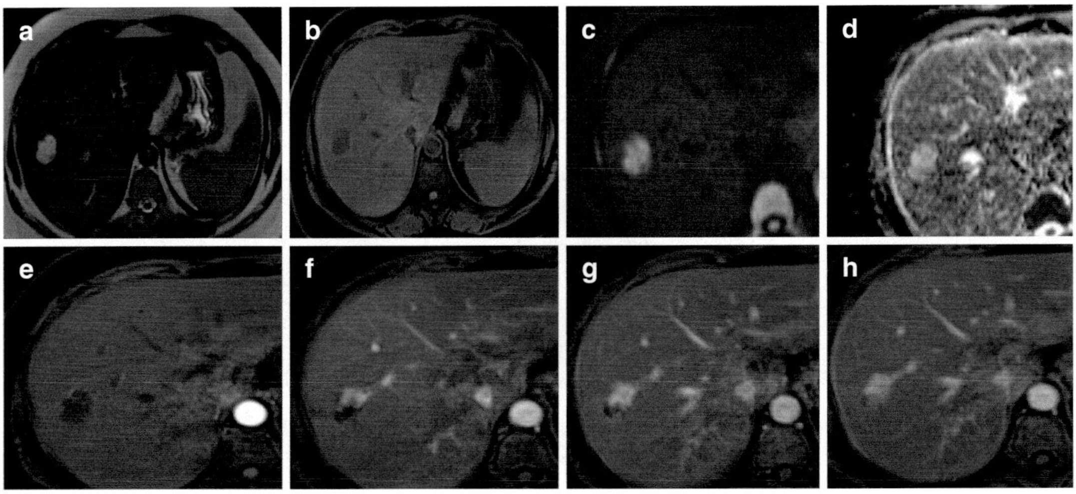

Fig. 4.13 Hepatic haemangioma on MRI. A circumscribed lesion is seen in segment VIII which is homogenously hyperintense on T2-W (**a**) and hypointense on T1-W (**b**) sequence, showing no diffusion restriction (**c**, DWI b-8000; **d**, ADC). The dynamic post-contrast MRI sequence (**e**–**h**) demonstrates the characteristic enhancement pattern of haemangioma; early peripheral discontinuous enhancement is followed by progressive, centripetal filling in the later phases

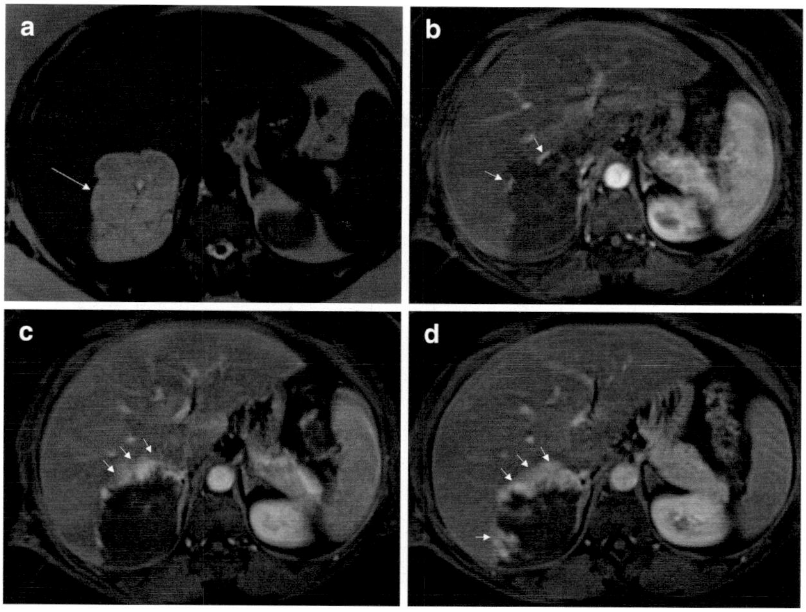

Fig. 4.14 Giant haemangioma. A well-defined lobulated lesion (arrow) measuring 8 × 6 cm is seen in segment VI of the liver, which is hyperintense on the T2-weighted image with fine T2-hypointense internal septa (**a**). On dynamic post-contrast MRI, the lesion shows areas of nodular peripheral enhancement in the arterial phase (**b**), with non-uniform, progressive enhancement and centripetal filling in the venous (**c**) and delayed (**d**) phases

enhancing components and centripetal filling in delayed phase images (Fig. 4.14) [84]. Radionuclide RBC scintigraphy is a valuable tool when there is a diagnostic dilemma with haemangiomas showing decreased activity on initial dynamic images followed by increased activity on delayed, blood pool images.

Rapidly Filling/Flash Haemangiomas

Rapidly filling haemangiomas are smaller in size (<1 cm) and account for 16% of all haemangiomas [75]. On ultrasound, they are typically hyperechoic with some showing unusual arterial flow on colour Doppler. They demonstrate a particular enhancement pattern on CT and MRI, with immediate homogenous complete enhancement in the arterial phase, which persists on venous and delayed phase images. The early arterial enhancement matches that of the aorta, and the lesion remains hyperattenuating/hyperintense on delayed phase images (Fig. 4.15) [85].

Other atypical imaging patterns in haemangioma including calcification, intralesional fat, hyalinisation and fluid-fluid levels are rare. A particular calcific pattern described is of multiple spotty calcifications within the lesion, which likely corresponds to phleboliths [75, 86]. Hyalinised haemangiomas do not show high signal intensity on T2-W images and often lack the early enhancement typical of classical haemangiomas [87]. Fluid-fluid level is seen in haemangiomas secondary to haemorrhage and is not specific as it can be seen in other benign and malignant vascular lesions as well.

4.6.2 Angiomyolipoma

Hepatic angiomyolipomas are rare mesenchymal liver tumours which can occur sporadically or in patients with tuberous sclerosis.

4.6.2.1 Pathology

They have varying amounts of smooth muscles, blood vessels and adipose tissue which account for their typical imaging appearance. They are characterised by HMB-45 positivity on immunohistochemical staining [88].

4.6.2.2 Imaging

US

The lesions are typically circumscribed and nonencapsulated, with intralesional macroscopic fat which accounts for a hyperechoic echo pattern.

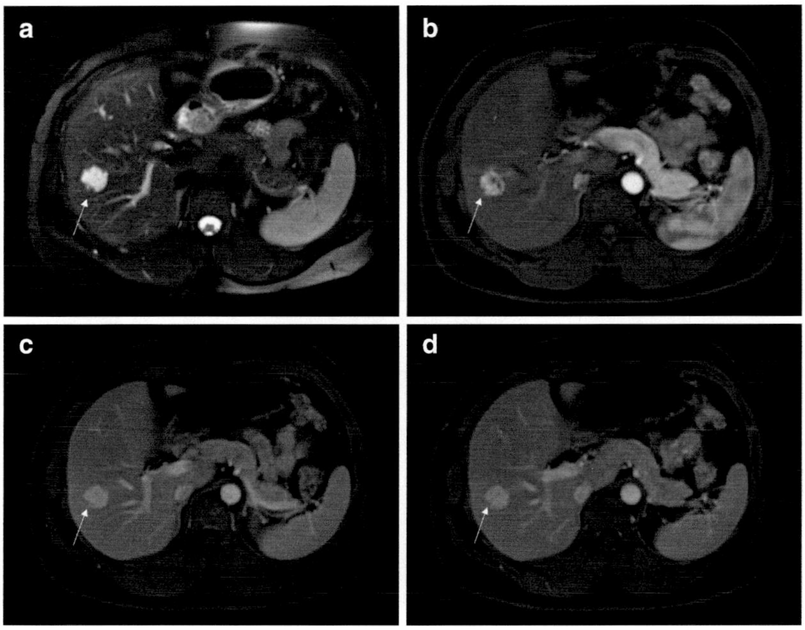

Fig. 4.15 Flash haemangioma on MRI. Axial T2-weighted image (**a**) shows a well-defined lobulated, hyperintense lesion in segment VII (arrow). This lesion shows immediate homogenous complete enhancement in the arterial phase (**b**), which persists in the venous (**c**) and delayed (**d**) phases. The enhancement matches that of the aorta in all phases, and the lesion remains hyperintense in the delayed phase

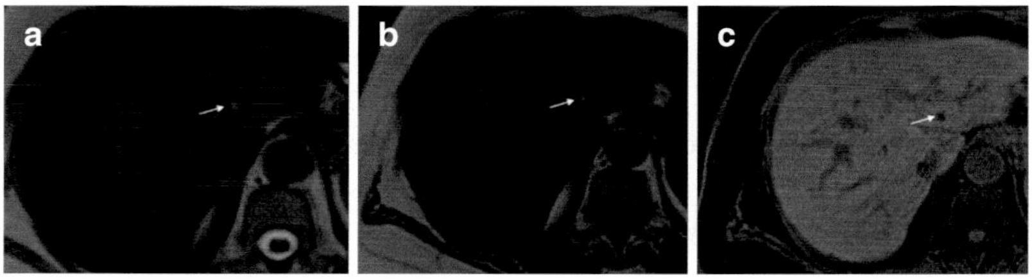

Fig. 4.16 Hepatic lipoma. Axial T2-W image (**a**) depicts a small T2 hyperintense lesion in segment III, adjacent to the ligamentum venosum. On T1-W water-suppressed sequence (**b**), the lesion is hyperintense, with a drop in signal on fat-suppressed sequence (**c**), suggestive of macroscopic fat

CT

There is variable enhancement with central vessels and areas of interspersed macroscopic fat seen depending on the composition.

MRI

The lesion typically has high signal intensity on T1-W and T2-W images with suppression of signal on fat-suppressed sequences. Microscopic fat can be demonstrated using chemical shift imaging. However, 50% of hepatic angiomyolipomas lack considerable fat content making differentiation from other vascular lesions of the liver difficult [89].

4.6.3 Lipoma

Hepatic lipomas are uncommon benign hepatic tumours characterised by intralesional fat. They have a non-specific imaging appearance on ultrasound and appear hyperechoic. Cross-sectional imaging features are diagnostic, like lipomas elsewhere in the body. They are homogenous circumscribed lesions with fat attenuation on CT showing no post-contrast enhancement. On MRI, there is high signal intensity on non-fat suppressed T1-W and T2-W images with signal drop on fat suppressed sequences (Fig. 4.16) [90].

4.6.4 Inflammatory Pseudotumour

Inflammatory pseudotumours are rare lesions composed of inflammatory cells and fibrous stroma. The exact etiopathogenesis remains unclear, although they have been speculated to occur secondary to hepatic infections [91]. Imaging features are nonspecific. They can be hypoechoic or hyperechoic on US with increased posterior acoustic enhancement and have multiple septa. On CT, the lesions are hypoattenuating with a varied degree of enhancement after contrast administration. On MRI, they are usually hyperintense on T2-W images and hypointense on T1-W images with a variable enhancement pattern [92].

4.6.5 Paragangliomas

The majority of paragangliomas are benign, typically occurring along the sympathetic chains due to their neural crest cell as a cell of origin. Intrahepatic paragangliomas have been described, although their imaging appearance is nonspecific. They are usually well circumscribed with areas of cystic changes. They typically have high signal intensity on T2-W images and show avid post-contrast enhancement [93].

4.6.6 Leiomyoma

Leiomyoma of the liver is an extremely rare lesion associated with human immunodeficiency virus infection. The imaging features are nonspecific. Post-contrast enhancement is present and can be in the form of rim enhancement or homogenous intense enhancement [94].

4.6.7 Fibromas

Fibromas are rare tumours composed of spindle cells and collagen which occur on the surface of the liver. No specific imaging pattern exists.

4.6.8 Lymphangioma

Hepatic lymphangioma is composed of multiple dilated lymphatic channels, usually associated with lymphatic malformation elsewhere in the body.

4.7 Mesenchymal Benign Liver Tumours of the Paediatric Population

4.7.1 Mesenchymal Hamartomas

Mesenchymal hamartoma is a benign cystic tumour of the liver seen in children younger than 2 years of age. It is more common in boys as compared to girls and is usually solitary [95].

4.7.1.1 Pathology

They are predominantly cystic lesions with a fibrous solid component composed of fibroblast-like mesenchymal cells, bile ducts and liver parenchyma. There is gelatinous mesenchymal tissue with remnants of normal liver parenchyma [96].

4.7.1.2 Clinical Features

Slow, progressive, painless abdominal distension is the typical imaging feature. Systemic symptoms develop when the lesion reaches a considerable size.

4.7.1.3 Imaging

On US, a well-circumscribed unilocular or multilocular cystic lesion is seen with internal septations of variable thickness. On CT and MRI, the imaging appearance is predominantly cystic with enhancement of the internal septa. The solid component appears as hypointense on T1-W and T2-W images. No calcification or haemorrhage is seen [1, 95].

4.7.2 Infantile Haemangioma

Infantile haemangiomas are the most common benign hepatic tumours of infants occurring more commonly in females as compared to males. It is usually diffuse with multiple lesions throughout the liver parenchyma. Focal and multifocal are other uncommon types [97].

4.7.2.1 Pathology

Infantile haemangiomas are composed of multiple vascular channels lined by endothelial cells with areas of haemorrhage, necrosis, thrombosis and calcification. Immature pleomorphic cells can be encountered in lesions with malignant potential [98].

4.7.2.2 Clinical Features

Typically, infants present with a palpable abdominal mass with features of congestive heart failure due to large arteriovenous shunting.

4.7.2.3 Imaging

Multiple variable-sized lesions are seen with imaging appearances like adult haemangiomas. However, calcifications are common (40–50% of cases), and there is characteristic narrowing of the abdominal aorta below the origin of the celiac axis with dilated celiac axis, common hepatic artery and prominent draining veins [99].

4.8 Benign Liver Tumours of Cholangiocellular Origin

4.8.1 Biliary Cystadenoma

Biliary cystadenomas are rare benign cystic neoplasms of biliary origin. They are typically encountered in women of the middle-aged group. They are premalignant tumours, with conversion to biliary cystadenocarcinoma, a well-recognised complication. They are usually solitary, with multifocality being rare [100].

4.8.1.1 Pathology

Biliary cystadenomas are cystic masses with the locules containing clear fluid or mucinous fluid, although serous, haemorrhagic and biliary contents can also be present. In 80% of cases, there can be ovarian stroma on histology [26].

4.8.1.2 Clinical Features

Clinical features are often non-specific. There can be jaundice in case of biliary system compression.

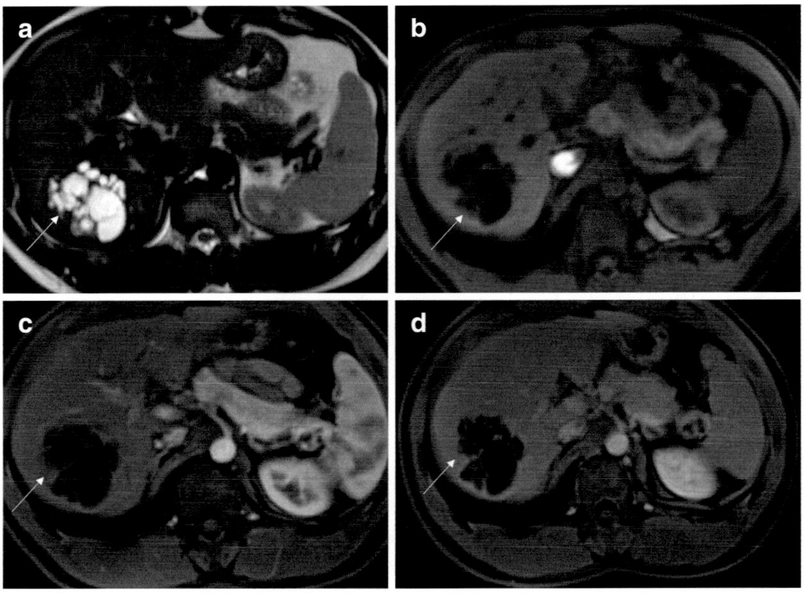

Fig. 4.17 Biliary cystadenoma. Axial T2-weighted MRI image shows a multilocular cystic lesion (arrow) in segment VII (**a**), with thin internal septations. The lesion is homogenously hypointense on the T1-weighted image (**b**). The septations show enhancement on arterial (**c**) and delayed (**d**) post-contrast images. No mural nodules are seen

4.8.1.3 Imaging

US

Biliary cystadenomas are circumscribed, multiloculated cystic lesions with thin internal septations. Vascularity can be seen within the septa on colour Doppler with enhancement of the septa on CE US [12].

CT

On CT, biliary cystadenoma appears as a well-defined hypodense multilocular lesion. Depending on the cystic content (mucinous or proteinaceous), the attenuation can vary. There is post-contrast enhancement of the internal septa and wall. Calcification is uncommonly seen along the septa. The presence of mural nodules, solid component and coarse calcification is more commonly associated with cystadenocarcinoma [101].

MRI

MRI signal intensity depends on the content of the cyst. However, predominantly, there is high signal intensity on T2-W and low-mixed signal intensity on T1-W images. There is enhancement of the septa on post-contrast administration (Fig. 4.17) [102].

4.8.2 Bile Duct Adenoma

It is a rare benign epithelial tumour derived from bile duct cells. Pathologically, there is a proliferation of ductules and fibrous stroma. On imaging, they are usually small (<1 cm) circumscribed lesions showing intense post-contrast enhancement which persists in the venous and delayed phases [76].

4.9 Conclusion

Benign hepatic lesions are of multiple etiologies. They may be incidentally detected and may have nonspecific clinical features. Imaging plays a crucial role in diagnosing and suggesting a reasonable differential diagnosis. However, due to atypical features of common lesions and the occurrence of uncommon hepatic tumours, diagnosis can be challenging. Patient history, relevant clinical data and a combination of various imaging modalities are often needed for arriving at the final diagnosis.

References

1. Anderson SW, Kruskal JB, Kane RA. Benign hepatic tumors and iatrogenic pseudotumors. Radiographics. 2009;29(1):211–29.
2. Ros PR, Erturk SM. Benign tumors of the liver. In: Gore RM, Levine MS, editors. Textbook of gastrointestinal radiology. 4th ed; 2015.
3. Iannaccone R, Federle MP, Brancatelli G, Matsui O, Fishman EK, Narra VR, Grazioli L, McCarthy SM, Piacentini F, Maruzzelli L, Passariello R, Vilgrain V. Peliosis hepatis: spectrum of imaging findings. AJR Am J Roentgenol. 2006;187(1):W43–52.
4. Heiken JP. Distinguishing benign from malignant liver tumours. Cancer Imaging. 2007;7(Special issue A):S1–14.
5. Grazioli L, Ambrosini R, Frittoli B, Grazioli M, Morone M. Primary benign liver lesions. Eur J Radiol. 2017;95:378–98.
6. Chernyak V, Fowler KJ, Kamaya A, Kielar AZ, Elsayes KM, Bashir MR, et al. Liver Imaging Reporting and Data System (LI-RADS) Version 2018: imaging of hepatocellular carcinoma in at-risk patients. Radiology. 2018;289(3):816–30.
7. Marin D, Furlan A, Federle MP, Midiri M, Brancatelli G. Imaging approach for evaluation of focal liver lesions. Clin Gastroenterol Hepatol. 2009;7(6):624–34.
8. D'Onofrio M, Crosara S, De Robertis R, Canestrini S, Mucelli RP. Contrast-enhanced ultrasound of focal liver lesions. AJRAm J Roentgenol. 2015;205(1):W56–66.
9. Jo PC, Jang HJ, Burns PN, Burak KW, Kim TK, Wilson SR. Integration of contrast-enhanced US into a multimodality approach to imaging of nodules in a cirrhotic liver: how I do it. Radiology. 2017;282(2):317–31.
10. Wilson SR, Burns PN. An algorithm for the diagnosis of focal liver masses using microbubble contrast-enhanced pulse-inversion sonography. AJR Am J Roentgenol. 2006;186(5):1401–12.
11. Moudgil S, Kalra N, Prabhakar N, Dhiman RK, Behera A, Chawla YK, Khandelwal N. Comparison of contrast enhanced ultrasound with contrast enhanced computed tomography for the diagnosis of hepatocellular carcinoma. J Clin Exp Hepatol. 2017;7(3):222–9.
12. Burrowes DP, Medellin A, Harris AC, Milot L, Wilson SR. Contrast-enhanced US approach to the diagnosis of focal liver masses. RadioGraphics. 2017;37(5):1388–400.

13. Strobel D, Seitz K, Blank W, Schuler A, Dietrich C, von Herbay A, Friedrich-Rust M, et al. Contrast-enhanced ultrasound for the characterization of focal liver lesions – diagnostic accuracy in clinical practice (DEGUM multicenter trial). Ultraschall Med. 2008;29(5):499–505.
14. Sahani DV, Kalva SP. Imaging the liver. Oncologist. 2004;9(4):385–97.
15. Hanson GJ, Michalak GJ, Childs R, McCollough B, Kurup AN, Hough DM, et al. Low kV versus dual-energy virtual monoenergetic CT imaging for proven liver lesions: what are the advantages and trade-offs in conspicuity and image quality? A pilot study. Abdom Radiol (NY). 2018;43(6):1404–12.
16. Foley WD, Mallisee TA, Hohenwalter MD, Wilson CR, Quiroz FA, Taylor AJ. Multiphase hepatic CT with a multirow detector CT scanner. AJR Am J Roentgenol. 2000;175(3):679–85.
17. Semelka RC, Martin DR, Balci NC. Focal lesions in normal liver. J Gastroenterol Hepatol. 2005;20(10):1478–87.
18. Neto JA, Elazzazzi M, Altun E, Semelka RC. When should abdominal magnetic resonance imaging be used? Clin Gastroenterol Hepatol. 2008;6(6):610–5.
19. Semelka RC, Martin DR, Balci NC. Magnetic resonance imaging of the liver: how I do it. J Gastroenterol Hepatol. 2006;21(4):632–7.
20. Vogl TJ, Kümmel S, Hammerstingl R, Schellenbeck M, Schumacher G, Balzer T. Liver tumors: comparison of MR imaging with Gd-EOB-DTPA and Gd-DTPA. Radiology. 1996;200(1):59–67.
21. Grazioli L, Bondioni MP, Haradome H, Motosugi U, Tinti R, Frittoli B, et al. Hepatocellular adenoma and focal nodular hyperplasia: value of gadoxetic acid-enhanced MR imaging in differential diagnosis. Radiology. 2012;262(2):520–9.
22. Ba-Ssalamah A, Fakhrai N, Matzek WK, Herneth AM, Stadler A, Bastati N, et al. Magnetic resonance imaging of liver malignancies. Top Magn Reson Imaging. 2007;18(6):445–55.
23. Mortelé KJ, Ros PR. Cystic focal liver lesions in the adult: differential CT and MR imaging features. RadioGraphics. 2001;21(4):895–910.
24. Mavilia MG, Pakala T, Molina M, Wu GY. Differentiating cystic liver lesions: a review of imaging modalities, diagnosis and management. J Clin Transl Hepatol. 2018;6(2):208–16.
25. Borhani AA, Wiant A, Heller MT. Cystic hepatic lesions: a review and an algorithmic approach. AJR Am J Roentgenol. 2014;203(6):1192–204.
26. Qian LJ, Zhu J, Zhuang ZG, Xia Q, Liu Q, Xu JR. Spectrum of multilocular cystic hepatic lesions: CT and MR imaging findings with pathologic correlation. Radiographics. 2013;33(5):1419–33.
27. Furlanetto A, Dei Tos AP. Squamous cell carcinoma arising in a ciliated hepatic foregut cyst. Virchows Arch. 2002;441(3):296–8.
28. Harty MP, Hebra A, Ruchelli ED, Schnaufer L. Ciliated hepatic foregut cyst causing portal hypertension in an adolescent. AJR Am J Roentgenol. 1998;170(3):688–90.
29. Fang SH, Dong DJ, Zhang SZ. Imaging features of ciliated hepatic foregut cyst. World J Gastroenterol. 2005;11(27):4287–9.
30. Itai Y, Ebihara R, Tohno E, Tsunoda HS, Kurosaki Y, Saida Y, Doy M. Hepatic peribiliary cysts: multiple tiny cysts within the larger portal tract, hepatic hilum, or both. Radiology. 1994;191(1):107–10.
31. Bazerbachi F, Haffar S, Sugihara T, Mounajjed TM, Takahashi N, Murad MH, Abu Dayyeh BK. Peribiliary cysts: a systematic review and proposal of a classification framework. BMJ Open Gastroenterol. 2018;5(1):e000204.
32. Zheng RQ, Zhang B, Kudo M, Onda H, Inoue T. Imaging findings of biliary hamartomas. World J Gastroenterol. 2005;11(40):6354–9.
33. Tohmé-Noun C, Cazals D, Noun R, Menassa L, Valla D, Vilgrain V. Multiple biliary hamartomas: magnetic resonance features with histopathologic correlation. Eur Radiol. 2008;18(3):493–9.
34. Zhao Y, Liu Y, Zhou L, Zhang XX, Li P, He Q. Clinical experience of liver transplantation in the treatment of peliosis hepatis. Hepatobiliary Pancreat Dis Int. 2022;21(1):83–5.
35. Calistri L, Rastrelli V, Nardi C, Maraghelli D, Vidali S, Pietragalla M, Colagrande S. Imaging of the chemotherapy-induced hepatic damage: yellow liver, blue liver, and pseudocirrhosis. World J Gastroenterol. 2021;27(46):7866–93.
36. Torabi M, Hosseinzadeh K, Federle MP. CT of nonneoplastic hepatic vascular and perfusion disorders. Radiographics. 2008;28(7):1967–82.
37. Maves CK, Caron KH, Bisset GS 3rd, Agarwal R. Splenic and hepatic peliosis: MR findings. AJR Am J Roentgenol. 1992;158(1):75–6.
38. Bioulac-Sage P, Balabaud C, Zucman-Rossi J. Subtype classification of hepatocellular adenoma. Dig Surg. 2010;27(1):39–45.
39. Zucman-Rossi J, Jeannot E, Nhieu JT, Scoazec JY, Guettier C, Rebouissou S, et al. Genotype-phenotype correlation in hepatocellular adenoma: new classification and relationship with HCC. Hepatology. 2006;43(3):515–24.
40. Grazioli L, Federle MP, Brancatelli G, Ichikawa T, Olivetti L, Blachar A. Hepatic adenomas: imaging and pathologic findings. Radiographics. 2001;21(4):877–92. discussion 892–4
41. Bioulac-Sage P, Laumonier H, Couchy G, Le Bail B, Sa Cunha A, Rullier A, et al. Hepatocellular adenoma management and phenotypic classification: the Bordeaux experience. Hepatology. 2009;50(2):481–9.
42. Tao LC. Oral contraceptive-associated liver cell adenoma and hepatocellular carcinoma: cytomorphology and mechanism of malignant transformation. Cancer. 1991;68(2):341–7.
43. Boulahdour H, Cherqui D, Charlotte F, Rahmouni A, Dhumeaux D, Zafrani ES, et al. The hot spot hepatobiliary scan in focal nodular hyperplasia. J Nucl Med. 1993;34(12):2105–10.
44. Katabathina VS, Menias CO, Shanbhogue AK, Jagirdar J, Paspulati RM, Prasad SR. Genetics and

imaging of hepatocellular adenomas: 2011 update. Radiographics. 2011;31(6):1529–43.
45. Rebouissou S, Amessou M, Couchy G, Poussin K, Imbeaud S, Pilati C, et al. Frequent in-frame somatic deletions activate gp130 in inflammatory hepatocellular tumours. Nature. 2009;457(7226):200–4.
46. Spannbauer MM, Trautwein C. Frequent in-frame somatic deletions activate gp130 in inflammatory hepatocellular tumors. Hepatology. 2009;49(4):1387–9.
47. Bioulac-Sage P, Rebouissou S, Sa Cunha A, Jeannot E, Lepreux S, Blanc JF, et al. Clinical, morphologic, and molecular features defining so-called telangiectatic focal nodular hyperplasias of the liver. Gastroenterology. 2005;128(5):1211–8.
48. Bluteau O, Jeannot E, Bioulac-Sage P, Marqués JM, Blanc JF, Bui H, et al. Bi-allelic inactivation of TCF1 in hepatic adenomas. Nat Genet. 2002;32(2):312–5.
49. Rebouissou S, Imbeaud S, Balabaud C, Boulanger V, Bertrand-michel J, Terce F, et al. HNF1alpha inactivation promotes lipogenesis in human hepatocellular adenoma independently of SREBP-1 and carbohydrate-response element- binding protein(ChREBP) activation. J Biol Chem. 2007;282(19):14437–46.
50. Chen YW, Jeng YM, Yeh SH, Chen PJ. P53 gene and Wnt signaling in benign neoplasms: beta-catenin mutations in hepatic adenoma but not in focal nodular hyperplasia. Hepatology. 2002;36(41):927–35.
51. Bioulac-Sage P, Laumonier H, Laurent C, Zucman-Rossi J, Balabaud C. Hepatocellular adenoma: what is new in 2008. Hepatol Int. 2008;2(3):316–21.
52. Paradis V, Champault A, Ronot M, Deschamps L, Valla DC, Vidaud D, Vilgrain V, Belghiti J, Bedossa P. Telangiectatic adenoma: an entity associated with increased body mass index and inflammation. Hepatology. 2007;46(1):140–6.
53. Wang W, Liu JY, Yang Z, Wang YF, Shen SL, Yi FL, et al. Hepatocellular adenoma: comparison between real-time contrast-enhanced ultrasound and dynamic computed tomography. Springerplus. 2016;5(1):95.
54. Horton KM, Bluemke DA, Hruban RH, Soyer P, Fishman EK. CT and MR imaging of benign hepatic and biliary tumors. Radiographics. 1999;19(2):431–51.
55. Tajima T, Honda H, Kuroiwa T, Yoshimitsu K, Irie H, Aibe H, et al. Radiologic features of intrahepatic bile duct adenoma: a look at the surface of the liver. J Comput Assist Tomogr. 1999;23(5):690–5.
56. Lewin M, Handra-Luca A, Arrivé L, Wendum D, Paradis V, Bridel E, Fléjou JF, et al. Liver adenomatosis: classification of MR imaging features and comparison with pathologic findings. Radiology. 2006;241(2):433–40.
57. Laumonier H, Bioulac-Sage P, Laurent C, Zucman-Rossi J, Balabaud C, Trillaud H. Hepatocellular adenomas: magnetic resonance imaging features as a function of molecular pathological classification. Hepatology. 2008;48(3):808–18.
58. Ponnatapura J, Kielar A, Burke LMB, Lockhart ME, Abualruz AR, Tappouni R, Let al. Hepatic complications of oral contraceptive pills and estrogen on MRI: controversies and update – adenoma and beyond. Magn Reson Imaging. 2019 ;60:110-121.
59. Ichikawa T, Federle MP, Grazioli L, Nalesnik M. Hepatocellular adenoma: multiphasic CT and histo-pathologic findings in 25 patients. Radiology. 2000;214(3):861–8.
60. Venturi A, Piscaglia F, Vidili G, Flori S, Righini R, Golfieri R, et al. Diagnosis and management of hepatic focal nodular hyperplasia. J Ultrasound. 2007;10(3):116–27.
61. Nguyen BN, Flejou JF, Terris B, Belghiti J, Degott C. Focal nodular hyperplasia of the liver: a comprehensive pathologic study of 305 lesions and recognition of new histologic forms. Am J Surg Pathol. 1999;23(12):1441–54.
62. Hussain SM, Terkivatan T, Zondervan PE, Lanjouw E, de Rave S, Ijzermans JN, et al. Focal nodular hyperplasia: findings at state-of-the-art MR imaging, US, CT, and pathologic analysis. Radiographics. 2004;24(1):3–17. discussion 18–9
63. Wanless IR, Mawdsley C, Adams R. On the pathogenesis of focal nodular hyperplasia of the liver. Hepatology. 1985;5(6):1194–200.
64. Vidili G, Piscaglia F, Ainora ME, Solinas G, Sagrini E, Gianstefani A, et al. Focal nodular hyperplasia: new findings at Doppler ultrasonography. Eur Rev Med Pharmacol Sci. 2020;24(23):12288–95.
65. Shirkhoda A, Farah MC, Bernacki E, Madrazo B, Roberts J. Hepatic focal nodular hyperplasia: CT and sonographic spectrum. Abdom Imaging. 1994;19(1):34–8.
66. Kang TW, Jeong WK, Kim YY, Min JH, Kim YK, Kim SH, Sinn DH, et al. Comparison of super-resolution US and contrast material-enhanced US in detection of the spoke wheel sign in patients with focal nodular hyperplasia. Radiology. 2021;298(1):82–90.
67. Carlson SK, Johnson CD, Bender CE, Welch TJ. CT of focal nodular hyperplasia of the liver. AJR Am J Roentgenol. 2000;174(3):705–12.
68. Mortelé KJ, Praet M, Van Vlierberghe H, Kunnen M, Ros PR. CT and MR imaging findings in focal nodular hyperplasia of the liver: radiologic-pathologic correlation. AJR Am J Roentgenol. 2000;175(3):687–92.
69. Hussain SM, Bijl MS, Zondervan PEI, Jzermans JN, Schalm SW, Krestin GP. Benign versus malignant hepatic nodules: findings at MR imaging with histopathologic correlation. RadioGraphics. 2002;22(5):1023–39.
70. Beets-Tan RG, Van Engelshoven JM, Greve JW. Hepatic adenoma and focal nodular hyperplasia: MR findings with superparamagnetic iron oxide-enhanced MRI. Clin Imaging. 1998;22(3):211–5.
71. Steiner PE. Nodular regenerative hyperplasia of the liver. Am J Pathol. 1959;35(5):943–53.

72. Ghabril M, Vuppalanchi R. Drug-induced nodular regenerative hyperplasia. Semin Liver Dis. 2014;34(2):240–5.
73. Siegelman ES, Outwater EK, Furth EE, Rubin R. MR imaging of hepatic nodular regenerative hyperplasia. J Magn Reson Imaging. 1995;5(6):730–2.
74. Krinsky GA, Lee VS, Theise ND, Weinreb JC, Rofsky NM, Diflo T, et al. Hepatocellular carcinoma and dysplastic nodules in patients with cirrhosis: prospective diagnosis with MR imaging and explantation correlation. Radiology. 2001;219(2):445–54.
75. Vilgrain V, Boulos L, Vullierme MP, Denys A, Terris B, Menu Y. Imaging of atypical hemangiomas of the liver with pathologic correlation. RadioGraphics. 2000;20(2):379–97.
76. Terkivatan T, Hussain SM, De Man RA, Ijzermans JN. Diagnosis and treatment of benign focal liver lesions. Scand J Gastroenterol Suppl. 2006;243:102–15.
77. Albitar HAH, Iyer V. Giant liver hemangioma with Kasabach-Merritt Syndrome. Am J Med. 2020;133(1):56–7.
78. Nelson RC, Chezmar JL. Diagnostic approach to hepatic hemangiomas. Radiology. 1990;176(1):11–3.
79. Moody AR, Wilson SR. Atypical hepatic hemangioma: a suggestive sonographic morphology. Radiology. 1993;188(2):413–7.
80. Quinn SF, Benjamin GG. Hepatic cavernous hemangiomas: simple diagnostic sign with dynamic bolus CT. Radiology. 1992;182(2):545–8.
81. Leslie DF, Johnson CD, MacCarty RL, Ward EM, Ilstrup DM, Harmsen WS. Single-pass CT of hepatic tumors: value of globular enhancement in distinguishing hemangiomas from hypervascular metastases. AJR Am J Roentgenol. 1995;165(6):1403–6.
82. Semelka RC, Brown ED, Ascher SM, Patt RH, Bagley AS, Li W, Edelman RR, Shoenut JP, Brown JJ. Hepatic hemangiomas: a multi-institutional study of appearance on T2-weighted and serial gadolinium-enhanced gradient-echo MR images. Radiology. 1994;192(2):401–6.
83. Soyer P, Dufresne AC, Somveille E, Scherrer A. Hepatic cavernous hemangioma: appearance on T2-weighted fast spin-echo MR imaging with and without fat suppression. AJR Am J Roentgenol. 1997;168(2):461–5.
84. Soyer P, Gueye C, Somveille E, Laissy JP, Scherrer A. MR diagnosis of hepatic metastases from neuroendocrine tumors versus hemangiomas: relative merits of dynamic gadolinium chelate-enhanced gradient-recalled echo and unenhanced spin-echo images. AJR Am J Roentgenol. 1995;165(6):1407–13.
85. Honda H, Matsuura Y, Onitsuka H, Murakami J, Kaneko K, Murayama S, Kanematsu T, Masuda K. Differential diagnosis of hepatic tumors (hepatoma, hemangioma, and metastasis) with CT: value of two-phase incremental imaging. AJR Am J Roentgenol. 1992;159(4):735–40.
86. Mitsudo K, Watanabe Y, Saga T, Dohke M, Sato N, Minami K, Shigeyasu M. Nonenhanced hepatic cavernous hemangioma with multiple calcifications: CT and pathologic correlation. Abdom Imaging. 1995;20(5):459–61.
87. Cheng HC, Tsai SH, Chiang JH, Chang CY. Hyalinized liver hemangioma mimicking malignant tumor at MR imaging. AJR Am J Roentgenol. 1995;165(4):1016–7.
88. Sturtz CL, Dabbs DJ. Angiomyolipomas: the nature and expression of the HMB45 antigen. Mod Pathol. 1994;7(8):842–5.
89. Prasad SR, Wang H, Rosas H, Menias CO, Narra VR, Middleton WD, Heiken JP. Fat-containing lesions of the liver: radiologic-pathologic correlation. Radiographics. 2005;25(2):321–31.
90. Martí-Bonmatí L, Menor F, Vizcaino I, Vilar J. Lipoma of the liver: US, CT, and MRI appearance. Gastrointest Radiol. 1989;14(2):155–7.
91. Horiuchi R, Uchida T, Kojima T, Shikata T. Inflammatory pseudotumor of the liver: clinicopathologic study and review of the literature. Cancer. 1990;65(7):1583–90.
92. Nam KJ, Kang HK, Lim JH. Inflammatory pseudotumor of the liver: CT and sonographic findings. AJR Am J Roentgenol. 1996;167(2):485–7.
93. Qiao HS, Feng XL, Yong L, Yong Z, Lian ZJ, Ling LB. The MRI of extraadrenal pheochromocytoma in the abdominal cavity. Eur J Radiol. 2007;62(3):335–41.
94. Navarro C, Hamidian Jahromi A, Donato M, Caliri N, Tempra A, Sangster G. Primary leiomyoma of the liver: case report and review of the literature. J La State Med Soc. 2015;167(3):129–33.
95. Stanley P, Hall TR, Woolley MM, Diament MJ, Gilsanz V, Miller JH. Mesenchymal hamartomas of the liver in childhood: sonographic and CT findings. AJR Am J Roentgenol. 1986;147(5):1035–9.
96. Kaude JV, Felman AH, Hawkins IF Jr. Ultrasonography in primary hepatic tumors in early childhood. Pediatr Radiol. 1980;9(2):77–83.
97. Shabbir Z, Javaid A, Din IU. Infantile hepatic hemangioma. J Pak Med Assoc. 2018;68(12):1846–7.
98. Dachman AH, Lichtenstein JE, Friedman AC, Hartman DS. Infantile hemangioendothelioma of the liver: a radiologic-pathologic-clinical correlation. AJR Am J Roentgenol. 1983;140(6):1091–6.
99. Keslar PJ, Buck JL, Selby DM. From the archives of the AFIP. Infantile hemangioendothelioma of the liver revisited. Radiographics. 1993;13(3):657–70.
100. Ishak KG. Benign tumors and pseudotumors of the liver. Appl Pathol. 1988;6(2):82–104.
101. Buetow PC, Buck JL, Pantongrag-Brown L, Ros PR, Devaney K, Goodman ZD, et al. Biliary cystadenoma and cystadenocarcinoma: clinical-imaging-pathologic correlations with emphasis on the importance of ovarian stroma. Radiology. 1995;196(3):805–10.
102. Stoupis C, Ros PR, Dolson DJ. Recurrent biliary cystadenoma: MR imaging appearance. J Magn Reson Imaging. 1994;4(1):99–101.

Hepatocellular Carcinoma and Other Malignant Hepatic Tumours

5

Sanchita Gupta, Manish Saini, and Kumble S. Madhusudhan

5.1 Introduction

Hepatic malignancies are the sixth most common cancer worldwide and the third leading cause of cancer-related mortality [1]. The ever-increasing incidence combined with the high associated morbidity and mortality makes malignant hepatic tumours a global health challenge that needs to be tackled at all levels of medical care, from prevention to diagnosis and treatment. Imaging of these tumours is critical in their management as they assist in the detection, characterisation, staging, assessing treatment response and identifying recurrence of these malignancies. The modalities available include ultrasonography (US) including elastography and contrast-enhanced ultrasonography (CEUS), computed tomography (CT), magnetic resonance imaging (MRI) and positron emission tomography–CT (PET-CT).

5.2 Hepatocellular Carcinoma

Hepatocellular carcinoma (HCC) is the most common primary hepatic malignancy, accounting for 90% of all diagnosed liver tumours [2]. Over the past decade, the incidence of HCC has been steadily increasing in the higher socio-economic index countries like the USA, Canada, Australia and many European countries along with a decline in traditionally higher incidence countries like China and sub-Saharan Africa, mainly due to the increase in the incidence of non-alcoholic fatty liver disease (NAFLD)–associated cirrhosis.

The incidence of HCC increases with advanced age and male sex. The presence of cirrhosis due to hepatitis B, hepatitis C, chronic alcohol intake and NAFLD is an important risk factor for HCC development. Other less common etiologies include hereditary hemochromatosis, glycogen storage disease, alpha-1-antitrypsin deficiency, primary biliary cirrhosis and autoimmune hepatitis. While all the aforementioned causes of cirrhosis may result in tumour development, the risk is higher for viral hepatitis. Chronic inflammation in the absence of cirrhosis in cases of hepatitis B, hepatitis C and non-alcoholic steatohepatitis (NASH) can also lead to the development of HCC, although at a much lower rate. Chronic contamination of food grains with aflatoxin (due to *Aspergillus* sp.) is also an important risk factor for the development of HCC, especially in tropical areas like sub-Saharan Africa.

S. Gupta · M. Saini · K. S. Madhusudhan (✉)
Department of Radiodiagnosis and Interventional Radiology, All India Institute of Medical Sciences, New Delhi, India

© The Author(s), under exclusive license to Springer Nature Singapore Pte Ltd. 2025

B. Sureka (ed.), *Hepato-Pancreatico Biliary Imaging*, https://doi.org/10.1007/978-981-95-1699-5_5

5.3 Hepatocarcinogenesis

Mature hepatocytes are generally considered to be the cells of origin for HCC. Hepatocarcinogenesis is a complex multistep process during which the accumulation of molecular alterations and consequent histological changes occur which often have specific imaging correlates [3]. Chronic hepatic injury results in the development of fibrosis and multiple non-neoplastic nodules called regenerative nodules (RNs). RNs are histologically similar to the surrounding liver parenchyma. As the insult continues, progressive molecular alterations occur in the RNs promoting their unchecked cell proliferation. This leads to the development of low-grade dysplastic nodules (LGDNs) which further progress to high-grade dysplastic nodules (HGDNs) and early HCC. The final step in this pathway is the development of progressed HCC (Fig. 5.1).

A few important molecular and histological changes occur during carcinogenesis, which form the basis of imaging features in these cases.

1. *Loss of cell transporter function*: Hepatocytes contain an uptake transporter, the organic anion transporting polypeptide 1B3 (OATP1B3) along the sinusoidal aspect. The OATP1B3 is responsible for the extraction of substances from the portal blood. These substrates after metabolism are subsequently excreted into the biliary canaliculi via multidrug resistance protein 1 (MDR1). There is a progressive reduction in the expression of the organic anion transporting polypeptide (OATP) during the process of hepatocarcinogenesis. This is reflected as reduced or a lack of uptake of hepatobiliary contrast agent in the hepatobiliary phase MRI [4].

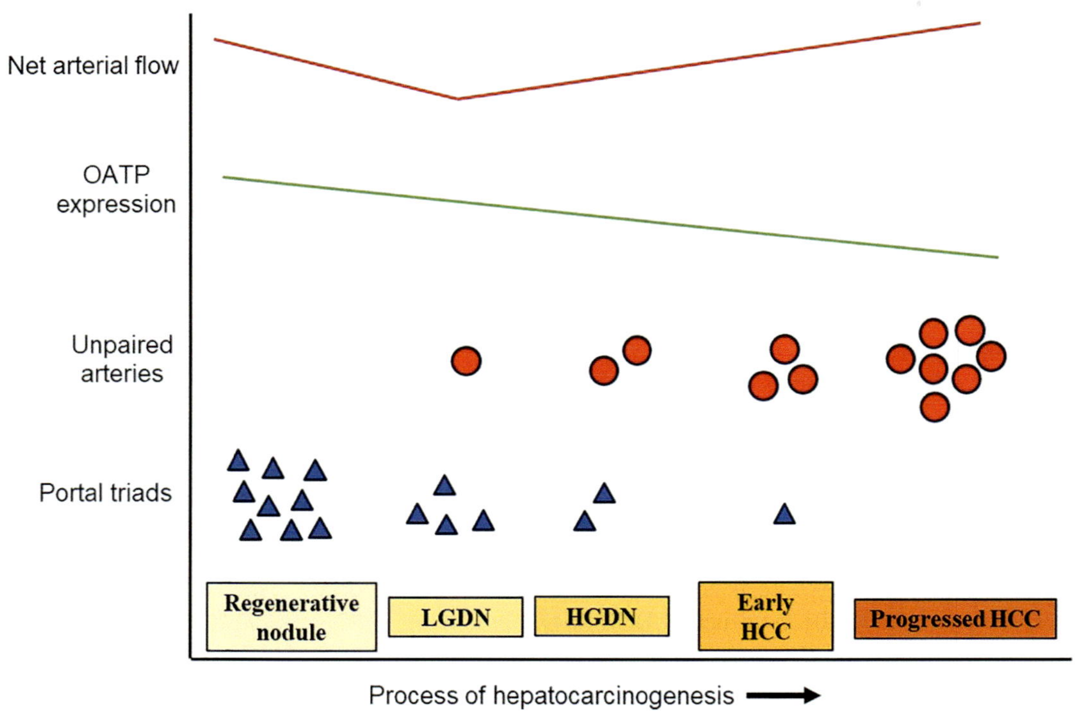

Fig. 5.1 Process of hepatocarcinogenesis. Cirrhotic or regenerative nodules transform into dysplastic nodules which then ultimately progress to HCC. During this multistep hepatocarcinogenesis, OATP expression decreases progressively as malignant transformation occurs. Intralesional blood flow initially decreases as portal triads are lost, followed by an increase in arterial flow in progressed HCC due to unpaired arteries. *HCC* hepatocellular carcinoma, *HGDN* high-grade dysplastic nodule, *LGDN* low-grade dysplastic nodule, *OATP* organic anion transporting polypeptide

2. *Increased cell density*: As the process progresses, the size of cells decreases with an associated increase in the number and density of cells within lesions. This causes restriction of diffusion of lesions on diffusion-weighted imaging (DWI).
3. *Neoangiogenesis*: During the phase of early carcinogenesis, there is a reduction in the number of portal triads leading to a decrease in arterial and portal venous flow in dysplastic nodules and early HCC which appear hypoenhancing compared to adjacent hepatic parenchyma. As the lesion becomes progressively more malignant, the development of new unpaired arteries occurs due to angiogenic factors which leads to increased arterial flow seen in progressed HCCs. This is shown as arterial phase hyperenhancement of the lesions [5].
4. *Capsule formation*: As lesions transform into overt malignancy, i.e. progressed HCC, they cause compression of the adjacent host parenchyma leading to the development of a capsule by hepatic mesenchymal cells. This capsule interferes with the invasion of HCC further into the hepatic parenchyma.
5. *Iron accumulation*: During early carcinogenesis, lesions (LGDN, HGDN) tend to accumulate iron due to the upregulation of transferrin receptors and appear as hypointense on both T1W and T2W images. This is later followed by iron loss or iron resistance in early and progressed HCCs as receptor expression decreases. Hence, loss of iron from a previously siderotic nodule may be a sign of malignant transformation. The phenomenon appears as the 'nodule within nodule' sign—the presence of isointense areas within a hypointense siderotic nodule on T2-weighted MRI, which is strongly suggestive of the presence of early HCC in a siderotic nodule [6].
6. *Fat accumulation*: Dysplastic nodules and early HCCs may accumulate fat, followed by fat loss as lesions transform into overt malignancy.

Key Point: Loss of intralesional iron in a previously siderotic nodules—sign of malignant transformation.

5.4 Ultrasound (US)

According to the current recommendations, US is an integral part of the 6-monthly screenings (along with tumour markers) in cirrhotics and patients at high risk of HCC. Operator dependence, inability to detect lesions <1 cm and lower ability to characterize lesions limit the usage of US. In high-risk patients undergoing screening for HCC on US, the identification of a lesion >10 mm in size, not benign in appearance, or the development of a new portal vein thrombus is an indication for multiphasic contrast-enhanced CT or MRI.

5.5 Contrast-Enhanced Ultrasound (CEUS)

CEUS may be performed as the second-line diagnostic investigation for the characterisation of indeterminate focal hepatic lesions detected on conventional US. Currently, second-generation microbubble contrast agents comprising sulfur hexafluoride gas stabilised by a shell of albumin, surfactant or phospholipid are used. Different dynamic phases are acquired after rapid intravenous administration of 2.4 ml of contrast agent followed by 5 ml of saline flush. The arterial phase starts at 10–20 s and lasts for 35–40 s after injection. The portal venous phase begins at 60 s and persists for ~2 min after injection. Enhancement and washout patterns during these phases help categorise lesions as either benign or malignant and ascertain the nature of malignancy, if present.

5.6 Multiphase Computed Tomography (MPCT)

MPCT and MRI are the recommended modalities of choice for the characterisation of hepatic lesions. A multi-detector CT system with ≥8 rows is recommended for scanning. Scans are acquired in multiple phases after administration of iodinated contrast agent (1.5–2 ml/kg body weight) at 4–5 ml/s followed by a 20–30 ml saline flush. Three essential phases are acquired as part of the HCC protocol: late arterial, portal venous and delayed phases.

The late arterial phase is optimal for the detection of hypervascular hepatic lesions like HCC. It is obtained at approximately 25–30 s after contrast injection or 15–20 s after bolus detection using the bolus tracking technique. This phase shows good enhancement of the hepatic artery and mild enhancement of the portal vein with minimally enhancing hepatic parenchyma and no enhancement of hepatic veins. It is extremely important to detect the presence of arterial enhancement which may be missed on the early arterial phase. The portal venous phase is acquired at 60–70 s after contrast injection and demonstrates the presence or absence of washout of contrast within hepatic lesions. It is characterised by the enhancement of the portal and hepatic veins along with the hepatic parenchyma. The delayed phase is acquired at 180 s after the contrast administration and may demonstrate washout in certain lesions. The capsule, when present, can be seen either in the portal venous phase or the delayed phase.

The early arterial phase is generally omitted as it frequently fails to demonstrate arterial enhancement in smaller HCCs. Similarly, a non-contrast scan also has no significant role in the HCC protocol, except in previously treated lesions (e.g. post-chemoembolization). Moreover, newer dual-energy CT scanners can produce virtual non-contrast images eliminating the need for a non-contrast scan.

Key Point: The *late arterial* phase is the most important phase during dynamic scanning for HCC detection.

5.7 Contrast-Enhanced MRI (CEMRI)

CEMRI is performed using gadolinium-based extracellular contrast or hepatobiliary contrast agents. Extracellular gadolinium–based contrast (like gadobutrol, gadoterate meglumine, gadodiamide) behaves like CT contrast, and hence, in such cases, MRI protocol consists of the late arterial, portal venous and delayed phases.

Hepatobiliary contrast agents are selectively taken up by hepatocytes using the OATP1B1 receptors and excreted into the biliary system via multidrug resistance (MDR) transporters. Two such agents are gadobenate dimeglumine (MultiHance; 3–5% excretion by the liver) and gadoxetate disodium (Eovist; 50% excretion by the liver), the latter not being available in India. The late arterial and portal venous phases for both are similar to those of extracellular contrast agents. With gadoxetate disodium, the hepatocyte uptake starts during the first pass through the liver leading to combined intracellular and extracellular components of enhancement at the 3–5-min delayed scan. Hence, gadoxetate does not provide a conventional delayed phase, and this phase of transition from an extracellular dominant to intracellular dominant enhancement is called a *transitional phase*. It is important to distinguish true washout (seen in the portal venous phase/delayed phase of extracellular agents) from pseudo-washout (seen only in the transitional phase, not in the portal venous phase) which may be due to hyperenhancement of hepatic parenchyma relative to the lesion during the transitional phase. The hepatobiliary phase is acquired at 20 min for Eovist and 60–90 min for MultiHance. As the uptake of gadobenate dimeglumine (MultiHance) by hepatocytes occurs late, there is no overlap between the delayed and hepatobiliary phases, with no resultant transitional phase. Lesions which lack hepatocytes or have OATP1B3 downregulation do not show uptake of these hepatobiliary agents and appear hypointense within the normal enhancing hepatic parenchyma. Multiple ancillary criteria are also described which can help upgrade or downgrade the Liver Imaging Reporting and Data System (LI-RADS) category.

5.8 Positron Emission Tomography and Computed Tomography (PET-CT)

While whole-body 18-fluoro-2-deoxyglucose (FDG) PET-CT plays an important role in oncology, it has a limited role in the imaging of primary hepatic malignancies due to the excellent sensitivity and specificity of CT and MRI. PET-CT may help in the differentiation between malignant and benign hepatic mass lesions. Generally, primary and secondary hepatic malignancies show high uptake on FDG-PET scans, while benign lesions generally show decreased uptake on FDG-PET. As FDG uptake is higher for poorly differentiated HCCs compared to well and moderately differentiated tumours, PET can help assess the degree of differentiation of tumours. Avid uptake on FDG-PET also serves as an independent poor prognostic marker in hepatic malignancies. One of the most important roles of FDG-PET is to rule out extrahepatic disease in HCC due to its high sensitivity for recognition of nodal involvement and extrahepatic metastases.

5.9 Liver Imaging Reporting and Data System (LI-RADS)

LI-RADS is a reporting system which standardises terminology, technique, interpretation and reporting of imaging in patients with HCC or at risk of development of HCC. It was developed by the American College of Radiology (ACR) in 2011 with the latest update in 2024 and is a part of the AASLD clinical practice guidelines. The criteria are not applicable to patients <18 years of age and those with cirrhosis due to congenital hepatic fibrosis or vascular disorders.

LI-RADS consists of four major criteria: non-rim arterial phase hyperenhancement (APHE), washout in the venous/delayed phase, enhancing capsule and threshold growth which when combined with lesion size helps assign a LI-RADS category (LR1 to LR5, LR-M, LR-TIV) to the lesions (Table 5.1). Non-rim APHE is described

Table 5.1 LI-RADS categories—observation definitions and management options

LI-RADS category	Definition	Examples	Management
LR-NC	Non-categorizable due to image omission/ degradation		Repeat diagnostic imaging/ alternative imaging, usually ≤3 months
LR-1	Definitely benign	Cyst, hemangioma, perfusion alteration, focal fat deposition/sparing, confluent hepatic fibrosis, hypertrophic pseudomass	Routine surveillance
LR-2	Probably benign		Routine surveillance
LR-3	Intermediate probability of malignancy		Repeat imaging in 3–6 months
LR-4	Probably HCC		MDD—Biopsy/treatment/ alternative imaging ≤3 months
LR-5	Definitely HCC		MDD—Staging and treatment Biopsy not needed to confirm diagnosis
LR-M	Probably or definitely malignant, but not HCC-specific	iCCA, cHCC-CCA, metastasis, lymphoma	MDD—Staging and treatment Biopsy for determining the type of malignancy
LR-TIV	Definite tumour in the vein	HCC, iCCA, cHCC-CCA	MDD—Staging and treatment Biopsy for determining the type of malignancy

Note: *cHCC-CCA* combined HCC Cholangiocarcinoma, *HCC* hepatocellular carcinoma, *iCCA* intrahepatic cholangiocarcinoma, *MDD* multidisciplinary discussion as arterial enhancement unequivocally greater than the surrounding hepatic parenchyma. Washout is described as the temporal reduction in the enhancement relative to the adjacent parenchyma on the venous or delayed phase. According to LI-RADS, an intrahepatic lesion ≥2 cm with APHE, venous washout and capsule formation on CT or MRI is categorised as an LR-5 lesion which is the sine qua non of a progressed HCC and does not require a histopathological diagnosis. Multiple ancillary criteria are also present which can help upgrade or downgrade the LI-RADS category.

5.10 Imaging Appearance

5.10.1 Regenerative Nodules (RNs)

RNs are similar to the adjacent cirrhotic parenchyma both in terms of molecular and pathological profile, and this also reflects in their imaging appearances. RNs typically range from 5 to 10 mm in size. Most lesions are isoechoic to adjacent cirrhotic liver parenchyma and show no focal abnormality on US, except for coarsened underlying hepatic echotexture and surface nodularity. Certain larger RNs may also appear hypoechoic with a surrounding thin, slightly echogenic rim compared to the adjacent hepatic parenchyma. On CEUS, these nodules are iso-enhancing to the adjacent hepatic parenchyma in all the phases. Lesions usually appear isodense on plain CT and are isointense on T2-weighted MRI with no APHE or venous/delayed phase washout (Fig. 5.2). The lesions show no diffusion restriction or hepatobiliary phase hypointensity (Fig. 5.3). RNs may also appear mildly hyperintense on the hepatobiliary phase relative to adjacent fibrotic hepatic scars which appear hypointense.

5.10.2 Low-Grade Dysplastic Nodules (LGDNs)

LGDN may be visualised as discrete hypo-hyperechoic nodular lesions in a cirrhotic liver (depending on the extent of fat in them). On CEUS, these lesions may show transient hypoenhancement with respect to the adjacent liver in the arterial phase (due to a decrease in arterial supply during early hepatocarcinogenesis), with iso-enhancement in the delayed phase. These nodules are generally isodense or hypodense to adjacent hepatic parenchyma on plain CT with no APHE or venous/delayed washout. Lesions appear hyperintense on T1-weighted MRI, likely due to the accumulation of paramagnetic substances, and iso-hypointense on T2-weighted MRI. T2 hyperintensity, diffusion restriction and hepatobiliary hypointensity—features that serve as ancillary features of malignancy—are generally not seen. Lesions also do not show any APHE or venous washout.

Deposition of a high amount of iron may occur within these nodules leading to the development of 'siderotic' nodules which appear markedly hypointense on T2-weighted MRI. Due to the resistance of malignant cells to iron, loss of iron in a previously siderotic nodule or appearance of an iron-poor nodule in a siderotic nodule may signify malignant transformation.

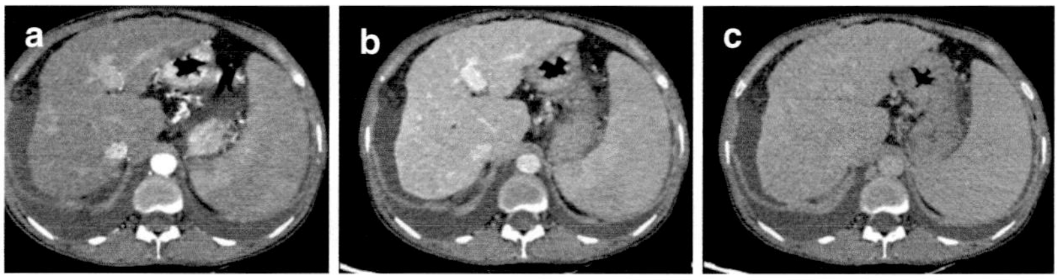

Fig. 5.2 A 38-year-old female with regenerative nodules. (**a**–**c**) Axial late arterial phase CT image (**a**) showed cirrhotic liver with a nodular outline and multiple isodense nodules scattered throughout the liver which remain isodense on both venous (**b**) and delayed (**c**) phase CT images, suggestive of regenerative nodules. Bilateral mild pleural effusion and ascites were also noted

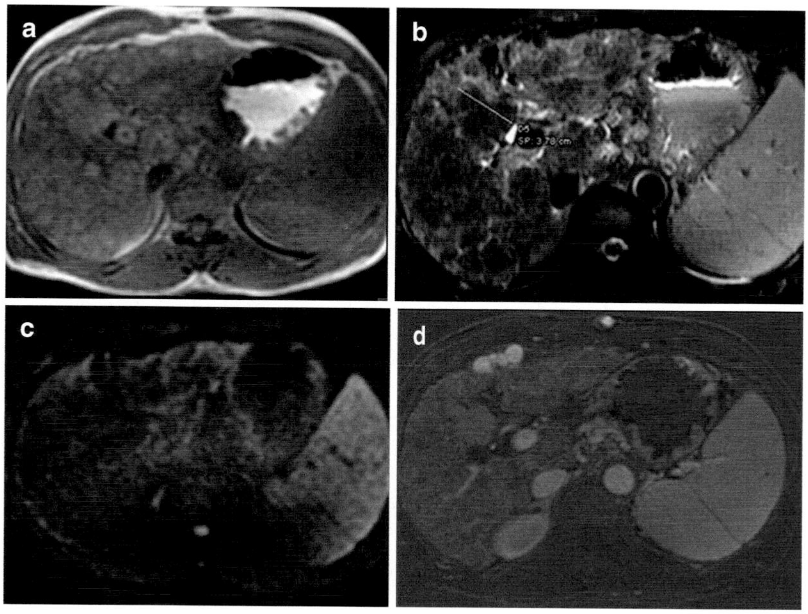

Fig. 5.3 A 45-year-old male with regenerative nodules. (**a**, **b**) Axial T1-weighted MRI (**a**) showed multiple iso-hyperintense nodules scattered in the liver which are iso-hypointense on T2-weighted MRI (**b**). (**c**) Axial high-b value (b-800) diffusion-weighted MRI showed no diffusion restriction in the nodules. (**d**) Axial post-contrast T1-weighted MRI did not show any arterial enhancement or washout of the nodules

5.10.3 High-Grade Dysplastic Nodules (HGDNs) and Early HCC

HGDN and early HCC are difficult to distinguish from each other on imaging, the difference mainly being the presence of stromal invasion on histopathology.

HGDN may be identified on US as hypoechoic nodules. These lesions generally do not show APHE on CEUS and become iso-enhancing in the delayed phase. They generally show iso-hyperintensity on T1-weighted MRI and iso-intensity on T2-weighted MRI with no diffusion restriction. Intralesional steatosis, seen as signal loss on opposed-phase T1-weighted MRI, may be present in HGDNs and early HCC. A few lesions may show APHE without any washout in the venous/delayed phase. The loss of the OATP receptor occurs early during the process of hepatocarcinogenesis, and thus, hepatobiliary phase hypointensity may be seen in HGDNs before the appearance of APHE (Fig. 5.4).

Early HCCs are defined as small (<2 cm), vaguely nodular lesions with no definite capsule formation. These lesions have little tendency to invade vessels or metastasise. On CEUS, these lesions may show APHE but without washout in the portal venous/delayed phase. These lesions show most of the ancillary features of malignancy on MRI—T2 hyperintensity, diffusion restriction and intralesional fat along with hepatobiliary phase hypointensity. APHE may also be seen in these lesions due to neoangiogenesis with or without venous phase washout (Fig. 5.5).

The *nodule-in-nodule* appearance is defined as the presence of an arterially enhancing nodule developing within a previously benign iso-enhancing nodule. This appearance is pathognomonic of an HCC.

Key Point: Hepatobiliary hypointensity is an early marker of malignant transformation of hepatic nodules.

5.10.4 Progressed HCC

These lesions are overtly malignant with a tendency to invade vessels and metastasise. Morphologically, they may appear as a well-defined nodule with a capsule or a diffusely infiltrating mass.

On CEUS, progressed HCCs show APHE with gradual washout (after 60 s) in the portal venous/late phase (c.f. rapid washout in <60 s in

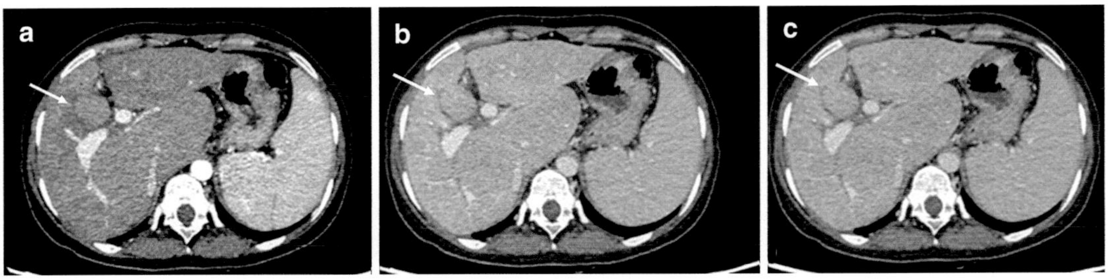

Fig. 5.4 A 25-year-old female with a high-grade dysplastic nodule in the liver. (**a–c**) Axial late arterial phase CT image (**a**) showed a hyperenhancing nodule in segment IVb of the liver (arrow) which becomes isodense to the adjacent parenchyma in the venous (**b**) and delayed (**c**) phase CT images (arrow)

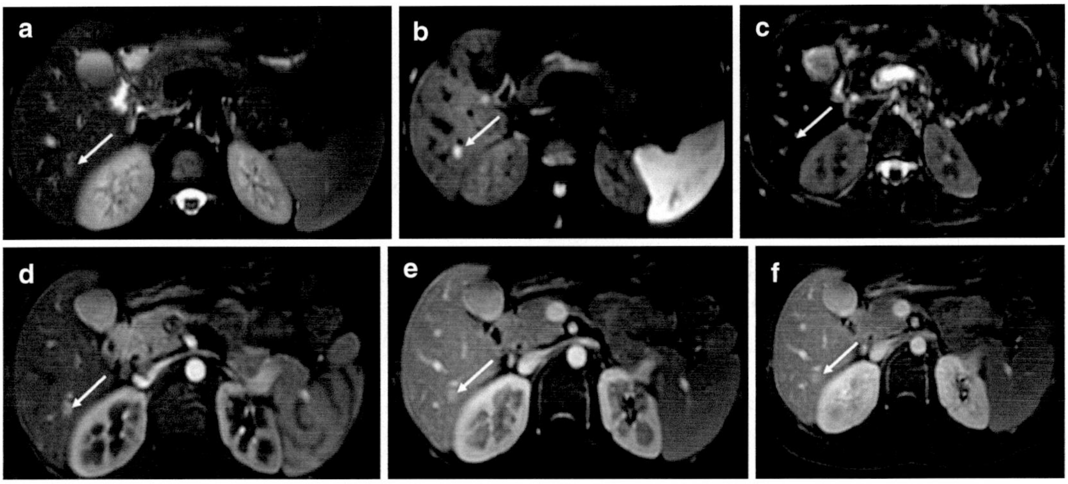

Fig. 5.5 A 27-year-old female with a high-grade dysplastic nodule/early HCC. (**a**) Axial T2-weighted MRI showed a hyperintense nodule in segment VI of the liver (arrow). (**b**, **c**) Axial high b-value (b-800) diffusion-weighted MRI (**b**) showed a hyperintense signal of the nodule with corresponding hypointensity on the ADC image (**c**) suggestive of true diffusion restriction (arrow). (**d–f**) Axial post-contrast late arterial phase T1-weighted MRI (**d**) showed non-rim arterial phase hyperenhancement (arrow) with the persistence of enhancement in venous (**e**) and delayed (**f**) phase images (arrow)

intrahepatic cholangiocarcinoma and hypervascular metastasis) (Fig. 5.6). Progressed HCCs appear hypodense on plain CT, iso-hypointense on T1-weighted MRI and moderately hyperintense on T2-weighted MRI with restricted diffusion on diffusion-weighted images (DWIs).

Dynamic contrast enhancement on CT/MRI exhibits non-rim APHE with venous/delayed phase washout and capsule formation. A combination of non-rim APHE with washout has 100% specificity for the diagnosis of HCC > 20 mm and 90% specificity for HCC between 10 and 19 mm in patients with cirrhosis and other risk factors for HCC. The presence of a capsule is also a feature of progressed HCC. This capsule should be visualised as a uniform smooth rim of hyperenhancement on the portal venous or delayed phase (Fig. 5.7). A 'mosaic appearance' is also seen in advanced HCC which is characterised by the presence of multiple compartments of heterogeneous signal intensity with septations and surrounded by an enhancing capsule (Fig. 5.8). Extracapsular extension, seen in the form of satellite nodules, is also frequently seen. These occur in the same venous drainage area as the primary tumour (within 2 cm), and each lesion, although small, can metastasise and invade vessels. Multifocal HCC may be seen in up to 74%

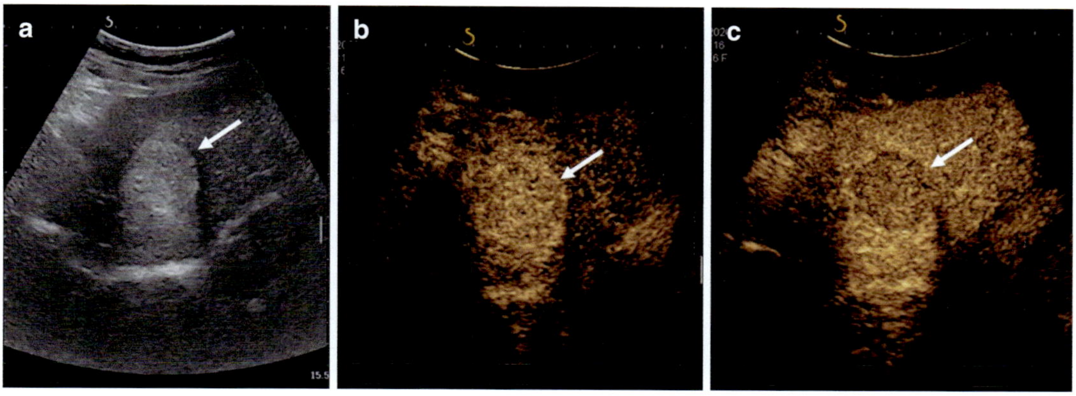

Fig. 5.6 A 40-year-old male with hepatocellular carcinoma. (**a**–**c**) Ultrasonography image of the liver (**a**) showed a well-defined echogenic lesion in the liver (arrow). The background liver shows coarse echotexture. On contrast-enhanced ultrasound (**b**), the lesion showed hyperenhancement (arrow) compared to the surrounding liver parenchyma with washout in the venous phase (**c**, arrow). This suggests a LI-RADS-5 lesion

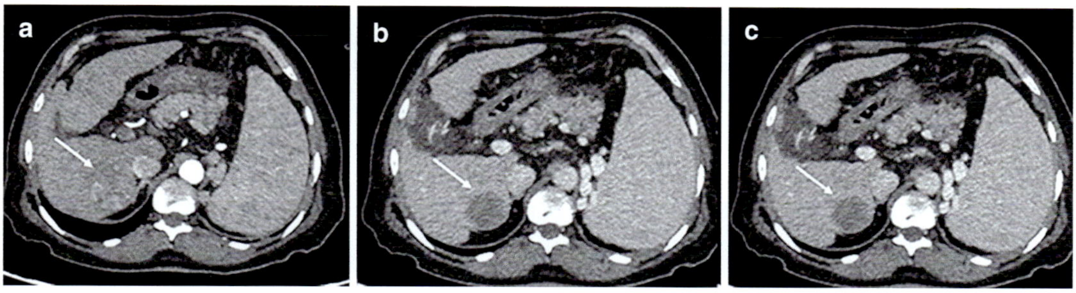

Fig. 5.7 A 56-year-old male with hepatocellular carcinoma. (**a**) Axial late arterial phase CT image showed cirrhotic liver with a non-rim arterial phase hyperenhancing lesion in the liver (arrow) with washout in the venous phase (**b**) and capsule formation in the delayed phase (**c**) images (arrow). These findings are suggestive of a LI-RADS-5 lesion

of patients with cirrhosis and are either multiple tumours of multicentric origin or multiple intrahepatic metastases from a single HCC (Fig. 5.9).

The portal vein (PV) is a common site of invasion by HCC and may be seen in 44–62% of cases [7]. The presence of a malignant PV thrombosis confers a poorer prognosis, with an increased risk of metastatic disease and acts as a contraindication to surgery and locoregional therapy. Consequently, it becomes essential to differentiate a malignant from a bland PV thrombus, a commonly seen entity in cirrhotic patients (5–20% depending on the severity of cirrhosis) [8]. Imaging appearance and differentiating features between malignant and bland thrombus are described in Table 5.2.

Infrequently, HCC may be associated with thrombosis of the hepatic veins which may extend to the inferior vena cava and the right atrium (1.4–4.9%) [9]. Invasion into the hepatic veins is a very poor prognostic marker, and a majority of the patients demonstrate metastatic disease to other organs. The presence of macrovascular invasion automatically upgrades these lesions into Barcelona Clinic Liver Cancer (BCLC) Stage C.

The infiltrative variety of HCC shows a diffuse, cirrhomimetic appearance with permeative margins without a dominant tumour nodule and may be difficult to differentiate from the underlying cirrhotic liver. It shows minimal APHE with variable washout patterns on dynamic contrast imaging. The lesion may show mild hyperintensity to the adjacent hepatic parenchyma on T2-weighted MRI and DWI. Frequently, the only clue to the diagnosis of infiltrative HCC is the

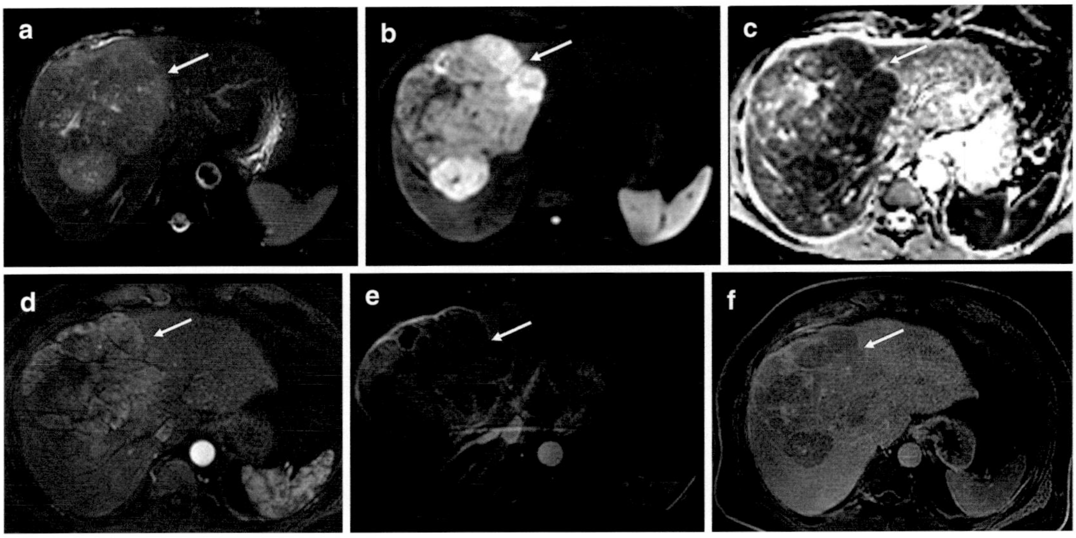

Fig. 5.8 A 72-year-old male with hepatocellular carcinoma (arrow). (**a**) Axial T2-weighted MRI showed a large heterogeneous hyperintense mass in the right lobe of the liver. (**b**) Axial high b-value (b-800) diffusion-weighted MRI showed a hyperintense signal of the mass with corresponding hypointensity on the ADC image (**c**) suggestive of true diffusion restriction. (**d**) Axial late arterial phase T1-weighted MRI showed non-rim arterial phase hyperenhancement with a mosaic pattern. (**e**) Axial delayed phase T1-weighted MRI showed washout and capsule. (**f**) Axial T1-weighted hepatobiliary phase MRI showed a hypointense signal of the lesion

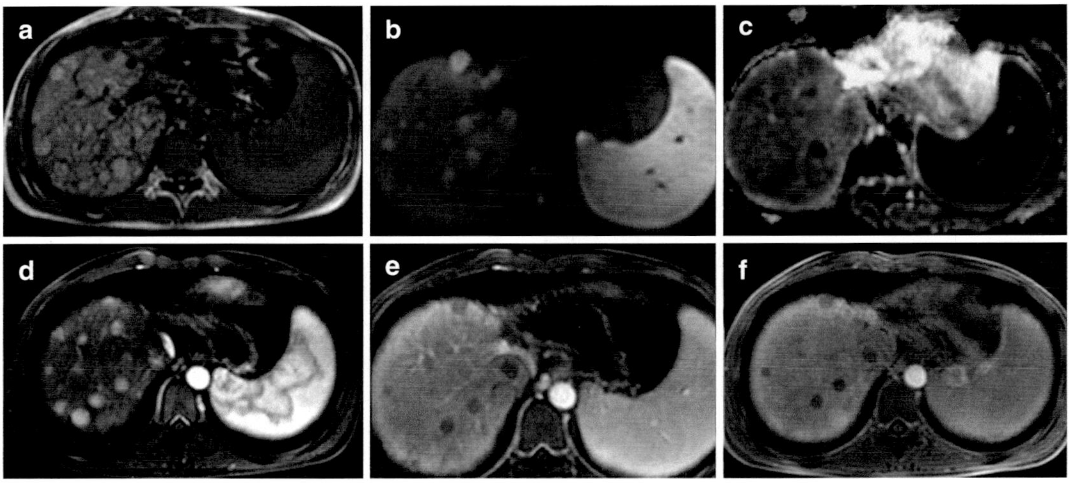

Fig. 5.9 A 22-year-old male with multifocal hepatocellular carcinoma. (**a**) Axial T1-weighted MRI showed multiple hyperintense nodules in the liver. (**b**) Axial high b-value (b-800) diffusion-weighted MRI showed hyperintense signal of the nodules with corresponding hypointensity on the ADC image (**c**) suggestive of true diffusion restriction. (**d**) Axial late arterial phase T1-weighted MRI showed non-rim arterial phase hyperenhancement with washout and capsule formation in venous (**e**) and delayed (**f**) phase images

presence of a malignant portal vein thrombus (Fig. 5.10).

The propensity to metastasise increases with the presence of vascular invasion. This can be macrovascular, seen in the form of an enhancing tumour in the vein or microvascular invasion. One of the most important determinants of prognosis is the presence of microvascular invasion (MVI) seen as perilesional enhancement on the arterial phase (corona enhancement), perilesional

Table 5.2 Imaging differences between malignant and bland portal vein thrombus

	Malignant PV thrombus	Bland PV thrombus
Incidence	Seen in 44–62% of HCC cases	5–20%, depending on the severity of cirrhosis
Conventional ultrasound	Echogenic soft tissue in the lumen Dilatation of main PV > 23 mm	Hypoechoic (acute) or echogenic (chronic) intraluminal soft tissue Main PV diameter < 20 mm
US Doppler	Internal vascularity with arterial spectral trace	No internal vascularity
CEUS	Enhancement of thrombus in the arterial phase with or without washout in the venous phase	No enhancement of the thrombus
CECT	Enhancing soft tissue within dilated PV may or may not show continuity with hepatic mass '*Thread and streak pattern*' of enhancement in the arterial phase Associated transient hepatic attenuation difference (THAD)	Non-opacification of the PV Hypo/non-enhancing thrombus Associated transient hepatic attenuation difference (THAD)
MRI	T2 hyperintense content within normal PV flow void PV diameter > 23 mm Associated transient hepatic intensity difference (THID) Diffusion restriction + Dynamic enhancement—Similar to that seen in CECT	T2 hyperintense content within normal PV flow void PV diameter < 20 mm May be associated with THID Diffusion restriction—In acute thrombus Dynamic enhancement—absent or minimal
PET-CT	Moderate to high ^{18}FDG avidity	No or slight ^{18}FDG avidity

Note: *CECT* contrast-enhanced computed tomography, *CEUS* contrast-enhanced ultrasound, *MRI* magnetic resonance imaging, *PET-CT* positron emission tomography-CT, *PV* portal vein, *US* ultrasonography

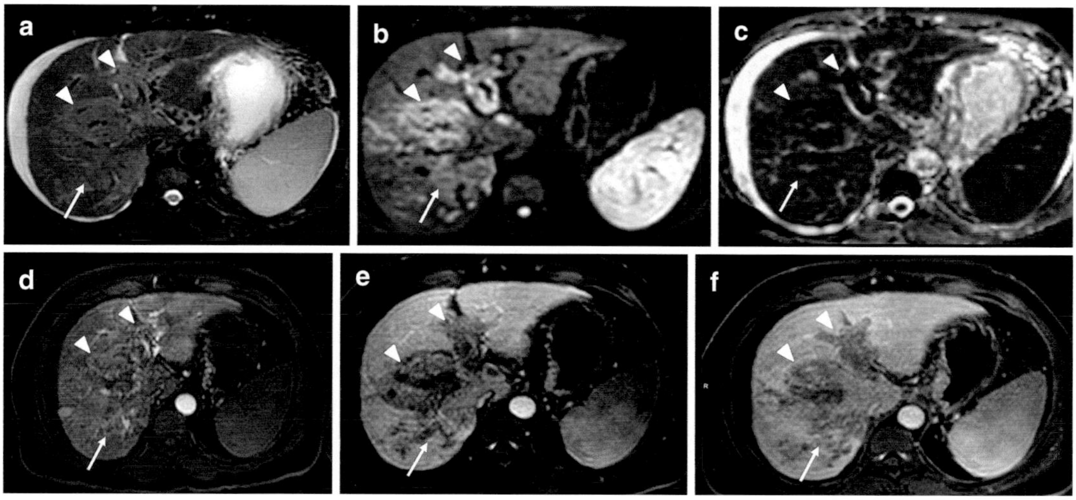

Fig. 5.10 A 43-year-old male with an infiltrative type of hepatocellular carcinoma. (**a**) Axial T2-weighted MRI showed an ill-defined hyperintense area in the right lobe of the liver (arrow) with extension along the portal vein (arrowheads). There is a nodular outline of the liver and mild perihepatic free fluid. (**b**, **c**) Axial high b-value (b-800) DWI (**b**) and ADC images (**c**) showed diffusion restriction in the lesion (arrow) and within the portal vein (arrowheads). (**d**) Axial late arterial phase T1-weighted MRI showed subtle heterogeneous enhancement of the lesion (arrow) with a 'thread and streak' pattern of enhancement in the portal vein (arrowheads) suggesting malignant tumour thrombus (tumour in vein). (**e**, **f**) The lesion showed heterogeneous enhancement in the venous (**e**) and delayed (**f**) phases, with tumour in the vein showing washout

hepatobiliary phase hypointensity, irregular tumour margins and a disrupted capsule.

HCC infrequently invades the bile duct, with an incidence between 0.53% and 12.9%, and is considered a poor prognostic marker due to the infiltrative nature of these malignancies [10]. HCCs may also extend up to the capsular surface and undergo spontaneous rupture in approximately 3–26% of cases with associated hemoperitoneum and resultant shock. Mortality occurs in 25–75% of these cases according to different studies [11].

Table 5.3 demonstrates MRI features that can help differentiate various nodules seen in a cirrhotic liver.

Key Point: Microvascular invasion is a poor prognostic marker, seen as perilesional enhancement in the arterial phase (corona enhancement), perilesional hepatobiliary phase hypointensity, irregular tumour margins and a disrupted capsule.

5.10.5 HCC Subtypes

Presently, lesions described as LR-5 on CT or MRI imaging in at-risk patients are unequivocally considered to be HCC, and there is no requirement for biopsy. However, up to 43% of LRM lesions turn out to be HCCs and have an atypical imaging appearance. As research is progressing, multiple molecular subtypes of HCC have been discovered, all of which portend different prognostic implications and may be identified due to atypical imaging appearance.

The 2019 fifth edition of the WHO classification states that almost 35% of all HCCs can be categorised into eight subtypes based on pathomolecular characteristics—steatohepatitic, clear cell, macrotrabecular-massive, scirrhous, chromophobe, fibrolamellar, neutrophil-rich and lymphocyte-rich. The remaining 65% of HCCs are classified as not-otherwise-specified HCC (NOS-HCC) [12]. A few imaging characteristics of the important HCC subtypes have been described below:

1. *Steatohepatitic HCC*: This is the most common subtype comprising ~5–20% of all HCCs. They generally occur in the presence of underlying NAFLD and NASH and are associated with a favourable prognosis. Lesions are generally smaller in size compared to other HCCs and show APHE, venous washout and intralesional fat in the background of a fatty liver. Intralesional fat can be recognised as areas of signal drop on opposed-phase T1-weighted MRI. Intralesional fat is also a common feature of early HCCs as inadequate tumour neoangiogenesis leads to hypoxia and consequent fatty metamorphosis. Progressed HCCs generally do not show any intralesional fat (Fig. 5.11). Thus, a lesion resembling a progressed HCC on dynamic contrast-enhanced imaging but showing intralesional fat and background features of NAFLD/NASH should raise suspicion of a steatohepatitic HCC.
2. *Macrotrabecular-massive HCC*: This pathological subtype comprises only 5% of all HCCs and is associated with a poor prognosis. Serum alpha-fetoprotein (AFP) levels are more than those seen in NOS-HCC. Histopathology requires at least 50% of the tumour area to be composed of a macrotrabecular pattern (cords >6 cells thick). Additionally, these lesions are also associated with an increase in hypoxia-related gene expression. On imaging, these lesions appear large with increased frequency of tumour in the vein along with large areas of intratumoural necrosis (>20%).
3. *Scirrhous HCC*: Pathologically characterised by dense fibrous stroma comprising >50% of the tumour, scirrhous HCCs represent only 4% of all HCCs. These lesions are positive for stem cell markers like cytokeratin-19 and show a worse prognosis than conventional HCC. The imaging characteristics follow the histology of the tumours, with central hypointensity on T2-weighted MRI, peripheral APHE with progressive central enhancement and targetoid appearance on DWI and hepatobiliary phase. The main imaging mimic is intrahepatic cholangiocarcinoma. However,

Table 5.3 MRI features to differentiate various nodules in a cirrhotic liver

Lesion	Conventional USG	CEUS	Dynamic enhancement (CT/MRI)			MRI			
			APHE	Washout (venous/ delayed)	Capsule formation	T1W	T2W	Diffusion restriction	HBP hypointensity
Regenerative nodule	Altered hepatic echotexture, isoechoic	Iso-enhancing on all phases	Absent	Absent	Absent	Iso-hyperintense	Iso-hypointense	Absent	Absent
Siderotic nodule	Echogenic	Iso-enhancing on all phases	Absent	Absent	Absent	Variable	Markedly hypointense	Absent	Present
LGDN	Hypo or hyperechoic (depending on fat content)	Iso-enhancing on all phases	Absent	Absent	Absent	Iso-hyperintense	Iso-hypointense	Absent	Present
HGDN	Hypo or hyperechoic (depending on fat content)	Iso-enhancing in all phases ± transient hypoenhancement in the arterial phase	May be present	Absent	Absent	Iso-hyperintense	Isointense	Absent	Present
Early HCC	Hypoechoic	Arterial enhancement, no washout	May be present	Absent	Absent	Variable	Hyperintense	Present	Present
Progressed HCC	Hypoechoic	Arterial enhancement, rapid washout (<60 s)	Present	Present	Present	Variable	Hyperintense	Present	Present

HCC hepatocellular carcinoma, *HGDN* high-grade dysplastic nodule, *LGDN* low-grade dysplastic nodule

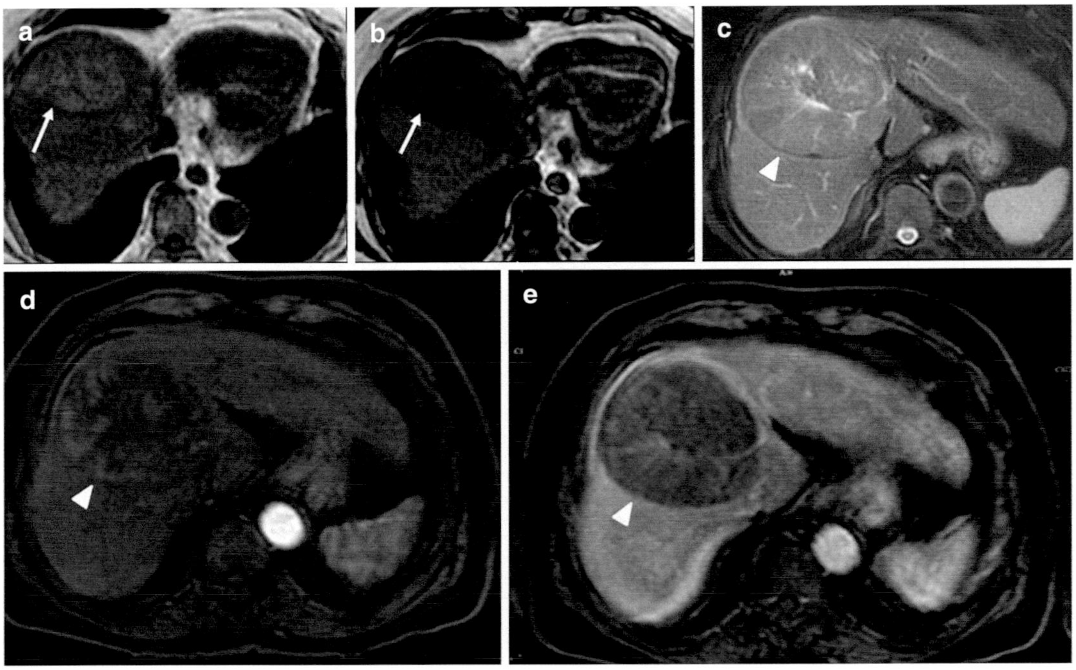

Fig. 5.11 A 69-year-old male with steatohepatitic variant of hepatocellular carcinoma. (**a**, **b**) Axial T1-weighted in-phase MRI (**a**) showed a well-defined mass in the right lobe of the liver with central hyperintensity (arrow), which showed loss of signal on opposed-phase T1-weighted MRI (**b**) suggestive of microscopic fat within the lesion. (**c**) Axial T2-weighted MRI showed a large heterogeneously hyperintense mass (arrowhead) with a central hyperintense scar. (**d**, **e**) Axial late arterial phase T1-weighted MRI (**d**) showed non-rim arterial phase hyperenhancement with washout and capsule formation in the delayed phase (**e**) (arrowhead) with enhancement of the central scar

the presence of a capsule, internal septa and central hypointensity suggests a diagnosis of HCC.

4. *Fibrolamellar HCC*: This is a rare HCC subtype (1%) typically seen in young patients in the absence of liver disease. It is associated with low levels of serum AFP. On imaging, they are well-defined lesions appearing hypointense on T1-weighted MRI and hyperintense on T2-weighted MRI with a central hypointense scar and calcification. On post-contrast images, it shows heterogeneous APHE with iso-hypointensity on the venous/delayed phases and a typically hypoenhancing central scar (Figs. 5.12 and 5.13). Lesions generally appear hypointense in the hepatobiliary phase. Appearance may mimic focal nodular hyperplasia (FNH). However, FNH generally shows iso-hyperintensity on the hepatobiliary phase with scars generally appearing hyperintense on T2-weighted MRI with enhancement on the delayed phase.

5.10.6 Treatment

The Barcelona Clinic Liver Cancer (BCLC) classification [13] (Fig. 5.14) is the most commonly used staging system for HCC which links tumour burden, liver function and patient performance status with prognosis and management.

In patients with preserved liver function and good performance status (0–1), very early stage (0) HCC is defined as a solitary HCC $\leq$ 2 cm with no vascular invasion or extrahepatic spread. In patients who are potential candidates for transplant, surgical resection may be considered the first option (in the absence of clinically significant portal hypertension (CSPH)) or liver transplant (LT)

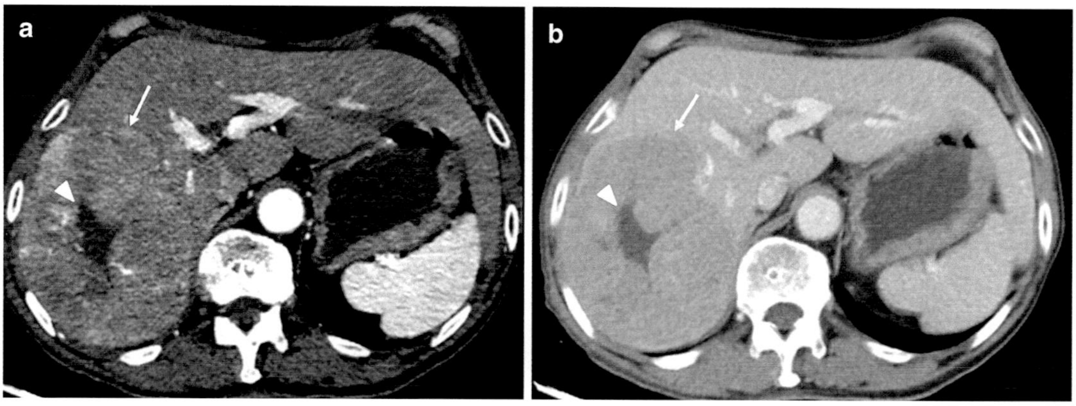

Fig. 5.12 A 72-year-old male with fibrolamellar carcinoma. (**a**) Axial late arterial phase CT image showed a non-cirrhotic liver with a well-defined non-rim arterial phase hyperenhancing lesion in the right lobe (arrow) with intralesional vascularity and central non-enhancing scar (arrowhead). (**b**) Axial venous phase CT image showed washout, with the lesion (arrow) becoming hypodense compared to the surrounding liver parenchyma

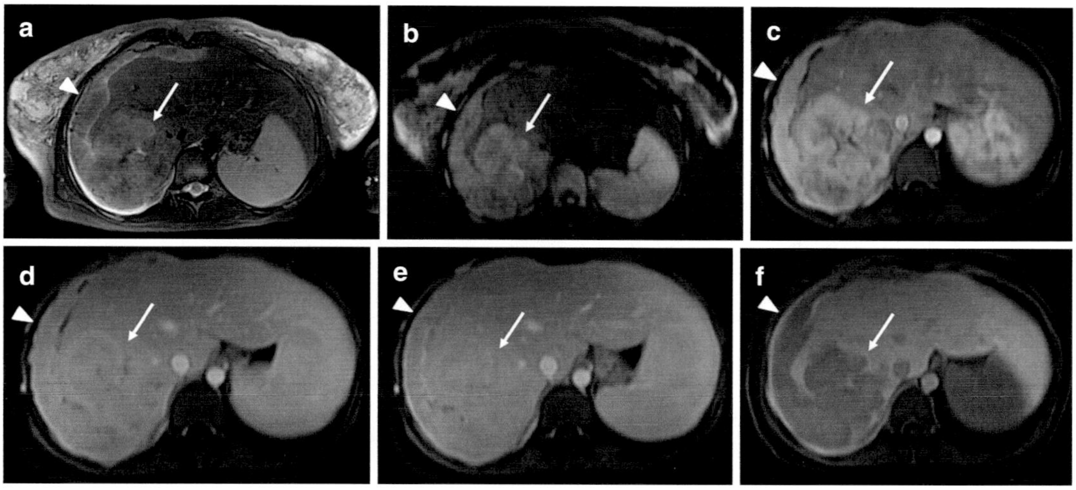

Fig. 5.13 A 26-year-old female with fibrolamellar carcinoma. (**a**, **b**) Axial T2-weighted MRI showed a well-defined lobulated heterogeneously hyperintense lesion (arrow) with a central hypointense scar in the liver with similar appearing soft tissue deposits along the hepatic surface; both the lesion and deposits showed diffusion restriction on diffusion-weighted MRI (**b**). (**c**–**e**) The lesions showed heterogeneous non-rim arterial hyperenhancement in the late arterial phase (**c**) and appeared iso-enhancing to the hepatic parenchyma in the venous (**d**) and delayed phases (**e**). (**f**) Axial T1-weighted hepatobiliary phase MRI showed a hypointense signal of the lesion (arrow) and the deposits (arrowhead)

depending on pathological features of increased recurrence risk. If a transplant is not feasible, ablation therapies comprising mainly radiofrequency ablation (RFA) or microwave ablation (MWA) are the preferred options. Transarterial chemoembolization (TACE) may be performed in cases of recurrence after ablation as a part of 'Tumour stage migration'.

Early stage (A) comprises solitary HCC irrespective of size or multifocal HCC up to 3 in number (none ≥3 cm) without vascular invasion, extrahepatic spread or cancer-related symptoms and with a preserved liver function. In solitary lesions ≤3 cm in size, ablation and resection show similar results in terms of survival. Thus, ablation may be chosen as it is minimally invasive and

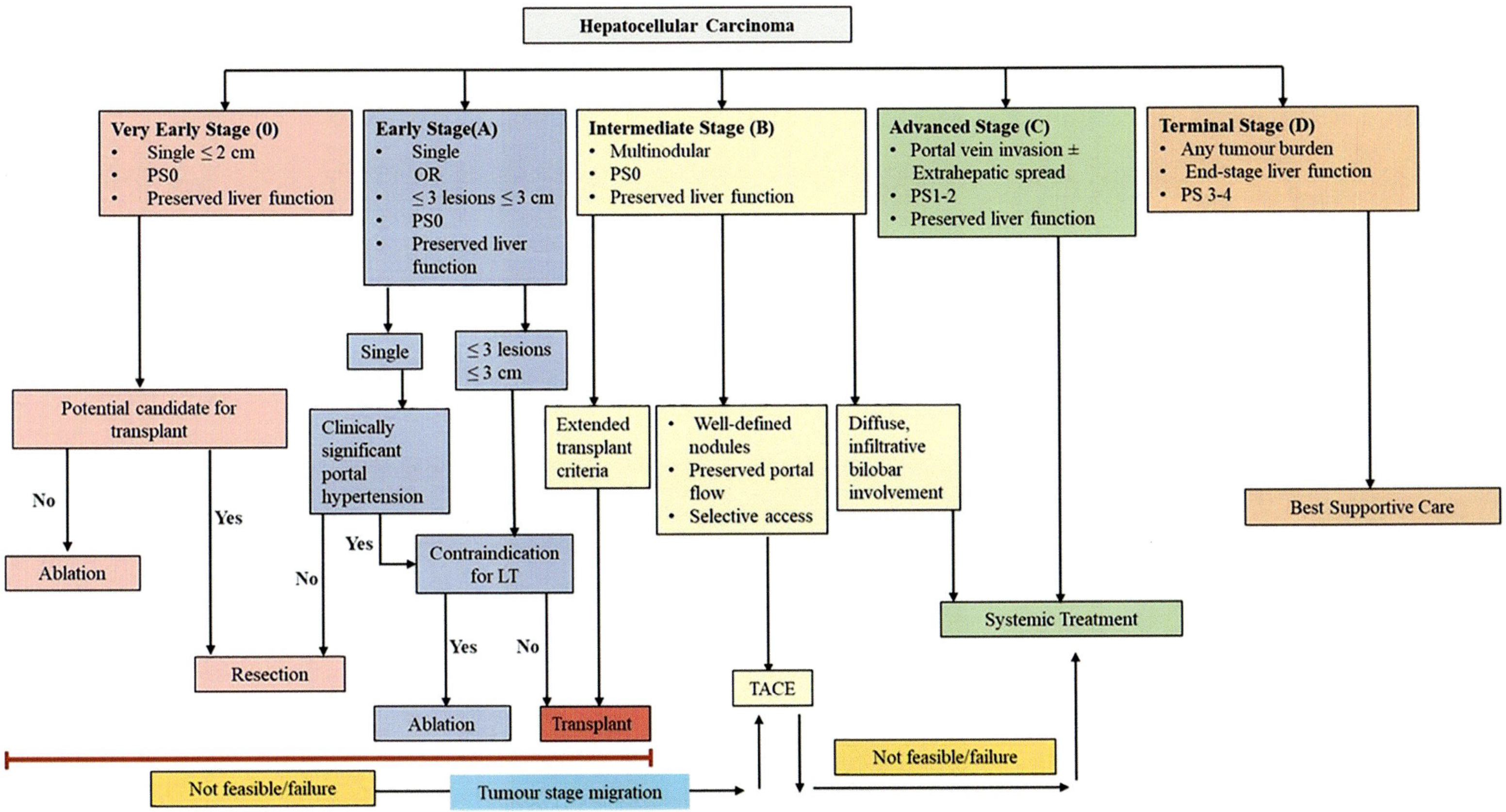

Fig. 5.14 BCLC staging and treatment strategy (2022). *LT* liver transplantation, *PS* performance status, *TACE* transarterial chemoembolization (Reproduced from BCLC Strategy for prognosis prediction and treatment recommendation: The 2022 update)

cheaper. In solitary lesions >3 cm, resection (without CSPH) or LT may be considered. Multifocal disease within Milan criteria (up to 3 lesions, each ≤3 cm) should undergo LT. If LT is not feasible, either ablation or TACE may be considered.

Intermediate stage HCC (BCLC-B) comprises patients with preserved liver function and performance status with large or multifocal HCC (> three tumours of any size, two to three tumours >3 cm in maximum dimension or a single tumour >5 cm) without macrovascular invasion or extrahepatic spread. These patients may be candidates for LT if they meet the institutional 'Extended Liver Transplant Criteria'. Patients who are not amenable to LT but have preserved portal flow and selective access to feeding arteries are candidates for TACE. If patients meet none of the criteria or present with diffuse infiltrative HCC, systemic chemotherapy may be started upfront.

The advanced stage (BCLC-C) is defined as patients with vascular invasion or extrahepatic spread with preserved liver function and performance status. This group of patients should be evaluated for the institution of systemic therapy at offset.

End-stage (BCLC-D) disease comprises patients with poor performance status (PS > 2) with or without deranged liver function who are not candidates for a LT. In such cases, symptomatic management and best supportive care must be provided.

5.10.7 Post-Treatment Changes and Detection of Recurrence

Follow-up imaging is essential to assess for treatment response after locoregional therapies for HCC like thermal ablation (radiofrequency ablation/microwave ablation), TACE, transarterial radioembolization (TARE) and stereotactic beam radiation therapy (SBRT).

Initial contrast-enhanced computed tomography/contrast-enhanced MRI (CECT/CE-MRI) is done at 3–4 weeks after thermal ablation or TACE to evaluate for treatment response, followed by 3-monthly imaging for the next 2 years to assess for tumour recurrence. Tumour size may not decrease after locoregional therapy, leading to overdiagnosis of lesions as a stable or progressive disease when using the usual response evaluation criteria in solid tumours (RECIST). The mRECIST (modified RECIST) compares the longest diameter of any remaining post-treatment arterially enhancing component within lesions to assess for response. The LI-RADS tumour response (LI-RADS TR) criteria are also used to assess for response in these cases.

After thermal ablation or TACE, non-viable tumours typically appear hypoenhancing to the adjacent hepatic parenchyma. A thin, uniform enhancing peripheral rim may be seen. Viable tumours may appear as peripheral nodular areas of arterial enhancement, a thick, irregular tumour rim or any disruption in the smooth, thin enhancing rim that is expected after treatment. Lesions generally appear hypointense on both T1- and T2-weighted MRI, but internal T1 hyperintensity may be seen in cases of intralesional haemorrhage or proteinaceous debris [14].

It is important to note that tumour size may paradoxically increase after TARE or SBRT due to oedema. Additionally, persistent solid APHE may also be seen after these therapies, generally up to 3 months for TARE and about 1 year for SBRT. Hence, unlike other locoregional therapies, the initial scan to detect tumour response to TARE/SBRT is done after 3 months. Temporal reduction in size and arterial enhancement serve as important markers of tumour response in these cases. Any increase in size or any new/increasing APHE within a lesion should be treated as local recurrence in these cases.

Key Point: Persistent arterial enhancement is commonly seen after locoregional therapy involving radiation (TARE/SBRT) and should not be confused with viable tumour.

5.11 Intrahepatic Cholangiocarcinoma (ICC)

Intrahepatic cholangiocarcinoma (ICC) is the second most common primary malignant hepatic mass lesion after HCC. Cholangiocarcinoma can

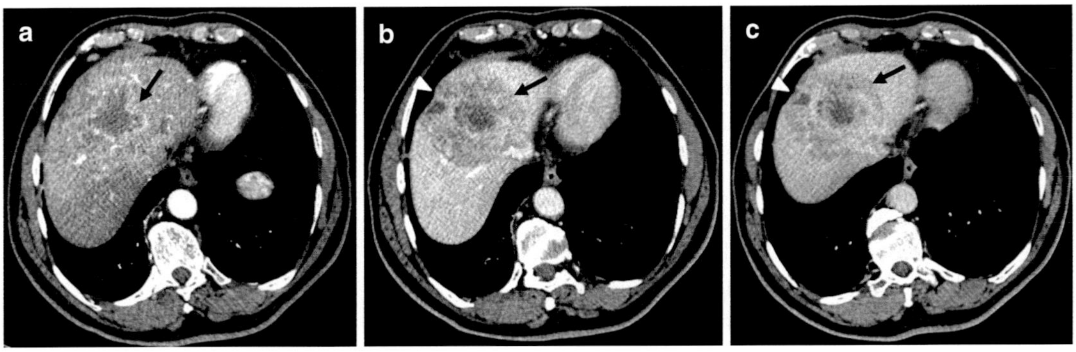

Fig. 5.15 A 35-year-old male with intrahepatic mass-forming cholangiocarcinoma. (**a**) Axial late arterial phase CT image showed a rim-arterial enhancing mass in the liver (arrow). The lesion (arrow) showed centripetal progressive enhancement in the venous (**b**) and delayed phases (**c**), with adjacent capsular retraction (arrowhead)

be categorised either based on location (intrahepatic, perihilar or extrahepatic distal) or gross morphology (mass-forming, periductal infiltrating, intraductal). ICC is defined as a tumour arising from the biliary epithelium of intrahepatic biliary radicals beyond the secondary confluence and constitutes only 10% of all cholangiocarcinoma [15]. The majority of ICC are of the mass-forming type on gross morphology (78%) followed by the periductal infiltrating type (16%) and intraductal growing (6%). Most lesions are well-differentiated adenocarcinomas with variable degrees of stromal fibrosis on histopathology.

Several risk factors are associated with the development of ICC-like infection with liver flukes or viral hepatitis, primary sclerosing cholangitis, hepatolithiasis, biliary cystic disease, alcohol abuse and tobacco use. Like HCC, chronic liver disease and cirrhosis are also risk factors for the development of ICC [16].

On US, mass-forming ICC appears as a well-defined hypoechoic mass which may be associated with adjacent biliary ductal dilatation. Periductal infiltrating and intraductal forms may not have any obvious abnormality on US except for focal biliary radical dilatation. On CEUS, ICCs may show heterogeneous or rim arterial phase hyperenhancement with rapid washout during the portal venous phase (<60 s). CECT and CE-MRI are the mainstays for the characterisation and assessment of the resectability of ICC.

Typically, mass-forming ICC appears hypodense on unenhanced CT with a thick, irregular rim APHE and progressive, centripetal enhancement during the venous and delayed phases (Fig. 5.15). They show irregular but well-defined margins associated with adjacent capsular retraction and peripheral ductal dilatation. Periductal infiltrating lesions show hyperenhancement compared to the adjacent hepatic parenchyma with associated irregular narrowing of biliary radicals and proximal ductal dilatation. Intraductal growing ICC appears as papillary/polypoidal lesions within a dilated bile duct with faint contrast enhancement compared to adjacent hepatic parenchyma [17].

On MRI, ICC appear as a well-defined, hypointense mass on T1-weighted images. Peripheral hyperintensity and areas of central hypointensity are seen on T2-weighted images which correspond to peripheral viable tumour cells and central fibrous stroma. A similar targetoid appearance is also seen on high b-value DWI. The arterial phase shows thick rim enhancement with progressive wash-in during the portal venous/delayed phase with no obvious capsule formation. ICCs lack OATP expression leading to a hypointense appearance on the hepatobiliary phase images (Fig. 5.16). However, some amount of contrast pooling may occur centrally in lesions with a large quantity of central fibrous stroma giving a 'targetoid appearance' on the hepatobiliary phase. Large lesions

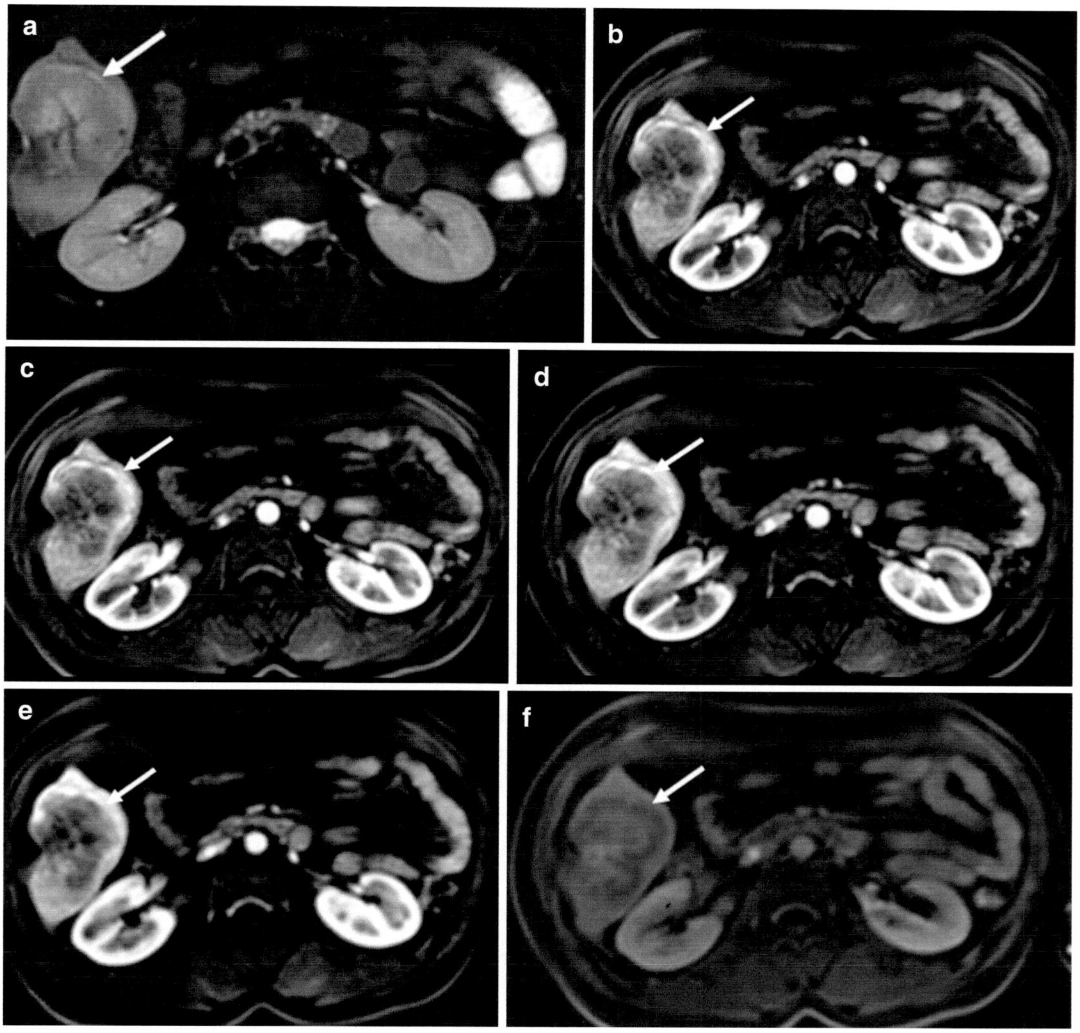

Fig. 5.16 A 35-year-old male with intrahepatic cholangiocarcinoma. (**a**, **b**) Axial T2-weighted MRI (**a**) showed a well-defined, heterogeneous hyperintense mass in the liver (arrow) with diffusion restriction on high b-value (b-800) DWI (**b**). Overlying capsular retraction is seen. (**c**–**f**) Axial late arterial T1-weighted MRI (**c**) showed peripheral enhancement of the lesion with progressive centripetal enhancement in subsequent venous (**d**) and delayed phases (**e**) and with targetoid appearance in the hepatobiliary phase (**f**)

frequently show portal vein invasion and adjacent satellite nodules. The 'targetoid' appearance on T2, DWI, late arterial phase and hepatobiliary phase when present is an important sign of distinguishing mass-forming ICC from HCC, especially in small (≤3 cm) hepatic lesions.

Periductal infiltrating lesions appear as ill-defined, T2 hyperintensity along the biliary radicles with associated ductal irregularity and narrowing. This soft tissue shows hyperenhancement compared to the adjacent hepatic parenchyma on the arterial and venous phases. Intraductal ICC appear as T2 hypointense papillary lesions within the dilated hyperintense biliary radicals, showing faint contrast enhancement.

ICC may exhibit atypical appearances, especially in cirrhotic livers where they frequently show homogeneous hyperenhancement in the arterial phase, particularly lesions <3 cm in size. The absence of venous phase washout in these cases is important as it helps distinguish them from HCCs. Moreover, small scirrhous HCCs may also show stromal fibrosis and a resultant targetoid appearance on DWI, similar to ICC [18].

Most observations that are categorised as LR-M under LI-RADS are ICC. As a result, the 'targetoid' appearance of an observation on dynamic contrast-enhanced scans, DWI or hepatobiliary phase is one of the criteria for its categorisation as LR-M.

Complete surgical resection is the only available curative treatment. The presence of extensive local involvement, vascular invasion, non-satellite hepatic metastasis, nodal disease beyond the porta, celiac axis or peripancreatic location and distant organ metastasis preclude resectability. Poor patient performance status and inadequate residual liver volume (<30% future liver remnant in patients with normal liver parenchyma) are also contraindications to surgical resection. In such cases, most patients present at a later stage with unresectable disease, only suitable for palliative therapy with a dismal prognosis.

Key Point: 'Targetoid' appearance on T2W, DWI or the arterial phase of dynamic contrast is highly suggestive of ICC.

5.11.1 Combined Hepatocellular-Cholangiocarcinoma (cHCC-CCA)

Combined hepatocellular-cholangiocarcinoma is a rare primary hepatic tumour with a 'biphenotypic' appearance on histology and features of hepatocytic and cholangiocytic differentiation. The incidence ranges from 0.4% to 14.2% with chronic viral hepatitis and cirrhosis being the major risk factors [19, 20]. The developmental pathophysiology of cHCC-CCA has evolved, and the conventionally accepted theory of them being collision tumours is outdated. Hepatic progenitor cells (HPCs) have been identified which reside in the canals of Herring, which may by the process of 'transdifferentiation' lead to the development of cHCC-CCA.

cHCC-CCAs frequently show mixed imaging features of both HCC and ICC. Dynamic contrast characteristics of any one component may be predominant with the ICC pattern being more prevalent. Lesions may show arterial phase enhancement and venous washout (HCC mimicker) or rim arterial enhancement with delayed progressive enhancement (ICC mimickers) (Fig. 5.17) [21]. A concordant high level of both AFP and CA-19-9 can improve diagnostic confidence. A diagnosis of cHCC-CCAs may also be sought if AFP or CA-19-9 levels are discordant with imaging findings. The majority of cHCC-CCAs are expected to fall into the LR-M category of LI-RADS with a 'targetoid' appearance having the maximum sensitivity for detection of these lesions since most of them are 'ICC mimickers'.

Surgery is the preferred option in patients with resectable disease. The risk of recurrence is higher in these patients compared to other liver tumours like HCC leading to poor prognosis. Unresectable cases may be treated with locoregional therapy like TACE or chemotherapy, the efficacy of both being debatable due to the dual nature of cancer cells [22].

5.11.2 Primary Hepatic Lymphoma (PHL)

Hepatic lymphoma is considered primary when the lymphoproliferative tissue is confined to the hepatic parenchyma without the involvement of other lymphoid tissue (distant nodes, spleen and bone marrow) for at least 6 months. PHL is rare and comprises only 0.4% of all extranodal non-Hodgkin's lymphoma, the majority being diffuse large B-cell lymphoma [23]. It affects middle-aged adults with a male-to-female ratio of 1.7:1. The incidence of PHL appears to be increased in patients with hepatitis C, hepatitis B, Epstein-Barr virus (EBV) and human immunodeficiency virus (HIV) [24].

PHL frequently presents as a solitary intrahepatic lesion without any mass effect on the adjacent biliary and portal radicles, described as an 'insinuating' appearance. Multiple nodules

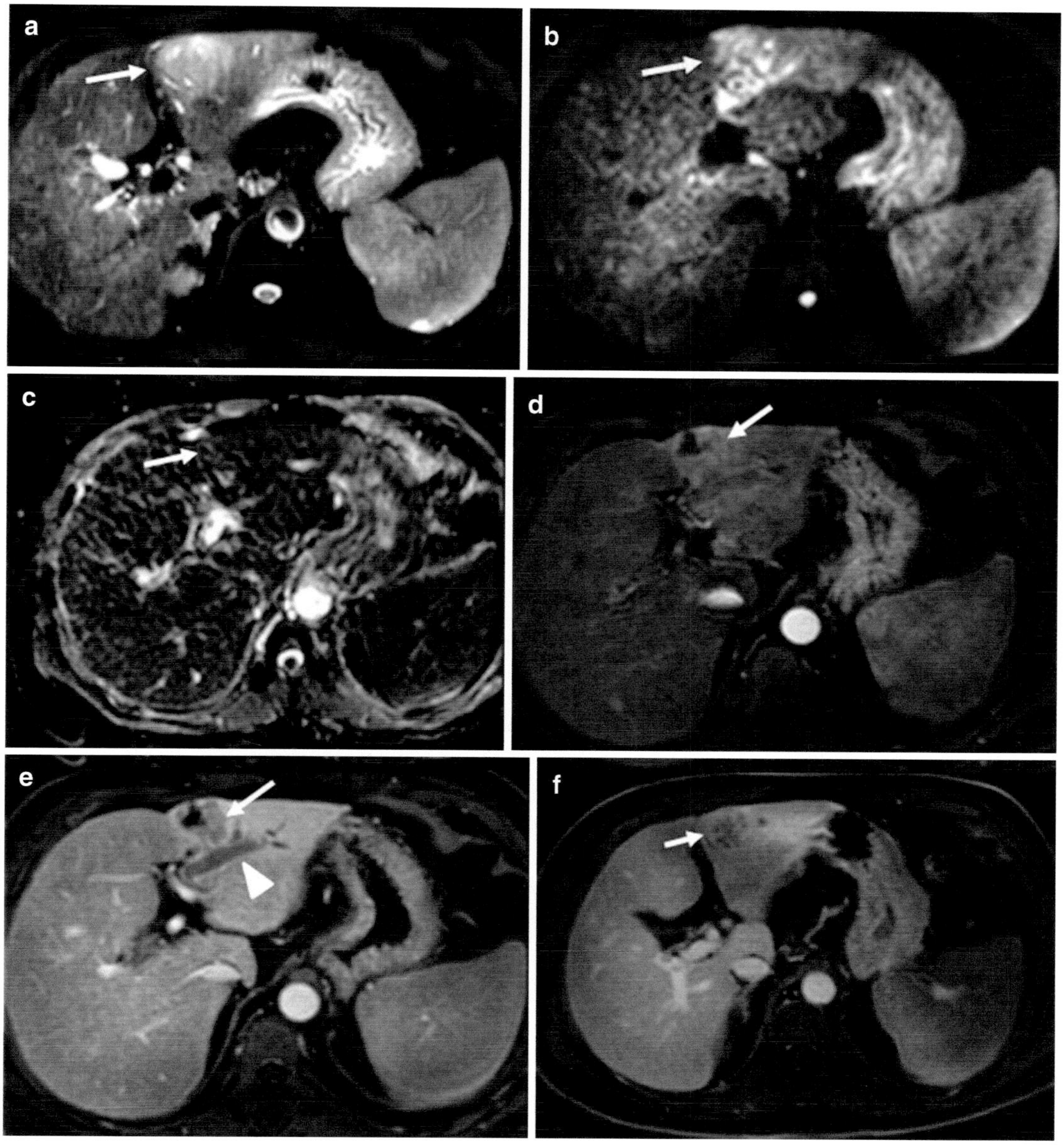

Fig. 5.17 A 62-year-old male with hepatocholangiocarcinoma. (**a**) Axial T2-weighted MRI showed a well-defined, heterogeneous mass in the liver (arrow). (**b**, **c**) Axial high b-value (b-800) DWI (**b**) showed a hyperintense signal in the lesion with corresponding hypointensity on the ADC image (**c**). (**d**) Axial late arterial phase T1-weighted MRI showed heterogeneous enhancement of the lesion (arrow). (**e**) Axial venous phase T1-weighted MRI showed washout in the hepatocellular component of the tumour (arrow). Note the associated malignant thrombosis of the left portal vein branch (arrowhead). (**f**) Axial delayed phase T1-weighted MRI showed filling in of contrast in the cholangiocarcinoma component (arrow)

(Fig. 5.18) and a diffuse infiltrative growth pattern may also be seen, but these appearances are more common in secondary hepatic lymphoma. US may show a large, hypoechoic mass without significant mass effect on the adjacent intrahepatic structures. Infrequently, multiple hypoechoic variable-sized lesions may be seen. Plain CT demonstrates a dominant, hypoattenuating lesion, which shows hypoenhancement compared to adjacent parenchyma after contrast

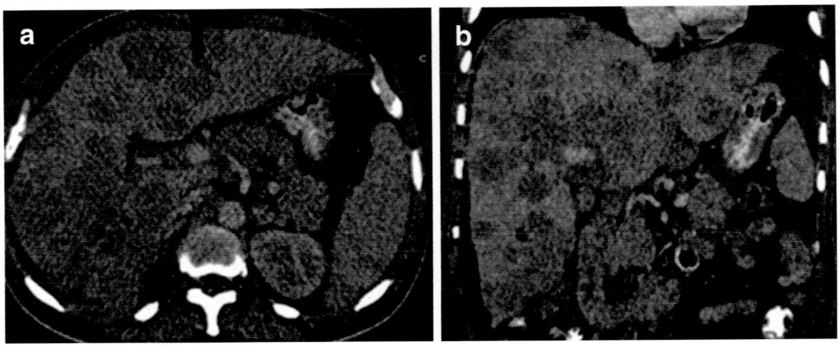

Fig. 5.18 A 43-year-old male with primary hepatic lymphoma. (**a**, **b**) Axial (**a**) and coronal (**b**) contrast-enhanced CT images in the venous phase showed multiple hypoenhancing solid lesions in both lobes of the liver. On biopsy, these lesions were confirmed as non-Hodgkin's lymphoma

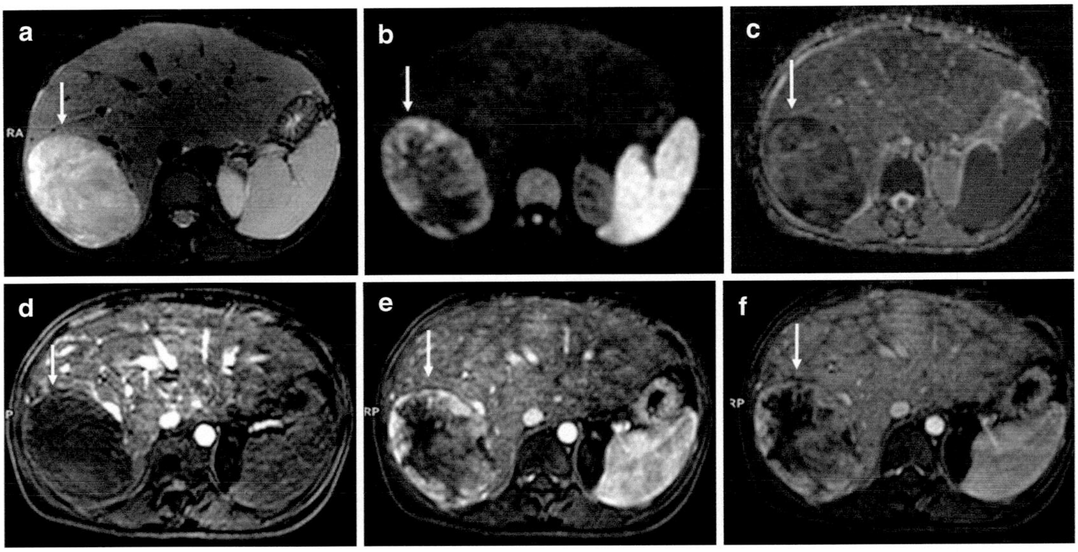

Fig. 5.19 A 32-year-old female with primary hepatic lymphoma. (**a**) Axial T2-weighted MRI showed a well-defined hyperintense mass in the liver (arrow). (**b**, **c**) Axial high b-value (b-800) diffusion-weighted image (**b**) showed hyperintense signal of the mass, predominantly along the periphery with corresponding hypointensity on the ADC image (**c**) suggestive of true diffusion restriction. (**d**–**f**) Axial T1-weighted contrast-enhanced dynamic MRI showed no arterial phase enhancement (**d**) with progressive heterogeneous enhancement in the venous (**e**) and delayed (**f**) phases

administration. Lymphoma usually appears homogeneously hypointense on T1-weighted MRI and hyperintense on T2-weighted MRI. Central areas of heterogeneity may be present due to necrosis. On dynamic contrast-enhanced images, lesions generally appear hypoenhancing to the hepatic parenchyma in all phases. A 'targetoid' rim peripheral enhancement has also been described in some cases (Fig. 5.19) [25, 26]. Diffusion restriction plays an important role in establishing the diagnosis as the lesions show low apparent diffusion coefficient (ADC) values compared to other benign and malignant hepatic lesions likely due to the hypercellular nature of the tumour [27]. Biopsy is however necessary for confirmation.

The absence of mass effect and arterial enhancement along with low serum AFP levels can help differentiate these lesions from HCC on imaging. Targetoid appearance may be similar to ICC; however, there is no associated capsular retraction or biliary radical dilatation. Secondary hepatic lymphomas are generally multifocal with homogeneous appearing lesions showing no areas of necrosis before chemotherapy along with associated enlarged nodes, splenomegaly or bowel involvement. PHL is chemosensitive, and chemotherapy is the treatment of choice.

Key Point: An 'insinuating' appearance with absence of mass effect on adjacent hepatic vasculature is characteristically seen in primary hepatic lymphoma.

5.11.3 Mucinous Cystic Neoplasms of the Liver (MCN-L)

Mucinous cystic neoplasms of the liver, previously known as biliary cystadenoma and cystadenocarcinoma, are a rare group of cystic hepatic neoplasms. The fifth edition of the WHO classification describes MCN-L as a cystic epithelial neoplasm lined with mucin-producing epithelium over a subepithelial layer of ovarian-like stroma and no associated biliary communication [28]. Most lesions are benign (90%) with invasive carcinoma seen in only 3–6% of cases. They are almost always seen in middle-aged females. Patients are generally symptomatic with a non-specific presentation of abdominal pain and fullness.

On US, MCN-L appears as a solitary, multiloculated cystic lesion, often in the left lobe of the liver. They may contain low-level echoes due to proteinaceous content, multiple septations and foci of calcification along them. Invasive forms may show mural nodules with wall thickening and nodularity. On CT, the lesion is multiloculated with hypodense fluid attenuation, well-defined margins and enhancing septations with or without calcification and mural nodules.

MCN-L may show variable signal intensity on T1-weighted MRI depending on proteinaceous content and debris. Lesions are hyperintense on T2-weighted MRI with hypointense septa with or without solid components. Post-contrast images show enhancement of septa and mural nodules, if any (Fig. 5.20) [29].

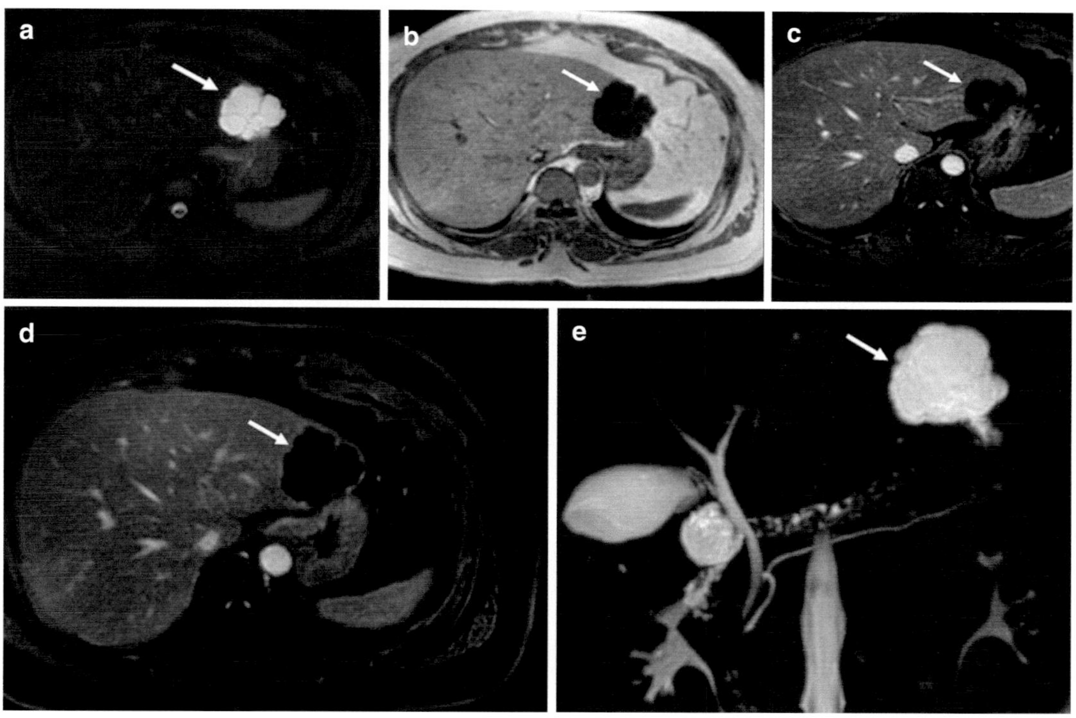

Fig. 5.20 A 50-year-old female with hepatic mucinous cystic neoplasm (biliary cystadenoma). (**a**, **b**) Axial T2-weighted MRI (**a**) showed a well-defined lobulated hyperintense lesion in the liver (arrow), appearing hypointense on T1-weighted MRI (**b**), with multiple hypointense septations. (**c**, **d**) Axial T1-weighted contrast-enhanced images showed peripheral and septal enhancement. (**e**) Thick slab coronal MRCP did not show any communication of the lesion with the biliary system

Cystic intraductal papillary neoplasm of the bile duct (IPNB) is an important differential. The presence of an intraductal mass, biliary communication and biliary dilatation are important features distinguishing a cystic IPMB from an MCN-L. Other cystic hepatic lesions like simple hepatic cysts, cystic metastasis, amoebic or pyogenic liver abscess and hydatid cysts may also mimic this lesion [30].

The presence of enhancing mural nodules or solid components >1 cm, wall enhancement and calcification points towards an invasive subtype of MCN. However, it remains difficult to confidently distinguish benign from malignant subtypes. Invasive components of the lesion may be missed in cases of percutaneous biopsy. Hence, complete surgical excision is the treatment of choice which is associated with a very low risk of recurrence [31].

5.12 Epithelioid Hemangioendothelioma

Epithelioid hemangioendothelioma (EHE) is a rare, low-intermediate grade, locally aggressive malignant vascular neoplasm. The liver is the most frequent site of involvement of EHE. Imaging appearance parallels the disease progression, with early disease consisting of multiple discrete nodules in the peripheral hepatic parenchyma, which later coalesce to form larger masses that may invade hepatic vasculature. EHE consists of a central fibrotic stroma surrounded by a zone of cellular proliferation and a peripheral thin avascular zone due to the occlusion of tiny vessels by the tumour [32].

On US, EHE often appears as multifocal, discrete, hypoechoic nodules in the periphery of the liver. Subcapsular lesions may be associated with focal capsular retraction. In cases of diffuse disease, focal lesions may not be identified on US, and only altered hepatic echotexture may be seen in areas of involvement. On unenhanced CT, they appear iso-hypodense, with or without associated calcification. On contrast CT, they appear as multiple hypoenhancing nodules or large confluent hypoenhancing areas in peripheral distribution. The nodules show peripheral enhancement (halo or target pattern) frequently in the arterial and venous phases with centripetal enhancement in the delayed phase.

On MRI, EHE appears hypointense on T1-weighted images and heterogeneously hyperintense on T2-weighted images. The multilayered histopathological appearance is visualised in the form of a concentric 'target sign' on T2-weighted (central hyperintensity surrounded by a thin rim hypointensity, with a bright halo around it) or post-contrast images (hypointense centre surrounded with an enhancing rim and thin zone of hypoenhancement) (Fig. 5.21). The 'lollipop' sign is the presence of a well-defined mass (candy) with an adjacent occluded vessel (stick) terminating just at the edge of the lesion [33].

Extrahepatic tumour extension beyond portal nodes, presence of metastasis, older age and male gender are poor prognostic markers. Surgery is the mainstay of treatment (resection vs transplant based on tumour burden).

Key Point: Epithelioid hemangioendotheliomas frequently appear as multiple peripheral lesions with associated capsular retraction and show '*target*' sign on T2-weighted and post-contrast MRI and '*lollipop*' sign on post-contrast images.

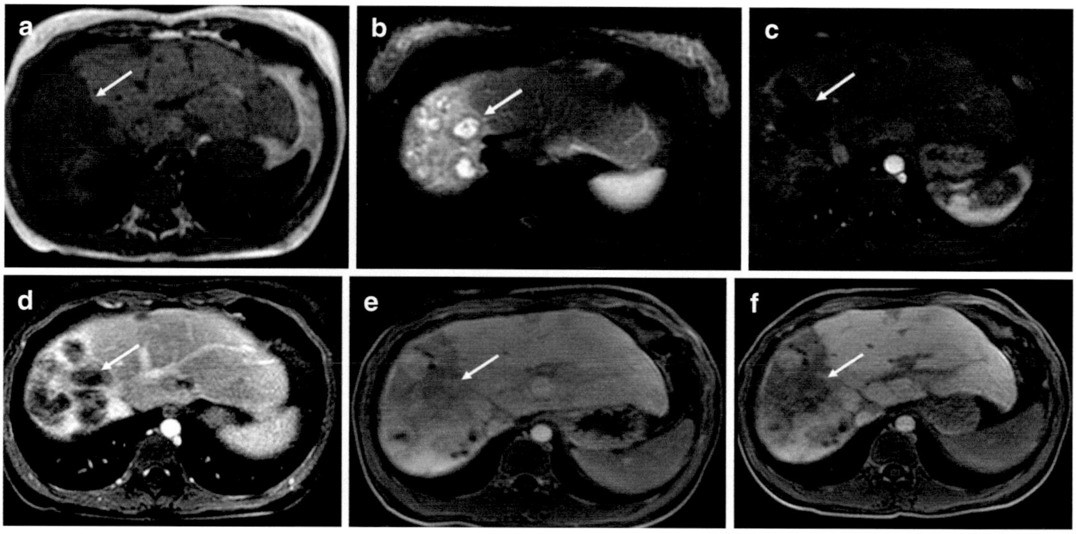

Fig. 5.21 A 26-year-old female with hepatic epithelioid hemangioendothelioma. (**a**) Axial T1-weighted MRI showed a geographic area of hypointensity in the right lobe of the liver (arrow). (**b**) Axial T2-weighted MRI showed multiple hyperintense lesions with a hypointense rim in the periphery of the right lobe of the liver (arrow). (**c**–**e**) Axial dynamic contrast-enhanced T1-weighted MRI showed peripheral enhancement in the late arterial phase (**c**) with progressive enhancement in the venous (**d**) and delayed (**e**) phases, giving a target appearance. (**f**) Axial T1-weighted hepatobiliary phase MRI shows no contrast uptake in the lesions. Note a smaller subcapsular lesion in segment 4A

5.13 Hepatic Angiosarcoma

Primary hepatic angiosarcoma is the most common malignant mesenchymal tumour involving the liver, but it only accounts for 2% of all hepatic malignancies. The lesions occur in the sixth–seventh decade with a distinct male predominance. Exposure to environmental toxins like thorotrast, vinyl chloride and anabolic steroids is an established risk factor for their development. However, a majority occur sporadically in the absence of any known risk factor [34].

Four morphological patterns have been recognised on imaging: multinodular, dominant mass, a combination of dominant mass with multiple nodules and diffuse infiltrative. Lesions appear predominantly hypodense on unenhanced CT with scattered areas of hyperdensity due to haemorrhage. Dynamic contrast enhancement shows the arterial phase ring enhancement with progressive centripetal fill-in.

On MRI, angiosarcoma appears predominantly hypointense on T1-weighted images with scattered areas of hyperintensity due to haemorrhage. On T2-weighted images, they appear heterogeneous and may be associated with blood fluid levels. Similar to CT, dynamic contrast MRI shows heterogeneous enhancement in the arterial and venous phases with progressive fill-in during the delayed phase (Fig. 5.22) [35, 36].

Common differentials include hypervascular hepatic masses like haemangioma, HCC and hypervascular metastasis. Unlike haemangiomas, these lesions are generally multifocal, do not follow the blood pool or show discontinuous nodular arterial enhancement. The lack of washout in the portal venous and delayed phases may help differentiate them from HCC and metastasis.

Tumour usually metastasizes to the spleen, lung or bones. The final diagnosis is confirmed on histopathology. Haemorrhage and rupture are common complications associated with image-guided biopsy in these cases. Surgical resection may be possible in cases with limited disease, but the prognosis is poor as a large percentage of patients have metastatic disease at the time of presentation.

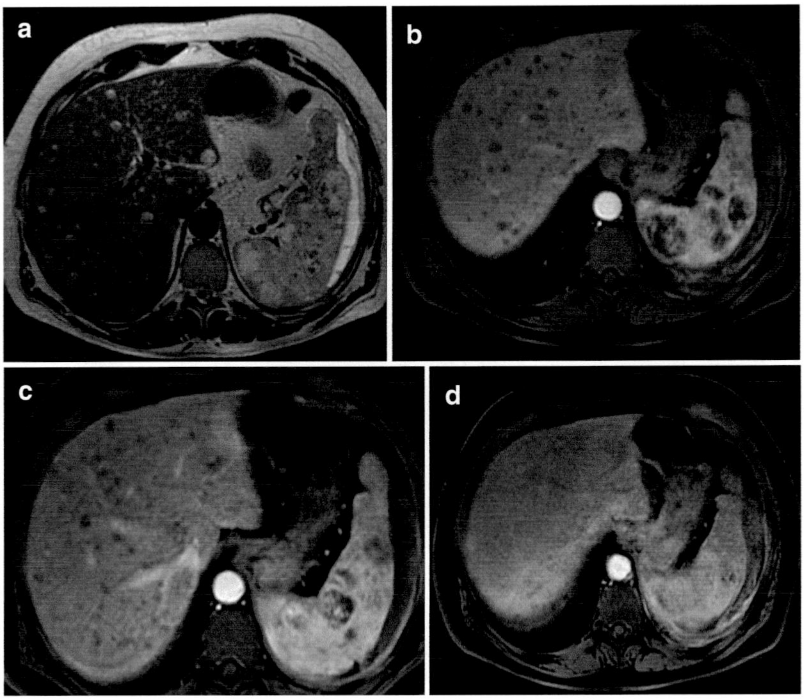

Fig. 5.22 A 51-year-old male with hepatic angiosarcoma. (**a**) Axial T2-weighted MRI showed multiple well-defined hyperintense lesions in the liver and spleen. (**b**) Axial late arterial phase T1-weighted MRI showed rim enhancement of the hepatic and splenic lesions. (**c**, **d**) Progressive enhancement of the lesions is seen on the axial T1-weighted venous (**c**) and delayed (**d**) phases

5.14 Malignant Mesenchymal Tumours

These are rare primary hepatic tumours which frequently present as a diagnostic dilemma. The list includes malignant fibrous histiocytoma, rhabdomyosarcoma, leiomyosarcoma, localised malignant mesothelioma and Kaposi sarcoma. Imaging appearances are variable, ranging from a non-specific appearance to typical findings which may predict pathological diagnosis. However, histopathology is crucial to establishing a final diagnosis in most of the cases.

5.15 Metastasis

Metastatic lesions are the most common malignant neoplasms involving the liver, occurring at a much greater incidence than primary hepatic tumours. The liver is also the most common site of metastasis, with most primaries being adenocarcinomas arising from the colorectum, pancreas and breast. The hepatic parenchyma is a dominant site of metastasis due to its rich blood supply from both the hepatic artery and the portal vein. Additionally, the fenestra of the sinusoidal epithelium provides a pathway for the extension of metastatic cells into the parenchyma. Primary tumours may also secrete certain liver trophic exosomes which help develop a ‘premetastatic niche’ leading to organ-specific metastasis.

The detection and characterisation of hepatic metastasis are essential for establishing a definitive treatment plan. Differentiation of these lesions from primary hepatic malignancies like HCC, identification of an unknown primary and detection of small metastatic foci and incidental lesions with a known primary are the current challenges that are faced in imaging.

Conventional US has low sensitivity (approximately ~69%) for the identification of hepatic metastasis due to poor spatial resolution and poor visualisation of small lesions, lesions in difficult locations and lesions in obese patients [37]. On grayscale US, metastatic lesions may show hypoechoic (most common), isoechoic or hyperechoic (mucinous adenocarcinoma, hypervascular) appearance. Frequently, lesions are multiple with well-defined margins and hypoechoic appearance. Isoechoic metastasis may be difficult to identify especially in the absence of mass effect. A 'target' or 'bull's eye' appearance comprising an echogenic centre surrounded by a hypoechoic halo is also a common imaging appearance in adenocarcinoma of the colon and lung.

CEUS improves the sensitivity (80–90%) of detection of metastasis, with rates comparable to those of CECT [38]. Majority of hepatic metastases are hypovascular (adenocarcinomas from colon, stomach, breast, lung; squamous cell carcinomas). They appear hypoechoic with a thin rim of enhancement in the arterial phase and appear hypoechoic in the venous/delayed phase. Hypervascular hepatic metastasis (neuroendocrine tumours, melanomas, sarcomas and renal, breast and thyroid neoplasms) show enhancement in the arterial phase with rapid washout (c.f. more delayed washout in HCC, typically >60 s) (Fig. 5.23) [39].

CECT shows a sensitivity of ~82% for the detection of hepatic metastasis. Acquisition of only the portal venous phase is generally considered sufficient for the evaluation of metastatic disease. The arterial phase may be acquired in cases with hypervascular primary tumours (Fig. 5.24). The majority of hypovascular metastases appear as well-circumscribed hypodense lesions with peritumoural enhancement in the arterial and portal venous phases (Fig. 5.25). Lesions generally become iso-dense in the delayed phase, providing no diagnostic information. The unenhanced phase may be useful in cases in which primary lesions contain calcifications. Virtual non-contrast images may be recreated from the dataset acquired on dual-energy CT.

MRI is currently considered the most sensitive modality (~93.1%) for the detection of hepatic metastasis, especially for lesions <10 mm. Lesions typically appear hypointense on T1-weighted images and hyperintense on

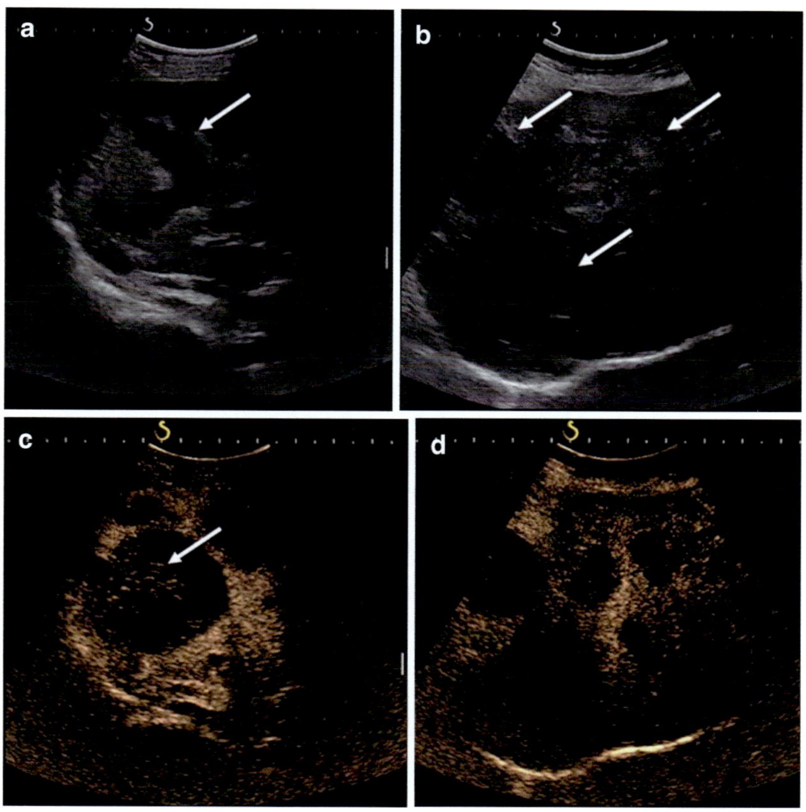

Fig. 5.23 A 54-year-old male with cystic hepatic metastasis from a pancreatic neuroendocrine tumour. (**a**, **b**) Grayscale ultrasound images showed multiple solid and cystic lesions (arrows) in both lobes of the liver. (**c**, **d**) Contrast-enhanced ultrasonography showed hypoenhancement of the lesions, with enhancement of the solid component in one of the lesions (arrow in **c**)

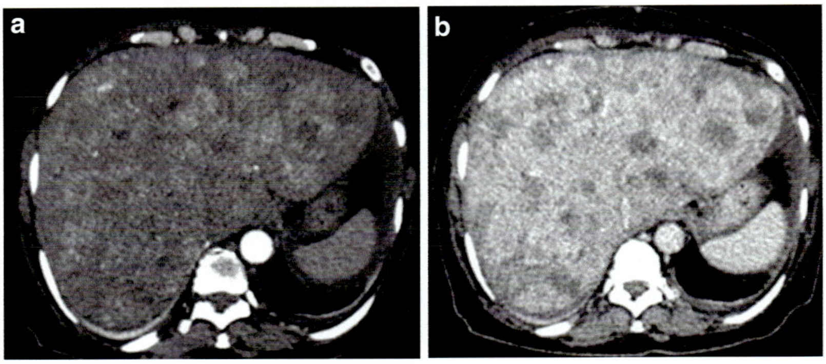

Fig. 5.24 A 62-year-old female with metastatic neuroendocrine tumour of the pancreas. (**a**, **b**) Axial late arterial phase CT image (**a**) showed a non-cirrhotic liver with multiple enhancing lesions, which showed washout in the venous phase (**b**), consistent with hypervascular metastases

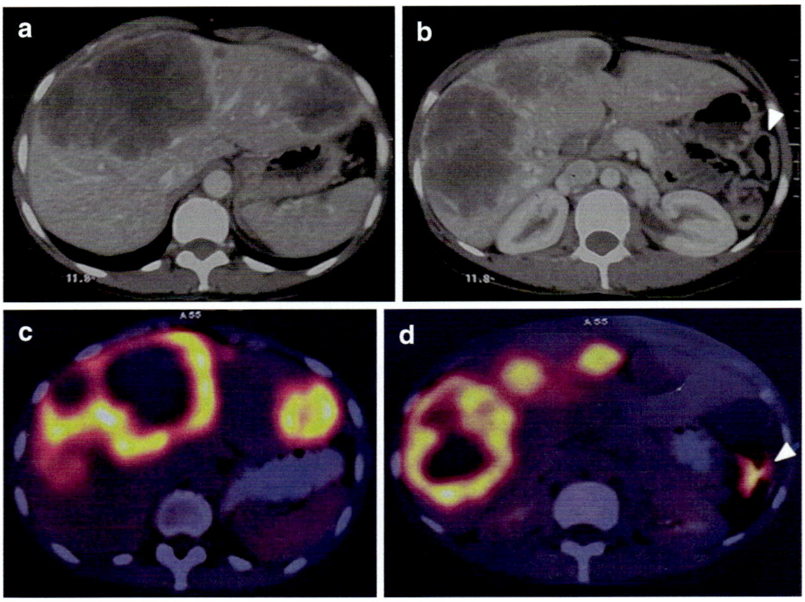

Fig. 5.25 A 55-year-old female with hypovascular metastasis from colon cancer. (**a**, **b**) Axial contrast-enhanced CT images (venous phase) showed multiple, irregular peripherally enhancing lesions in the liver. (**c**, **d**) Axial ^{18}FDG PET-CT images show avid uptake in the liver lesions. The primary malignancy is seen in the splenic flexure as circumferential wall thickening (arrowhead in **b**) with avid FDG uptake (arrowhead in **d**)

T2-weighted images. Hypovascular metastasis may also show peripheral T2 hypointensity with central hyperintensity ('target' appearance). The addition of DWI and the use of hepatobiliary phase (HBP) contrast agents have improved the sensitivity for the detection of hepatic metastasis (82.2% for only DWI, 91.2% for HBP imaging and 95% for combined DWI with HBP imaging) [40]. Metastatic lesions show restricted diffusion with low ADC values due to their hypercellular nature. Since there is the absence of hepatocytes in these metastatic tumours, they appear as hypointense areas in the hepatobiliary phase.

The imaging appearance of metastatic lesions often follows that of the primary malignancy. Hypervascular metastasis from hypervascular primaries shows arterial phase enhancement with washout in the delayed phase. The absence of underlying cirrhosis along with the presence of a primary tumour may help differentiate them from HCC. Cystic appearance of metastasis may be due to necrosis within lesions (neuroendocrine tumour, gastrointestinal stromal tumour, sarcoma, squamous cell carcinoma), primary tumour with cystic component (intraductal papillary mucinous carcinoma of pancreas, ovarian serous/mucinous carcinoma) and histological nature of primary (mucinous adenocarcinoma colon, ovary, endometrial carcinoma). These lesions show a fluid signal on T2-weighted images with irregular and nodular contrast enhancement of their wall. T1 hyperintensity may be due to the presence of melanin (e.g. malignant melanoma), haemorrhage or protein content. Metastasis from pancreatic adenocarcinoma may appear as isolated arterioportal shunts, signifying metastasis even in the absence of an obvious nodular lesion [41].

The sensitivity of PET-CT for hepatic metastasis is lower than that of DWI/CEMRI, especially for small lesions. However, PET-CT shows improved sensitivity for the detection of extrahepatic metastatic burden compared to conventional imaging which may upstage tumours.

Table 5.4 concisely demonstrates the salient imaging features of common primary hepatic malignancies and of hepatic metastasis discussed above.

Table 5.4 Salient imaging features of common primary hepatic malignancies on CECT/CE-MRI

Malignant tumours	T2WI	Diffusion restriction	Dynamic enhancement			HBP	Comments
			Late arterial	Venous	Delayed		
HCC	Hyperintense	Present	Non-rim APHE	Washout	Washout ± capsule	Hypointensity	Nodule within nodule, mosaic attenuation
ICC	Hyperintense, targetoid	'Targetoid' restriction present	Rim APHE	Progressive centripetal enhancement	Progressive centripetal enhancement, no capsule	Targetoid hypointensity	Capsular retraction, biliary radical dilatation
cHCC-ICC	Hyperintense	Present	Areas of rim and non-rim APHE	Washout in areas of non-rim APHE	Progressive enhancement in areas of rim APHE	Hypointensity	A mixture of dynamic enhancement of HCC and ICC
PHL	Hyperintense	Strongly present	Rim APHE ±	Progressive centripetal enhancement	Progressive centripetal enhancement	Hypointensity	Usually solitary, insinuating appearance
MCN-L	Hyperintense with hypointense septations	Absent	Rim enhancement, septal enhancement Nodules and solid areas in the malignant type			Hypointense	No communication with the biliary system
EHE	Multifocal, peripheral hyperintense lesions	'Targetoid' restriction present	Heterogeneous or rim enhancement	Progressive centripetal fill in		Targetoid appearance	Target sign, lollipop sign, capsular retraction ±
Angiosarcoma	Heterogeneously hyperintense, fluid-fluid levels	Present	Rim enhancement	Progressive centripetal fill in		Isointense	Often associated with splenic lesions
Metastasis (hypovascular)	Hyperintense	Present	Peritumoural enhancement	Hypoenhancing	Iso-enhancing	Hypointense	Variable dynamic enhancement depending on primary tumour appearance

5.16 Conclusion

The liver is a frequently involved site in both primary and secondary malignancies. As advances continue in all aspects of the management of these malignancies, from diagnostic to therapeutic, most cases require multidisciplinary teamwork for comprehensive treatment. The radiologist stands at the forefront, leading the way for early identification and characterisation of lesions and guiding the treating physician/surgeon regarding treatment options, especially as evidence for endovascular and percutaneous interventional procedures increases.

References

1. Sung H, Ferlay J, Siegel RL, et al. Global cancer statistics 2020: GLOBOCAN estimates of incidence and mortality worldwide for 36 cancers in 185 countries. CA Cancer J Clin. 2021;71(3):209–49.
2. Galle PR, Forner A, Llovet JM, et al. EASL clinical practice guidelines: management of hepatocellular carcinoma. J Hepatol. 2018;69(1):182–236.
3. Llovet JM, Kelley RK, Villanueva A, et al. Hepatocellular carcinoma. Nat Rev Dis Primer. 2021;7(1):6.
4. Fujita N, Nishie A, Asayama Y, et al. Hyperintense liver masses at hepatobiliary phase gadoxetic acid–enhanced MRI: imaging appearances and clinical importance. RadioGraphics. 2020;40(1):72–94.
5. Choi JY, Lee JM, Sirlin CB. CT and MR imaging diagnosis and staging of hepatocellular carcinoma: part I. Development, growth, and spread: key pathologic and imaging aspects. Radiology. 2014;272(3):635–54.
6. Mitchell DG, Rubin R, Siegelman ES, Burk DL, Rifkin MD. Hepatocellular carcinoma within siderotic regenerative nodules: appearance as a nodule within a nodule on MR images. Radiology. 1991;178(1):101–3.
7. Zhang ZM, Lai ECH, Zhang C, et al. The strategies for treating primary hepatocellular carcinoma with portal vein tumor thrombus. Int J Surg. 2015;20:8–16.
8. Hepatobiliary Disease Study Group, Chinese Society of Gastroenterology, Chinese Medical Association. Consensus for management of portal vein thrombosis in liver cirrhosis (2020, Shanghai). J Dig Dis. 2021;22(4):176–86.
9. Xia Y, Zhang J, Ni X. Diagnosis, treatment and prognosis of hepatocellular carcinoma with inferior vena cava/right atrium tumor thrombus (Review). Oncol Lett. 2020;20(4):101.
10. Wu JY, Huang LM, Bai YN, et al. Imaging features of hepatocellular carcinoma with bile duct tumor thrombus: a multicenter study. Front Oncol. 2021;11:723455.
11. Yan J, Li T, Deng M, Fan H. Ruptured hepatocellular carcinoma: what do interventional radiologists need to know? Front Oncol. 2022;12:927123.
12. Loy LM, Low HM, Choi JY, Rhee H, Wong CF, Tan CH. Variant hepatocellular carcinoma subtypes according to the 2019 WHO Classification: an imaging-focused review. Am J Roentgenol. 2022;219(2):212–23.
13. Reig M, Forner A, Rimola J, et al. BCLC strategy for prognosis prediction and treatment recommendation: the 2022 update. J Hepatol. 2022;76(3):681–93.
14. Mendiratta-Lala M, Masch WR, Shampain K, et al. MRI assessment of hepatocellular carcinoma after local-regional therapy: a comprehensive review. Radiol Imaging Cancer. 2020;2(1):e190024.
15. Seo N, Kim DY, Choi JY. Cross-sectional imaging of intrahepatic cholangiocarcinoma: development, growth, spread, and prognosis. Am J Roentgenol. 2017;209(2):W64–75.
16. Brindley PJ, Bachini M, Ilyas SI, et al. Cholangiocarcinoma. Nat Rev Dis Primer. 2021;7(1):65.
17. Kovač JD, Janković A, Đikić-Rom A, Grubor N, Antić A, Dugalić V. Imaging spectrum of intrahepatic mass-forming cholangiocarcinoma and its mimickers: how to differentiate them using MRI. Curr Oncol. 2022;29(2):698–723.
18. Kim JH, Joo I, Lee JM. Atypical appearance of hepatocellular carcinoma and its mimickers: how to solve challenging cases using gadoxetic acid-enhanced liver magnetic resonance imaging. Korean J Radiol. 2019;20(7):1019.
19. Taguchi J, Nakashima O, Tanaka M, Hisaka T, Takazawa T, Kojiro M. A Clinicopathological study on combined hepatocellular and cholangiocarcinoma. J Gastroenterol Hepatol. 1996;11(8):758–64.
20. Goodman ZD, Ishak KG, Langloss JM, Sesterhenn IA, Rabin L. Combined hepatocellular-cholangiocarcinoma. A histologic and immunohistochemical study. Cancer. 1985;55(1):124–35.
21. Kim TH, Kim H, Joo I, Lee JM. Combined hepatocellular-cholangiocarcinoma: changes in the 2019 World Health Organization Histological Classification System and potential impact on imaging-based diagnosis. Korean J Radiol. 2020;21(10):1115.
22. Leoni S, Sansone V, De Lorenzo S, et al. Treatment of combined hepatocellular and cholangiocarcinoma. Cancers. 2020;12(4):794.
23. Freeman C, Berg JW, Cutler SJ. Occurrence and prognosis of extranodal lymphomas. Cancer. 1972;29(1):252–60.
24. Dhamija E, Madhusudhan KS, Das P, et al. Primary hepatic diffuse large B-cell lymphoma: unusual presentation and imaging features. Curr Probl Diagn Radiol. 2015;44(3):290–3.

25. Rajesh S, Bansal K, Sureka B, Patidar Y, Bihari C, Arora A. The imaging conundrum of hepatic lymphoma revisited. Insights Imaging. 2015;6(6):679–92.
26. Alves AMA, Torres US, Velloni FG, Ribeiro BJ, Tiferes DA, D'Ippolito G. The many faces of primary and secondary hepatic lymphoma: imaging manifestations and diagnostic approach. Radiol Bras. 2019;52(5):325–30.
27. Colagrande S, Calistri L, Grazzini G, et al. MRI features of primary hepatic lymphoma. Abdom Radiol. 2018;43(9):2277–87.
28. Nakanuma Y, Klimstra DS, Zen Y, Komuta M. Mucinous cystic neoplasm of the liver and biliary system. In: WHO classification of tumours. 5th ed. Lyon: IARC; 2020.
29. Lee MH, Katabathina VS, Lubner MG, et al. Mucin-producing cystic hepatobiliary neoplasms: updated nomenclature and clinical, pathologic, and imaging features. RadioGraphics. 2021;41(6):1592–610.
30. Chenin M, Paisant A, Lebigot J, et al. Cystic liver lesions: a pictorial review. Insights Imaging. 2022;13(1):116.
31. Hutchens JA, Lopez KJ, Ceppa EP. Mucinous cystic neoplasms of the liver: epidemiology, diagnosis, and management. Hepatic Med Evid Res. 2023;15:33–41.
32. Jang JK, Thomas R, Braschi-Amirfarzan M, Jagannathan JP. A review of the spectrum of imaging manifestations of epithelioid hemangioendothelioma. Am J Roentgenol. 2020;215(5):1290–8.
33. Liu X, Yu H, Zhang Z, et al. MRI appearances of hepatic epithelioid hemangioendothelioma: a retrospective study of 57 patients. Insights Imaging. 2022;13(1):65.
34. Singh G, Mills C, Asadi K, Testro A. Hepatic angiosarcoma as a cause of acute liver failure. BMJ Case Rep. 2018;2018:bcr2018225896.
35. Thapar S, Rastogi A, Ahuja A, Sarin S. Angiosarcoma of the liver: imaging of a rare salient entity. J Radiol Case Rep. 2014;8(8):24–32.
36. Koyama T, Fletcher JG, Johnson CD, Kuo MS, Notohara K, Burgart LJ. Primary hepatic angiosarcoma: findings at CT and MR imaging. Radiology. 2002;222(3):667–73.
37. Lincke T, Zech CJ. Liver metastases: detection and staging. Eur J Radiol. 2017;97:76–82.
38. Cantisani V. Liver metastases: Contrast-enhanced ultrasound compared with computed tomography and magnetic resonance. World J Gastroenterol. 2014;20(29):9998.
39. D'Onofrio M, Crosara S, De Robertis R, Canestrini S, Mucelli RP. Contrast-enhanced ultrasound of focal liver lesions. Am J Roentgenol. 2015;205(1):W56–66.
40. Canellas R, Patel MJ, Agarwal S, Sahani DV. Lesion detection performance of an abbreviated gadoxetic acid–enhanced MRI protocol for colorectal liver metastasis surveillance. Eur Radiol. 2019;29(11):5852–60.
41. Ozaki K, Higuchi S, Kimura H, Gabata T. Liver metastases: correlation between imaging features and pathomolecular environments. RadioGraphics. 2022;42(7):1994–2013.

Diffuse Liver Diseases

6

Mohit Gupta, Dhawal Arora, Vijay Chidambaram, Ashok Katti, and Ankur Arora

6.1 Diffuse Liver Diseases

Diffuse liver disorders can be broadly classified into storage, vascular, inflammatory/infectious or neoplastic disorders. The pathophysiology is frequently a metabolic or a haemodynamic cause affecting liver parenchyma and causing hepatocyte injury, resulting in liver fibrosis which if untreated progresses to cirrhosis and its complications [1–5]. Imaging plays an important role in the assessment of these disorders, with different imaging modalities aiding in providing morphological and functional characteristics of the underlying disorders [1, 2]. Moreover, imaging can help in detecting and quantifying chronic fibrotic changes which are the end result of all the diffuse liver disorders leading to cirrhosis [4]. Although on its own, imaging may not always be diagnostic, nevertheless, in many disorders, the specific radiological features on CT or MR can be sufficient to clinch the diagnosis, thereby avoiding the need for histologic confirmation.

M. Gupta · V. Chidambaram
Department of Radiology, Royal Liverpool University Hospital, Liverpool University Hospitals NHS Foundation Trust, Liverpool, UK
e-mail: Mohit.Gupta@liverpoolft.nhs.uk; Vijay.Chidambaram@liverpoolft.nhs.uk

D. Arora
Department of Radiology, Royal Liverpool University Hospital, Liverpool University Hospitals NHS Foundation Trust, Liverpool, UK

Department of Radiology, Salford Royal Hospital, Manchester, UK
e-mail: Dhawal.Arora@nhs.net

A. Katti
Department of Radiology, Aintree University Hospital, Liverpool University Hospitals NHS Foundation Trust, Liverpool, UK
e-mail: Ashok.Katti@liverpoolft.nhs.uk

A. Arora (✉)
Department of Radiology, Royal Gwent Hospital, Aneurin Bevan University Health Board, Newport, South Wales, UK
e-mail: Ankur.Arora@wales.nhs.uk

6.2 Storage Diseases

6.2.1 Fatty Liver Disease

Fatty liver encompasses a spectrum of disorders that result from triglyceride accumulation within hepatocytes. Population-wide studies in different countries have indicated the prevalence of fatty liver at around 25%; there is no sex predilection [6, 7]. The major risk factors for developing a fatty liver are alcohol use, diabetes mellitus, alcohol intake, obesity and medications. Over the recent past, non-alcoholic fatty liver disease (NAFLD) has emerged as the commonest cause of hepatic steatosis—it is associated with obesity and/or metabolic syndrome [7, 8].

Hepatic steatosis has become one of the common radiological findings seen on cross-sectional imaging in today's world. In most cases, fatty

© The Author(s), under exclusive license to Springer Nature Singapore Pte Ltd. 2025
B. Sureka (ed.), *Hepato-Pancreatico Biliary Imaging*, https://doi.org/10.1007/978-981-95-1699-5_6

liver is asymptomatic and is diagnosed incidentally on radiological examination. In a minority, it may present with non-specific symptoms such as abdominal fullness and right upper quadrant pain.

The heterogeneous nature of fat distribution within the liver makes histology less specific for the diagnosis of fatty liver [8]. Imaging, therefore, helps in the non-invasive diagnosis and management of hepatic steatosis [9].

US, owing to its easy accessibility and cost-effectiveness, is often used as an initial screening tool. The lipid droplets within hepatocytes cause an increased scatter of the US beam. This results in the liver parenchyma appearing more echogenic relative to the renal cortex or spleen (Fig. 6.1) [10]. Increased scatter also reduces the transmission of the US beam, and as a result, the diaphragm and intrahepatic vessels appear poorly delineated. However, unfortunately, increased echogenicity of the liver is non-specific and can be seen in other metabolic or storage disorders. US is also not able to accurately quantify fatty changes and distinguish fibrosis from steatosis.

An unenhanced CT scan is used for the detection of fatty liver. There are usually two accepted criteria to diagnose fatty liver. The first criterion is to ascertain the average attenuation of the liver. The normal liver usually has an average 60–70 HU attenuation value, whereas in the underlying steatotic liver, the attenuation decreases to less than 40 HU. Another criterion is to compare the attenuating properties of the liver and spleen. The attenuation of the liver should be 10HU less than the spleen [10, 11]. Reduction in hepatic attenuation results in the intrahepatic vessels appearing brighter than the background liver (Fig. 6.2).

Contrast-enhanced CT has poor sensitivity in diagnosing fatty liver. The time of acquisition of scan, contrast volume and cardiac perfusion all affect the attenuation of the liver and spleen. Therefore, the comparison between attenuation values of spleen and liver cannot be reliably used for the diagnosis of fatty liver [11, 12]. Few studies have shown that the difference in attenuation values of the liver and spleen of more than 18 to 25 can be considered as a sensitive marker for the underlying fatty liver [12]. Newer techniques such as dual-energy CT (DECT) are also being used for better characterization of fat distribution [13].

MR is the most useful and specific imaging tool to diagnose fatty liver [10, 11, 13]. Different techniques are used to determine underlying steatosis; they include chemical shift imaging, gradient echo with fat suppression, frequency selective imaging and MR spectroscopy. The Dixon chemical shift method exploits the physical properties of water and fat under the magnetic field to assess fatty infiltration. The method uses the precession frequency differences between water and fat molecules in in-and-out-of phases. In the normal liver, there is no difference in images in both phases. However, in a fatty liver, the affected liver shows a signal drop on out-of-phase imaging (Fig. 6.3). This helps in easy qualitative measurement of hepatic fat. The sequence unfortunately is easily affected by the presence of iron and other paramagnetic substances which can limit its diagnostic accuracy.

The most common appearance of fatty liver is diffuse hepatic involvement. Localized, heterogeneous or multifocal fatty lesions can be seen sometimes (Fig. 6.4). They may give a

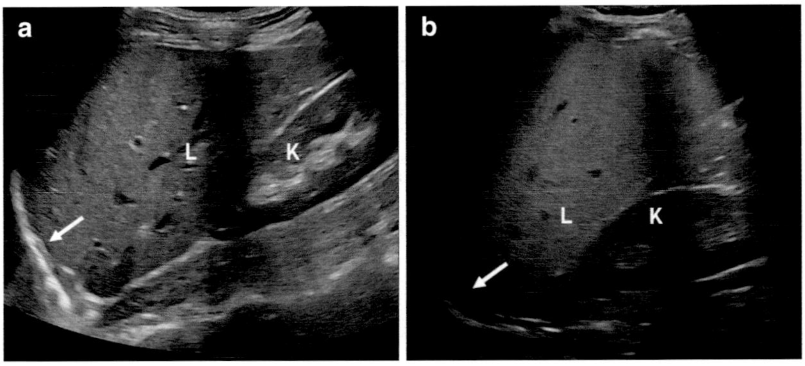

Fig. 6.1 (**a**) Normal liver (L) appears isoechoic to the right kidney cortex (K) with clear visualization of the diaphragm (arrow). (**b**) Liver appearing brighter than the right kidney due to diffuse steatosis, with suboptimal visualization of the diaphragm (arrow)

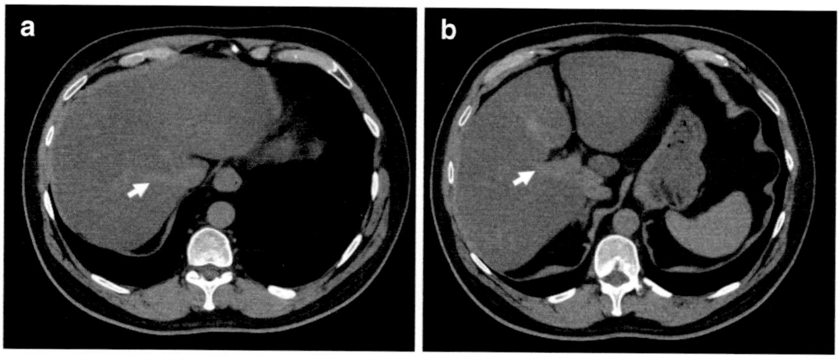

Fig. 6.2 (**a** and **b**) Unenhanced CT demonstrating a hypodense fatty liver. Intrahepatic vessels (arrow) appear brighter than the background liver due to diffuse background steatosis. The liver attenuation (28 HU) was significantly lower than that of the spleen (51 HU)

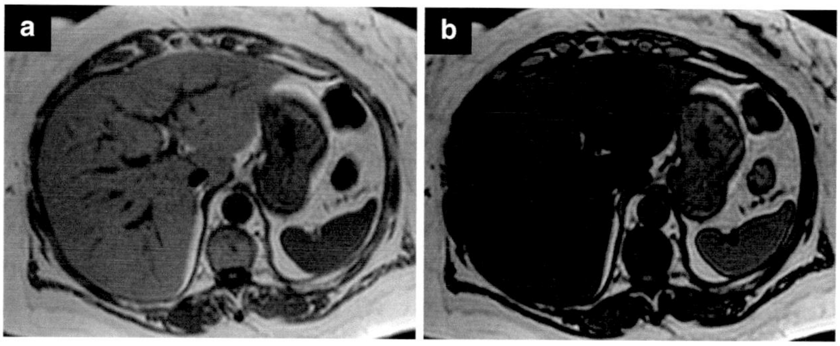

Fig. 6.3 (**a** and **b**) In-phase and opposed-phase images of the liver demonstrating marked signal drop on the latter suggestive of diffuse (homogeneous) hepatic steatosis

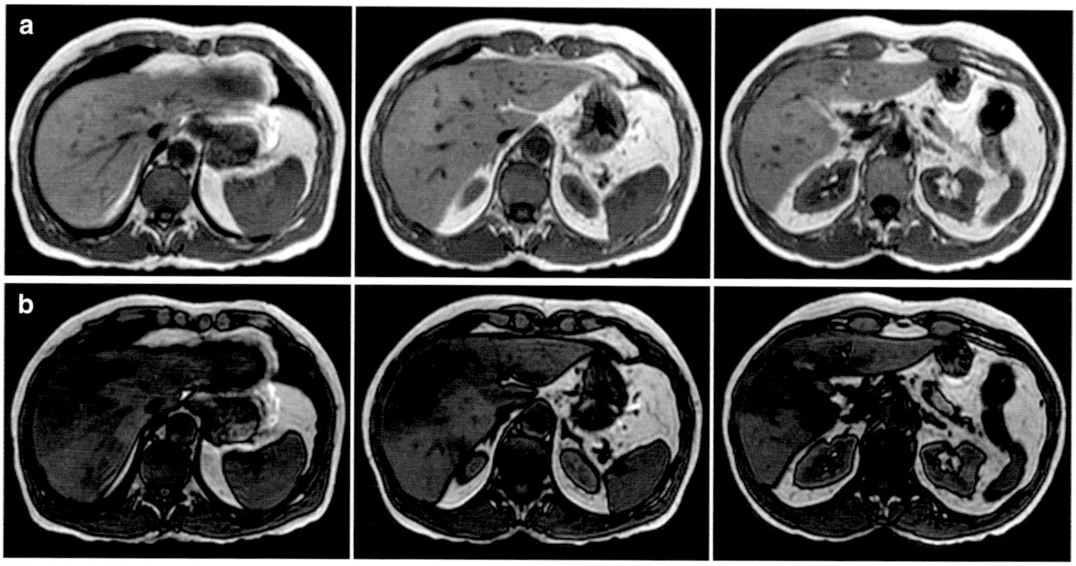

Fig. 6.4 (**a** and **b**) In-phase and opposed-phase images of the liver demonstrating heterogeneous signal drop on the opposed-phase in keeping with heterogeneous steatosis

false impression of mass lesion(s). In these cases, MRI with a gradient echo sequence is extremely helpful for confirming fatty infiltration and excluding masses.

MR spectroscopy gives a more accurate assessment of liver fat [11]. In MR spectroscopy, the strength of proton signals from different tissue types at precession frequency is measured, and the values are reported as peaks. In a normal liver, there is only a single peak of water, but in the case of fatty liver, the hydrogen molecules generate two different peaks. The heights of fat peaks give a quantitative assessment of fat content within the liver. The patient should be fasted at the time of MR spectroscopy to avoid the effect of food in the stomach cavity.

6.2.2 Haemochromatosis

Haemochromatosis is an iron overload disorder causing abnormal absorption of iron from the gut, leading to a progressive increase in the body's iron stores. Although the liver is the most frequently affected organ, it is not uncommon to see clinical and imaging features in the heart, pancreas, skin, endocrine glands and bones [1, 2].

Since haemochromatosis is a multi-organ disorder, the patient may present with varying clinical presentations, such as hepatomegaly (90%), hyperpigmented skin (90%), arthralgia (50%), diabetes (30%) and heart failure or arrhythmia (15%). In addition, there is an increased risk of malignancy in these patients with hepatocellular carcinoma recognized as a documented complication for advanced cases of haemochromatosis [14].

Raised serum ferritin and transferring saturation index are reliable markers for the diagnosis of haemochromatosis [14]. However, these tests have low sensitivity and specificity. False-positive results can be seen in alcohol excess and false-negative results in young individuals with haemochromatosis.

The key imaging features of hepatic iron overload are increased organ density on CT and reduced signal intensity on MRI [1, 2]. Non-contrast CT features suggest a marked homogeneous increase in liver density (up to or more than 72 HU) with apparent low attenuation of intrahepatic portal vessels and hepatic veins relative to hepatic parenchyma. Colluding factors such as associated fat deposition causing a decrease in hepatic attenuation reduce the sensitivity of CT [14]. Additionally, the minimal threshold for hepatic iron accumulation is 5 times the normal hepatic iron for its detection on CT, further compromising its sensitivity. Similarly, Wilson's disease, gold deposition, type IV glycogen storage or long-term amiodarone therapy causing an increase in hepatic attenuation decrease the specificity of the modality. Non-contrast CT is really important because iron accumulation cannot be satisfactorily demonstrated in the background of enhancing hepatic parenchyma [1, 2]. Dual-energy CT can help in the quantification of iron overload.

MRI is the modality of choice for the diagnosis of iron overload with high sensitivity and specificity [1–5, 14–16]. Although hepatic biopsy is the gold standard, MRI is emerging as a non-invasive alternative for the evaluation of iron overload, determination of the severity of disease and monitoring of therapy. The superparamagnetic effect of iron ions results in shortening of relaxation time on T1, T2 and T2* sequences. This presents as a loss of signal which is proportional to iron deposition. Hepatic iron concentration can be estimated using gradient in-and-out-of-phase sequences (Fig. 6.5). These demonstrate loss of signal on the in-phase sequence as compared to the out-of-phase sequence (reverse of what is seen in fat deposition) [5, 14].

The key differentiating feature is the iron deposition pattern. Predominant liver involvement is consistent with non-RES deposition and is suggestive of primary haemochromatosis. Predominant spleen and bone marrow involvement with lesser extent of liver involvement is consistent with RES deposition which is suggestive of secondary haemochromatosis.

There are two methods which have been successfully implemented in the quantification of hepatic iron overload. One is the signal intensity ratio method which measures the signal intensity

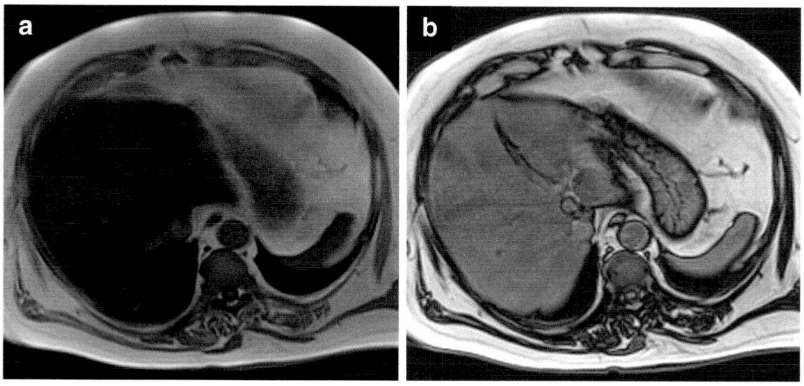

Fig. 6.5 (**a**) In-phase and (**b**) opposed-phase images in a 48-year-old patient with iron overload due to haemochromatosis. The liver shows signal loss on the in-phase

of the liver and another tissue and gives the proportion of these to quantify hepatic iron overload. The other one is the relaxometry method which measures the signal intensity of the liver across multiple echo times and calculates T2 or T2* values. T2 and T2* values are inversely related to iron concentration. Therefore, R or R* (1000/T2 or T2*) values are directly related and increase linearly with hepatic iron concentration. These are of great importance in the evaluation of hepatic iron overload. A T2* value less than 18 ms is considered consistent with iron overload. A recent study suggested that an R2* value cutoff of 147.1 Hz/T2* value of 6.8 ms can help in the determination of moderate and severe iron overload from absent and mild iron overload [15]. The GRE sequence with T2* weighting and progressively longer echo times is particularly sensitive in identifying and evaluating mild to moderate iron overload. It is detected as a lower signal intensity of the iron-loaded hepatic parenchyma than the paraspinal musculature in contrast to the higher signal of normal hepatic parenchyma than paraspinal musculature. This proves to be an excellent internal control (3). A recent study has successfully evaluated the correlation between liver-to-muscle (L/M) signal intensity and hepatic iron concentration. It has been suggested that a highly weighted GRE sequence has a high sensitivity of 89% and a specificity of 80% in the validation group, with an L/M ratio less than 0.88. This technique allowed them to detect an iron overload greater than 60 micromol/g (normal value <36 micromol/g) [16].

In the clinical setting, either a vendor software platform or a manual assessment can be done. There are multiple freely available softwares to help the radiologist in calculating the liver iron concentrations. The most common of these is the MRQuantif from the group from Rennes (https://imagemed.univ-rennes1.fr/en). A periodic audit with patients who have also had a biopsy would give an indication of the degree of accuracy of the results.

US is not a suitable modality for the diagnosis of hepatic iron overload but is useful to determine long-term features such as cirrhosis or portal hypertension caused by haemochromatosis [15]. Hepatocellular carcinoma is a complication of advanced haemochromatosis in almost 35% of patients. US is also widely used for surveillance and HCC detection (Fig. 6.6) [1].

6.2.3 Amyloidosis

Amyloidosis is an umbrella term used for diseases in which tissue damage occurs secondary to extracellular deposition of abnormally folded fibrillar proteins called amyloid. Hepatic involvement in amyloidosis is uncommon, wherein the abnormal extracellular proteins cause tissue damage by local mass effect on the hepatocytes and their resultant destruction [1].

Hepatic amyloidosis is usually asymptomatic [1]. Patients may have non-specific symptoms of abdominal pain due to liver enlargement, whilst others may present with deranged liver enzymes. Imaging findings are non-specific. As amyloido-

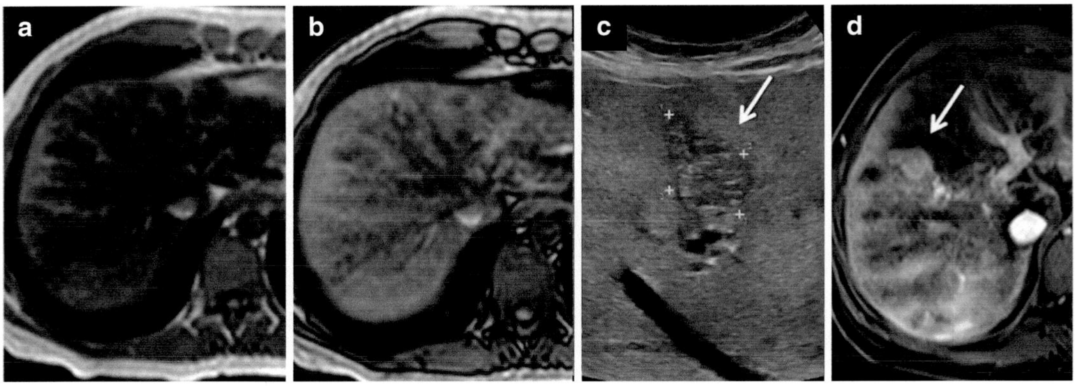

Fig. 6.6 (**a**) In-phase and (**b**) opposed-phase images in a 29-year-old patient with hepatic iron overload. (**c**) A focal hypoechoic lesion was picked up on US surveillance. (**d**) On post-contrast MRI, this exhibited arterial hyperenhancement favouring an HCC

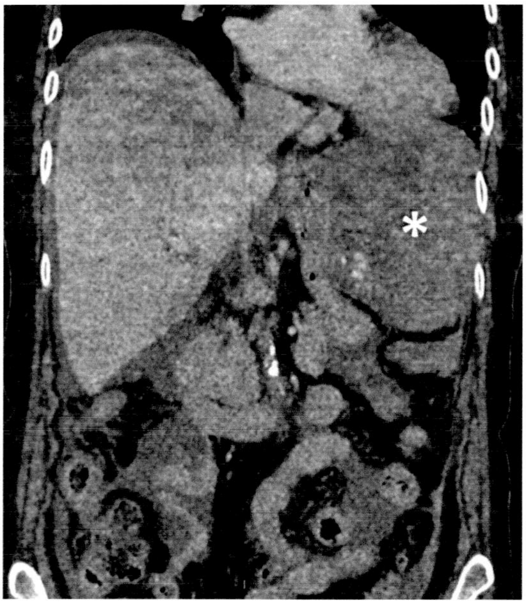

Fig. 6.7 Coronal CT demonstrating an enlarged, slightly heterogeneous liver in a 77-year-old lady, a known case of multi-organ amyloidosis, who presented with spontaneous atraumatic splenic rupture (asterisk)

sis is an infiltrative disorder, hepatomegaly is a common finding seen in almost all patients with amyloidosis [1, 5]. The liver often shows heterogeneous appearances on US, CT and MRI. Splenomegaly is commonly present along with hepatomegaly (Fig. 6.7) [17, 18].

On CT, the liver parenchyma may have lower attenuation, giving the appearance of fatty liver. On MRI, the liver is diffusely involved and shows low signal change on both T1- and T2-weighted images with no signal drop on opposed-phase chemical shift imaging, thus aiding differentiation from fatty liver or haemochromatosis [17, 18]. The liver can progressively develop an irregular outline and may show triangular hypertrophy, i.e. apex towards the falciform ligament.

6.2.4 Wilson's Disease

Wilson's disease, aka hepatolenticular degeneration, is a rare autosomal recessive disorder characterized by increased intestinal uptake of copper, leading to accumulation of its toxic levels in the liver, cornea and brain [1].

Within the liver, copper predominantly accumulates in the periportal region and along the hepatic sinusoids. This eventually results in the inflammatory reaction leading to acute hepatitis with steatosis. This is followed by the development of chronic hepatitis leading to hepatic fibrosis and macronodular cirrhosis as end-stage [19]. Very rarely, malignant transformation into hepatocellular carcinoma may occur [20]. Liver manifestations are more common in the younger age group, often in individuals presenting in the first and second decades of life. Presentation with neurological symptoms usually occurs in the third decade of life, but these individuals have usually developed hepatic disease as well by the time of presentation [20].

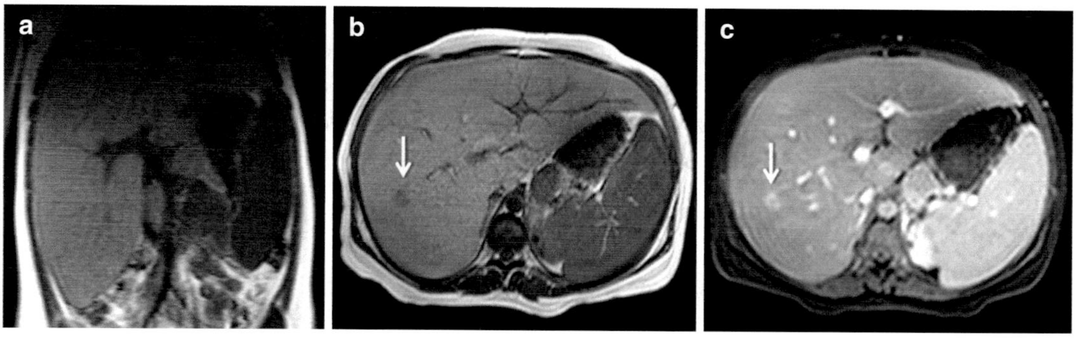

Fig. 6.8 (**a**) Coronal T1W MRI demonstrating massive hepatomegaly in a 16-year-old girl with type IB GSD. (**b** and **c**) Pre- and post-contrast T1W images demonstrating an enhancing adenoma (arrow), picked up on one of the annual surveillance scans

US, CT and MRI findings usually represent non-specific features such as fatty infiltration, hepatomegaly, features of acute or chronic hepatitis and, in advanced cases, cirrhosis. Hepatic attenuation may be increased secondary to the accumulation of copper, resulting in a hyperdense liver on an unenhanced CT scan. However, in patients with concurrent steatosis, the cancelling effect of fat and copper may result in no change in attenuation [12]. There are no specific MRI findings, although early disease may be characterized by the presence of multiple hepatic nodules that are T2 hypointense and T1 hyperintense. This is secondary to the paramagnetic effect of ionic copper [21]. The role of imaging is primarily for the monitoring and surveillance of liver cirrhosis rather than for diagnosing Wilson's disease.

6.2.5 Glycogen Storage Diseases

Glycogen storage disorders are inherited as autosomal recessive genetic diseases, characterized by a deficiency of one of the enzymes responsible for the synthesis, metabolism or storage of glycogen. The most common glycogen storage diseases are type I and type II with an overall incidence of 1 in 100,000 and 1 in 40,000 live births (in the United States) [22, 23].

Glycogen storage diseases have hepatomegaly as one of the cardinal features. Diagnosis of glycogen storage disorder should be excluded in children presenting with hepatomegaly and associated hypoglycaemia, growth retardation or disproportionate distribution of body fat [12].

On imaging, the deposition of glycogen in hepatocytes is seen as increased echogenicity on ultrasound and increased hepatic attenuation on CT. On MRI, it is seen as a homogeneously increased signal intensity relative to bone marrow on the T1W sequence [21]. Patients are at risk for developing hepatic adenoma/adenomatosis (multiple adenomas), cirrhosis and hepatocellular carcinoma. Imaging plays a more important role in screening for these changes rather than in diagnosing glycogen storage disorders (Fig. 6.8).

6.3 Infectious/Inflammatory Diseases

A variety of inflammatory and infectious diseases can lead to diffuse liver involvement. The majority demonstrate overlapping features ranging from hepatomegaly to multiple small liver lesions in the form of granulomas or abscesses [1].

The most prevalent of these are viral infections [2]. They can present with acute hepatitis, but they can also present with liver fibrosis/cirrhosis and may go on to develop HCC. Less common conditions include fungal infections, especially candidiasis, which leads to multiple micro-abscesses in the liver. Granulomatous diseases such as tuberculosis, sarcoidosis and histoplasmosis can cause hepatomegaly or small granuloma/tuberculoma formations, which appear as small hypodense lesions with variable enhancement. Calcifications can be seen in healed tuberculosis and histoplasmosis. Parasitic infections, especially schistosomiasis, lead to periportal fibrosis and characteristic calcified septa lying perpendicular to the liver capsule, described as the 'turtleback' appearance. Bacterial infections such as pyogenic and amoebic liver abscesses usually present as focal liver abscesses which combined with clinical symptoms make the diagnosis straightforward.

6.3.1 Viral Hepatitis

Acute viral hepatitis is the most common cause of acute liver disease. Most of the viral hepatitides are caused by hepatotropic viruses: A, B, C, E and G. Other viruses like herpes virus, adenovirus and coxsackievirus can also cause acute hepatitis in immunosuppressed individuals. Viral hepatitis is usually diagnosed with clinical features, biochemistry and serologic positivity. Imaging findings are non-specific and are mainly used for ruling out other differentials which can present with a similar clinical picture.

The most common imaging manifestation is hepatomegaly accompanied by periportal oedema and gallbladder wall oedema (Fig. 6.9). Periportal lymphadenopathy can be seen. Liver parenchymal attenuation and enhancement are generally heterogeneous on CT. MRI also shows non-specific findings of hepatomegaly and enhancement of the liver capsule, often accompanied by periportal oedema tracking along portal channels on T2-weighted images [24, 25].

Other diseases such as TB, candidiasis, histoplasmosis and some inflammatory disorders like sarcoidosis can also show diffuse involvement of the liver. These disorders also present with non-specific hepatomegaly. These diseases have been discussed elsewhere in the book.

6.3.2 Hepatic Fibrosis and Liver Cirrhosis

Chronic inflammatory changes/hepatitis can progress to the early stage of reversible hepatic fibrosis and eventually the advanced stage of fibrosis if untreated. Hepatic fibrosis is seen as coarse parenchymal echogenicity on ultrasound. Sonographic appearance of early fibrosis is non-specific; however, the sensitivity improves in the advanced stage of fibrosis which shows parenchymal heterogeneity and surface nodularity. Portal hypertension is an associated finding. Elastography techniques such as point shear wave elastography (pSWE), shear wave elastography (SWE) and vibration-controlled transient elastography (VCTE) are highly accurate in detecting hepatic fibrosis [26] but unfortunately are operator-dependent.

On CT, fibrosis/cirrhosis can be seen as a heterogeneous, irregular/nodular hepatic surface, widened fissures, segmental atrophy with compensatory hypertrophy and associated features of portal hypertension. It can be helpful in the evaluation of complications such as oesophageal varices, ascites or hepatocellular carcinoma. The sensitivity and specificity of the CT scan for diagnosing hepatic cirrhosis are 77.1–84.3% and 52.9–67.6%, respectively.

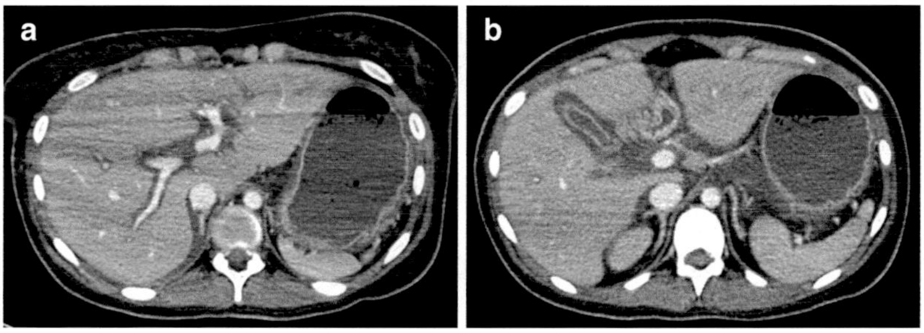

Fig. 6.9 (**a** and **b**) Axial CT images demonstrating florid periportal oedema and oedematous gallbladder in a 19-year-old female presenting with acute severe viral hepatitis

Conventional MRI is more accurate than the CT scan for diagnosing early fibrosis. Newer techniques such as susceptibility weighted imaging (SWI), diffusion-weighted imaging (DWI), perfusion imaging, texture analysis, hepatocellular function imaging, t1-p imaging and MR elastography (MRE) are showing an increasing role in the evaluation of hepatic fibrosis [27, 28]. MRE shows high sensitivity and specificity of 98% and 99%, respectively, in the detection of hepatic fibrosis and differentiating NAFLD or NASH prior to the development of hepatic fibrosis. Hepatic stiffness increases with advancing stages of fibrosis and can be easily differentiated from normal stiffness, i.e <2.5 kPa. Studies have suggested that it is not influenced by associated features of cirrhosis such as ascites, obesity or hepatic steatosis. It can however prove unreliable in patients with iron deposition disorders. Upcoming MRI techniques like magnetic transfer ratio (MTR), T1ρ imaging and texture analysis are being developed as supplementary tools in these patients.

A major complication of chronic liver fibrosis or cirrhosis is hepatocellular carcinoma. Imaging surveillance is key for its timely detection and optimal treatment and also for following up patients post-treatment (Fig. 6.10).

6.3.3 Sarcoidosis

Hepatic involvement in sarcoidosis, a systemic autoimmune (granulomatous) disorder, is not uncommon and has been reported in 11–80% of patients with sarcoidosis, but progression to chronic hepatitis and cirrhosis is relatively uncommon [29, 30]. Diagnosis of hepatic sarcoidosis is challenging and often dependent on a combination of biochemical, imaging and histological findings [29].

The most common imaging manifestations on CT or MRI are hepatomegaly followed by multiple hypodense hepatic nodules ranging up to 2 cm, often accompanied by splenic granulomas, splenomegaly and abdominal adenopathy [1, 5].

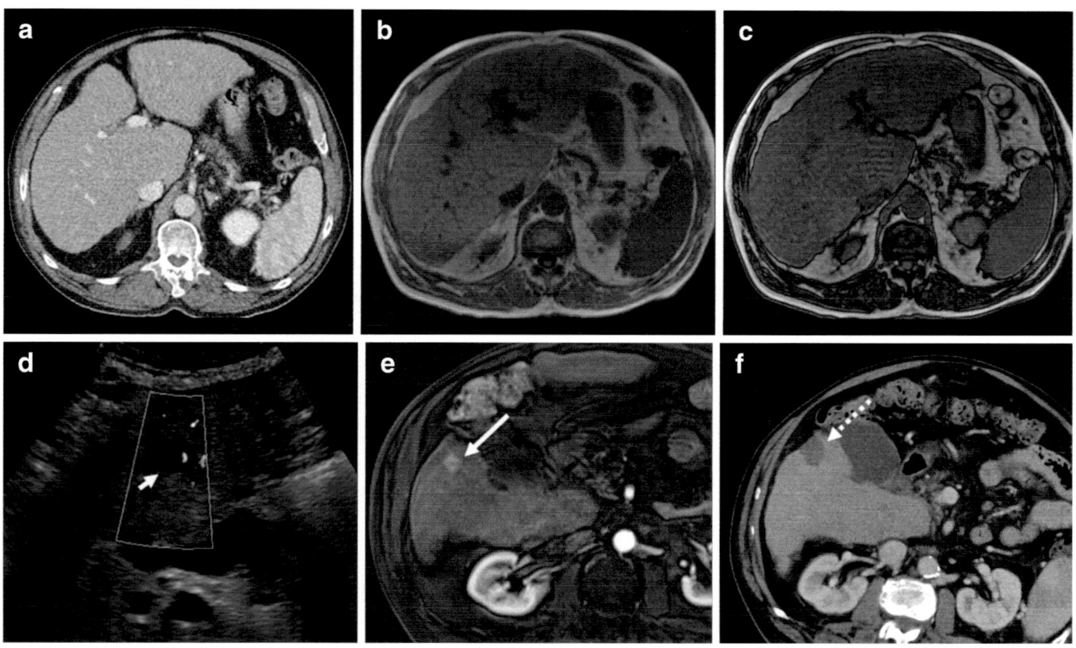

Fig. 6.10 (**a**) Axial CT demonstrating a dysmorphic liver with an undulating contour and enlarged caudate lobe. (**b** and **c**) In- and opposed-phase MRI shows diffuse steatosis and micronodular change. (**d**) US surveillance detected a new hypoechoic nodule (short arrow). (**e**) MRI demonstrates arterial hyperenhancement (long arrow) and washout (not shown) in keeping with HCC. (**f**) Post-microwave-ablation CT ensures there's no residual disease

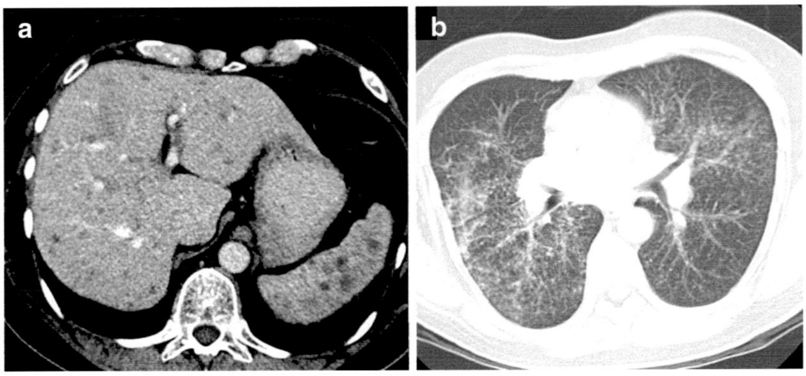

Fig. 6.11 (**a** and **b**) Axial abdominal CT in a 66-year-old male showing numerous randomly scattered hepatosplenic hypodense nodules (sarcoid granulomas). (**b**) CT thorax performed a year prior shows typical changes of pulmonary sarcoidosis (bilateral peri-fissural and peribronchovascular nodules)

The presence of classical perilymphatic nodular change in the lungs, the most common organ involved in sarcoidosis, can be a helpful diagnostic clue (Fig. 6.11). However, one has to be wary of lymphoma, metastases and candidiasis which can have overlapping imaging manifestations.

Once the disease has progressed to chronic liver disease, the presence of large central regenerative nodules accompanied by wedge-shaped subcapsular areas of parenchymal loss on MRI has been shown to be helpful in suggesting the diagnosis [31].

6.4 Vascular Disorders

Disease processes that lead to abnormal hepatic perfusion can also manifest as diffuse liver disease [2, 5].

6.4.1 Congestive Hepatopathy

Chronic cardiovascular conditions leading to heart failure create a state of elevated central venous pressure. This leads to passive congestion within the liver parenchyma with elevated hepatic venous pressure. This chronically elevated hepatic pressure state is also termed as congestive hepatopathy (CH) and has a tendency to cause hepatic fibrosis and cirrhosis in the long term [5, 32].

Persistently raised hepatic venous pressure leads to dilatation of hepatic sinusoids, perisinusoidal oedema and haemorrhage. This leads to hepatocyte atrophy with subsequent development of fibrosis. Liver dysfunction does not happen till late in CH; therefore, imaging plays an important role in the early recognition of CH [32].

US shows hepatomegaly along with dilation of the inferior vena cava (IVC) and hepatic veins. There is a loss of respiratory variations in IVC with loss of the normal triphasic pattern of flow in hepatic veins on Doppler. This is due to increased resistance in the flow towards the heart [32, 33]. On CT and MRI, hepatomegaly, contrast reflux into distended IVC and hepatic veins and mosaic liver parenchymal enhancement are features that suggest CH (Fig. 6.12). Phase-contrast MRI can be used to determine the vascular flow and the direction of the flow.

In long-standing CH, hepatic to hepatic shunts can develop (Fig. 6.13). Extrahepatic features of cardiac findings like cardiomegaly, effusion or restrictive cardiomyopathy are generally helpful in confirming the diagnosis.

6.4.2 Budd-Chiari Syndrome

Budd-Chiari syndrome is characterized by hepatic venous outflow obstruction leading to portal hypertension, ascites and progressive liver failure [2]. It has both acute and chronic presenta-

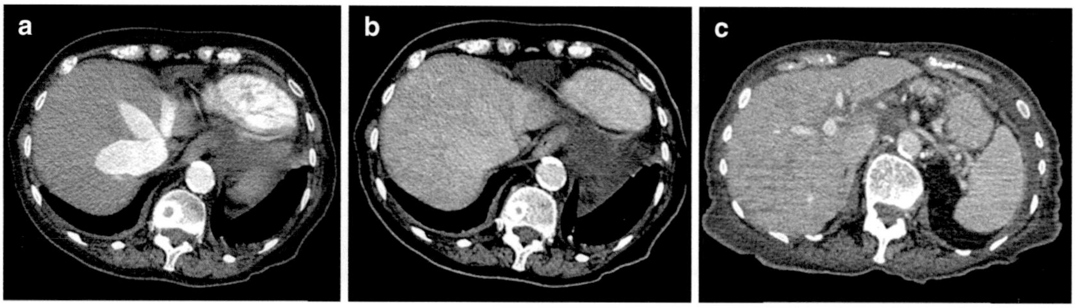

Fig. 6.12 (**a** and **b**) Arterial and PV axial CT images demonstrating contrast reflux into IVC-hepatic veins and mosaic parenchymal enhancement in a 77-year-old lady with longstanding cardiac disease. (**c**) Patient progressed to cardiac cirrhosis at age 80, note dysmorphic liver with mosaic enhancement on CT

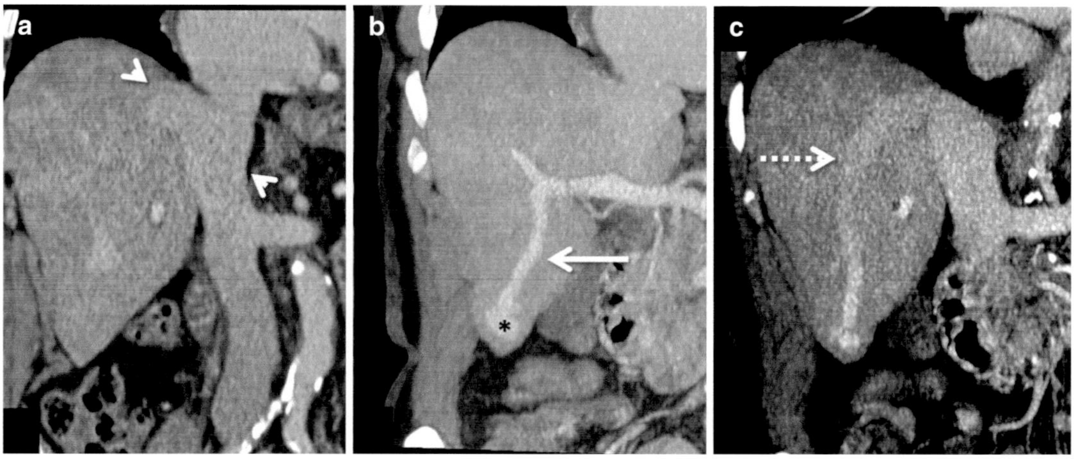

Fig. 6.13 (**a**) Coronal MPR demonstrating distended IVC-hepatic veins (arrowheads) in a 73-year-old lady with CH. (**b** and **c**) Coronal MIP shows an intrahepatic veno-venous shunt (asterisk) connecting the right hepatic vein (dotted arrow) with the right PV (arrow)

tions [5]. The classic triad of clinical manifestations includes hepatomegaly, ascites and abdominal pain.

Ultrasound shows hepatomegaly, thrombosis of the hepatic veins/IVC and associated features of portal hypertension. Colour Doppler shows absent or reversal flow in the hepatic veins.

On CT and MRI, there is a classic 'mottled' appearance of the liver (Fig. 6.14). Post-contrast CT also shows the classic 'flip-flop' phenomenon of enhancement characterized by delayed enhancement of the peripheral liver [34]. Chronic disease presents with (caudate lobe enlargement) and atrophy of the peripheral liver and features of portal hypertension. Hepatic veins are non-visualized/constricted with multiple intrahepatic collaterals seen appearing as enhancing 'comma-shaped' structures.

6.4.3 Arteriovenous Malformation

Hepatic arterio-venous (AV) malformations are rare. These may be caused either iatrogenically or in hereditary conditions such as haemorrhagic telangiectasia (HHT) [2]. HHT is characterized by AV malformations between the hepatic artery and the hepatic vein or the hepatic artery and the portal-venous system and can diffusely involve the liver.

HHT presents as multiple asterisk-like vascular abnormalities (telangiectasias) distributed throughout the hepatic parenchyma. There is enlargement

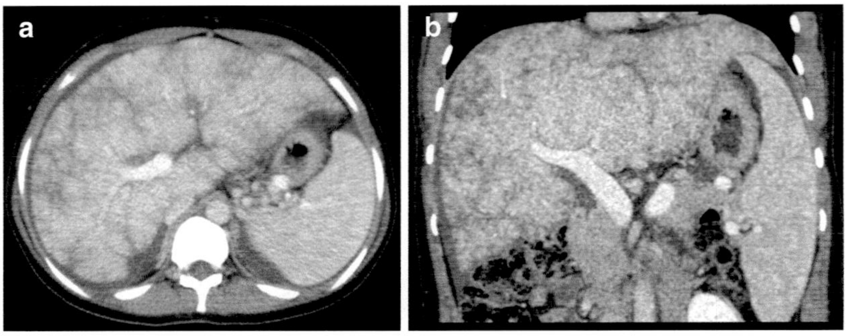

Fig. 6.14 (**a**) Axial CT and coronal MPR images demonstrating classical 'mottled' liver in a 30-year-old lady with Budd-Chiari syndrome. (**b**) There are signs of portal hypertension as evidenced by splenic enlargement and ascites

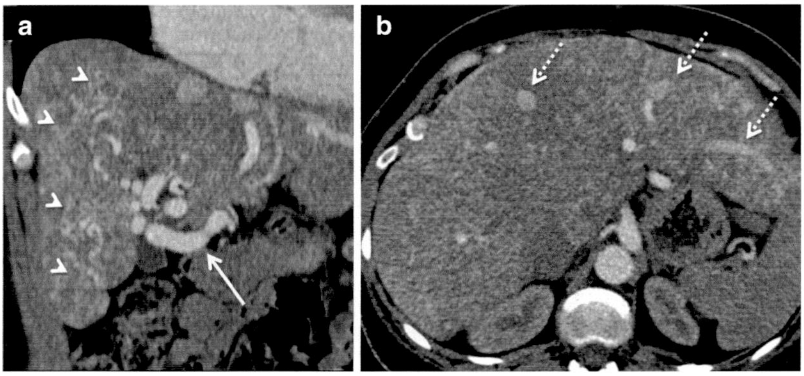

Fig. 6.15 (**a**) Coronal MPR demonstrating innumerable hepatic telangiectasias (arrowheads) in a 55-year-old lady with HHT. The hepatic artery is unusually dilated and ectatic (arrow). (**b**) Axial CT shows opacification of the hepatic veins (dotted arrows) on the arterial phase scan suggestive of AV shunting (arrow)

of the hepatic artery and an increased number of tortuous vessels at the hepatic hilum. Early opacification of the HV or PV on arterial phase scan suggests underlying AV malformations (Fig. 6.15) [35].

Increased arterial perfusion leads to secondary nodular hypertrophy which may mimic a malignant hepatic lesion. However, these nodules do not show any washout and become isodense to background liver parenchyma on the portal-venous and equilibrium phases. In cases where doubt persists, the use of hepatobiliary contrast can solve the query as these (FNH-like) nodules retain contrast on delayed images [35].

6.5 Neoplastic Disorders

6.5.1 Metastatic Disease

Metastases are the most common malignant hepatic lesions and can sometimes diffusely infiltrate the liver [1]. Diffuse metastatic infiltration is most frequently seen secondary to malignant neuroendocrine cancers, pancreatic carcinoma, colonic adenocarcinoma and breast carcinoma [36].

On US, CT and MR imaging, the appearances can be varied with conglomerate/coalescent (Fig. 6.16), infiltrative, cystic and occasionally calcified appearances. They are typically hypovascular and show ring/peripheral enhancement in the arterial phase, followed by progressive thick rind enhancement in the venous phase. Hypervascular metastases show diffuse enhancement on the arterial phase and are typically seen with neuroendocrine tumours, renal cell carcinoma, thyroid carcinoma, melanoma, etc.

Diffuse metastatic infiltration can be subtle at initial presentation and may not be readily discernible, but the presence of subtle parenchymal heterogeneity and/or architectural, contour or vascular distortion should prompt further assessment with MRI. Diffusion-weighted imaging is of paramount importance [36].

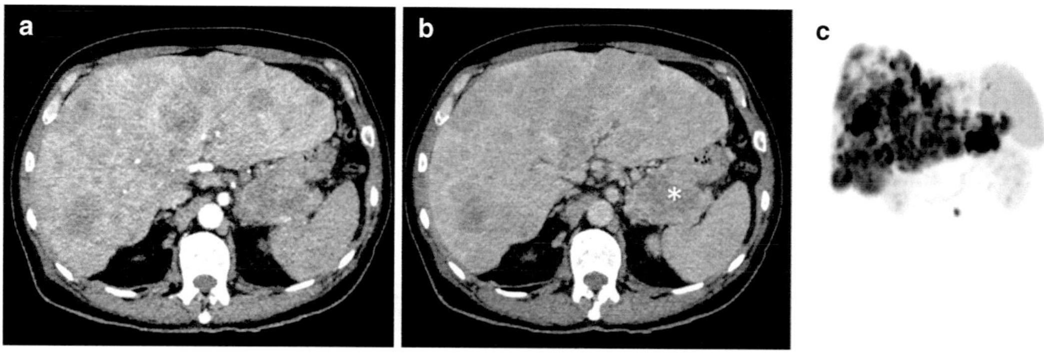

Fig. 6.16 (**a** and **b**) Arterial and PV axial CT slices demonstrating extensive diffuse metastatic infiltration of the liver in a 50-year-old male with a pancreatic tail neuroendocrine cancer (asterisk). (**c**) DOTATAE Gallium PET-CT confirming bilobar liver metastases

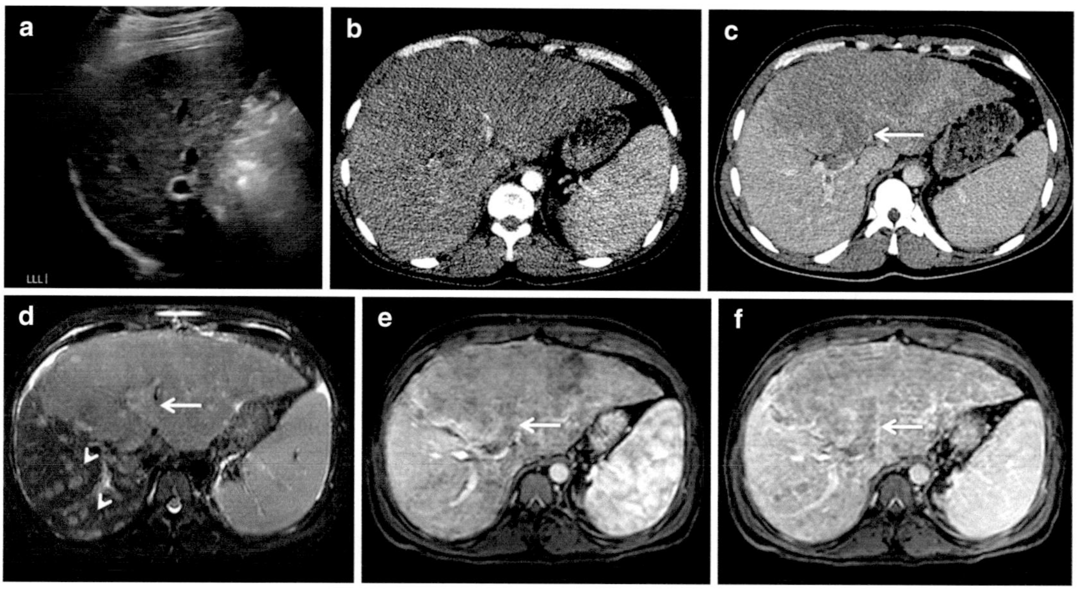

Fig. 6.17 (**a**) Liver US in a 25-year-old male showing a heterogeneous left liver lobe, but with no discrete lesion shown. (**b** and **c**) Axial arterial and PV CT showing a mass permeating the left liver lobe with no discernible arterial enhancement, but there is a washout appearance on the PV phase. Of note is an expansile PV thrombus (arrow). (**d**) Axial T2W MRI shows the thrombus to be of similar signal intensity to the neighbouring mass. Additional lesions are seen in the right lobe (asterisk). (**e** and **f**) The thrombus enhances similar to the left lobe infiltrative HCC (arrow)

6.5.2 Primary Liver Tumours

Primary hepatic malignancies such as hepatocellular carcinoma (HCC) can rarely present with diffuse involvement of the liver either in the form of multicentric HCC nodules or as an infiltrative HCC. Infiltrative HCC is a unique variety of HCC, wherein innumerable tiny tumour nodules infiltrate multiple hepatic segments, the entire lobe or the whole of the liver [37].

The tumour is often not easy to distinguish from the background heterogeneous cirrhotic liver, particularly on US and CT. Moreover, the typical arterial phase enhancement is often lacking, although it may show vague washout appearances on the venous phase (Fig. 6.17). The most helpful imaging finding is the presence of an expansile thrombus within the intra- and extrahepatic PV branches, seen in 68–100%. On CT and

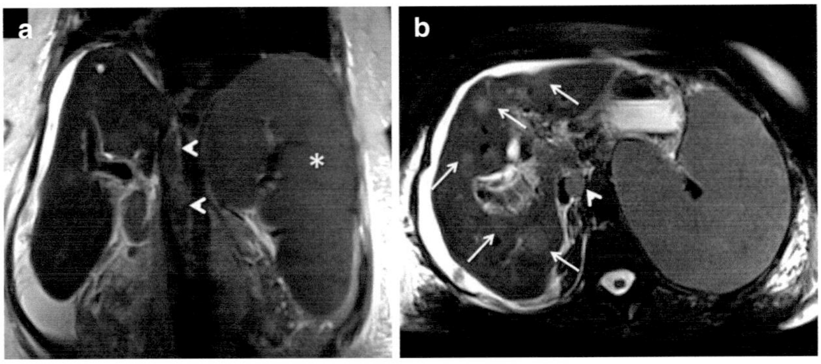

Fig. 6.18 (**a** and **b**) Coronal and axial T2W MRI in a 56-year-old female with non-Hodgkin lymphoma demonstrating an enlarged liver with multifocal nodular lesions (arrows). Note the massively enlarged spleen (asterisk) and enlarged retroperitoneal nodes (arrowhead)

MRI, the thrombus often shows heterogeneous enhancement similar to the adjacent tumour [37].

6.5.3 Lymphoma

Hepatic involvement is mostly secondary, with primary liver lymphoma being a rare disease. The imaging manifestations are largely non-specific, ranging from nodular lesions, diffuse infiltration to a mixed infiltrative and nodular pattern (Fig. 6.18). In an appropriate clinical setting, the presence of ancillary findings such as splenomegaly, lymphadenopathy or periportal mass can serve as helpful diagnostic clues [1, 38].

6.6 Drug-Induced Diffuse Liver Disease

A variety of drugs and toxins have been implicated in causing diffuse liver injury. Although less common, it remains a significant concern which needs proper monitoring and surveillance to prevent liver failure in these patients [39, 40].

The list of drugs that can cause liver damage is wide and long. Anesthetics (halothane, enflurane), anticonvulsants (phenytoin), analgesics (acetaminophen), hormonal derivatives (danazol), antidepressant or antianxiety drugs (amitriptyline, amineptine), antimicrobials (isoniazid, amoxicillin, sulfamethoxazole-trimethoprim), hypolipidemic agents (nicotinic acid, gemfibrozil), drugs for inflammatory bowel disease (sulfasalazine), combined antiretroviral therapy (cART), cardiovascular drugs (quinidine, amiodarone) and various classes of chemotherapy drugs (methotrexate, cisplatin, gemcitabine, etc.) have all been associated with parenchymal liver disease. The common mechanisms of liver injury are hepatic steatosis, cholestatic injury, vascular injury in the form of Budd-Chiari syndrome and sinusoidal obstruction syndrome [39].

6.6.1 Amiodarone Hepatotoxicity

Amiodarone is commonly used for acute and chronic dysrhythmias and is known to deposit in the reticuloendothelial system, mostly in the liver but also in the spleen. Amiodarone and its toxic metabolite '*desethylamiodarone*' cause hepatocyte damage.

Hepatotoxicity is a major concern while initiating amiodarone therapy. Studies have suggested that there is an increased risk of hepatotoxicity with high-dose usage and long-term treatments. In most of the patients, hepatotoxicity is detected incidentally during routine testing of hepatic function tests [40].

An increase in average CT (HU) density is the most common finding (Fig. 6.19). Studies have suggested that there is a significant correlation between blood *desethylamiodarone* and hepatic hyperattenuation. Hence, amiodarone should be considered a differential possibility in cases with hepatic hyperattenuation. The only definitive treatment is discontinuation of drugs.

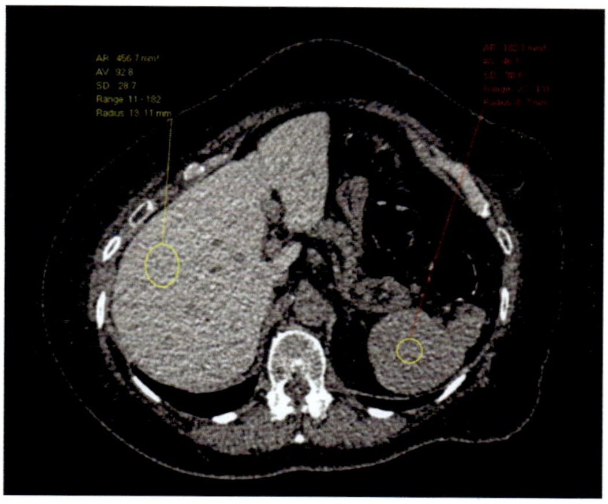

Fig. 6.19 Axial unenhanced CT in a 70-year-old lady demonstrating hyperattenuating liver secondary to amiodarone. The average liver attenuation was 92.8 HU (normally 55 HU)

6.7 Conclusion

With the growing incidence and detection of liver diseases globally, awareness of the diagnostic imaging features of common and uncommon aetiologies of diffuse liver diseases is critical for their timely detection and treatment. If untreated, chronic liver injury can evolve into cirrhosis, thus putting the patient at risk of liver cancer and other cirrhosis-related complications. Imaging not only plays an essential role in the diagnostic pathway but also in disease monitoring, particularly to screen for malignancy.

References

1. Ros PR. Chapter 22: Imaging of diffuse and inflammatory liver disease. In: Hodler J, Kubik-Huch RA, von Schulthess GK, editors. Diseases of the abdomen and pelvis 2018–2021: diagnostic imaging – IDKD Book [Internet]. Cham: Springer; 2018.
2. Schneider G, Grazioli L, Saini S. Imaging of diffuse liver disease. In: Schneider G, Grazioli L, Saini S, editors. MRI of the liver. Milano: Springer; 2003. https://doi.org/10.1007/978-88-470-2946-0_6.
3. Tubay M, Jesinger R. Imaging of diffuse liver disease. Curr Radiol Rep. 2017;5:26. https://doi.org/10.1007/s40134-017-0222-z.
4. Chundru S, Kalb B, Arif-Tiwari H, Sharma P, Costello J, Martin DR. MRI of diffuse liver disease: characteristics of acute and chronic diseases. Diagn Interv Radiol. 2014;20(3):200–8. https://doi.org/10.5152/dir.2014.13170.
5. Chundru S, Kalb B, Arif-Tiwari H, Sharma P, Costello J, Martin DR. MRI of diffuse liver disease: the common and uncommon etiologies. Diagn Interv Radiol. 2013;19(6):479–87. https://doi.org/10.5152/dir.2013.13148.
6. Mitra S, De A, Chowdhury A. Epidemiology of non-alcoholic and alcoholic fatty liver diseases. Transl Gastroenterol Hepatol. 2020;5:16. https://doi.org/10.21037/tgh.2019.09.08.
7. Abeysekera KWM, Fernandes GS, Hammerton G, Portal AJ, Gordon FH, Heron J, Hickman M. Prevalence of steatosis and fibrosis in young adults in the UK: a population-based study. Lancet Gastroenterol Hepatol. 2020;5(3):295–305. https://doi.org/10.1016/S2468-1253(19)30419-4.
8. Noureddin M, Lam J, Peterson MR, Middleton M, Hamilton G, Le TA, Bettencourt R, Changchien C, Brenner DA, Sirlin C, Loomba R. Utility of magnetic resonance imaging versus histology for quantifying changes in liver fat in nonalcoholic fatty liver disease trials. Hepatology. 2013;58(6):1930–40. https://doi.org/10.1002/hep.26455.
9. Joy D, Thava VR, Scott BB. Diagnosis of fatty liver disease: is biopsy necessary? Eur J Gastroenterol Hepatol. 2003;15(5):539–43. https://doi.org/10.1097/01.meg.0000059112.41030.2e.
10. Hamer OW, Aguirre DA, Casola G, Lavine JE, Woenckhaus M, Sirlin CB. Fatty liver: imaging patterns and pitfalls. Radiographics. 2006;26(6):1637–53. https://doi.org/10.1148/rg.266065004.
11. Zhang YN, Fowler KJ, Hamilton G, Cui JY, Sy EZ, Balanay M, Hooker JC, Szeverenyi N, Sirlin CB. Liver fat imaging – a clinical overview of ultrasound, CT, and MR imaging. Br J Radiol. 2018;91(1089):20170959. https://doi.org/10.1259/bjr.20170959.
12. Johnston RJ, Stamm ER, Lewin JM, Hendrick RE, Archer PG. Diagnosis of fatty infiltration of the liver on contrast enhanced CT: limitations of liver-minus-spleen attenuation difference measurements. Abdom Imaging. 1998;23(4):409–15. https://doi.org/10.1007/s002619900370.
13. Boll DT, Merkle EM. Diffuse liver disease: strategies for hepatic CT and MR imaging. Radiographics. 2009;29(6):1591–614. https://doi.org/10.1148/rg.296095513.
14. Queiroz-Andrade M, Blasbalg R, Ortega CD, Rodstein MA, Baroni RH, Rocha MS, Cerri GG. MR imaging findings of iron overload. Radiographics. 2009;29(6):1575–89. https://doi.org/10.1148/rg.296095511.
15. İdilman İS, Akata D, Özmen MN, Karçaaltıncaba M. Different forms of iron accumulation in the liver on MRI. Diagn Interv Radiol. 2016;22(1):22–8. https://doi.org/10.5152/dir.2015.15094.
16. Gandon Y, Olivié D, Guyader D, Aubé C, Oberti F, Sebille V, Deugnier Y. Non-invasive assessment of hepatic iron stores by MRI. Lancet.

2004;363(9406):357–62. https://doi.org/10.1016/S0140-6736(04)15436-6.
17. Kim SH, Han JK, Lee KH, Won HJ, Kim KW, Kim JS, Park CH, Choi BI. Abdominal amyloidosis: spectrum of radiological findings. Clin Radiol. 2003;58(8):610–20. https://doi.org/10.1016/s0009-9260(03)00142-9.
18. Özcan HN, Haliloğlu M, Sökmensüer C, Akata D, Özmen M, Karçaaltıncaba M. Imaging for abdominal involvement in amyloidosis. Diagn Interv Radiol. 2017;23(4):282–5. https://doi.org/10.5152/dir.2017.16484.
19. Cheon JE, Kim IO, Seo JK, Ko JS, Lee JM, Shin CI, Kim WS, Yeon KM. Clinical application of liver MR imaging in Wilson's disease. Korean J Radiol. 2010;11(6):665–72. https://doi.org/10.3348/kjr.2010.11.6.665.
20. Patil M, Sheth KA, Krishnamurthy AC, Devarbhavi H. A review and current perspective on Wilson disease. J Clin Exp Hepatol. 2013;3(4):321–36. https://doi.org/10.1016/j.jceh.2013.06.002.
21. Tani I, Kurihara Y, Kawaguchi A, Nakajima Y, Ishikawa T, Maeyama S, Tanaka R. MR imaging of diffuse liver disease. AJR Am J Roentgenol. 2000;174(4):965–71. https://doi.org/10.2214/ajr.174.4.1740965.
22. Shieh JJ, Terzioglu M, Hiraiwa H, Marsh J, Pan CJ, Chen LY, Chou JY. The molecular basis of glycogen storage disease type 1a: structure and function analysis of mutations in glucose-6-phosphatase. J Biol Chem. 2002;277(7):5047–53. https://doi.org/10.1074/jbc.M110486200.
23. Dasouki M, Jawdat O, Almadhoun O, Pasnoor M, McVey AL, Abuzinadah A, Herbelin L, Barohn RJ, Dimachkie MM. Pompe disease: literature review and case series. Neurol Clin. 2014;32(3):751–76., ix. https://doi.org/10.1016/j.ncl.2014.04.010.
24. Bächler P, Baladron MJ, Menias C, Beddings I, Loch R, Zalaquett E, Vargas M, Connolly S, Bhalla S, Huete Á. Multimodality imaging of liver infections: differential diagnosis and potential pitfalls. Radiographics. 2016;36(4):1001–23. https://doi.org/10.1148/rg.2016150196.
25. Mortelé KJ, Segatto E, Ros PR. The infected liver: radiologic-pathologic correlation. Radiographics. 2004;24(4):937–55. https://doi.org/10.1148/rg.244035719.
26. Honda Y, Yoneda M, Imajo K, Nakajima A. Elastography techniques for the assessment of liver fibrosis in non-alcoholic fatty liver disease. Int J Mol Sci. 2020;21(11):4039. https://doi.org/10.3390/ijms21114039.
27. Willatt JM, Hussain HK, Adusumilli S, Marrero JA. MR Imaging of hepatocellular carcinoma in the cirrhotic liver: challenges and controversies. Radiology. 2008;247(2):311–30. https://doi.org/10.1148/radiol.2472061331.
28. Idilman IS, Li J, Yin M, Venkatesh SK. MR elastography of liver: current status and future perspectives. Abdom Radiol (NY). 2020;45(11):3444–62. https://doi.org/10.1007/s00261-020-02656-7.
29. Ryland KL. Hepatic sarcoidosis: incidence, monitoring, and treatment. Clin Liver Dis. 2020;16:208–11. https://doi.org/10.1002/cld.1002.
30. Shah N, Mitra A. Gastrointestinal and hepatic sarcoidosis: a review article. Clin Liver Dis. 2021;17:301–7. https://doi.org/10.1002/cld.1055.
31. Ferreira A, Ramalho M, de Campos RO, Heredia V, Roque A, Vaidean G, Semelka RC. Hepatic sarcoidosis: MR appearances in patients with chronic liver disease. Magn Reson Imaging. 2013;31(3):432–8. https://doi.org/10.1016/j.mri.2012.08.005.
32. Wells ML, Venkatesh SK. Congestive hepatopathy. Abdom Radiol (NY). 2018;43(8):2037–51. https://doi.org/10.1007/s00261-017-1387-x.
33. Wells ML, Fenstad ER, Poterucha JT, Hough DM, Young PM, Araoz PA, Ehman RL, Venkatesh SK. Imaging findings of congestive hepatopathy. Radiographics. 2016;36(4):1024–37. https://doi.org/10.1148/rg.2016150207.
34. Cura M, Haskal Z, Lopera J. Diagnostic and interventional radiology for Budd-Chiari syndrome. Radiographics. 2009;29(3):669–81. https://doi.org/10.1148/rg.293085056.
35. Harwin J, Sugi MD, Hetts SW, Conrad MB, Ohliger MA. The role of liver imaging in hereditary hemorrhagic telangiectasia. J Clin Med. 2020;9(11):3750. https://doi.org/10.3390/jcm9113750.
36. Sica GT, Ji H, Ros PR. CT and MR imaging of hepatic metastases. AJR Am J Roentgenol. 2000;174(3):691–8. https://doi.org/10.2214/ajr.174.3.1740691.
37. Reynolds AR, Furlan A, Fetzer DT, Sasatomi E, Borhani AA, Heller MT, Tublin ME. Infiltrative hepatocellular carcinoma: what radiologists need to know. Radiographics. 2015;35(2):371–86. https://doi.org/10.1148/rg.352140114.
38. Rajesh S, Bansal K, Sureka B, Patidar Y, Bihari C, Arora A. The imaging conundrum of hepatic lymphoma revisited. Insights Imaging. 2015;6(6):679–92. https://doi.org/10.1007/s13244-015-0437-6.
39. McGettigan MJ, Menias CO, Gao ZJ, Mellnick VM, Hara AK. Imaging of drug-induced complications in the gastrointestinal system. Radiographics. 2016;36(1):71–87. https://doi.org/10.1148/rg.2016150132.
40. Kojima S, Kojima S, Ueno H, Takeya M, Ogawa H. Increased density of the liver and amiodarone-associated phospholipidosis. Cardiol Res Pract. 2009;2009:598940. https://doi.org/10.4061/2009/598940.

7 Imaging and Interventions in Budd-Chiari Syndrome

Sreedhara Bettadahally Chaluvashetty, Prabhjyot Singh Chowhan, and Naveen Kalra

7.1 Introduction

Budd-Chiari syndrome (BCS) is defined as the obstruction of the outflow of the hepatic venous system which may occur at any level between the hepatic venules and the inferior vena cava (IVC)—right atrium junction, irrespective of the cause of obstruction. Outflow obstruction caused by cardiac disorders and veno-occlusive disease of the liver is not included in this definition [1]. As far as pathophysiology is concerned, obstruction of the venous outflow from the liver leads to congestion and stasis, causing elevation of pressure within the sinusoids and a resultant hypoxic damage to hepatocytes and the sinusoidal endothelium. Hepatocyte necrosis then ensues along with gradually increasing centrilobular fibrosis, nodular regenerative hyperplasia and finally cirrhosis [2, 3]. However, liver function can be preserved if the pressure within the sinusoids is brought down by re-establishing the outflow system, forming a portosystemic shunt or by the formation of venous collaterals. Therefore, it is important to understand the underlying causative factors, clinical features and baseline liver function for choosing the best management plan for patients which may vary from conservative therapy to endovascular management to liver transplantation.

Radiological evaluation plays a key role in diagnosing and classifying BCS. It may be particularly important in patients with non-specific clinical features, wherein it may provide the initial clues to the underlying disease. In addition, imaging is also an integral part of the routine follow-up of BCS patients.

7.2 Hepatic Venous System: Normal Anatomy and Doppler Study

By convention, there are three major hepatic veins (HVs) that drain into the IVC. The middle hepatic vein (MHV) is responsible for draining segments IVa, IVb, V and VIII. The largest of the three HVs—the right hepatic vein (RHV)—is responsible for the drainage of segments V, VI and VII, while segments II and III are drained by the left hepatic vein (LHV). In approximately 65–85% of the population, the LHV and MHV merge prior to joining the IVC [4, 5].

Hepatic venous anatomy variations may be observed in around 16–33% of the population [6]. Accessory HVs that drain independently into the IVC constitute the commonest variant. The inferior right HV (that drains segment VI of the liver) is the commonest accessory HV and is seen in 18% of people [7]. This information is of vital

S. B. Chaluvashetty · P. S. Chowhan · N. Kalra (✉)
Department of Radiodiagnosis and Imaging, PGIMER, Chandigarh, India

© The Author(s), under exclusive license to Springer Nature Singapore Pte Ltd. 2025

B. Sureka (ed.), *Hepato-Pancreatico Biliary Imaging*, https://doi.org/10.1007/978-981-95-1699-5_7

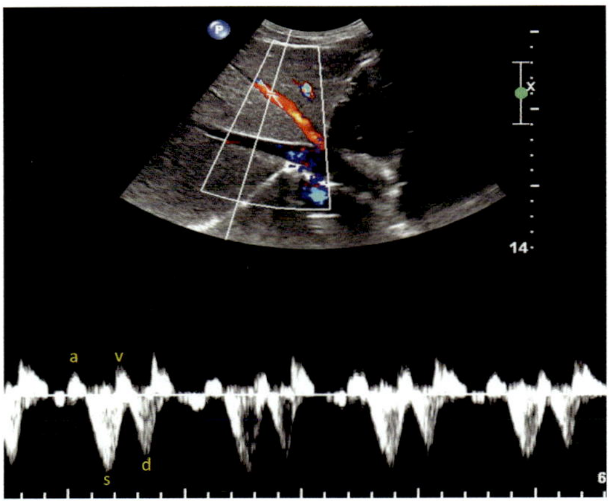

Fig. 7.1 Normal spectral Doppler waveform of hepatic veins with its four components

importance prior to planning any endovascular or surgical procedure.

There are four components of a normal HV waveform—the A wave, an antegrade S wave, a V wave and an antegrade D wave (Fig. 7.1) [8]. The retrograde A wave occurs due to the contraction of the atrium. During the S wave (which corresponds to ventricular contraction), the tricuspid valve annulus moves towards the apex, causing the blood to flow from the liver to the right atrium due to the creation of negative pressure. In patients with a healthy heart, this is the phase during which there is the greatest amount of antegrade flow.

The V wave is associated with atrial overfilling. The tricuspid valve starts returning to its natural position once the ventricular contraction starts decreasing in intensity, resulting in a decrease in velocity of the blood flow towards the heart. The V wave's peak may lie below, at or above the baseline, based on whether there is transient retrograde flow, transient equilibrium with no flow or antegrade flow throughout, respectively.

The D wave starts with the opening of the tricuspid valve. During diastole, blood flows passively in an antegrade fashion from the liver to the right atrium. In healthy patients, the velocity of this flow is less than that during the S wave.

Patient factors play a key role in the HV spectral Doppler waveform appearance, and one must always take the Doppler tracings during end inspiration or quiet respiration.

This is because during these two states, the venous return to the heart is good, and it produces a normal waveform. When performing a Valsalva manoeuvre and during end-expiration, nearly monophasic waveforms are generated because of lesser blood return to the right heart, resulting in blunted waveforms.

7.3 Epidemiology and Classification of BCS

Worldwide, BCS is not a very common liver disease. Two Asian and four European epidemiological studies were included in a recent meta-analysis that revealed a prevalence and incidence of around 2.40–33.10 per million and 0.168–4.09 per million every year, respectively [9]. Notably, well-designed epidemiological studies are lacking from India and China, and the two Asian studies included in the meta-analysis were conducted in Japan [10] and South Korea [11], respectively. However, China and India probably have a greater number of BCS patients, taking into view that single-centre studies from these two nations frequently involve hundreds of BCS cases [12, 13]. Furthermore, inadequate knowledge and low-quality diagnostic equipment may be responsible for the underdiagnosis of BCS in some parts of Asian countries. This often leads to missed or delayed diagnosis of BCS, thereby resulting in inaccurate epidemiological data. Therefore, establishing a high index of suspicion is important based on the patient demographics, history, clinical signs and symptoms and biochemical parameters.

As far as classification is concerned, BCS may be classified based on the underlying cause, the level of obstruction and/or the duration of symptoms. Based on the aetiology, it may be classified into primary (obstruction due to a primary venous thrombosis, stenosis or web) and secondary types. Hematologic abnormalities (e.g. myeloproliferative disorders (MPDs), inherited deficiencies of protein C, protein S and antithrombin III, etc.) account for most of the cases of BCS. The other causative factors include consumption of oral contraceptive pills, pregnancy and the immediate postpartum period. Secondary BCS occurs due to space-occupying lesions that may exert extraluminal compression or due to malignant tumours that invade the vessels. In some patients, it is tough to work out the aetiology, and in some, multiple factors are involved in the development of the outflow occlusion. In the West, HV thrombosis is the commonest type of obstruction with MPDs being the most common cause. However, in the Asian countries, there are significant regional variations that are reported in the clinical features, type and cause of obstruction.

Depending on the site of obstruction, BCS may be classified into three types (Table 7.1) [14].

Depending on the acuteness of venous obstruction, its extent and also on whether or not collateral circulation has formed, patients with BCS can have a fulminant, acute, subacute or chronic presentation. The hallmark features include abdominal pain, ascites, hepatomegaly and dilated superficial abdominal wall vessels. In the East, the majority of patients have a chronic presentation, while in the West, acute presentation is more common, and patients come with abdominal pain, hepatomegaly, ascites and jaundice. Liver transaminases may be significantly elevated, reaching up to five to ten times the normal values. Around 15% of the patients do not have the typical symptoms and are diagnosed while getting evaluated for abnormal liver function tests [15, 16]. When all three HVs are blocked acutely, BCS may present as a fulminant liver failure.

Table 7.1 Classification of BCS based on the site of obstruction

Type 1	Obstruction of the IVC with or without secondary HV occlusion
Type 2	Obstruction of major HVs
Type 3	Obstruction of small centrilobular venules

7.4 Radiological Features of BCS

Doppler ultrasonography, due to its wide availability, is usually the initial diagnostic test to be performed. It also carries the advantage of being a non-invasive modality with sensitivity and specificity rates of >80% for identifying BCS [17]. However, the one disadvantage of Doppler is that its accuracy relies on the patient's body habitus as well as the observer's experience. Cross-sectional imaging is reliable in establishing both direct and indirect evidence of BCS and may be conducted for confirmation and also to facilitate multidisciplinary discussions. MRI gives the benefit of being radiation-free and, hence, is preferable in the young and in patients who require repeated imaging. The gold standard test for evaluating the HVs is still direct venography [18]. It is, however, not usually performed as the first test due to its invasive nature and may be performed when non-diagnostic results are obtained with non-invasive imaging. Venography also allows one to carry out a transjugular liver biopsy in the same sitting in case of patency of one of the HVs and also precisely delineates the anatomy prior to the treatment. In the subsequent sections, we shall be discussing the imaging features of BCS based on the duration of the disease under the subheadings of parenchymal and vascular changes.

7.5 Acute BCS

7.5.1 Parenchymal Changes

An acute obstruction of HV outflow leads to an increase in pressure within the sinusoids with slowing or reversal of the inflow from the portal vein (PV). Since venous collaterals do not develop in the acute form, hepatocyte necrosis occurs rather quickly. The liver turns heterogeneous and shows delayed peripheral enhancement on contrast-enhanced cross-sectional imaging. On the arterial phase imaging, the peripheral areas of the liver appear hypodense on CECT and hypointense on contrast-enhanced MRI (Fig. 7.2). In addition, in comparison with the rest of the liver, the caudate lobe shows greater enhancement. This phenomenon is explained by the caudate lobe's independent drainage directly into the IVC. In the portal venous phase, a 'flip-flop' pattern may be observed, in which the central liver shows lower attenuation (as a result of washout), while the peripheral portion of the liver shows gradually rising attenuation due to accumulation of contrast from capsular veins.

7.5.2 Vascular Changes

An acute thrombus will appear hypoechoic on ultrasonography and will cause luminal expansion. On Doppler, it will not show any flow. After some days, it becomes echogenic and is associated with retraction of the involved HV lumen. On cross-sectional imaging, the thrombus may be seen as hypointensity (on MRI) or hypodensity (on CT) within the HVs. Doppler ultrasonography is usually the best modality to pick up stenosis since it permits evaluation of haemodynamic effects which may be seen as colour aliasing and a focal rise in flow velocity. In a study conducted by Rossi et al., it was seen that contrast-enhanced ultrasound was better than both grayscale and Doppler for picking up and characterizing HV thrombosis [19]. IVC webs may be visualized on ultrasound as hyperreflective linear foci that are best seen in deep inspiration. On direct venography and MR venography, these may be seen as thin dome-shaped linear filling defects.

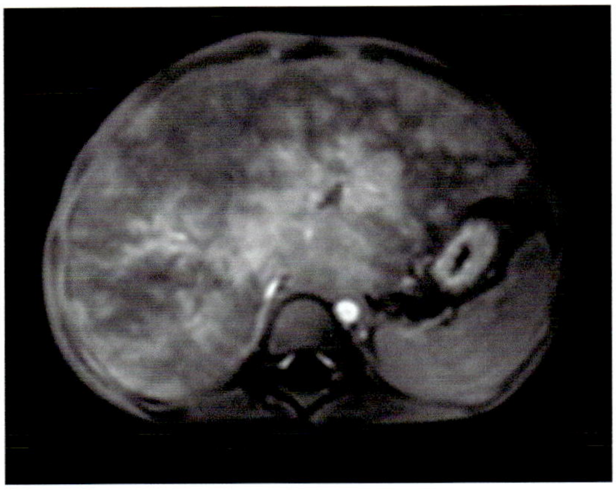

Fig. 7.2 Post-contrast arterial phase axial T1-weighted MR image in a known case of Budd-Chiari syndrome showing hypointense signal in the periphery of the liver as compared to the central portion

During evaluation for suspected BCS patients, it is also important to assess the inferior right hepatic and caudate veins. The inferior right HV is the main vessel draining segment VI of the liver. In patients with an occluded RHV, this vein enlarges and starts acting as the main outflow of the right lobe. A caudate vein size ≥3 mm should raise a possibility of BCS in the appropriate clinical setting (Fig. 7.3) [20].

The portal venous flow is also altered in BCS and is typically slowed. Reversal of flow in the main portal vein may be seen as a result of the simultaneous occlusion of all three main HVs. In such scenarios, the PV acts as the liver's outflow vein, and on Doppler, hepatofugal flow may be appreciated.

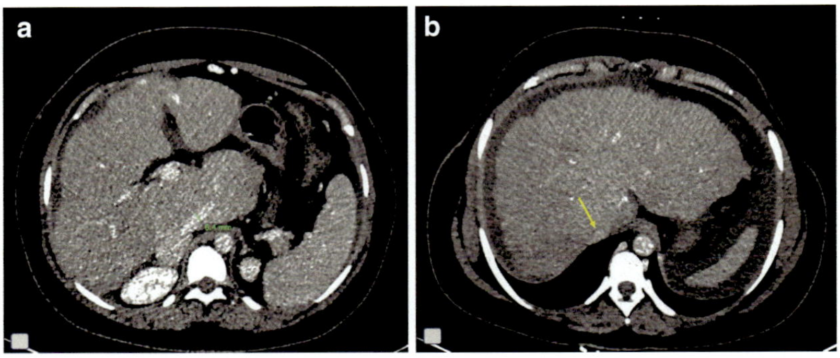

Fig. 7.3 (**a**) Axial portal venous phase CECT image in a 17-year-old known case of chronic BCS showing enlarged caudate vein. (**b**) Axial section at a higher level showing a significantly attenuated IVC (yellow arrow). Note the nodular outline and heterogeneous attenuation of the liver

7.6 Subacute BCS

Having an insidious onset, this form could take around 3–4 months to become symptomatic.

Volume redistribution and collateral development are the important imaging features in this form of BCS. The radiological features overlap with those of chronic BCS, and therefore, clinical presentation needs consideration in order to make this differentiation [21].

7.7 Chronic BCS

7.7.1 Parenchymal Changes

Histologically, this form shows bridging fibrosis between the HVs and portal tracts, and radiologically, one can appreciate contour irregularities, right lobe atrophy with hypertrophy of the caudate and left lobe (Fig. 7.4) along with the development of regenerative nodules. Parenchymal oedema is usually not a feature of this form of BCS. Furthermore, the 'flip-flop' enhancement pattern becomes more subtle. Collateral vessels and some amount of ascites are other findings that may be picked up in chronic BCS. Although non-visualization of HVs is considered a characteristic feature of BCS, patent HVs may sometimes not get visualized in the background of a cirrhotic parenchyma. Therefore, when performing ultrasonography in cases with severe parenchymal changes, Doppler is useful for detecting flow within the HVs that are otherwise not visualized on grayscale.

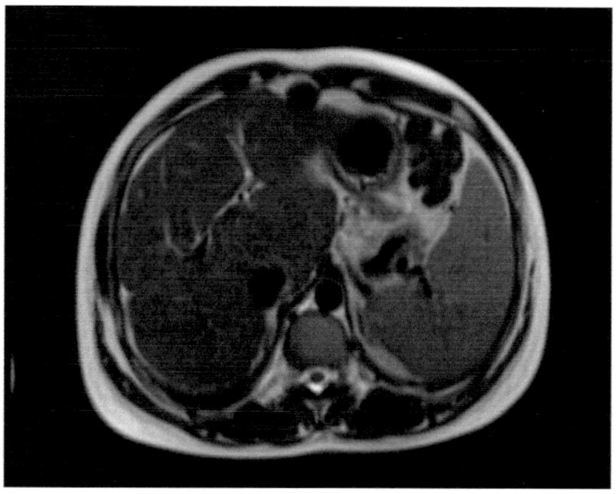

Fig. 7.4 Axial T2-weighted MR image of a 33-year-old chronic BCS patient showing marked caudate lobe hypertrophy

As aforementioned, the development of regenerative nodules is a typical feature of chronic BCS. These nodules are often multiple and vary in size from 5 mm to 4 cm. In chronic BCS, there are areas of insufficient blood supply that become atrophic. As a result, compensatory nodular hyperplasia ensues in the regions with adequate blood supply. These regenerative nodules have a predominant arterial supply and, thus, show marked arterial hyperenhancement. Hepatocellular carcinoma (HCC) may arise in the setting of chronic BCS and accounts for around 0.7% of all HCCs [22]. Radiological differentiation of HCC from regenerative nodules can become difficult at times. However, regenerative nodules tend to be multiple and smaller in size (usually <4 cm) and are disseminated throughout the liver with normal serum alpha-fetoprotein (AFP) levels.

7.7.2 Vascular Changes

Thrombosis of the HVs is not quite directly appreciable in chronic BCS. The hallmark of this phase is the formation of small, bridging intra- and extrahepatic veno-venous collaterals. The intrahepatic ones (Figs. 7.5 and 7.6) bridge the non-occluded segments of the HVs with either a normal vein, an accessory vein or with the caudate lobe vein. These vessels have typical appearances, e.g. 'hockey-stick', 'comma', 'undulated', 'h-shaped' or 'inverted U-shaped', and can be identified on both grayscale and Doppler ultrasonography. On spectral analysis, these collaterals show flat waveforms.

The extrahepatic collaterals in BCS develop mainly in the retroperitoneum, and the sites are different from those seen in cirrhosis. These collaterals can be assessed in four groups. The most frequently collateralized routes are the left renal–hemiazygous pathway (Fig. 7.7) and the vertebrolumbar azygous pathway (Fig. 7.8). The other commonly seen collaterals are the inferior

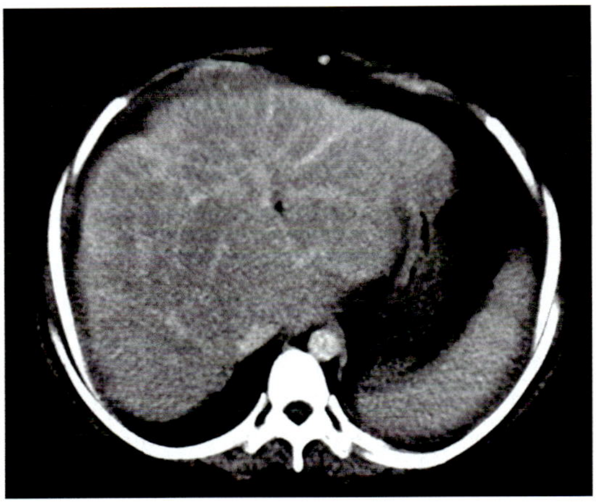

Fig. 7.5 Axial CECT image of a patient with BCS showing intrahepatic veno-venous collaterals

phrenic-pericardiophrenic collaterals and superficial abdominal wall collaterals between the superior and inferior epigastric veins (Fig. 7.9).

Features of portal hypertension may also be seen in patients with chronic BCS. The portal and splenic veins will commonly be dilated and may show reduced or hepatofugal flow. Multiple collaterals may be seen in the periportal and peripancreatic locations and also near the splenic hilum. Oesophageal and rectal varices may also be seen.

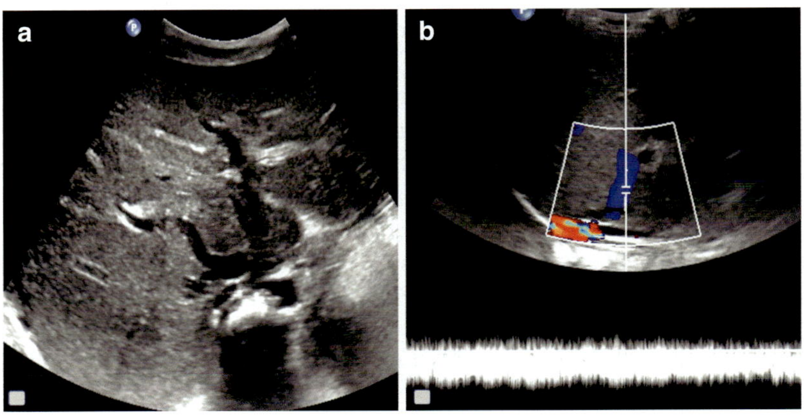

Fig. 7.6 Grayscale and Doppler images of another BCS patient showing characteristic 'U-shaped' intrahepatic collaterals. Note the flat waveform on spectral analysis of the intrahepatic collateral vessel

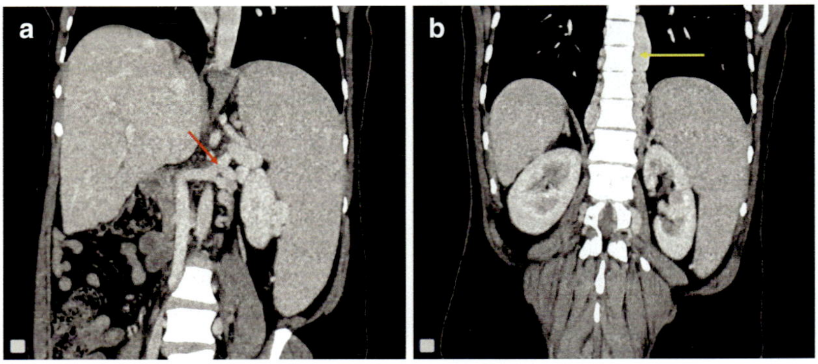

Fig. 7.7 Coronal reformatted images of CECT abdomen showing left renal hemiazygous pathway. A collateral is seen arising from the left renal vein (red arrow in (**a**)) and draining into an enlarged hemiazygous vein (yellow arrow in (**b**)). Also note the gross splenomegaly

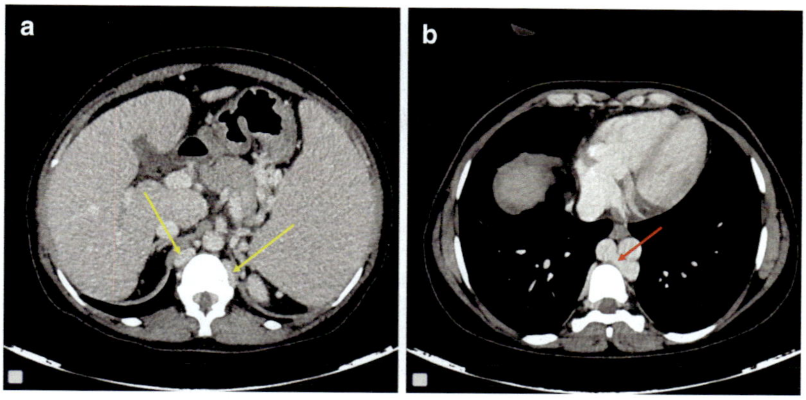

Fig. 7.8 Axial CECT abdomen images displaying vertebrolumbar azygous pathway. (**a**) Dilated and tortuous lumbar veins are seen (yellow arrows) draining into the azygous and hemiazygous veins. (**b**) Hemiazygous vein seen draining into the azygous vein (red arrow)

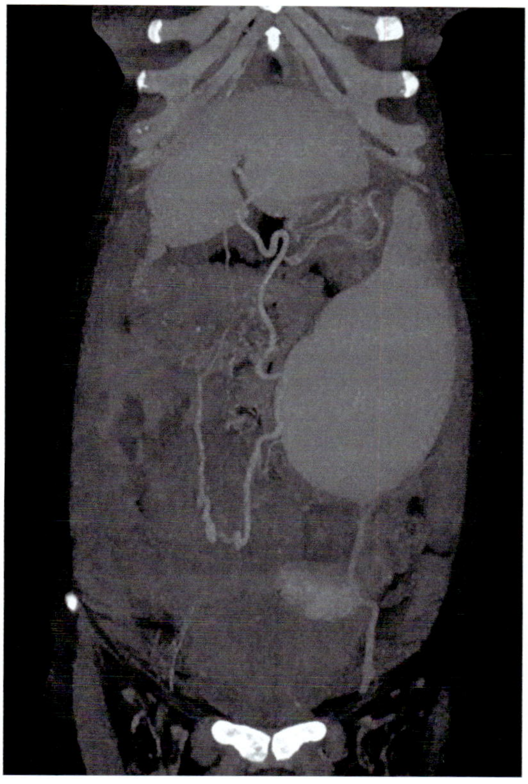

Fig. 7.9 Coronal maximum-intensity projection (MIP) image of CECT abdomen in a known case of chronic BCS displaying anterior abdominal wall collaterals. Communications of superior and inferior epigastric veins and superficial epigastric veins are seen

7.8 Nodules in BCS

One of the important complications of chronic BCS is the formation of focal hepatic lesions. Morphologically, these lesions represent a spectrum of entities ranging from benign to malignant nodules. The etiopathogenesis of these nodules is quite different from each other. However, the diagnosis of such nodules remains challenging due to considerable overlap in radiological features, and thus, patients may end up requiring tissue sampling in the form of biopsies.

7.9 Large Regenerative Nodules (LRNs)

The commonest nodules found in BCS patients are benign regenerative nodules. Different names have been given in literature to depict these nodules including adenomatous hyperplastic nodules, regenerative macronodules and FNH-like lesions. The pathogenesis of these nodules is not very clear. Alterations in the hepatic microcirculation and hepatocellular growth factors may contribute to their formation. Portocaval shunts created surgically may also contribute to the pathogenesis of these nodules. As described earlier, such regenerative nodules are often >10 in number, small (<4 cm) and hypervascular. On MRI (Fig. 7.10), LRNs show iso- to hypointense signal on T2-weighted images and appear hyperintense on T1-weighted images. On dynamic contrast imaging using the subtraction software, these nodules show intense arterial phase enhancement due to their increased arterial supply. These nodules increase in number progressively during the successive phases of dynamic MRI. Furthermore, the enhancement of these nodules persists until the late venous phase.

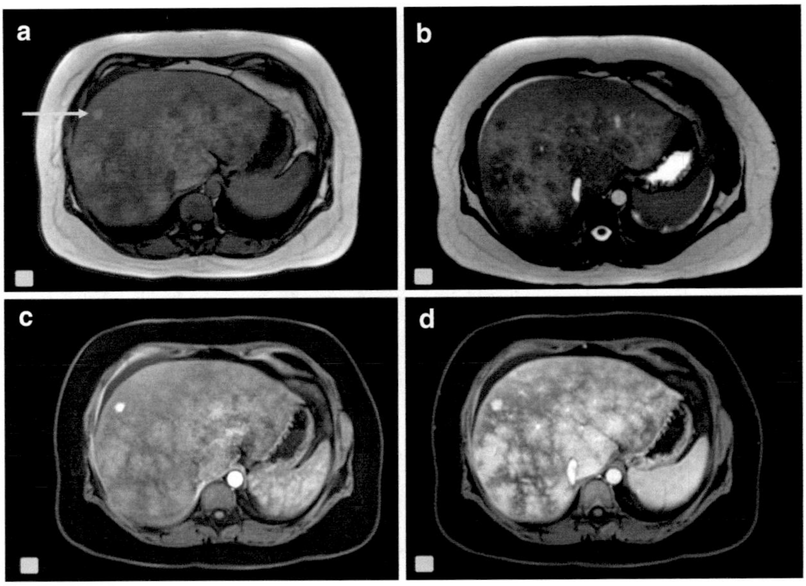

Fig. 7.10 Axial MR images of a patient with BCS showing a regenerative nodule. (**a**) T1-weighted image showing a small hyperintense nodule in segment VIII of the liver. (**b**) On T2-weighted imaging, the nodule shows hypointense signal. (**c**) The nodule shows hyperintense signal on post-contrast arterial phase images and (**d**) the enhancement persists into the portal venous phase

7.10 Hepatocellular Adenomas (HCAs)

These are benign hepatocellular proliferative lesions that are classically seen in normal livers of young women receiving oral contraceptive pills. Their late recognition may be because of issues in terminology, since, for a long time, a diagnosis of HCA has required a normal background liver. In a multi-centric collaborative study of 32 BCS cases, adenomas were noted in seven patients, mostly associated with LRNs and FNH-like nodules [23]. Ibarolla et al. [24] also reported 24 nodules in a series of four BCS patients which included six cases of hepatocellular adenomas diagnosed in two patients, in association with LRNs.

7.11 Hepatocellular Carcinomas

When compared with other vascular diseases of the liver, BCS patients are at a higher risk of developing HCC, with combined prevalence reaching up to 15.4% [25]. Studies have shown that HCCs occurring in BCS patients are usually greater in size than regenerative nodules with a median size of >4 cm [26, 27]. Just like LRNs, HCC forms in a background of extensive fibrosis (Fig. 7.11) and can also be multifocal. It is critical to note that an incorrect diagnosis of HCC may lead to unnecessary liver transplantation. Therefore, accurate tissue analysis is needed, including additional staining (reticulin) and immunophenotypical markers suggestive of malignancy, such as glypican-3.

It has been shown that in the imaging workup for HCCs, the typical features of arterial phase hyperenhancement and washout on portal phase are less valuable in the setting of BCS [28]. In a study that analyzed 49 BCS patients with 253 focal liver lesions (12 HCCs and 241 benign lesions), washout was seen in approximately 2/3 and 1/3 of benign and malignant lesions, respectively [29]. In such cases, AFP levels have been shown to perform well for discriminating LRN from HCC [26, 27, 29]. In addition, MR signal characteristics may also help in the differentiation. HCCs will appear hypointense on T1-weighted images and hyperintense on T2-weighted images as opposed to the appearance of benign nodules. Furthermore, diffusion restriction is usually a feature of malignant liver nodules.

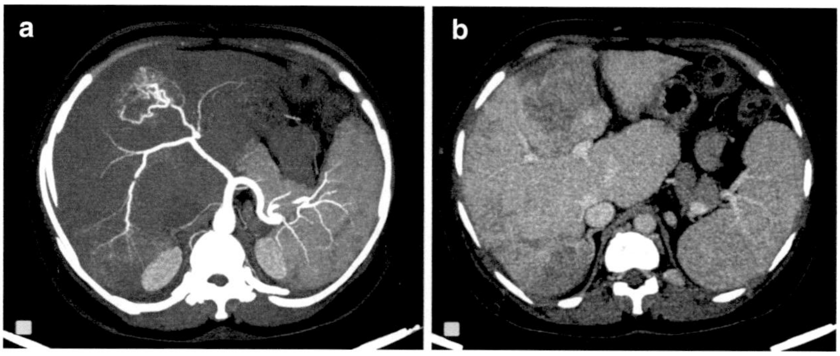

Fig. 7.11 HCCs in a known case of BCS. (**a**) Axial arterial phase maximum-intensity projection (MIP) image showing two hypervascular lesions in segments IV and VII of the liver. (**b**) Corresponding venous phase images showing washout of contrast from the two lesions. Also note the hypertrophied caudate lobe and dilated caudate lobe vein

7.12 Role of Venography in BCS

Inferior venocavography and hepatic venography are the gold standard diagnostic tests for BCS. At present, these tests are usually conducted to guide therapeutic interventional procedures. Multiple factors may alter the efficacy of these venographic tests, including the type of access, catheter site, amount of contrast administered, direction of flow in the IVC and the presence (or absence) of collaterals. As a result, there could be a significant disparity between the patient's actual haemodynamics and the information gathered from the venographic images. Thus, one must always perform a Doppler to complement the venography findings.

Venography shows the site and extent of the obstruction in the HVs and/or the IVC and also allows one to measure the intraluminal pressure necessary to assess the effects of treatment. It also provides the option of performing a simultaneous liver biopsy via the transvenous approach. A characteristic 'spider web appearance' has been described in chronic HV occlusion. This appearance arises because of the innumerable collateral vessels that are interconnected with each other. Due to caudate lobe hypertrophy, the IVC may be compressed in its retrohepatic segment. Inhomogeneous prolonged intense hepatogram with fine mottling may also be seen.

There are, however, certain limitations of direct venography that cannot be ignored [30]. Firstly, a technical failure leading to non-cannulation of the HVs may incorrectly be interpreted as HV occlusion, thus leading to an overdiagnosis of thrombosis/stenosis. Secondly, it is not possible to visualize the portion of the IVC that is distal to the site of obstruction due to diversion of contrast into the collaterals. Thus, a double catheter study may be required to assess the IVC below and above the level of obstruction. Lastly, the small intrahepatic collaterals may not be well detected with IVC graphy on multiple occasions.

Recently, MR venography has shown great potential in overcoming many of the limitations of IVC graphy. It can accurately depict the site and cause of obstruction with clear delineation of the IVC both above and below the obstruction. MR also performs excellently for the detection of both intra- and extrahepatic collaterals, PV obstruction and detection of tumour thrombi within the HVs and the IVC.

7.13 Interventions in Budd-Chiari Syndrome

7.13.1 Principles of Management

The current recommended therapeutic strategies for BCS are largely based on retrospective studies, expert guidelines and a few prospective studies [15, 31, 32]. Large randomized controlled trials to evaluate the different therapeutic strategies are lacking due to low incidence and varied stages of presentation. Goals of management include treatment of the underlying disease, correction of hepatic venous outflow tract obstruction and management of portal hypertension complications, taking into consideration the clinical stage of presentation. Thus, an individualized multidisciplinary stepwise strategy based on the invasiveness of intervention is proposed to achieve good long-term results [33, 34]. Initial medical therapy is aimed at treating the underlying prothrombotic disorder with anticoagulation and managing the complications of portal hypertension medically. The second line of management is to treat hepatic outflow tract obstruction with interventional radiology procedures like angioplasty, stenting and derivative techniques like transjugular intrahepatic portosystemic shunt (TIPS). Surgical decompressive techniques like mesoatrial and mesocaval shunts are considered when TIPS is not feasible. Liver transplantation is indicated in patients who fail to respond to the aforementioned treatment modalities and/or those who present with acute or fulminant liver failure. Several prognostic indices have been developed to assess the severity of disease, identify patients at risk of disease progression and predict mortality or outcome (Clichy score, New Clichy score, Child-Pugh score, MELD, Rotterdam score, BCS-TIPS score and AIIMS-HVOTO score). However, due to the unpredictable accuracy of these scores, there are currently no recommendations for universal usage of these indices [33, 35].

7.13.2 Medical Management

Anticoagulation is the first line of management once the diagnosis of BCS is made and is indicated in all patients irrespective of the underlying disease, even in patients who are initially asymptomatic [33–35]. It is aimed at achieving recanalization of thrombosed veins and preventing further thrombus formation or progression. Since there is a lack of a BCS-specific anticoagulation scheme, the current recommendation follows the anticoagulation regimen used in the treatment of deep vein thrombosis. Unfractionated heparin or low molecular weight heparin (LMWH) for the first 5–7 days in the acute setting and vitamin K agonists (VKAs) for lifelong administration are recommended, aimed at maintaining the international normalized ratio (INR) between 2 and 3. LMWH is preferred in pregnant patients. Currently, data on direct-acting oral anticoagulation (DAOC) is sparse with retrospective cohort studies identifying its safety, suggesting that it can be considered in those with maintained liver function. However, these drugs are not yet registered for the management of BCS, and hence, cautious usage is advised, especially in patients with associated renal failure [34]. The presence of gastroesophageal varices is not a contraindication to anticoagulation and should be considered after primary and secondary prophylaxis to manage variceal bleed as indicated [33].

In addition to anticoagulation, targeted therapies should also be considered for underlying prothrombotic disorders like myeloproliferative disorders and paroxysmal nocturnal haemoglobinuria. Haematological consultation is advised for the evaluation and management of underlying prothrombotic disorders [33]. The portal hypertension complications like ascites, variceal bleeding and other complications are managed like in cirrhotic patients.

7.13.3 Thrombolysis

There is currently limited experience with thrombolysis in BCS, with best results noted in those with recent and incomplete thrombosis, and managed by local and early infusion in combination with interventional procedures like angioplasty and stenting to restore venous outflow as evidenced by Sharma et al. [36]. Thrombolysis of the involved HVs can be performed by administering thrombolytic agents directly into HVs or mechanically by using balloon catheters. The technique for thrombolysis depends on the age of the thrombus, with pharmacological thrombolysis preferred in hyper-acute thrombus and combined pharmaco-mechanical thrombolysis reserved for those with long-standing older thrombi. Since there is a significant risk of major bleeding in the background of universal anticoagulation in BCS, thrombolysis should be attempted in selected cases [35].

7.13.4 Angioplasty and Stenting

A subset of BCS is due to segmental stenosis of HVs/IVC and membranous occlusion of the IVC, especially in Asian cohorts which can be managed by percutaneous angioplasty alone, thus restoring normal physiological hepatic outflow. Long-term favourable outcomes after angioplasty recanalization have been reported from large series [37, 38] with a recent meta-analysis revealing an 88.6% 5-year survival rate after recanalization [39]. However, frequent restenosis following angioplasty is well known, reported in up to 50% of patients within 1 year [40]. A recent RCT that compared angioplasty alone with routine stenting at the initial procedure reported a significantly reduced restenosis in patients who underwent routine stenting, without severe stent-related complications [41]. Stenting is associated with minimal risk of fracture and misplacement but can make future TIPS or liver transplantation more challenging. Hence, an individualized case-based approach with a stepwise management strategy based on the location and length of stenosis is recommended [42].

7.13.5 Technique of Angioplasty and Stenting

Transjugular, transfemoral and/or percutaneous transhepatic access routes are used based on the location and severity of stenosis. For membranous occlusion of the vena cava (MOVC) or segmental IVC stenosis, angioplasty is performed either through jugular or femoral venous access (Fig. 7.12), while a combined approach is used in resistant cases. Wide-bore, long sheaths (9–12Fr, 30–65 cm in length) are preferred for venous access as these provide a long, straight and stable pathway with better coaxial catheter control and manipulation. Initial recanalization attempts are made with standard 0.035-inch hydrophilic guidewires with angled and straight tips. In resistant cases, combined transfemoral and transjugular access is used for sharp recanalization with a TIPS puncture needle and a stiffening cannula.

For HV recanalization, the transjugular approach is preferred due to the favourable obtuse angle between the IVC and HVs. In our practice, we use a stepwise approach of transjugular access with an attempt at recanalization by using smooth tip guidewires followed by sharp recanalization using a TIPS puncture needle under ultrasound and fluoroscopy guidance to target the normal lumen of the HVs. In case of failure, percutaneous transhepatic access under ultrasound guidance is attempted (Fig. 7.13), and a balloon within the IVC can be used as a marker for sharp recanalization through the percutaneous route. Whenever a percutaneous approach is attempted, false tracking into the pericardial recess or capsular puncture should always be kept in mind, and cone beam CT may be used to confirm the location of the guidewire before balloon dilatation of the tract (Fig. 7.14). Once the occlusion or stenosed segment is crossed, the guidewire is snared across from the transjugular route, and further interventions are carried out through this route. If snaring is not successful, angioplasty is carried out through the transhepatic route; however, the access tract needs to be embolized with gel foam or coils to avoid the risk of haemoperitoneum. For accessory hepatic vein or collateral vein recanalization, the approach is chosen based on the angle of confluence with the IVC [35].

Most of the studies and expert consensus guidelines suggest a stepwise approach, with primary angioplasty followed by stenting as a bailout technique in case of residual stenosis or significant pressure gradient across the stenosed segments. Primary stenting is recommended in cases of occlusion rather than stenosis, and in cases of long-segment stenosis where the restenosis rate is high. The stent should always extend at least 1 cm beyond the margins of occluded/stenosed segments both proximally and distally. In a recent RCT by Wang et al. [41], patients were randomly divided into two

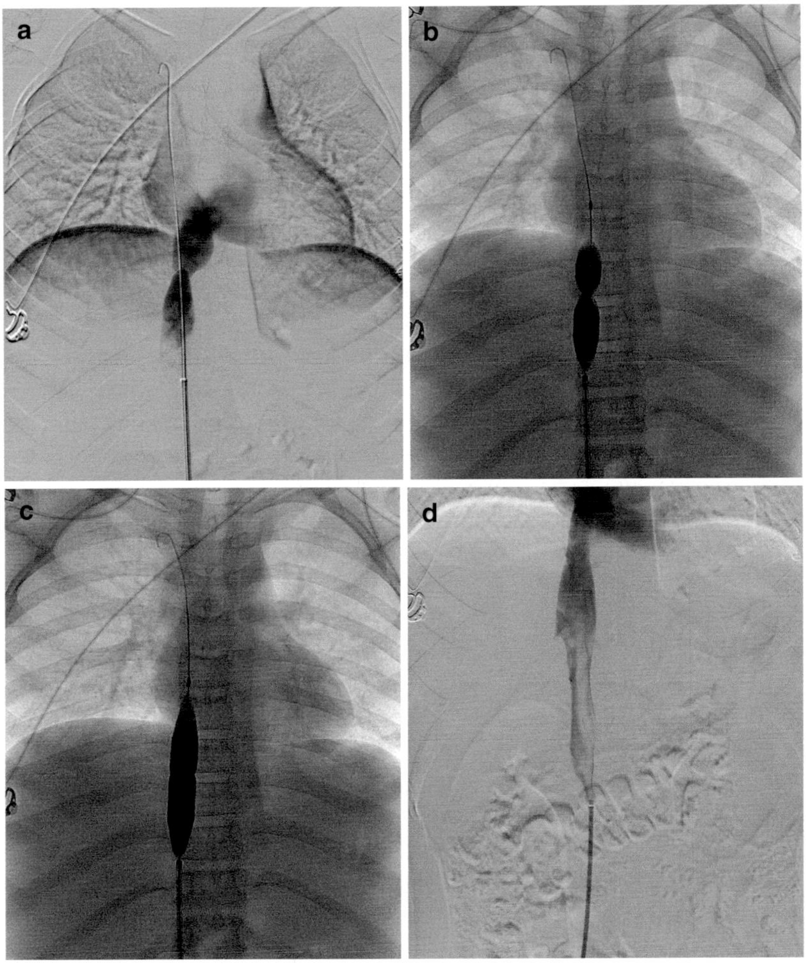

Fig. 7.12 Transfemoral venoplasty in a case of membranous occlusion of vena cava (MOVC). (**a**) DSA image showing stenosis of the retrohepatic IVC with a shelf-like filling defect suggestive of IVC web. (**b**) Venoplasty across the site of narrowing; note the formation of waist at the level of the IVC web. (**c**) Fluoro spot showing complete inflation of the balloon with effacement of the waist. (**d**) Post plasty venogram showing luminal gain with disappearance of the circumferential stenosis

groups—an angioplasty-only group ($n = 45$) and an angioplasty-plus-routine-stenting group ($n = 43$). During the median follow-up period of 27 months, the primary stenting group had a significantly higher proportion of patients free of restenosis (42 of 43 patients) compared to the angioplasty-only group (27 of 45 patients; $p < 0.0001$). In a retrospective study by Huang et al. [43], the long-term outcome of endovascular management for MOVC and segmental obstruction of the vena cava (SOVC) was compared. They concluded that balloon angioplasty alone could be sufficient for those with MOVC. However, for those with segmental obstruction, stenting was strongly recommended. Yang et al. [44], in their study of 38 BCS cases with MOVC, reported a successful outcome after balloon angioplasty without stent placement in all patients except one over a follow-up period of 8 years.

7.13.6 Follow-Up and Assessment of Treatment Response

Since BCS is associated with prothrombotic disorders, lifelong anticoagulation is advised, and INR should be maintained in the range of 2–3. Immediately after stenting or angioplasty, these patients should be started on LMWH, bridging with warfarin and lifelong anticoagulation thereafter. Post-intervention short-term follow-up is recommended at 1, 3 and 6 months with ultrasound and Doppler evaluation and every 6 months

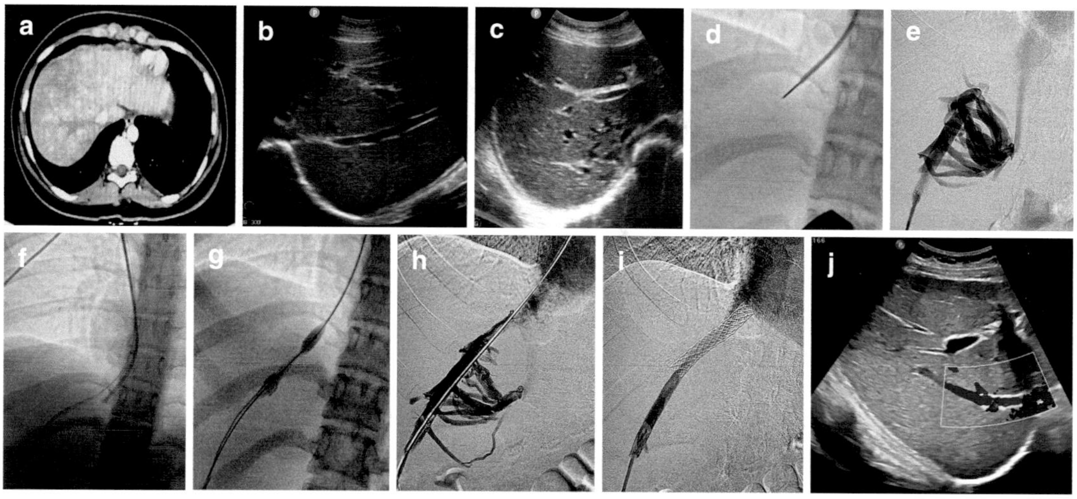

Fig. 7.13 RHV stenting in chronic BCS. (**a**–**c**) Axial CECT and USG image shows short segment RHV stenosis with intrahepatic veno-venous collateral. (**d**) Shows unsuccessful transjugular attempt to cannulate RHV. (**e**) Shows USG guided percutaneous access to RHV with complete occlusion and collaterals. (**f**–**h**) Crossing the occlusion through percutaneous approach with residual stenosis and collaterals after balloon angioplasty. (**i**) Post stenting run shows adequate dilatation. (**j**) USG-Doppler image 2 months post procedure shows good flow across the stent with reduced collaterals

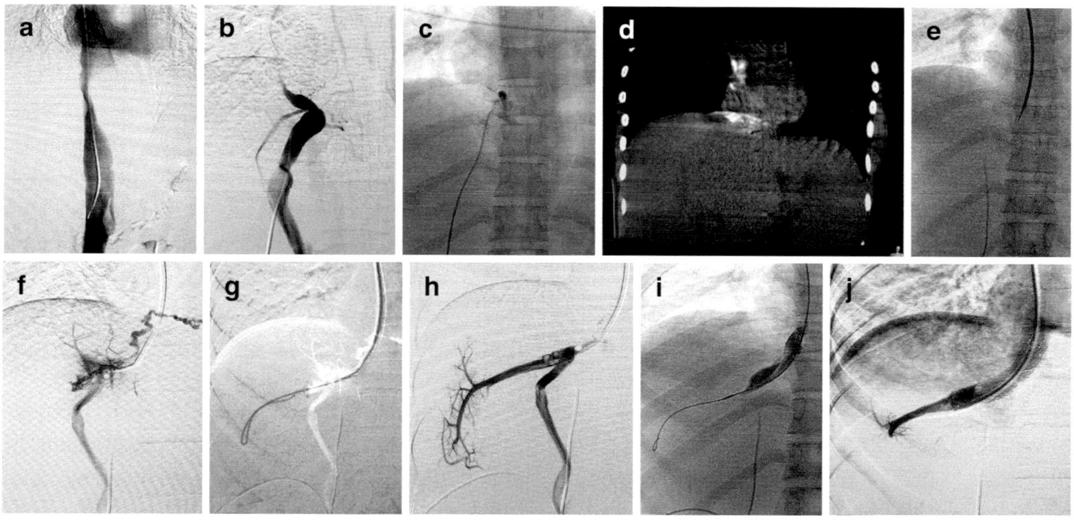

Fig. 7.14 A case of chronic BCS with short segment complete occlusion of right hepatic vein. (**a**) IVC gram showing narrowing of the retrohepatic segment secondary to extrinsic compression by the enlarged caudate lobe. No obvious collaterals were seen. Multiple attempts were made to cannulate the RHV via the transjugular route. However, these were unsuccessful. (**b**) Percutaneous access taken into one of the tributaries of the MHV. (**c, d**) Inadvertent intra-pericardial entry. As the course of guidewire was not along the IVC, the wire was withdrawn and contrast injected which showed spillage into the pericardial space. Cone beam CT confirmed the same. (**e**–**h**) RHV was finally cannulated using sharp recanalization via the transjugular route. (**i**) Angioplasty performed across the occluded segment followed by deployment of a self-expanding bare metallic stent. (**j**) Final run showing good luminal gain with establishment of forward flow across the RHV and resolution of collaterals

thereafter. In case of an inconclusive Doppler study, cross-sectional imaging is suggested, and venography is limited to symptomatic patients with features of re-occlusion or outflow obstruction on Doppler studies.

A good clinical response to intervention is defined by restoration of adequate blood flow across the occluded/stenosed segments and improvement in clinical symptoms as well as biochemical parameters (liver function tests including resolution of ascites and variceal bleed). Clinical improvement after interventions usually occurs within 2–4 weeks, whereas it takes 1–2 months in patients treated with anticoagulation alone for various reasons, and response may be delayed up to 5 months in 30% of patients who are slow responders [45, 46].

In case of restenosis or thrombosis of stents, recanalization should be attempted with thrombolysis and angioplasty based on the chronicity of presentation. However, persisting symptoms, failure to discontinue diuretics and no improvement in liver function tests are indicators of treatment failure and derivative techniques like TIPS/direct intrahepatic portosystemic shunt (DIPS) and surgical shunts should be considered in such patients. Liver transplantation is the last resort when all the above options fail.

7.13.7 TIPS

In comparison to surgical shunts, TIPS is a less invasive treatment of portal decompression and has shown very good long-term results, reducing the requirement for surgical shunts and liver transplantation [38, 47]. In a prospective multicentre study of 157 BCS patients by Seijo et al., 62 underwent TIPS, and only four cases needed liver transplantation, while just 2% underwent surgical shunting [32]. However, TIPS may not be technically feasible in a subset of BCS patients with complete HV obstruction, in which case a direct intrahepatic portosystemic shunt (DIPS) connecting the PV and the IVC is an acceptable alternative. A meta-analysis of 29 retrospective studies on 2255 BCS cases managed by endovascular techniques evaluated the outcomes of recanalization procedures and TIPS. Recanalization procedures had a success rate of 93.1% with a 5-year survival of 88.6%, while TIPS had a success rate of 96.4% and 5-year survival of 72.1% [39].

7.13.8 Indications and Technique of TIPS

As the current recommendations suggest a stepwise approach based on invasiveness of the intervention, TIPS is indicated in those patients who fail to respond to the first line of medical therapy and the second line of interventions like angioplasty and stenting. TIPS is also indicated in cases with progressive liver failure and in those with blockade of all three HVs. Some authors indicate early TIPS for BCS with the rationale of reducing chronic ischaemic insult that would otherwise lead to hepatic fibrosis and liver failure eventually [48, 49]. However, this approach has not been validated yet by other comparative studies and hence has not been adopted universally. Other authors propose early TIPS only in cases that develop signs of portal hypertension and recommend that medical management as sole treatment should be reserved only for asymptomatic or mildly symptomatic patients, as compensation by intrahepatic collateral vessels is adequate [50, 51]. Jaundice or prior history of encephalopathy is not a contraindication for TIPS. Right heart failure and severe pulmonary hypertension remain absolute contraindications for TIPS irrespective of underlying disease.

Preprocedural evaluation for TIPS includes prothrombotic disease work-up, assessment of coagulation, liver and renal function tests and cross-sectional imaging to evaluate liver parenchyma and venous anatomy. For patients with pre-existing coagulopathy, a recommended threshold of platelet count $>30 \times 10^9$/L and INR of <2.5 is suggested. Patients on anticoagulation need to withhold their medications before the procedure, as TIPS is a high-bleeding-risk procedure [52]. In patients with massive hydrothorax or ascites, fluid may need to be drained as it compromises respiratory function and may distort the anatomy of the cavo-atrial junction. Care should be taken to avoid reactionary pulmonary oedema, circulatory or renal impairment associated with large volume paracentesis, and albumin replacement or gradual drainage should be considered.

In patients with BCS, due to blockage of HVs, performing TIPS is more challenging and requires expertise. If cannulation of HVs is unsuccessful, then portal vein access is done directly from the IVC using a TIPS puncture needle, an approach known as DIPS (direct intrahepatic portosystemic shunt) (Fig. 7.15). The ideal puncture of the IVC is done at the level of HVs or within 6 cm of the cavo-atrial junction. Transabdominal ultrasound and fluoroscopic guidance are used to gain portal vein access, with technical modifications in difficult cases by using wires or snares within the PV as a target. Recent advances like intravascular ultrasound (IVUS) and intracardiac echocardiography are also used for guidance. In case of co-existing IVC stenosis or occlusion, IVC stenting should be considered first followed by TIPS stent through the interstices of the IVC stent. For TIPS, covered stents are preferred over bare metal stents owing to increased stent patency and reduced incidence of shunt thrombosis or failure, as reported by multiple studies. A 10-mm stent is recommended for TIPS, aimed at reducing the portosystemic gradient to less than 12 mm Hg with reduced risk of hepatic encephalopathy or decompensation [35].

7.13.9 Complications, Anticoagulation, and Post-Procedure Follow-Up

Acute complications include vascular injuries, liver laceration, intraparenchymal or subcapsular haematoma and haemoperitoneum, and most of them can be managed conservatively with a low incidence of mortality due to TIPS. Long-term complications include hepatic encephalopathy (<25%), shunt dysfunction (in up to 40%) and post-TIPS liver failure in rare instances due to portal flow diversion, causing a reduction of liver perfusion with possible progression of liver failure. BCS is associated with thrombosis of TIPS stents, and hence, it is suggested to start anticoagulation with LMWH 6–12 h after the procedure and conversion

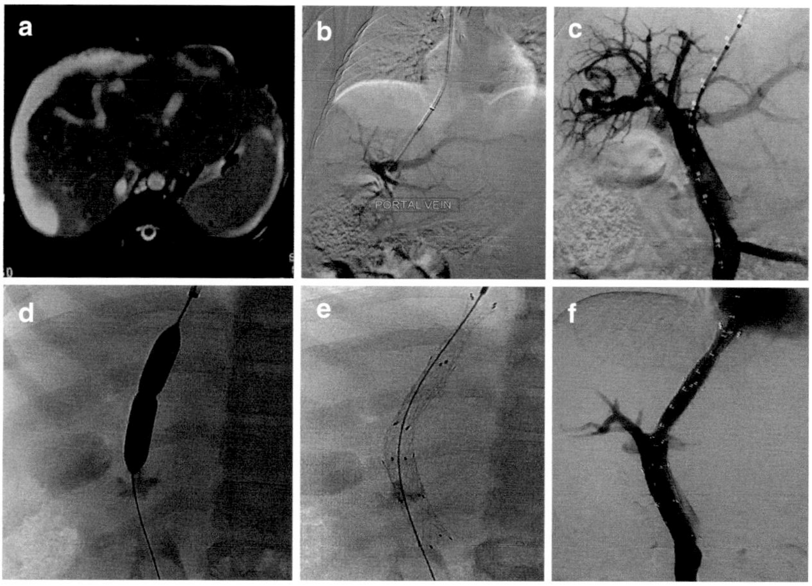

Fig. 7.15 Type II chronic BCS in a 32-year-old lady. (**a**) T2W axial image shows intrahepatic veno-venous collateral with non-visualized hepatic veins and changes of chronic BCS. IVC is normal. (**b**–**f**) DSA images show transjugular approach to left branch of portal vein with balloon plasty of the tract and stent graft placement, with good flow across the graft

to long-term anticoagulation with VKAs. Patients are regularly followed up with a colour Doppler study for stent patency at 1, 3 and 6 months and at 6–12 months interval thereafter [35].

Liver stiffness measurement (LSM) using ultrasound elastography is one of the promising tools to assess response to interventions in BCS. LSM reflects liver fibrosis as well as liver congestion and is correlated with HVPG in chronic liver disease [53]. Few studies have demonstrated the utility of LSM in assessing response to interventions wherein the values reduced following interventions suggesting good response [54, 55]. However, further studies are required to determine the efficacy of LSM in predicting long-term outcome following interventions.

7.13.10 Liver Transplantation

Liver transplantation (LT) is indicated as a primary intervention in patients with BCS presenting with acute liver failure or advanced decompensated liver cirrhosis and as a last therapeutic approach in patients who do not respond to medical management or interventions like TIPS and stenting of HVs and the IVC. In the setting of BCS with acute liver failure, TIPS may still be attempted while the patient is waiting for a transplant or when a transplant is not feasible. The BCS-TIPS Prognostic Index score is a TIPS-specific score to identify patients of BCS who could have a poor outcome following TIPS with very low 1-year survival [12]. Based on this study, patients with a BCS-TIPS PI score of >7 may be considered for liver transplantation. However, this has not been validated, and no clear consensus exists on its usefulness. The 5-year survival following LT is estimated to be around 71% in a large European study [56], which is similar to TIPS (78% without requiring liver transplant), reinforcing the benefit of a stepwise approach and saving organs for other indications of LT [47]. Since most often the patients of BCS have underlying prothrombotic disorders and the incidence of HV thrombosis following LT is in the range of 20%, long-term anticoagulation therapy is suggested.

7.14 Conclusion

Imaging plays an important role in the diagnosis of BCS, whereas radiological interventions remain the mainstay in the management of BCS. While the vascular changes are well seen on Doppler ultrasonography, cross-sectional imaging, especially MRI, is required for the evaluation of the liver parenchyma and the various nodules seen in BCS. Radiological interventions like angioplasty and stenting help to achieve anatomical recanalization of the hepatic outflow vein. TIPS is indicated in patients who fail to respond to these interventions, with good overall survival similar to LT. Hence, a stepwise approach from less invasive (anticoagulation) to more invasive (liver transplant) therapy is recommended.

References

1. Janssen HLA, Garcia-Pagan J-C, Elias E, Mentha G, Hadengue A, Valla D-C, et al. Budd-Chiari syndrome: a review by an expert panel. J Hepatol. 2003;38(3):364–71.
2. McCuskey RS. Morphological mechanisms for regulating blood flow through hepatic sinusoids. Liver. 2000;20(1):3–7.
3. McCuskey RS, Reilly FD. Hepatic microvasculature: dynamic structure and its regulation. Semin Liver Dis. 1993;13(1):1–12.
4. Sahani D, Mehta A, Blake M, Prasad S, Harris G, Saini S. Preoperative hepatic vascular evaluation with CT and MR angiography: implications for surgery. Radiographics. 2004;24(5):1367–80.
5. Barbaro B, Soglia G, Alvaro G, Vellone M, Giuliante F, Nuzzo G, et al. Hepatic veins in presurgical planning of hepatic resection: what a radiologist should know. Abdom Imaging. 2013;38(3):442–60.
6. Burk KS, Singh AK, Vagefi PA, Sahani D. Pretransplantation imaging workup of the liver donor and recipient. Radiol Clin North Am. 2016;54(2):185–97.
7. Cheng YF, Huang TL, Chen CL, Chen TY, Huang CC, Ko SF, et al. Variations of the middle and inferior right hepatic vein: application in hepatectomy. J Clin Ultrasound. 1997;25(4):175–82.
8. McGahan JP, Goldberg BB. Diagnostic ultrasound: a logical approach. Ultrasound Q. 1998;14(3):189.
9. Li Y, De Stefano V, Li H, Zheng K, Bai Z, Guo X, et al. Epidemiology of Budd-Chiari syndrome: a systematic review and meta-analysis. Clin Res Hepatol Gastroenterol. 2019;43(4):468–74.

10. Okuda H, Yamagata H, Obata H, Iwata H, Sasaki R, Imai F, et al. Epidemiological and clinical features of Budd-Chiari syndrome in Japan. J Hepatol. 1995;22(1):1–9.
11. Ki M, Choi HY, Kim K-A, Kim BH, Jang ES, Jeong S-H. Incidence, prevalence and complications of Budd-Chiari syndrome in South Korea: a nationwide, population-based study. Liver Int. 2016;36(7):1067–73.
12. Shalimar, Kumar A, Kedia S, Sharma H, Gamanagatti SR, Gulati GS, et al. Hepatic venous outflow tract obstruction: treatment outcomes and development of a new prognostic score. Aliment Pharmacol Ther. 2016;43(11):1154–67.
13. Ding P-X, Han X-W, Liu C, Zhang Y, Cheng A-L, Wu Y, et al. Long-term outcomes of individualized treatment strategy in treatment of type I Budd-Chiari syndrome in 456 patients. Liver Int. 2019;39(8):1577–86.
14. Ludwig J, Hashimoto E, McGill DB, van Heerden JA. Classification of hepatic venous outflow obstruction: ambiguous terminology of the Budd-Chiari syndrome. Mayo Clin Proc. 1990;65(1):51–5.
15. Darwish Murad S, Plessier A, Hernandez-Guerra M, Fabris F, Eapen CE, Bahr MJ, et al. Etiology, management, and outcome of the Budd-Chiari syndrome. Ann Intern Med. 2009;151(3):167–75.
16. Hadengue A, Poliquin M, Vilgrain V, Belghiti J, Degott C, Erlinger S, et al. The changing scene of hepatic vein thrombosis: recognition of asymptomatic cases. Gastroenterology. 1994;106(4):1042–7.
17. Bolondi L, Gaiani S, Li Bassi S, Zironi G, Bonino F, Brunetto M, et al. Diagnosis of Budd-Chiari syndrome by pulsed Doppler ultrasound. Gastroenterology. 1991;100(5 Pt 1):1324–31.
18. DeLeve LD, Valla D-C, Garcia-Tsao G. Vascular disorders of the liver. Hepatology. 2009;49(5):1729–64.
19. Rossi S, Rosa L, Ravetta V, Cascina A, Quaretti P, Azzaretti A, et al. Contrast-enhanced versus conventional and color Doppler sonography for the detection of thrombosis of the portal and hepatic venous systems. Am J Roentgenol. 2006;186(3):763–73.
20. Bargalló X, Gilabert R, Nicolau C, García-Pagán JC, Bosch J, Brú C. Sonography of the caudate vein: value in diagnosing Budd-Chiari syndrome. Am J Roentgenol. 2003;181(6):1641–5.
21. Bansal V, Gupta P, Sinha S, Dhaka N, Kalra N, Vijayvergiya R, et al. Budd-Chiari syndrome: imaging review. Br J Radiol. 2018;91(1092):20180441.
22. Takayasu K, Muramatsu Y, Moriyama N, Wakao F, Makuuchi M, Takayama T, et al. Radiological study of idiopathic Budd-Chiari syndrome complicated by hepatocellular carcinoma. A report of four cases. Am J Gastroenterol. 1994;89(2):249–53.
23. Sempoux C, Paradis V, Komuta M, Wee A, Calderaro J, Balabaud C, et al. Hepatocellular nodules expressing markers of hepatocellular adenomas in Budd-Chiari syndrome and other rare hepatic vascular disorders. J Hepatol. 2015;63(5):1173–80.
24. Ibarrola C, Castellano VM, Colina F. Focal hyperplastic hepatocellular nodules in hepatic venous outflow obstruction: a clinicopathological study of four patients and 24 nodules. Histopathology. 2004;44(2):172–9.
25. Ren W, Qi X, Yang Z, Han G, Fan D. Prevalence and risk factors of hepatocellular carcinoma in Budd-Chiari syndrome: a systematic review. Eur J Gastroenterol Hepatol. 2013;25(7):830–41.
26. Zhang R, Qin S, Zhou Y, Song Y, Sun L. Comparison of imaging characteristics between hepatic benign regenerative nodules and hepatocellular carcinomas associated with Budd-Chiari syndrome by contrast enhanced ultrasound. Eur J Radiol. 2012;81(11):2984–9.
27. Moucari R, Rautou P-E, Cazals-Hatem D, Geara A, Bureau C, Consigny Y, et al. Hepatocellular carcinoma in Budd-Chiari syndrome: characteristics and risk factors. Gut. 2008;57(6):828–35.
28. Vilgrain V, Paradis V, Van Wettere M, Valla D, Ronot M, Rautou P-E. Benign and malignant hepatocellular lesions in patients with vascular liver diseases. Abdom Radiol N Y. 2018;43(8):1968–77.
29. Van Wettere M, Purcell Y, Bruno O, Payancé A, Plessier A, Rautou P-E, et al. Low specificity of washout to diagnose hepatocellular carcinoma in nodules showing arterial hyperenhancement in patients with Budd-Chiari syndrome. J Hepatol. 2019;70(6):1123–32.
30. Kalra N, Gorsi U, Khandelwal N. Imaging and interventions in hepatic venous outflow tract obstruction. In: Gupta AK, Khandelwal N, Garg A, editors. Diagnostic radiology: gastrointestinal and hepatobiliary imaging. 4th ed. New Delhi: Jaypee Brothers Medical Publishers (P) Ltd.; 2017. p. 336–52.
31. Plessier A, Sibert A, Consigny Y, Hakime A, Zappa M, Denninger M-H, et al. Aiming at minimal invasiveness as a therapeutic strategy for Budd-Chiari syndrome. Hepatology. 2006;44(5):1308–16.
32. Seijo S, Plessier A, Hoekstra J, Dell'era A, Mandair D, Rifai K, et al. Good long-term outcome of Budd-Chiari syndrome with a step-wise management. Hepatology. 2013;57(5):1962–8.
33. Simonetto DA, Singal AK, Garcia-Tsao G, Caldwell SH, Ahn J, Kamath PS. ACG clinical guideline: disorders of the hepatic and mesenteric circulation. Am J Gastroenterol. 2020;115(1):18–40.
34. Hernández-Gea V, De Gottardi A, Leebeek FWG, Rautou P-E, Salem R, Garcia-Pagan JC. Current knowledge in pathophysiology and management of Budd-Chiari syndrome and non-cirrhotic non-tumoral splanchnic vein thrombosis. J Hepatol. 2019;71(1):175–99.
35. Shukla A, Shreshtha A, Mukund A, Bihari C, Eapen CE, Han G, et al. Budd-Chiari syndrome: consensus guidance of the Asian Pacific association for the study of the liver (APASL). Hepatol Int. 2021;15(3):531–67.
36. Sharma S, Texeira A, Texeira P, Elias E, Wilde J, Olliff SP. Pharmacological thrombolysis in Budd Chiari syndrome: a single Centre experience and review of the literature. J Hepatol. 2004;40(1):172–80.

37. Han G, Qi X, Zhang W, He C, Yin Z, Wang J, et al. Percutaneous recanalization for Budd-Chiari syndrome: an 11-year retrospective study on patency and survival in 177 Chinese patients from a single center. Radiology. 2013;266(2):657–67.
38. Eapen CE, Velissaris D, Heydtmann M, Gunson B, Olliff S, Elias E. Favourable medium term outcome following hepatic vein recanalisation and/or transjugular intrahepatic portosystemic shunt for Budd Chiari syndrome. Gut. 2006;55(6):878–84.
39. Zhang F, Wang C, Li Y. The outcomes of interventional treatment for Budd-Chiari syndrome: systematic review and meta-analysis. Abdom Imaging. 2015;40(3):601–8.
40. Valla D-C. Primary Budd-Chiari syndrome. J Hepatol. 2009;50(1):195–203.
41. Wang Q, Li K, He C, Yuan X, Luo B, Qi X, et al. Angioplasty with versus without routine stent placement for Budd-Chiari syndrome: a randomised controlled trial. Lancet Gastroenterol Hepatol. 2019;4(9):686–97.
42. Magaz M, Soy G, García-Pagán JC. Budd-Chiari syndrome: anticoagulation, TIPS, or transplant. Curr Hepatol Rep. 2020;19(3):197–202.
43. Huang Q, Shen B, Zhang Q, Xu H, Zu M, Gu Y, et al. Comparison of long-term outcomes of endovascular management for membranous and segmental inferior vena cava obstruction in patients with primary Budd–Chiari syndrome. Circ Cardiovasc Interv. 2016;9(3):e003104.
44. Yang XL, Cheng TO, Chen CR. Successful treatment by percutaneous balloon angioplasty of Budd-Chiari syndrome caused by membranous obstruction of inferior vena cava: 8-year follow-up study. J Am Coll Cardiol. 1996;28(7):1720–4.
45. Mukund A, Pargewar SS, Desai SN, Rajesh S, Sarin SK. Changes in liver congestion in patients with Budd-Chiari syndrome following endovascular interventions: assessment with transient elastography. J Vasc Interv Radiol. 2017;28(5):683–7.
46. Shukla A, Bhatia SJ. Outcome of patients with primary hepatic venous obstruction treated with anticoagulants alone. Indian J Gastroenterol. 2010;29(1):8–11.
47. Garcia-Pagán JC, Heydtmann M, Raffa S, Plessier A, Murad S, Fabris F, et al. TIPS for Budd-Chiari syndrome: long-term results and prognostics factors in 124 patients. Gastroenterology. 2008;135(3):808–15.
48. Rosenqvist K, Sheikhi R, Eriksson L-G, Rajani R, Rorsman F, Sangfelt P, et al. Endovascular treatment of symptomatic Budd–Chiari syndrome—in favour of early transjugular intrahepatic portosystemic shunt. Eur J Gastroenterol Hepatol. 2016;28(6):656–60.
49. Mancuso A. An update on the management of Budd-Chiari syndrome: the issues of timing and choice of treatment. Eur J Gastroenterol Hepatol. 2015;27(3):200–3.
50. Khan F, Mehrzad H, Tripathi D. Timing of transjugular intrahepatic portosystemic stent-shunt in Budd–Chiari syndrome: a UK hepatologist's perspective. J Transl Intern Med. 2018;6(3):97–104.
51. Sun Y, Ma X, Feng L, Guan S, Wang Z-W. Compensation by collateral circulation determines invasive therapeutic indications for patients with Budd-Chiari syndrome. Gut. 2012;61(12):1779–80.
52. Patel IJ, Rahim S, Davidson JC, Hanks SE, Tam AL, Walker TG, et al. Society of Interventional Radiology Consensus Guidelines for the periprocedural management of thrombotic and bleeding risk in patients undergoing percutaneous image-guided interventions—part II: recommendations: endorsed by the Canadian Association for Interventional Radiology and the cardiovascular and Interventional Radiological Society of Europe. J Vasc Interv Radiol. 2019;30(8):1168–1184.e1.
53. Song J, Ma Z, Huang J, Liu S, Luo Y, Lu Q, et al. Comparison of three cut-offs to diagnose clinically significant portal hypertension by liver stiffness in chronic viral liver diseases: a meta-analysis. Eur Radiol. 2018;28(12):5221–30.
54. Xu P, Lyu L, Ge H, Sami MU, Liu P, Hu C, et al. Segmental liver stiffness evaluated with magnetic resonance elastography is responsive to endovascular intervention in patients with Budd-Chiari syndrome. Korean J Radiol. 2019;20(5):773–80.
55. Wang H-W, Shi H-N, Cheng J, Xie F, Luo Y-K, Tang J. Real-time shear wave elastography (SWE) assessment of short- and long-term treatment outcome in Budd-Chiari syndrome: a pilot study. PLoS One. 2018;13(5):e0197550.
56. Mentha G, Giostra E, Majno PE, Bechstein WO, Neuhaus P, O'Grady J, et al. Liver transplantation for Budd-Chiari syndrome: a European study on 248 patients from 51 centres. J Hepatol. 2006;44(3):520–8.

8 Autoimmune Liver Diseases: Clinical and Imaging Perspective

Yashwant Patidar and Vinod Arora

Abbreviations

2-OADC	2-Oxo-acid dehydrogenase complex
AIH	Autoimmune hepatitis
AILD	Autoimmune liver disease
ANA	Antinuclear
Anti SLA	Anti-soluble liver antigen
ASC	Autoimmune sclerosing cholangitis
ASMA	Anti-smooth muscles antibodies
AZA	Azathioprine
BCOADC-E2	Branched-chain 2-OADC E2 subunit
ERCP	Endoscopic retrograde cholangiopancreatography
FXR	Farnesoid X receptor
OGDC-E2	2-Oxoglutaric acid dehydrogenase complex E2 subunit
PBC	Primary biliary cholangitis
PDC-E2	Pyruvate dehydrogenase complex E2 subunit
PPAR-α	Peroxisome proliferator activated receptor-α
PSC	Primary sclerosing cholangitis
UDCA	Ursodeoxycholic acid

Y. Patidar (✉)
Department of Interventional Radiology, Institute of Liver and Biliary Sciences, New Delhi, India

V. Arora
Department of Hepatology, Institute of Liver and Biliary Sciences, New Delhi, India

8.1 Introduction

The autoimmune liver disease comprises broadly three diseases confined to the liver: autoimmune hepatitis (AIH), primary biliary cholangitis (PBC) and primary sclerosing cholangitis (PSC) [1]. These diseases may affect people of all ages and usually have a chronic course and will require life-long follow-up [1]. Autoimmune hepatitis is characterised by chronic hypergammaglobulinemia, the presence of autoantibodies and elevated IgG [2]. Primary biliary cholangitis is a disease of small intrahepatic bile ducts, characterised by the presence of antimitochondrial antibodies (AMAs), and is usually a disease of middle-aged females [3]. Primary sclerosing cholangitis is a chronic inflammatory cholangiopathy, which usually affects males and is associated with inflammatory bowel disease in up to 80% of patients [4]. It is associated with the structuring and destruction of medium and small intrahepatic bile ducts. Similarly, in the paediatric population, autoimmune diseases of the liver include autoimmune hepatitis and autoimmune sclerosing cholangitis. Autoimmune sclerosing cholangitis is an immune-mediated destruction of bile ducts, characteristically seen in older males at prepubertal age [5].

© The Author(s), under exclusive license to Springer Nature Singapore Pte Ltd. 2025

B. Sureka (ed.), *Hepato-Pancreatico Biliary Imaging*, https://doi.org/10.1007/978-981-95-1699-5_8

8.2 Pathogenesis

There is a genetic predisposition to autoimmunity, which, in combination with the environmental factors, leads to an immune response and hepatic/biliary injury [6]. The immune response to injury, the response of hepatic and biliary epithelia and the effect of cholestasis determine the outcome in AIH, PSC and PBC. HLA DR8 in PBC, HLA-B * 08 in PSC and DRB1 * 03-DRB1 * 04 in AIH are the risk-conferring HLA haplotype in different autoimmune liver diseases [7]. The environment also influences the outcome in autoimmune liver disease, such as nitrofurantoin and minocycline, which trigger autoimmune hepatitis [8]. Some bacteria, such as *E. coli*, have an overlap with mitochondrial proteins and may contribute to pathogenesis in PBC [9]. Xenobiotics such as dyes and chemicals have been implicated as pathogenic in inciting the injury [10]. T-cell-mediated destruction is central to the pathogenesis of AIH. This may be secondary to loss of central tolerance which may explain the increased prevalence of AIH in AIRE deficiency and autoimmune polyendocrinopathy-candidiasis-ectodermal dystrophy [11]. In PBC, loss of tolerance to mitochondrial antigen directed against the lipoic acid residue triggers the biliary destruction. Xenobiotic-induced modification of the lipoic acid residue of pyruvate dehydrogenase E2 complex plays a role in PBC [12]. Similarly, in PSC, there is a clear T-cell infiltrate; however, no specific auto-antigen has been identified. Recruitment of Th-1 and Th-17 cells into the hepatic sinusoids is mechanistically important [13]. All autoimmune liver diseases (AILDs) are linked to abnormalities in the Th-17 pathway. A higher proportion of Th-17 cells and proinflammatory cytokines linked to it (IL-17 and TNF-α) are increased correspondingly. IL-12 and IL-23 are produced by antigen-presenting cells and are key parts of the Th-17 pathway [14]. Bile ducts, apart from being a victim of the immune-mediated injury, also have a role in disease progression. Cholangiocyte with altered apoptosis may act as a self-antigen, and increased senescence may be noted instead of undergoing apoptosis, which may lead to increased chemokine synthesis (CX3CL1 and CXCL8), resulting in immune cell recruitment [15]. Cholangiocytes also express toll-like receptor which recruits the inflammatory cells such as NK cells, T cells and macrophages, resulting in the disruption of the tight junction between cholangiocytes [16]. Lymphocytes from the gut are activated and recruited to the liver with the help of an expression molecule via VAP-1 which recruits lymphocytes to the area of inflammation [17]. These diseases are a result of complex interaction between the genetic and environmental exposure, leading to biliary and chronic inflammation of hepatobiliary cells.

We will be discussing in brief the disease aforementioned.

8.3 Autoimmune Hepatitis

AIH occurs in all age groups and ethnic groups, with Alaskan natives having a high prevalence of icteric hepatitis [18] and African Americans having accelerated progression and a higher rate of recurrence following liver transplant [19]. Female predominance is noted in adults and children with a bimodal age of presentation (10–30 years and 40–60 years of age). Diagnosis of AIH is characterised by interface hepatitis, elevated aspartate and alanine transaminases, presence of autoantibodies and elevated immunoglobulin G levels [20]. Viral hepatitis, drug-induced liver injury and Wilson's disease may mimic autoimmune hepatitis.

It is broadly classified into two types: In type I, antinuclear antibodies (ANAs) and anti-smooth muscle antibodies (ASMAs) are noted, while in type II, anti-liver-kidney microsome (LKM) antibodies are noted. These autoantibodies are negative in up to 20% of cases, i.e. seronegative AIH [21]. In acute stage, autoantibodies may be negative. In AIH, ANAs are the most common antibody seen in up to 80% of patients, ASMAs can be seen in up to 63%, and anti-LKM is seen in 3% of the adult population [21]. A total of 49% of patients have ANA/ASMA/anti-LKM as an isolated antibody, while 51% may have a combination of the antibodies. Anti-soluble liver antigen (anti-SLA) can be seen in 7–22% of patients with type I AIH; however, it has the highest specificity for the diagnosis of AIH. The presence of anti-SLA is usually associated with severe disease and relapse following withdrawal of medicine [22].

8.4 Histology

The histological hallmark is interface hepatitis, which is followed by plasma cell infiltration (66%), lobular inflammation (47%) and centrilobular necrosis in around 29% of patients [23]. Rosetting can be seen in around 33% of patients, while emperipolesis is also commonly noted. Non-alcoholic steatohepatitis can be seen in up to 17–30% of patients, which needs to be identified as an increased risk of liver-related mortality [24].

AIH-acute liver failure (ALF) usually affects the centrilobular zone. Central perivenulitis (65%), plasma cell inflammatory infiltrate and hepatic necrosis may be noted [25].

8.5 Clinical Features

Easy fatiguability is the most common presentation seen in around 85% of patients. Other features of chronic liver disease may be present. Acute AIH or AIH-ALF may present as hepatic encephalopathy in 3–6% of patients [26].

Concurrent autoimmune disease may be seen alongside AIH. Autoimmune thyroiditis can be seen in up to 10–18% of patients with type I AIH, while thyroid disorders, diabetes and alopecia can be seen in type II AIH.

8.6 Radiological Features

The role of imaging is to rule out other causes of chronic hepatitis and to evaluate complications of cirrhosis and autoimmune involvement of other organs. On USG and CT scan, imaging findings are non-specific and may range from hepatomegaly to cirrhosis. Hence, MRI is the imaging of choice.

In early disease, patchy areas of hyperintensity are seen in T2W MRI sequences (Fig. 8.1a). Early enhancement is also seen in these areas. The findings suggest active inflammation, which is transient and non-specific [27].

As the disease further progresses, areas of confluent hepatic fibrosis may develop with associated capsular retraction and surface nodularity (Fig. 8.1b). Areas of fibrosis appear hypointense on all MRI sequences and show delayed enhancement.

End-stage disease is characterised by global cirrhosis with a shrunken liver. Unlike other causes of cirrhosis, there is atrophy of the caudate lobe. Regenerative and dysplastic nodules may develop in the cirrhotic liver; however, the development of hepatocellular carcinoma is a rare event [28].

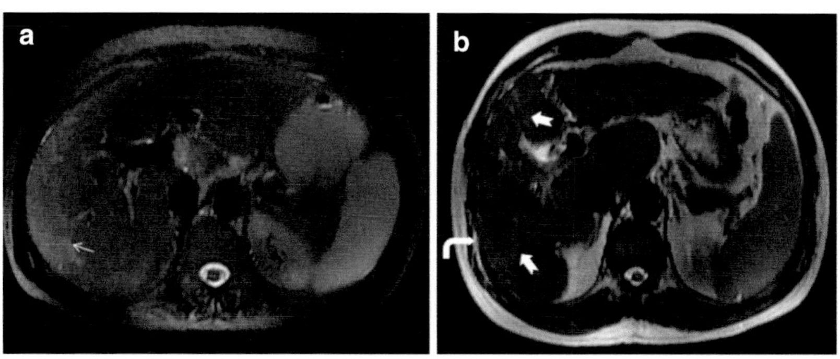

Fig. 8.1 Imaging findings in biopsy-proven cases of AIH. (**a**): Early inflammation is characterized by patchy reticular hyperintensities in T2-weighted sequences (white arrow) and hepatomegaly. No evidence of surface nodularity is seen. (**b**): A different patient in the later stages of the disease shows areas of confluent fibrosis (white block arrows) with subtle capsular retraction (white curved arrow). The liver appears cirrhotic

8.7 Treatment

The aim of the treatment is to control symptoms, slow down the progression of the disease, prevent fibrosis and cirrhosis and reduce hepatic inflammation. Normalisation of aspartate aminotransferase/alanine aminotransferase (AST/ALT) and serum immunoglobulin G level is the ideal goal after the treatment [26].

Except for patients with inactive disease, all patients should receive treatment.

Prednisone or prednisolone (40–60 mg/d; 1–2 mg/kg/d in children to a max. of 40–60 mg/d) in combination with azathioprine (AZA) is the mainstay of the treatment. Azathioprine is not recommended in decompensated cirrhotics, icteric AIH or severe acute hepatitis. Steroids are gradually tapered off to 5–10 mg/d in combination with the steroid-sparing agent to minimise the adverse events. Budesonide may be used in combination with AZA in patients with AIH. However, the use of budesonide is not recommended in cirrhotic patients, and no trials are available for AIH-ALF. It is used in a dosage of 9 mg/d in combination with AZR, gradually tapered to 3–6 mg/d. Sustained normalisation of AST/ALT and IgG over 2 years may be an indication to stop treatment. Relapses are common and may be seen in up to 60–80% of cases, and histological remission at 2 years confirmed by liver biopsy reduces the relapse to 28% [22, 26].

Liver transplant may be indicated in 2–4% of AIH-related ALF/cirrhosis in Europe and up to 5% in the USA. Recurrence post-transplant can be seen in up to 8–12% of cases in the first year and reaches 36%–68% after 5 years [29].

8.8 Primary Biliary Cholangitis

Previously known as primary biliary cirrhosis, it is a chronic cholestatic liver disease. PBC is characterised by anti-mitochondrial antibody which can be seen in 90% of patients [30]. These are the enzymes located on the inner membrane of the mitochondria: 2-oxo-acid dehydrogenase complex (2-OADC), which includes the pyruvate dehydrogenase complex E2 subunit (PDC-E2), the branched-chain 2-OADC E2 subunit (BCOADC-E2), the 2-oxoglutaric acid dehydrogenase complex E2 subunit (OGDC-E2) and dihydrolipoamide dehydrogenase-binding protein (E3BP). The most common variant of AMA is M-2 which is specific for the diagnosis [31].

Diagnosis of PBC is confirmed by the presence of autoantibodies, elevation of cholestatic liver enzymes and typical liver histology. However, a biopsy is not mandatory for the confirmation of diagnosis. Antinuclear antibodies such as sp100 and gp210 are detectable in patients with AMA-negative PBC [12].

Histologically, it is a disease of intrahepatic small and medium-sized bile ducts. Infiltration around the small interlobular bile ducts, known as chronic non-suppurative cholangitis, and granuloma are seen in histology. Nakanuma's classification is used for staging and grading the disease [32].

In a large fraction of the population, it is usually asymptomatic. Fatigue (70%) and pruritus (20–70%) are the most common symptoms, followed by jaundice. Sicca syndrome, osteopenia and osteoporosis, hyperlipidemia and metabolic syndrome are the most common manifestations [33].

8.9 Radiological Features

Inflammation involving the interlobular bile ducts seen in the early stages manifests as hyperintensity in T2-weighted sequences and hypointensity in T1-weighted sequences. These changes are seen surrounding the intrahepatic portal vein branches (along the portal triads) [34] (Fig. 8.2a).

Periportal inflammation is a non-specific finding and may be seen in varied aetiologies. Abdominal lymphadenopathy (periportal, portocaval), however, is a more specific imaging finding [35].

In later stages of the disease, there is the development of periportal fibrosis with hepatocellular depletion. Multiple small (5–10 mm) nodules with low signal in both T1W and T2W sequences

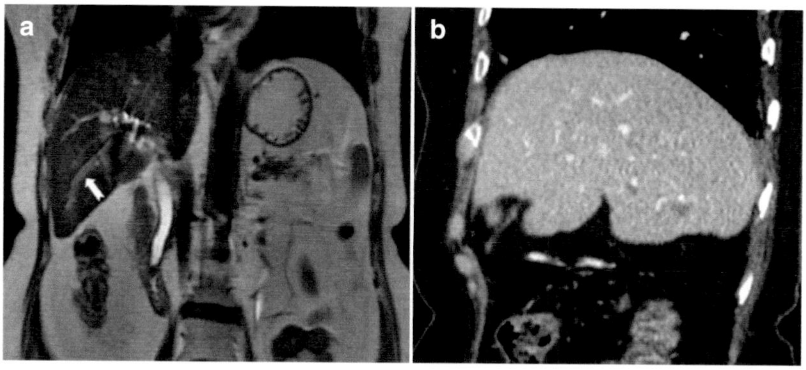

Fig. 8.2 Imaging findings in biopsy-proven cases of primary biliary cholangitis. (**a**): Periportal hyperintensity (white block arrow) is seen in T2-weighted sequences suggestive of periportal inflammation. (**b**): A different patient showing the more classic 'periportal halo sign' with non-enhancing hypodense nodules seen in the periportal region

are seen along the portal triads. This produces the more specific 'periportal halo sign' [36] (Fig. 8.2b).

8.10 Treatment

Ursodeoxycholic acid (UDCA) is the mainstay of treatment of PBC. UDCA is given at a dosage of 13–15 mg/kg body weight, and with elevated liver enzymes, it is recommended. A total of 20–30% may have an incomplete response to UDCA and usually have a poor prognosis. Multiple criteria have been proposed to assess the response to UDCA [12]. In patients who are non-responsive to UDCA, obetocholic acid is the farnesoid X receptor (FXR) agonist. OCA has been proposed as a second therapy for the management of PBC [37]. Other drugs that can be used are fibrates, which are peroxisome proliferator–activated receptor-α (PPAR-α) agonists, resulting in bile acid synthesis and upregulation of bile acid transporters. Benzafibrates in combination with UDCA have been shown to decrease the ALP levels and increase the expected LT-free survival.

Female sex, young age and anti-gp210 positivity are associated with poor prognosis. Intractable pruritus and decompensated liver disease are the common indications for transplant. AMA is positive after liver transplant, and recurrence can be seen up to 25% 5 years following transplant [38].

8.11 Primary Sclerosing Cholangitis

It is a chronic cholestatic disease characterised by intra- and extrahepatic bile duct injury. There is inflammatory bile duct destruction and fibrosis resulting in bile duct stricturing, cholestasis and leading to biliary cirrhosis [4]. Median survival from diagnosis to liver transplant or death is usually around 10 years.

It is closely associated with inflammatory bowel disease which can be seen in up to 2/3 of the patients [39]. Typical presentation is in a young male in the 3rd–fourth decade of life with a history of ulcerative colitis or Crohn's disease and abnormal liver function test. Genome-based wide association studies have reported 23 risk loci key to the pathogenesis of the disease [40].

8.11.1 Clinical Presentation

Diagnosis of PSC requires the exclusion of other causes of secondary cholangitis. Magnetic resonance cholangiopancreatography (MRCP) helps in making a diagnosis with a sensitivity and specificity of 0.86 and 0.94, respectively [41].

It is important to distinguish between the PSC and autoimmune pancreatitis which is characterised by elevated IgG4 levels, pancreatic findings, involvement of other organs, bile duct or ampullary biopsy with an IgG4 level of more than 10 per high power field.

Small duct PSC in presence of normal MRCP, while the clinical features are suggestive of the same. It is usually confirmed by biopsy [42].

The Ludwig score is used for the prognosis, and poor survival is associated with an increased Ludwig score.

Approximately 50% of the patients report having symptoms, with fatigue, pruritus and pain being the most common ones. Poor quality of life from recurrent cholangitis and pruritus may be an indication for liver transplant.

Bile cultures in patients with PSC show a wide range of bacteria, with or without intervention. Prophylactic antibiotics should be administered before any procedure. In advanced disease or recurrent cholangitis, rotational antibiotics may be indicated [43].

8.12 Dominant Stricture

Clinically significant stenosis is detected at the time of endoscopic retrograde cholangiopancreatography (ERCP). It is defined as $\leq$1.5 mm in the common bile duct or $\leq$ 1 mm in the hepatic duct within 2 cm of the hilum [44]. The same definition is not valid for MRCP.

8.13 Radiological Features

Initial inflammation produces irregular nodular enhancing wall thickening and mural irregularities involving the CBD and intrahepatic ducts. The duct wall inflammation appears echogenic on USG and hyperintense on T2-weighted sequences in MRI. On CT, soft tissue density thickening or an intraluminal mass may be seen.

In later stages, with the development of fibrosis, there is narrowing of the biliary tree. Since there is non-uniform involvement of the biliary tree, a 'beaded appearance' is classically described with alternate areas of narrowing and mild dilatation seen along the biliary tree (Fig. 8.3). Ductal diverticulae as well as intraductal webs may develop. Cholangiogram is the investigation of choice; however, it is an invasive procedure. MRCP is a non-invasive and efficient modality to depict these changes [45].

In advanced stages, the strictures may cause complete obliteration of intrahepatic biliary radicles, leading to a pruned tree appearance (Fig. 8.3). Since there is more pronounced involvement of the intrahepatic biliary duct bifurcations, there is development of obtuse angulation between the central and peripheral ducts.

Biliary duct stricture leads to cholestasis and the development of a number of complications like cholangitis, cholelithiasis, choledocholithiasis and carcinoma gallbladder. Hence, an annual survey is essential in these patients. Gall bladder polyps seen on USG in the setting of PSC have to be considered malignant.

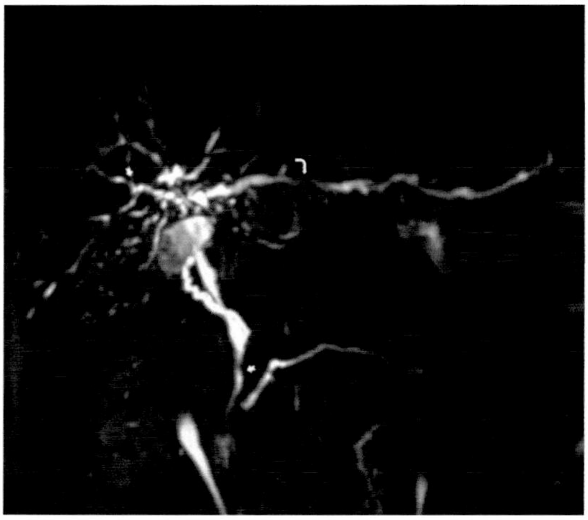

Fig. 8.3 Imaging findings in a biopsy-proven case of primary sclerosing cholangitis. Thick slab MRCP images depicting multiple short segment narrowing (white block arrows) involving both intrahepatic and extrahepatic biliary tree with a characteristic 'beaded appearance'. There is peripheral tapering of the intrahepatic biliary radicals (white arrows) with 'pruned tree' appearance. A 'dominant' stricture as seen involving the left hepatic duct (white curved arrow) should always raise a suspicion of underlying cholangiocarcinoma

Long-standing cholestasis may lead to the development of secondary biliary cirrhosis and portal hypertension. USG and CT may be used to evaluate the changes associated with cirrhosis and portal hypertension. There is marked caudate lobe hypertrophy which appears more hyperdense on CT as compared to the rest of the atrophied segments. Left lobe atrophy is an odd finding seen in cirrhosis associated with PSC which helps differentiate it from other causes of cirrhosis.

8.14 Medical Management

UDCA is the most common drug used in PSC. It is used in the dosage of 13–15 mg/kg/d and is associated with a reduction of liver enzymes but with no change in time to death, progression to mortality or death. Other drugs that may be used but still do not have a defined role are obeticholic acid (OCA) and cilofexor, a non-steroidal FXR receptor agonist. ERCP and stenting may help in the management of dominant strictures. Short duration of stenting is preferred over long stenting.

8.15 Cholangiocarcinoma in PSC

It usually complicates PSC. Rapid onset of weight loss, jaundice and abdominal pain may be the symptoms suggestive of complicated cholangiocarcinoma (CCA) on the background of PSC. Histology, Ca19.9, brush cytology and histology may help in the diagnosis of cholangiocarcinoma.

CCA is the most common malignancy noted in PSC. The annual incidence of cholangiocarcinoma is 0.6% per year in PSC, and the cumulative risk in patients with PSC is 16–20% [46]. Dominant strictures have a higher risk of developing CCA. CCA poses a higher risk of mortality with a median survival of 80% at 1 year. Resection or liver transplant is the curative option for the management of CCA complicating PSC. For the unresectable one, median survival is 5–12 months with or without chemotherapy [47].

8.16 Liver Transplant in PSC

Since PSC is a progressive disease, 40% of the patients will require a transplant. Decompensated cirrhosis and recurrent cholangitis are indications for liver transplant. Long-term outcome is usually good in PSC; however, 20% of the patients may have recurrence of disease post-transplant [48]. Active IBD confers a risk of post-transplant recurrence of the disease.

8.17 Autoimmune Sclerosing Cholangitis

Autoimmune sclerosing cholangitis (ASC) is characterised by inflammation of intrahepatic and extrahepatic bile ducts, bile duct dilatation and narrowing and obliteration, leading to bile duct damage and periductal fibrosis [49]. Small duct disease is diagnosed by features of histological features of cholangitis and normal MRCP. Features of sclerosing cholangitis resemble those of AIH. It is characterised by positive ANA, ASMA and high immunoglobulin G level. It is usually predominant in females seen in up to 79% of adults. Interface hepatitis along with periductal inflammation and onion duct fibrosis usually forms the histological hallmark of ASC. Steroids and azathioprine along with UDCA form the management of PSC [50]. In the King's College prospective study, biochemical response is seen with a combination of steroid and azathioprine; however, the disease progressed in 50% of patients owing to the progression of cholestatic disease. Liver transplantation may be indicated in decompensated chronic liver disease and recurrent cholangitis; however, a high probability of recurrence is noted in as high as 71% of patients.

8.18 Conclusion

Autoimmune liver diseases are a broad spectrum of diseases consisting of autoimmune hepatitis, primary biliary cholangitis, primary sclerosing cholangitis, AIH-PBC overlap, AIH-PSC overlap and autoimmune sclerosing cholangitis. Genetic and environmental factors along with defects in central tolerance in immunity play a major role in the pathogenesis of autoimmune liver diseases. Serological markers and liver biopsy help in making an early diagnosis and management of the patient. Steroids, azathioprine and UDCA are the mainstay of the treatment in the management of these diseases. In refractory cases with AIH, an anti-CD20 depleting antibody such as rituximab may be offered. OCA may be beneficial in UDCA-refractory PBC. Newer therapies such as faecal microbiota transplant may require further clinical trials.

References

1. Carbone M, Neuberger JM. Autoimmune liver disease, autoimmunity and liver transplantation. J Hepatol. 2014;60:210–23.
2. Manns MP, Czaja AJ, Gorham JD, Krawitt EL, Mieli-Vergani G, Vergani D, Vierling JM. American Association for the Study of Liver Diseases. Diagnosis and management of autoimmune hepatitis. Hepatology. 2010 Jun;51(6):2193–213.
3. European Association for the Study of the Liver. EASL clinical practice guidelines: management of cholestatic liver diseases. J Hepatol. 2009 Aug;51(2):237–67.
4. Karlsen TH, Folseraas T, Thorburn D, Vesterhus M. Primary sclerosing cholangitis – a comprehensive review. J Hepatol. 2017 Dec;67(6):1298–323.
5. Terziroli Beretta-Piccoli B, Vergani D, Mieli-Vergani G. Autoimmune sclerosing cholangitis: evidence and open questions. J Autoimmun. 2018 Dec;95:15–25.
6. Floreani A, Leung PS, Gershwin ME. Environmental basis of autoimmunity. Clin Rev Allergy Immunol. 2016;50:287–300.
7. Van Gerven NM, de Boer YS, Zwiers A, Verwer BJ, Drenth JP, van Hoek B, et al. HLA-DRB1*03:01 and HLA-DRB1*04:01 modify the presentation and outcome in autoimmune hepatitis type-1. Genes Immun. 2015;16:247–52.
8. Bjornsson E, Talwalkar J, Treeprasertsuk S, Kamath PS, Takahashi N, Sanderson S, et al. Drug-induced autoimmune hepatitis: clinical characteristics and prognosis. Hepatology. 2010;51:2040–8.
9. Bogdanos DP, Baum H, Vergani D, Burroughs AK. The role of E. Coli infection in the pathogenesis of primary biliary cirrhosis. Dis Markers. 2010;29(6):301–11.
10. Gilbert KM. Xenobiotic exposure and autoimmune hepatitis. Hepat Res Treat. 2010;2010:248157.
11. Liberal R, Longhi MS, Mieli-Vergani G, Vergani D. Pathogenesis of autoimmune hepatitis. Best Pract Res Clin Gastroenterol. 2011 Dec;25(6):653–64.
12. Louie JS, Grandhe S, Matsukuma K, Bowlus CL. Primary biliary cholangitis: a brief overview. Clin Liver Dis (Hoboken). 2020;15(3):100–4.
13. Gochanour E, Jayasekera C, Kowdley K. Primary sclerosing cholangitis: epidemiology, genetics, diagnosis, and current management. Clin Liver Dis (Hoboken). 2020;15(3):125–8.
14. Lafdil F, Miller AM, Ki SH, Gao B. Th17 cells and their associated cytokines in liver diseases. Cell Mol Immunol. 2010;7(4):250–4. https://doi.org/10.1038/cmi.2010.5.
15. Gulamhusein AF, Hirschfield GM. Primary biliary cholangitis: pathogenesis and therapeutic opportunities. Nat Rev Gastroenterol Hepatol. 2020 Feb;17(2):93–110.
16. Banales JM, Huebert RC, Karlsen T, Strazzabosco M, LaRusso NF, Gores GJ. Cholangiocyte pathobiology. Nat Rev Gastroenterol Hepatol. 2019;16(5):269–81.
17. Shetty S, Lalor PF, Adams DH. Lymphocyte recruitment to the liver: molecular insights into the pathogenesis of liver injury and hepatitis. Toxicology. 2008;254(3):136–46.
18. Gatselis NK, Zachou K, Koukoulis GK, Dalekos GN. Autoimmune hepatitis, one disease with many faces: etiopathogenetic, clinico-laboratory and histological characteristics. World J Gastroenterol. 2015;21(1):60–83.
19. Lim KN, Casanova RL, Boyer TD, Bruno CJ. Autoimmune hepatitis in African Americans: presenting features and response to therapy. Am J Gastroenterol. 2001 Dec;96(12):3390–4.
20. Mieli-Vergani G, Vergani D, Czaja AJ, Manns MP, Krawitt EL, Vierling JM, Lohse AW, Montano-Loza AJ. Autoimmune hepatitis. Nat Rev Dis Primers. 2018;4:18017.
21. Cancado EL, Abrantes-Lemos CP, Terrabuio DR. The importance of autoantibody detection in autoimmune hepatitis. Front Immunol. 2015;6:222.
22. Mack CL, Adams D, Assis DN, Kerkar N, Manns MP, Mayo MJ, Vierling JM, Alsawas M, Murad MH, Czaja AJ. Diagnosis and Management of Autoimmune Hepatitis in adults and children: 2019 practice guidance and guidelines from the American Association for the Study of Liver Diseases. Hepatology. 2020 Aug;72(2):671–722.
23. de Boer YS, van Nieuwkerk CM, Witte BI, Mulder CJ, Bouma G, Bloemena E. Assessment of the histopathological key features in autoimmune hepatitis. Histopathology. 2015 Feb;66(3):351–62.
24. De Luca-Johnson J, Wangensteen KJ, Hanson J, Krawitt E, Wilcox R. Natural history of patients presenting with autoimmune hepatitis and coincident nonalcoholic fatty liver disease. Dig Dis Sci. 2016 Sep;61(9):2710–20.
25. Stravitz RT, Lefkowitch JH, Fontana RJ, et al. Autoimmune acute liver failure: proposed

clinical and histological criteria. Hepatology. 2011;53(2):517–26.
26. Czaja AJ. Diagnosis and management of autoimmune hepatitis: current status and future directions. Gut Liver. 2016;10(2):177–203.
27. Semelka RC, Chung J, Hussain SM, et al. Chronic hepatitis: correlation of early patchy and late linear enhancement patterns on gadolinium-enhanced MR images with histopathology—initial experience. J Magn Reson Imaging. 2001;13:385–91.
28. Park SZ, Nagorney DM, Czaja AJ. Hepatocellular carcinoma in autoimmune hepatitis. Dig Dis Sci. 2000;45:1944–8.
29. Tanaka T, Sugawara Y, Kokudo N. Liver transplantation and autoimmune hepatitis. Intractable Rare Dis Res. 2015;4(1):33–8.
30. Hu CJ, Zhang FC, Li YZ, Zhang X. Primary biliary cirrhosis: what do autoantibodies tell us? World J Gastroenterol. 2010;16(29):3616–29.
31. Poyatos E, Morandeira F, Climent J, Mas V, Castellote J, Bas J. Detection of anti-mitochondrial 2-oxoacid dehydrogenase complex subunit's antibodies for the diagnosis of primary biliary cholangitis. Clin Immunol. 2021;268:108749.
32. Lewis J. Pathological patterns of biliary disease. Clin Liver Dis (Hoboken). 2017;10(5):107–10.
33. Reshetnyak VI. Primary biliary cirrhosis: clinical and laboratory criteria for its diagnosis. World J Gastroenterol. 2015;21(25):7683–708.
34. Kobayashi S, Matsui O, Gabata T, et al. MRI findings of primary biliary cirrhosis: correlation with Scheuer histologic staging. Abdom Imaging. 2005;30:71–6.
35. Blachar A, Federle MP, Brancatelli G. Primary biliary cirrhosis: clinical, pathologic, and helical CT findings in 53 patients. Radiology. 2001;220(2):329–36.
36. Wenzel JS, Donohoe A, Ford KL III, et al. Primary biliary cirrhosis: MR imaging findings and description of MR imaging periportal halo sign. Am J Roentgenol. 2001;176:885–9.
37. Manne V, Kowdley KV. Obeticholic acid in primary biliary cholangitis: where we stand. Curr Opin Gastroenterol. 2019 May;35(3):191–6.
38. Montano-Loza AJ, Hansen BE, Corpechot C, Roccarina D, Thorburn D, Trivedi P, et al. Factors associated with recurrence of primary biliary cholangitis after liver transplantation and effects on graft and patient survival. Gastroenterology. 2019 Jan;156(1):96–107.e1.
39. Mertz A, Nguyen NA, Katsanos KH, Kwok RM. Primary sclerosing cholangitis and inflammatory bowel disease comorbidity: an update of the evidence. Ann Gastroenterol. 2019;32(2):124–33.
40. Ellinghaus D, Folseraas T, Holm K, Ellinghaus E, Melum E, Balschun T, et al. Genome-wide association analysis in primary sclerosing cholangitis and ulcerative colitis identifies risk loci at GPR35 and TCF4. Hepatology. 2013 Sep;58(3):1074–83.
41. Weber C, Kuhlencordt R, Grotelueschen R, Wedegaertner U, Ang TL, Adam G, et al. Magnetic resonance cholangiopancreatography in the diagnosis of primary sclerosing cholangitis. Endoscopy. 2008 Sep;40(9):739–45.
42. Björnsson E. Small-duct primary sclerosing cholangitis. Curr Gastroenterol Rep. 2009 Feb;11(1):37–41.
43. Chapman MH, Thorburn D, Hirschfield GM, Webster GGJ, Rushbrook SM, et al. British Society of Gastroenterology and UK-PSC guidelines for the diagnosis and management of primary sclerosing cholangitis. Gut. 2019 Aug;68(8):1356–78.
44. Aljiffry M, Renfrew PD, Walsh MJ, Laryea M, Molinari M. Analytical review of diagnosis and treatment strategies for dominant bile duct strictures in patients with primary sclerosing cholangitis. HPB (Oxford). 2011;13(2):79–90.
45. Wiesner RH, LaRusso NF. Clinicopathologic features of the syndrome of primary sclerosing cholangitis. Gastroenterology. 1980;79:200–6.
46. Tyson GL, El-Serag HB. Risk factors for cholangiocarcinoma. Hepatology. 2011;54(1):173–84.
47. Ethun CG, Lopez-Aguiar AG, Anderson DJ, et al. Transplantation versus resection for hilar Cholangiocarcinoma: an argument for shifting treatment paradigms for Resectable disease. Ann Surg. 2018;267(5):797–805.
48. Wiesner RH. Liver transplantation for primary sclerosing cholangitis: timing, outcome, impact of inflammatory bowel disease and recurrence of disease. Best Pract Res Clin Gastroenterol. 2001 Aug;15(4):667–80.
49. Giorgio AD, Vergani D, Mieli-Vergani G. Cutting edge issues in juvenile sclerosing cholangitis. Dig Liver Dis. 2021;54:417–27. S1590-8658(21)00342-X
50. Kumar N, Poddar U, Yadav R, Lal H, Pani K, Yachha SK, Srivastava A, Pandey R. Autoimmune Sclerosing cholangitis in children: a prospective case-control study. Pediatr Gastroenterol Hepatol Nutr. 2021 Mar;24(2):154–63.

Acute Biliary Conditions

9

Lorenzo Costa, Marco Gasparetto, and Giulia A. Zamboni

9.1 Introduction

Acute biliary pathologies are one of the most common causes of emergency department visits in the adult population. They commonly present with acute right upper quadrant pain, nausea or vomiting, and/or jaundice, resulting in significant morbidity and mortality. Etiologies include inflammation with or without infection and non-inflammatory disorders.

Imaging plays an important role in the diagnosis of biliary disorders, identifying the underlying etiology, and evaluating the severity of the disease. In particular, complicated acute cholecystitis and acute suppurative cholangitis often require an immediate surgical approach or an endoscopic/percutaneous interventional approach.

Imaging of biliary disease often requires a multimodality imaging approach, including ultrasonography (US), color or power Doppler US, computed tomography (CT), and MR, including MR cholangiopancreatography.

Ultrasound (US) is the primary imaging modality used to evaluate acute right upper quadrant pain but may not always allow characterization of the cause of biliary disease. Both magnetic resonance cholangiopancreatography (MRCP) and CT allow detailed evaluation of the biliary system. Endoscopic retrograde cholangiopancreatography (ERCP) is nowadays typically reserved for therapeutic intervention.

9.2 Cholelithiasis

9.2.1 Introduction

Cholelithiasis is caused by intermittent obstruction of the cystic duct or neck of the gallbladder by a gallstone.

It is estimated that approximately 10–20% of the population in Western societies is affected by cholelithiasis and that one-third of those with gallstones will develop related complications, such as cholecystitis.

The "5-F rule" helps to remember the principal risk factors of cholelithiasis: ***fair*** (prevalent in the Caucasian population) [1], ***fat*** (BMI >30 kg/m^2 and hyperlipidemia) [2], ***female*** (estrogen cause more cholesterol to be excreted into bile), ***fertile*** (women with one or more children), and ***forty*** (age ≥ 40 years).

Other risk factors include rapid weight loss (e.g., after bariatric surgery), parenteral nutrition, loss of bile salts (terminal ileitis or after ileal resection), and diabetes.

L. Costa
Department of Radiology, Santa Chiara Hospital, APSS Trento, Italy

M. Gasparetto · G. A. Zamboni (✉)
Institute of Radiology, University of Verona, Verona, Italy
e-mail: giulia.zamboni@univr.it

© The Author(s), under exclusive license to Springer Nature Singapore Pte Ltd. 2025

B. Sureka (ed.), *Hepato-Pancreatico Biliary Imaging*, https://doi.org/10.1007/978-981-95-1699-5_9

Symptomatic cholelithiasis (biliary colic) typically presents with right upper quadrant abdominal pain that occurs after eating, nausea, and emesis. Any indication of possible biliary obstruction, enzyme elevation, or dilated common bile duct should prompt further work-up for choledocholithiasis.

Elective laparoscopic cholecystectomy is recommended only for symptomatic cholelithiasis.

9.3 Imaging

9.3.1 Ultrasound

Ultrasound (US) remains the method of choice for the detection of gallstones, with high sensitivity and accuracy (>95%) [3], depending on the experience of the ultrasound operator.

Patients need to fast before their ultrasound to ensure the best sensitivity.

There are different characteristic findings of gallstones at US; the most specific is the presence of posterior shadowing (Fig. 9.1a) [4]. Other important echographic signs are the highly reflective echo from the anterior surface of the gallstone and the mobility of the gallstone (helps to exclude other pathologies related to the gallbladder walls, such as tumors); dilatation of the biliary tree is an indirect sign suggesting the presence of a common bile duct (CBD) stone (choledocholithiasis).

9.3.2 Computed Tomography

Computed tomography (CT) is not routinely used. Calcified gallbladder stones are the only stones visualized on CT images (Fig. 9.1b). Pure cholesterol stones and other gallstones are isodense to the bile and not easily detectable.

However, CT is helpful when looking for complications, such as cholecystitis.

9.3.3 Magnetic Resonance Cholangiopancreatography

If there is a suspected stone in the common bile duct based on ultrasound results, magnetic resonance cholangiopancreatography (MRCP) is the next step. Gallstones appear as filling defects in the gallbladder and duct system, with an associated dilated biliary tree proximal to the level of obstruction.

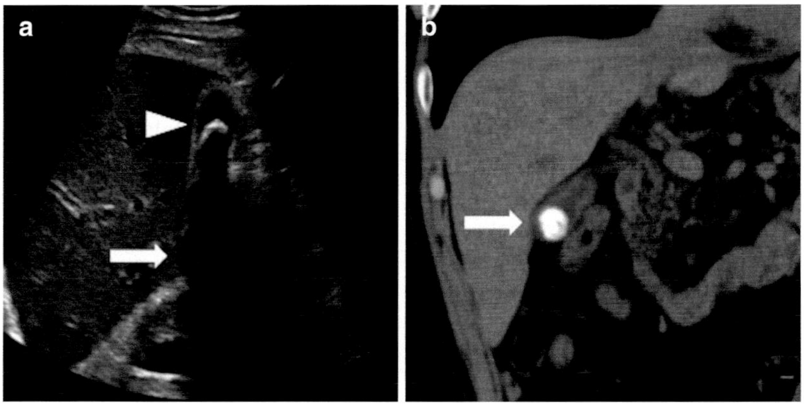

Fig. 9.1 Abdominal ultrasound (US) and computed tomography (CT) of the same patient with a calcified gallstone. (**a**): Note the presence of the posterior shadowing (arrow) and the highly reflective echo from the anterior surface of the gallstone (arrowhead). (**b**): CT confirmed the presence of a large calcified gallbladder stone in the fundus of the gallbladder (arrow). CT visualizes only calcified stones; pure cholesterol stones and other gallstones are isodense to bile and not clearly detectable

9.4 Acute Cholecystitis

9.4.1 Intro

Acute cholecystitis (AC) is an acute inflammatory disease of the gallbladder.

Obstruction of the cystic duct results in overdistension of the gallbladder (GB) and an increase in intraluminal pressure. This increased pressure, bile breakdown products (lysolecithin), and prostaglandins create ischemic damage to the mucosa and lead to chemical cholecystitis with an accumulation of inflammatory infiltrate and gallbladder wall edema. Albeit uncommon in the first 48 h, the risk of bacterial infection tends to increase to 70% within the first week unless treated.

An estimated 90–95% of cases are caused by an obstruction in the cystic duct or gallbladder neck due to cholelithiasis. The mortality in patients with acute cholecystitis is 0–10% and tends to be higher in elderly patients [5].

Clinical findings may include acute severe right upper quadrant abdominal pain, positive Murphy's sign, fever, nausea and emesis, and focal tenderness directly overlying the gallbladder.

Leukocytosis is the most common laboratory abnormality, seen in up to 60% of patients, and a positive bacterial culture has been reported in one-half to two-thirds of patients with AC. High total bilirubin and alkaline phosphatase levels are uncommon in patients with uncomplicated AC and should instead raise concerns for cholangitis.

Complications are more commonly seen in patients of advanced age, those with multiple comorbidities, and those with a delayed presentation. Gangrenous cholecystitis with subsequent perforation is the most common complication. Other common complications include emphysematous cholecystitis, gallbladder empyema, hemorrhagic cholecystitis, pericholecystic abscess, gallstone ileus, and Mirizzi syndrome.

9.4.2 Ultrasound

When AC is clinically suspected, ultrasound (US) tends to be the first choice imaging modality owing to its wide availability, speed, real-time imaging, absence of ionizing radiation, rapid identification of gallstones and biliary ductal dilatation, and ability to identify AC complications or alternative diagnoses. The sensitivity of sonography for this condition ranges from 80% to 100%, and the specificity ranges from 60% to 100% [6]. The presence of one or more impacted stones in the GB neck or cystic duct (cholelithiasis) found in addition to a positive sonographic Murphy sign (maximal tenderness with transducer pressure over the GB) is the most specific sonographic finding of AC (Fig. 9.2). Other imaging findings include gallbladder wall thickening (>3–5 mm), pericholecystic fluid, GB distension (>4 cm transverse and 10 cm in length), and echogenic bile (sludge) (Fig. 9.3).

9.4.3 Computed Tomography

Computed tomography (CT), commonly used to evaluate abdominal pain when diagnoses other than AC are contemplated, is also especially useful for AC complication detection. Typical CT findings in AC include gallbladder distention, mural thickening, mucosal hyperenhancement, pericholecystic fat stranding, pericholecystic fluid, and gallstones with a sufficient attenuation difference from bile to be visualized. A significant fraction of mixed cholesterol or pigment stones is so similar in attenuation to bile as not to be reliably identified. Even larger isodense gallstones may be invisible on CT. Typically, an increased enhancement of the hepatic parenchyma of the gallbladder fossa (CT rim sign) is found. Gallbladder mural thickening—the most common but the least specific finding—may be seen in a variety of other conditions, such as hepatitis, hypoproteinemia, heart failure, and acute pyelonephritis [7].

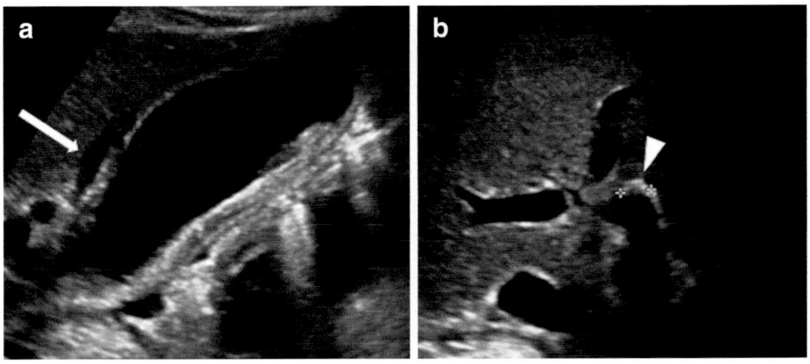

Fig. 9.2 A 55-year-old woman with right upper quadrant abdominal pain. (**a**): Sagittal image of the gallbladder shows a distended GB with mild wall thickening and pericholecystic free fluid (arrow). (**b**): Transverse oblique sonogram of the cystic duct shows an obstructing stone (arrowhead) with posterior shadowing. There was a positive sonographic "Murphy sign"

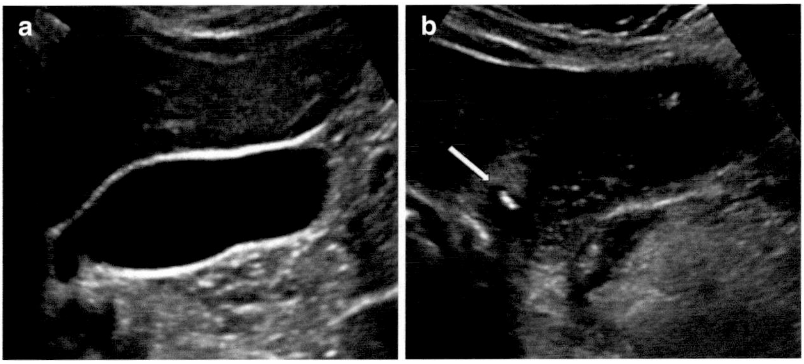

Fig. 9.3 Oblique coronal US images show (**a**) a normal gallbladder (GB) and (**b**) a thickened GB wall with an impacted calculus in the neck of the GB (arrow) in a patient with acute cholecystitis

9.4.4 Magnetic Resonance

Although magnetic resonance imaging (MRI), like CT, is not a first-line imaging modality in the evaluation of right upper quadrant pain, the reported sensitivity and specificity for AC for MRI are similar to those of US. Despite the good diagnostic performance, the cost, scan times, and availability limit its use for this purpose. At the same time, MRI is recommended for patients with suspected biliary obstruction secondary to choledocholithiasis or Mirizzi syndrome [8]. Imaging findings are analogous to those observed on sonography and CT, including gallbladder wall thickening, mural or mucosal hyperenhancement, pericholecystic fluid, and adjacent soft tissue inflammatory changes, abnormally increased gallbladder distention, and cholelithiasis (hypointense intraluminal foci on T2-weighted imaging sequences) (Fig. 9.4). Hyperenhancement of adjacent liver parenchyma on contrast-enhanced fat-saturated T1-weighted images may be noted, similar to CT. MR cholangiopancreatography (MRCP) may show an impacted stone in the gallbladder neck or cystic duct and can evaluate the extrahepatic bile ducts, which may not be optimally visualized sonographically in nonmobile or obese patients. MR is also preferred to CT in pregnant patients after an inconclusive US [9].

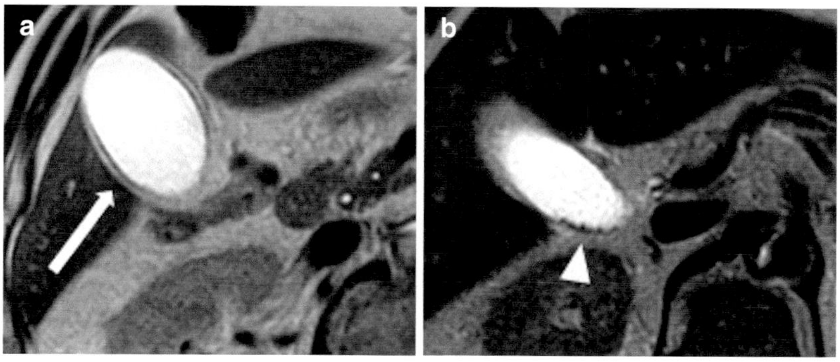

Fig. 9.4 An 85-year-old man with acute cholecystitis caused by cystic duct obstruction due to an impacted calculus. MR imaging was performed because the cause of the suspected acute cholecystitis could not be determined with US. **a, b,** Axial T2-weighted images show (**a**) diffuse hyperintense thickening of the gallbladder wall (arrow) with (**b**) multiple stones (arrowhead) in the gallbladder neck

9.5 Acalculous Cholecystitis

9.5.1 Intro

Up to 5–10% of patients with AC, especially those in critical care units, do not have stones in the gallbladder; inflammation of the gallbladder in this group of patients without any cystic duct obstruction is known as acute acalculous cholecystitis (AAC) and is associated with high morbidity and mortality if not managed promptly [10]. This condition is traced back to a gradual increase in bile viscosity leading to the eventual functional obstruction of the cystic duct. AAC complications include gangrenous cholecystitis, perforation, and pericholecystic abscess.

Patients with AAC demonstrate a variable clinical presentation depending on the underlying predisposing conditions. Vague abdominal pain, leukocytosis, and unexplained fever with associated jaundice in a critically ill patient in the intensive care unit should raise suspicion for AAC, and US should be performed immediately.

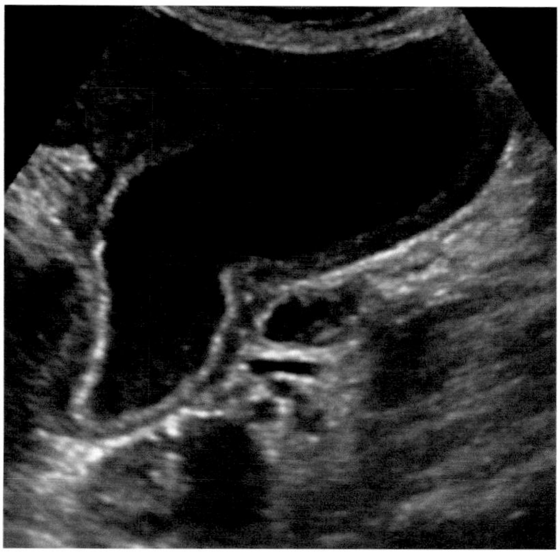

Fig. 9.5 Acalculous cholecystitis in an intensive care unit patient with sepsis. Sagittal image of the GB shows a distended GB with wall thickening and bile sludge. No gallstones were visualized

9.5.2 Ultrasound

The sonographic findings are nonspecific and include GB wall thickening, pericholecystic fluid, and GB distension (in the absence of gallstones) (Fig. 9.5). Sonographic Murphy sign is frequently hard to assess in patients with altered mental status or medicated or sedated due to underlying conditions.

9.5.3 Computed Tomography

CT may reveal similar imaging findings as well as pericholecystic inflammatory stranding with adjacent liver hyperemia. MRI is not commonly performed in patients with acalculous cholecystitis, mostly due to the difficulty in performing MRI studies in critically ill patients.

9.6 Acute Cholecystitis Complications

9.6.1 Gangrenous Cholecystitis

Gangrenous cholecystitis (GC) results from ischemia and necrosis of the GB wall due to increased intraluminal pressure and occurs in 2–29% of patients with acute calculous cholecystitis [11]. It is associated with higher morbidity and mortality rates than uncomplicated acute cholecystitis. Elderly patients and patients with a history of diabetes mellitus and white blood cell count >15,000 cells/mL are at an increased risk of having gangrenous changes at presentation. Discriminating between acute uncomplicated cholecystitis and gangrenous cholecystitis, a potentially clinically difficult task, is key since the medical and surgical treatment in the two cases may differ. Imaging plays a significant part in the distinction.

GC is manifested sonographically by sloughed mucosal membranes, focal wall bulge, ulceration, and disruption. It is associated with an increased risk of GB perforation. Sonographic Murphy sign is negative in the majority of GC patients. Specific CT findings that suggest gangrenous cholecystitis include foci of gas within the gallbladder wall, intraluminal membranes, irregular mural enhancement or hypoenhancement, focal mural defects, and pericholecystic abscesses (Fig. 9.6).

9.6.2 Emphysematous Cholecystitis

Emphysematous cholecystitis is determined by secondary infection of the gallbladder wall with gas-forming organisms. Affected patients are more frequently diabetic (30–50%), male, and in the 40–60 age group. Involved bacterial organisms include *Clostridium* species, *Escherichia coli*, *Staphylococcus aureus*, and *Streptococcus species*.

Emphysematous cholecystitis can be first diagnosed through abdominal radiography. Radiographs showing curvilinear lucencies within the gallbladder wall or an air-fluid level within the gallbladder lumen are specific for this entity in the setting of suspected cholecystitis. Sonographically, gas in the GB lumen or wall appears as curvilinear echogenic reflectors, which may have dirty shadowing and ring-down artefacts. This appearance must be carefully distinguished from a gallbladder packed with stones or calcification in the gallbladder wall

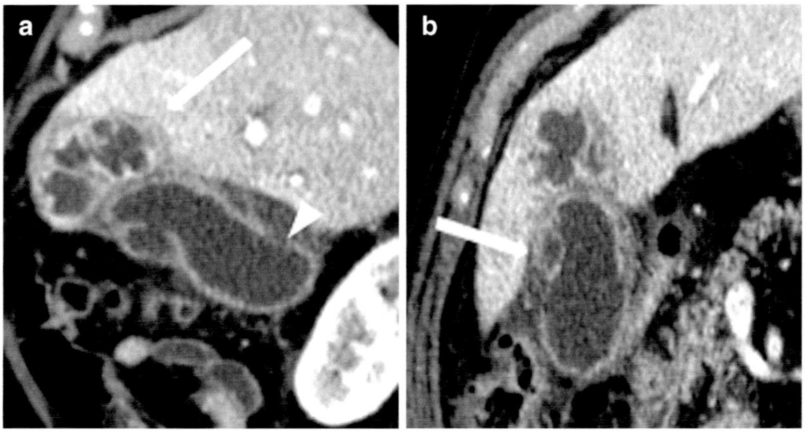

Fig. 9.6 Gangrenous cholecystitis in a 79-year-old man with malaise, fever, and leukocytosis without right upper quadrant pain. (**a**): Sagittal contrast-enhanced CT image shows gallbladder wall thickening, pericholecystic inflammation with focal mucosal defects (arrowhead) and hepatic abscess (arrow). (**b**): Coronal contrast-enhanced CT image shows intramural abscesses (arrow), a sign of gangrenous cholecystitis. The patient underwent urgent cholecystectomy, which confirmed gangrenous cholecystitis with mucosal ulcers and mural abscesses

(porcelain gallbladder). In difficult cases, CT is most sensitive for confirming gas in the gallbladder wall or lumen (low-attenuation foci). It also allows distinction between gas and wall calcifications, as is seen with a porcelain gallbladder. Additional findings may be similar to those observed in acute uncomplicated cholecystitis. On MRI, areas of signal void within the gallbladder wall or lumen may be observed, corresponding to foci of intramural or intraluminal gas. Complications of emphysematous cholecystitis include gangrenous change, perforation, and pericholecystic abscess formation. Due to the risk of perforation, the treatment is cholecystectomy, although percutaneous cholecystostomy can be used temporarily in patients too ill to undergo surgery.

9.6.3 Suppurative Cholecystitis

Empyema of the gallbladder is the most severe complication of acute cholecystitis. This condition ensues when purulent material fills and distends the gallbladder lumen, with an estimated incidence of 5 to 15% of AC patients. Patients with empyema of the gallbladder have symptoms similar to acute cholecystitis. Tenderness in the right upper quadrant and a positive Murphy sign are the predominant presenting symptoms. With the worsening of the disease, high fever, chills, and signs of systemic sepsis follow.

Imaging findings of suppurative cholecystitis are nonspecific and akin to those seen in acute uncomplicated cholecystitis. Echogenic (at sonography) or high-attenuation (at CT) material consistent with pus is identified within the distended gallbladder lumen and is indistinguishable from sludge. MRI can help in distinguishing pus from sludge using heavily T2-weighted sequences, which may display a fluid-fluid level with a dependent layering of purulent bile [12].

Suppurative cholecystitis is a surgical emergency that requires timely treatment with antibiotics and urgent aspiration/removal of the gallbladder to decrease septic shock risk.

9.6.4 Gallbladder Perforation

Gallbladder perforation is a severe complication of acute cholecystitis, potentially occurring in up to 10% of cases [13]. The associated mortality rate is 19–24%. Perforation has been classified into three types: type I, acute perforation into the free peritoneal cavity; type II, subacute perforation with abscess formation; and type III, chronic perforation with fistula formation between the gallbladder and another viscus. The most common site of perforation is the gallbladder fundus. Small areas of gallbladder perforation may be difficult to detect on imaging. A focal defect in the gallbladder wall may be visualized on sonography, CT, or MRI (Fig. 9.7). An extraluminal gallstone is a specific imaging finding pointing to perforation. More frequently, findings of perforation are nonspecific and include pericholecystic fluid, gallbladder lumen collapse, and pericholecystic abscess.

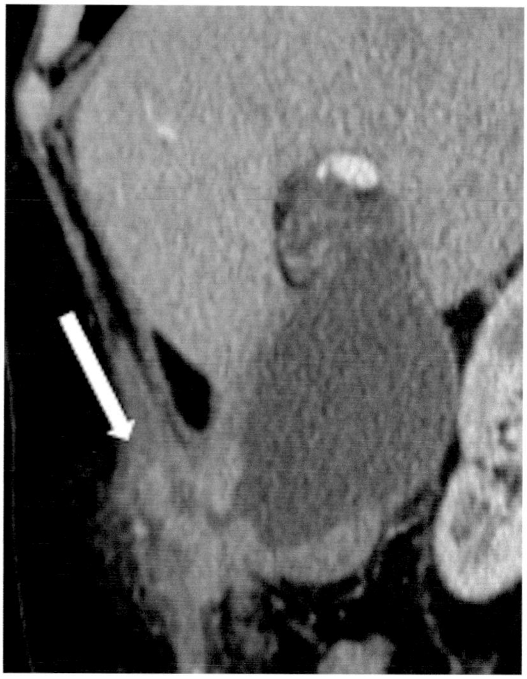

Fig. 9.7 Perforated cholecystitis in a 64-year-old woman presenting with abdominal pain at the emergency department Sagittal CT image shows gallbladder wall thickening with a wall defect in the fundus of the gallbladder and an abscess in the anterior abdominal wall (arrow)

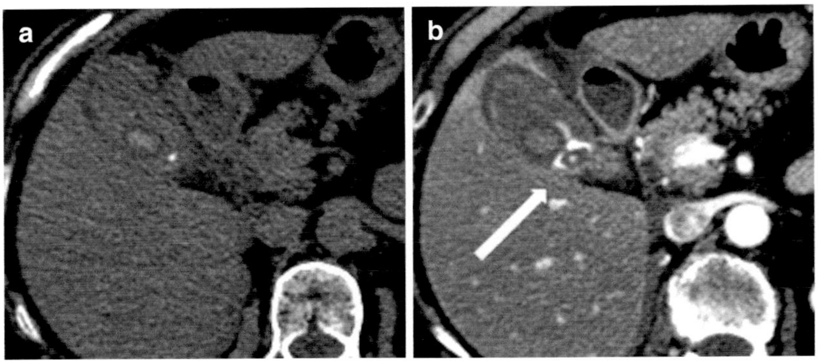

Fig. 9.8 Hemorrhagic cholecystitis in a 69-year-old woman with right upper quadrant pain. (**a**): Axial unenhanced CT image shows abnormally high-attenuation material within an abnormally distended gallbladder lumen. Gallbladder wall edema is also present. (**b**): Axial contrast-enhanced CT image in arterial phase shows active bleeding in the gallbladder lumen (arrow). Hyperenhancement of the gallbladder fossa indicates transient reactive hyperemia of hepatic parenchyma (CT rim sign)

9.6.5 Pericholecystic Abscess

Acute cholecystitis is complicated with pericholecystic abscess formation reportedly in 3–19% of cases. Abscesses take the form of intramural and pericholecystic rim-enhancing fluid collections. Extension of the pericholecystic abscess into the adjacent hepatic parenchyma will appear like a complex cystic lesion. Rim enhancement is typical, although not always present. Intralesional gas is not common.

9.6.6 Hemorrhagic Cholecystitis

Hemorrhagic cholecystitis, a rare entity with a high mortality rate, is the final stage of acalculous cholecystitis. In this condition, the formation of a pseudoaneurysm of the cystic artery and its consequent rupture leads to frank hemorrhage/acute bleeding into the gallbladder that may present clinically with an acute onset of biliary colic, jaundice, melena, and hematemesis. Hemorrhagic cholecystitis typically appears on sonography and CT with imaging findings indicating acute cholecystitis. In addition, sonography may show echogenic material within the gallbladder lumen. On CT, high-attenuation blood products are present within the gallbladder wall or lumen (Fig. 9.8). Cystic artery pseudoaneurysm is also occasionally seen. Complications of hemorrhagic cholecystitis include gallbladder wall perforation and associated hemoperitoneum. Treatment typically involves cholecystectomy and IV antimicrobial therapy.

9.7 Mirizzi Syndrome

Mirizzi syndrome is determined by an impacted stone in the gallbladder neck or cystic duct (CD) causing biliary obstruction with dilatation of the intrahepatic bile ducts. A cholecystocholedochal fistula may form as a consequence of recurrent inflammation around the impacted gallstone in the cystic duct [14]. Obstructive jaundice observed in combination with abdominal pain and fever is the most common clinical presentation. There are no pathognomonic features on history and physical examination, further complicating clinical diagnosis.

In 1989, Csendes et al. classified Mirizzi syndrome into four types:

- Type I—obstruction of CD by stone impacted in the gallbladder neck or cystic duct (10% to 51%).
- Type II—cholecystobiliary fistula with erosion of less than 1/3 of the circumference of the CD (15% to 41%).
- Type III—erosion of up to 2/3 of the circumference of the CD (3% to 44%).
- Type IV—complete destruction of the CD wall (1% to 4%).

In 2007, Csendes added one more type to his classifications, the Mirizzi type V, that corresponds to any type of Mirizzi associated with bilioenteric fistula with or without gallstone ileus. Type V could be present in up to 29%.

Sonography and CT in Mirizzi syndrome display a gallstone located within the gallbladder neck or cystic duct and dilatation of the intrahepatic bile ducts with a normal calibre common bile duct (CBD). MRI and MRCP can show an extrinsic compression of the common hepatic duct, a gallstone in the cystic duct, dilation of the intrahepatic ducts, and a common hepatic duct with a normal distal common bile duct. The added benefit of MRI/MRCP is that it can facilitate the distinction between Mirizzi syndrome and different gallbladder pathologies, including gallbladder malignancy [15].

9.8 Choledocholithiasis

Choledocholithiasis is defined as the presence of gallstones within the common bile duct.

The incidence of choledocholithiasis has been estimated as 5% to 20% in patients with cholelithiasis [16].

Bile duct stones can be broadly classified into two types according to the site of origin: primary and secondary. Primary ductal stones develop de novo in the intrahepatic ducts or common duct, typically in the setting of bile stasis resulting from conditions such as cystic fibrosis or periampullary diverticula. Secondary ductal stones originate from the gallbladder and result from the passage of gallstones into the common bile duct. Choledocholithiasis is seen more commonly in its secondary form because of the existence of cholelithiasis.

Clinical symptoms are similar to those of cholelithiasis, with right upper quadrant abdominal pain and nausea often accompanied by Jaundice. Stones in the common bile duct can also be the cause of different associated conditions, as acute gallstone pancreatitis and acute cholangitis. Sometimes patients could also have no symptoms, and the diagnosis is only suspected from laboratory values and imaging findings.

9.9 Imaging

9.9.1 Ultrasound (US)

The radiological diagnosis is very similar to that of cholelithiasis, with imaging showing a dilated biliary tree and the presence of stones in the CBD.

Ultrasound is the primary imaging modality and may demonstrate a dilated common bile duct (>6 mm).

9.9.2 Magnetic Resonance Cholangiopancreatography

Magnetic resonance cholangiopancreatography (MRCP), a second-level imaging study, has higher sensitivity and specificity than ultrasound and is often used as a confirmatory diagnostic test [17] (Fig. 9.9).

9.9.3 ERCP/PTC

Before MRI, the gold standard for identifying common duct stones was endoscopic retrograde cholangiopancreatogram (ERCP). ERCP still has a fundamental role in the management of choledocholithiasis for clearance of common bile duct stones followed by laparoscopic cholecystectomy [18].

A percutaneous transhepatic cholangiogram (PTC) is normally used when ERCP is not possible.

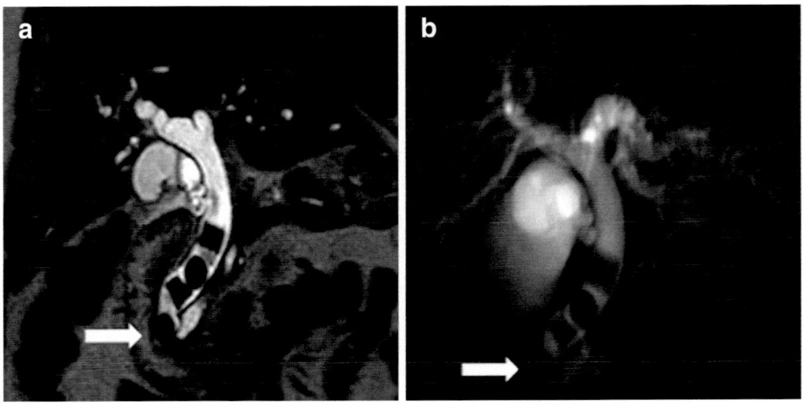

Fig. 9.9 Coronal T2-HASTE MRI (**a**) and CPRM (**b**): dilation of the biliary tree and the main pancreatic duct caused by multiple calculi of variable shapes inside the CBD, one of them impacted at the Ampulla of Vater (arrow). Gallstones are not directly visualized; they appear rather as filling defects inside the CDB

9.10 Acute Cholangitis

Acute cholangitis is a bacterial infection of the biliary system caused by biliary obstruction.

The prevalence of this condition is strictly related to that of choledocholithiasis.

It is much more prevalent in native Americans (60%–70%) and Hispanics but less common in Asians and African Americans [19].

The most frequently isolated pathogens are *Escherichia coli*, *Klebsiella* species, *Enterococcus* species, and *Enterobacter* species.

The most common etiology is choledocholithiasis [20]. Other causes of obstruction include benign or malignant stricture of the bile duct or hepatic ducts, such as pancreatic cancer, ampullary cancer, porta hepatis tumor, primary sclerosing cholangitis, Mirizzi syndrome, and strictured bilioenteric anastomoses [21]. Post-endoscopic retrograde cholangiopancreatography (ERCP) acute cholangitis can also occur in a minority of cases (about 2.5% of cases) [22].

The syndrome is characterized by fever, jaundice, and abdominal pain (= Charcot's triad, present in 15–70% of patients), hypotension, and altered mental status (= Reynold's pentad, present in only 4–8% of patients).

Cholangitis is a life-threatening condition, and if not promptly treated, it can rapidly escalate into septic shock.

The treatment of cholangitis is based on resuscitation, antibiotics, and biliary drainage. ERCP or percutaneous transhepatic biliary drainage should be urgently performed for biliary decompression. For patients with choledocholithiasis, definitive management includes cholecystectomy to avoid recurrence.

9.10.1 Ultrasound

Sonography is a relatively inexpensive and widely available method of imaging, often used as the primary imaging modality. Ultrasound may demonstrate dilation of the biliary tree; nevertheless, it is not always possible to recognize the cause of cholangitis. In fact, in the setting of acute cholangitis, the sensitivity for detecting choledocholithiasis is reduced.

9.10.2 Computed Tomography and Magnetic Resonance Cholangiopancreatography

CT, MRI, and MRCP are reliable modalities for the diagnosis, with the advantage of their noninvasive nature. MRI does not use radiation and is normally preferred over CT for studying biliary ducts with the advantage of visualizing noncalcific gallstones causing acute cholangitis. MRCP can depict dilation of intra- and extrahepatic bile ducts, as well as the presence of gallstones (Figs. 9.10 and 9.11).

In 85% of the cases, there is associated wall thickening with enhancement of intrahepatic biliary duct walls. This latter condition is best seen with gadolinium-enhanced delayed phase fat-suppressed sequences [23].

MRI allows also the detection of related complications, such as liver abscesses and portal vein thrombosis.

9.10.3 ERCP/PTC

ERCP is the gold standard for the diagnosis of cholangitis; it can easily detect dilatation of bile ducts, as well as the presence of calculi [24].

The other advantage of ERCP is that this technique may also be performed as a therapeutic procedure for biliary drainage in cholangitis [25]. When endoscopic decompression fails, percutaneous transhepatic cholangiography (PTC) is the preferred modality [26].

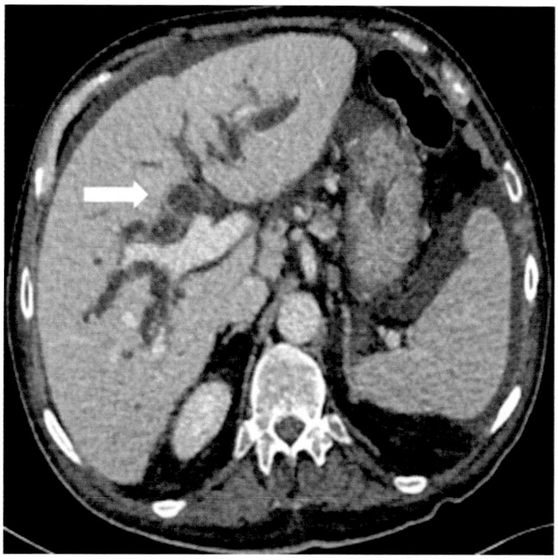

Fig. 9.10 CECT shows the classic signs of AC in this patient with a pancreatic adenocarcinoma: dilation of intrahepatic bile ducts with wall thickening and enhancement of duct walls (arrow). Note the presence ad ascites surrounding the liver and the spleen

9.11 Gallstone Pancreatitis

Acute pancreatitis is an inflammatory condition of the pancreas characterized by abdominal pain and elevated levels of pancreatic enzymes in the blood.

Gallstones (including microlithiasis) are the most common cause of acute pancreatitis, accounting for 35–65% of cases worldwide [27].

The most common symptom of pancreatitis is severe epigastric abdominal pain radiating to the back. Laboratory values with elevated serum levels of amylase and lipase are usually diagnostic.

All patients with acute pancreatitis should be managed with intravenous fluid resuscitation and bowel rest.

The management of gallstone pancreatitis includes ERCP and endoscopic sphincterotomy (ES) for removal of the obstructing stone and reestablishment of biliary drainage. Elective laparoscopic cholecystectomy helps to avoid recurrences.

9.11.1 Ultrasound/Magnetic Resonance Cholangiopancreatography

The identification of gallstones and dilatation of the extrahepatic biliary tree on ultrasound or MRCP support the diagnosis of gallstone pancreatitis.

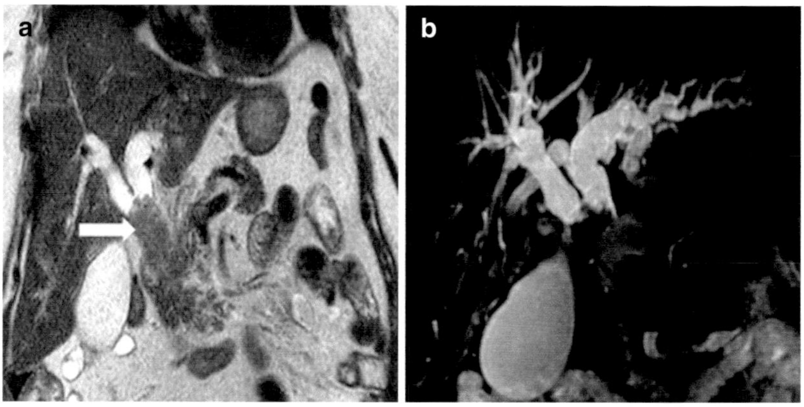

Fig. 9.11 T2-HASTE coronal plane (**a**) and MRCP (**b**) showing dilation of intrahepatic bile ducts due to the presence of a mass inside the common hepatic duct (cholangiocarcinoma) (arrow). This patient presented with fever, jaundice, and abdominal pain; MRI findings confirmed the condition of acute cholangitis

9.11.2 Computed Tomography

CT allows direct visualization of the pancreas and identification of pancreatic edema. This technique is also useful in the detection of complications, including pseudocysts, abscesses, hemorrhage, and necrosis [28]. Pancreatic necrosis is detected on scans performed at least 48–72 h after the onset of an attack of acute pancreatitis as a lack of parenchymal enhancement. However, CT is often less sensitive than transabdominal ultrasound in the identification of gallstones.

9.12 Gallstone Ileus

Gallstone ileus is a bowel obstruction due to an ectopic gallstone, a rare complication of chronic recurrent cholecystitis in which a fistulous tract is created between the biliary and enteric systems [29].

It occurs in 0.3% to 0.5% of patients with cholelithiasis, especially elderly females [30].

Recurrent episodes of cholecystitis associated with cholelithiasis can cause inflammatory changes of the gallbladder walls, which tend to become necrotic, developing a fistulous tract from the gallbladder into the small bowel.

Stones greater than 2 cm can obstruct the small bowel at the ileocecal valve.

The most common site for bilio-enteric fistula is the duodenum because of its proximity to the gallbladder; small bowel and transverse colon have also been reported as involved.

The typical site of obstruction is at the terminal ileum and the ileocecal valve because of their small intraluminal diameter.

An uncommon site of obstruction is the stomach where the stone can migrate proximally causing a gastric outlet obstruction; this phenomenon is also known as Bouveret syndrome.

The diagnosis is difficult, as this condition usually presents with nonspecific signs. The symptoms normally indicate a small bowel obstruction, with nausea, emesis, constipation, and abdominal pain.

Laboratory values are nonspecific, with patients often severely dehydrated with electrolyte and metabolic alterations secondary to the obstruction.

Imaging is very useful for obtaining a correct diagnosis.

Computed tomography is the gold standard, showing signs of small bowel obstruction, pneumobilia (due to the bilio-enteric fistula), and the presence of ectopic gallstones. Most commonly, surgery is required to relieve the obstruction by removing the impacted gallstone.

9.13 Imaging

9.13.1 Ultrasound

Ultrasound can show pneumobilia, cholelithiasis, or choledocholithiasis, but the distortion by bowel gas due to the bowel obstruction makes a diagnosis by ultrasound difficult.

9.13.2 Abdominal X-Ray

Abdominal radiographs are the primary imaging modality, showing Rigler's triad (with sensitivity from 40% to 70%) consists of a partial or complete intestinal obstruction, pneumobilia, and the direct visualization of the ectopic gallstone (Fig. 9.12a).

9.13.3 Computed Tomography

CT has the highest sensitivity, being the gold standard for diagnosis; for this reason, if there is a clinical suspicion but negative x-ray findings, a CT scan should be performed.

Different common signs can be detected, such as gallbladder wall thickening, pneumobilia, intestinal obstruction, and direct visualization of the obstructing gallstones (Fig. 9.12b).

Other diagnostic tests, such as hepatobiliary iminodiacetic acid (HIDA) scan, MRCP, and EGDS, may be necessary only in doubtful cases.

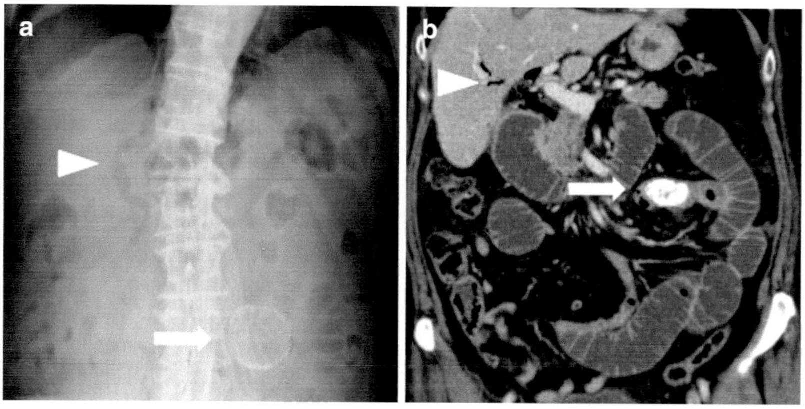

Fig. 9.12 Supine abdominal X-ray (A-XR) and contrast-enhanced computed tomography (CECT) in gallstone ileus with atypical localization of the impacted stone. (**a**): A calcified round gallstone is projected over the left flank (arrow) in combination with air seen in the biliary tree—pneumobilia (arrowhead). (**b**): CECT shows a large calcified gallstone (arrow) impacted in jejunal loops causing a dilation of the small bowel upstream. Note the presence of the pneumobilia (arrowhead)

9.14 Sphincter of Oddi Dysfunction

Sphincter of Oddi dysfunction (SOD) is a benign, non-calculus obstructive disease of the sphincter of Oddi.

Biliary SOD seems to be more prevalent in post-cholecystectomy patients. Among post-cholecystectomy patients, the prevalence of SOD has been reported to be up to 14% in symptomatic patients but only 1% overall.

Symptoms resemble pre-operative biliary pain, with right upper quadrant post-prandial pain, in the absence of evidence of gallstones or cholecystitis. The cause of this condition is thought to be elevated pressures of the sphincter of Oddi, causing emptying issues.

The diagnosis is by exclusion, as laboratory values and imaging studies are typically normal. Non-invasive testing for other possible etiologies should be considered initially to rule out more common conditions, such as musculoskeletal pain, functional abdominal pain, and peptic ulcer disease.

ERCP cholangiography with sphincter of Oddi manometry (SOM) is the gold standard for the diagnosis; a basal pressure greater than 40 mmHg is diagnostic [31].

ERCP with sphincterotomy is also used as the standard care for the treatment of SOD.

Secretin-enhanced magnetic resonance cholangiopancreatography (S-MRCP) improves the visualization of the pancreaticobiliary ductal system and is a good noninvasive option to ERCP.

Secretin is a gastrointestinal peptide that stimulates pancreatic duct epithelial cells to produce a bicarbonate-rich fluid.

An initial breath-hold oblique coronal fat-suppressed heavily T2-weighted long-TE HASTE image encompassing the pancreas is acquired. After an IV dose of human secretin (normally 0.2 μg/kg) is administered, the same sequence study in the same plane is repeated (every 30 s to 1 min for the next 10 to 15 min).

The S-MRCP examination is considered abnormal when the main pancreatic duct diameter on the final sequence remains dilated by greater than 1 mm compared with the baseline measurement [32].

HIDA scans allow following of the transit of a radioisotope as it passes from the hilum of the liver down the biliary tract to the duodenum. A delay in transit suggests sphincter of Oddi dysfunction.

Evaluation of the CBD by ultrasound measurement after a fatty meal is also useful. The test is positive when the CBD expands at least 2 mm from baseline fasting measurement.

9.15 Bile Leak/Biloma

A biloma is a well-demarcated collection of bile outside the biliary tree resulting from a bile leak due to an injury. Traumatic and iatrogenic injuries are the usual causes.

Bile leaks are most commonly associated with hepatobiliary surgery or invasive procedures such as open or laparoscopic cholecystectomy (the most common, with an incidence of bile duct injuries in the range of 0.3%–0.6%0.8), hepatic resection, hepatic transplantation, liver biopsy, and percutaneous transhepatic cholangiography. Blunt abdominal trauma may result in the formation of bilomas days after the trauma.

The presenting symptoms of bile leaks/bilomas are abdominal fullness and dull right upper quadrant abdominal discomfort, as most bilomas are intrahepatic or located in the right subphrenic or subhepatic region. These collections can evolve with a superimposed infection; in these cases, the patients can present with septic shock.

Laboratory studies may demonstrate leukocytosis with neutrophilia, and liver function tests may suggest obstructive disease.

US is often the initial imaging modality used in the case of biloma, demonstrating a cystic lesion, but CT is normally required.

Smaller bilomas can often be conservatively managed with periodic monitoring, whereas larger bilomas often require intervention.

The therapy is based on drainage of the collection and endoscopic sphincterotomy, to decrease the tone of the sphincter of Oddi and divert the bile flow away from the leak site.

9.16 Imaging

9.16.1 Computed Tomography

CT is normally used as a first-line imaging modality in the setting of hepatic injury.

It may show a well-circumscribed, water-attenuation perihepatic or intraparenchymal fluid collection, suggestive of a biloma (Fig. 9.13).

9.16.2 Ultrasound

US has been advocated as a fast and convenient imaging modality, especially in liver trauma. Perihepatic and/or intrahepatic fluid collections may suggest a biliary leak.

9.16.3 Scintigraphy

Hepatobiliary scintigraphy with Tc99 diisopropyl iminodiacetic acid (DISIDA) scan can help detect active bile leaks. Progressive accumulation

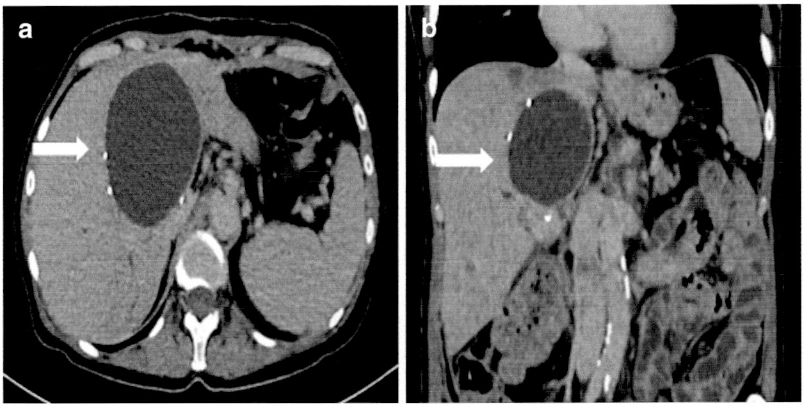

Fig. 9.13 Contrast-enhanced computed tomography (CECT) axial (**a**) and coronal (**b**) planes of a patient who underwent cholecystectomy. Note the presence of a water-attenuation intraparenchymal fluid collection consisting of a biloma (arrow) due to iatrogenic injury

of the radiotracer in an intrahepatic or perihepatic collection is diagnostic [33].

9.16.4 MRI

The typical MRI finding is a well-circumscribed perihepatic or intrahepatic bilious collection with high signal intensity on T2-weighted imaging. This technique may become more sensitive after the administration of a hepatobiliary contrast agent. Hepatobiliary contrasts allow obtaining dynamic biliary imaging during the hepatobiliary phase. A delayed enhanced scan using one of these agents may confirm the bilious nature of an intrahepatic or perihepatic collection and increase the diagnostic accuracy in localizing the bile leak [34].

Bibliography

1. Pavel S, Thijs CT, Potocky V, Knipschild PG. Fair, and still a sun lover: risk of gallstone formation. J Epidemiol Community Health. 1992;46(4):425–7.
2. Hung SC, Liao KF, Lai SW, Li CI, Chen WC. Risk factors associated with symptomatic cholelithiasis in Taiwan: a population-based study. BMC Gastroenterol. 2011;11:111.
3. Tse F, Barkun JS, Romagnuolo J, Friedman G, Bornstein JD, Barkun AN. Nonoperative imaging techniques in suspected biliary tract obstruction. HPB. 2006;8(6):409–25.
4. Crade M, Taylor KJ, Rosenfield AT, de Graaff S, Minihan P. Correlation of Cholecystosonography. Am J Roentgenol. 1978;131:227–9.
5. Shakespear JS, Shaaban AM, Rezvani M. CT findings of acute cholecystitis and its complications. AJR Am J Roentgenol. 2010;194(6):1523–9.
6. Smith EA, Dillman JR, Elsayes KM, Menias CO, Bude RO. Cross-sectional imaging of acute and chronic gallbladder inflammatory disease. AJR Am J Roentgenol. 2009;192(1):188–96.
7. Chawla A, Bosco JI, Lim TC, Srinivasan S, Teh HS, Shenoy JN. Imaging of acute cholecystitis and cholecystitis-associated complications in the emergency setting. Singapore Med J. 2015;56(8):438–43.
8. Katabathina VS, Zafar AM, Suri R. Clinical presentation, imaging, and management of Acute Cholecystitis. Tech Vasc Interv Radiol. 2015;18(4):256–65.
9. Oppenheimer DC, Rubens DJ. Sonography of acute Cholecystitis and its mimics. Radiol Clin North Am. 2019;57(3):535–48.
10. Hanbidge AE, Buckler PM, O'Malley ME, Wilson SR. From the RSNA refresher courses: imaging evaluation for acute pain in the right upper quadrant. Radiographics. 2004;24(4):1117–35.
11. Fagan SP, Awad SS, Rahwan K, Hira K, Aoki N, Itani KM, et al. Prognostic factors for the development of gangrenous cholecystitis. Am J Surg. 2003;186(5):481–5.
12. Watanabe Y, Nagayama M, Okumura A, Amoh Y, Katsube T, Suga T, et al. MR imaging of acute biliary disorders. Radiographics. 2007;27(2):477–95.
13. Derici H, Kara C, Bozdag AD, Nazli O, Tansug T, Akca E. Diagnosis and treatment of gallbladder perforation. World J Gastroenterol. 2006;12(48):7832–6.
14. Ibrarullah M, Mishra T, Das AP. Mirizzi syndrome. Indian J Surg. 2008;70(6):281–7.
15. Kim PN, Outwater EK, Mitchell DG. Mirizzi syndrome: evaluation by MRI imaging. Am J Gastroenterol. 1999;94(9):2546–50.
16. Collins C, Maguire D, Ireland A, Fitzgerald E, O'Sullivan GC. A prospective study of common bile duct calculi in patients undergoing laparoscopic cholecystectomy: natural history of Choledocholithiasis revisited. Ann Surg. 2004;239(1):28–33.
17. O'Connor OJ, O'Neill S, Maher MM. Imaging of biliary tract disease. Am J Roentgenol. 2011;197(4):551–8.
18. Demehri FR, Alam HB. Evidence-based management of common gallstone-related emergencies. J Intensive Care Med. 2016;31(1):3–13.
19. Shaffer EA. Epidemiology of gallbladder stone disease. Best Pract Res Clin Gastroenterol. 2006;20(6):981–96.
20. Kimura Y, Takada T, Kawarada Y, Nimura Y, Hirata K, Sekimoto M, et al. Definitions, pathophysiology, and epidemiology of acute cholangitis and cholecystitis: Tokyo guidelines. J Hepato-Biliary-Pancreat Surg. 2007;14(1):15–26.
21. Mosler P. Diagnosis and Management of Acute Cholangitis. Curr Gastroenterol Rep. 2011;13(2):166–72.
22. Kimura Y, Takada T, Strasberg SM, Pitt HA, Gouma DJ, Garden OJ, et al. TG13 current terminology, etiology, and epidemiology of acute cholangitis and cholecystitis. J Hepatobiliary Pancreat Sci. 2013;20(1):8–23.
23. Bader TR, Braga L, Beavers KL, Semelka RC. MR imaging findings of infectious cholangitis. Magn Reson Imaging. 2001;19(6):781–8.
24. Lee NK, Kim S, Lee JW, Kim CW, Kim GH, Kang DH, et al. Discrimination of suppurative cholangitis from nonsuppurative cholangitis with computed tomography (CT). Eur J Radiol [Internet] 2009;69(3):528–35. [cited 2021 Jul 13]. Available from: http://www.ejradiology.com/article/S0720048X0700589X/fulltext
25. Tohda G, Dochin M, Ohtani M. Efficacy and safety of emergency endoscopic retrograde cholangiopancreatography for acute cholangitis in the elderly retrospective study. World J Gastroenterol [Internet] 2016;22(37):8382–8. Available from: http://www.

wjgnet.com/esps/HelpDesk: http://www.wjgnet.com/esps/helpdesk.aspx:8382-8388: Availablefrom: http://www.wjgnet.com/1007-9327/full/v22/i37/8382.htm. https://doi.org/10.3748/wjg.v22.i37.8382.
26. Tsujino T, Sugita R, Yoshida H, Yagioka H, Kogure H, Sasaki T, et al. Risk factors for acute suppurative cholangitis caused by bile duct stones. Eur J Gastroenterol Hepatol [Internet]. 2007;19(7) Available from: https://journals.lww.com/eurojgh/Fulltext/2007/07000/Risk_factors_for_acute_suppurative_cholangitis.12.aspx
27. Gullo L, Migliori M, Oláh A, Farkas G, Levy P, Arvanitakis C, et al. Acute pancreatitis in five European countries: etiology and mortality. Pancreas [Internet]. 2002;24(3) Available from: https://journals.lww.com/pancreasjournal/Fulltext/2002/04000/Acute_Pancreatitis_in_Five_European_Countries_.3.aspx
28. Baron RL, Stanley RJ, Lee JKT, Koehler RE, Levitt RG. Computed tomographic features of biliary obstruction. Am J Roentgenol. 1983;140(6):1173–8.
29. Artioli G, Muri M, Praticò FE, Marcantoni EA, Gazzani SE, Lana S, et al. Gallstone ileus: literature review. Acta Biomed. 2016;87(1):40–4.
30. Chang L, Chang M, Chang HM, Chang AI, Chang F. Clinical and radiological diagnosis of gallstone ileus: a mini review. Emerg Radiol. 2018;25(2):189–96. https://doi.org/10.1007/s10140-017-1568-5.
31. Drossman DA. The functional gastrointestinal disorders and the Rome III process. Gastroenterology. 2006;130(5):1377–90.
32. Fusaroli P, Kypraios D, Caletti G, Eloubeidi MA. Pancreatico-biliary endoscopic ultrasound: a systematic review of the levels of evidence, performance and outcomes. World J Gastroenterol. 2012;18(32):4243–56.
33. Singh AK, Nachiappan AC, Verma HA, Uppot RN, Blake MA, Saini S, et al. Postoperative imaging in liver transplantation: what radiologists should know. Radiographics. 2010;30(2):339–51.
34. Kantarcı M, Pirimoglu B, Karabulut N, Bayraktutan U, Ogul H, Ozturk G, et al. Non-invasive detection of biliary leaks using Gd-EOB-DTPA-enhanced MR cholangiography: comparison with T2-weighted MR cholangiography. Eur Radiol. 2013;23:2713–22.

Approach to Cholangiopathies

10

Anu Eapen, Kirthi Sathyakumar, and D. Jayavelu Hariram Prasad

10.1 Cholangiopathies

The term 'cholangiopathy' refers to a chronic disorder which affects the 'cholangiocytes' or bile duct epithelial cells. The small cholangiocytes lining the intrahepatic bile ducts and the large cholangiocytes lining the extrahepatic bile ducts have varying functions, depending on their location in the biliary tree. These include production and transport of bile, remodelling of bile duct epithelium and repair of liver cell damage [1]. An injury or insult to cholangiocytes may evoke a series of responses in cholangiocytes which can eventually lead to periportal fibrosis, ductopaenia and biliary cirrhosis [1, 2]. Table 10.1

Several of the cholangiopathies mentioned in Table 10.1 have distinct imaging findings, and these are discussed below.

A. Eapen (✉) · K. Sathyakumar · D. Jayavelu Hariram Prasad
Christian Medical College, Vellore, India

© The Author(s), under exclusive license to Springer Nature Singapore Pte Ltd. 2025
B. Sureka (ed.), *Hepato-Pancreatico Biliary Imaging*, https://doi.org/10.1007/978-981-95-1699-5_10

Table 10.1 Classification of cholangiopathies. (Adapted from Cheung et al. Ref. 3)

Congenital	Immune-mediated	Idiopathic	Infectious	Malignant	Other
Alagille's syndrome	Allograft rejection (acute and chronic)	Biliary atresia	AIDS cholangiopathy	Cholangiocarcinoma	Drug induced
Caroli syndrome	Graft versus host disease	Idiopathic ductopenia (child & adult)	Bacterial cholangitis (e.g. *E. coli*, *Klebsiella*)		Vascular/ ischaemic (post-transplant narrowing of hepatic artery/ vasculitis)
Cystic fibrosis	Primary biliary cholangitis	IgG4-related cholangitis	Parasitic cholangitis (e.g. *Ascaris lumbricoides*, *Opisthorchis viverrini*, *Fasciola hepatica*)		
MDR3 deficiency		Primary sclerosing cholangitis			
Polycystic liver disease		Sarcoidosis			

10.2 Idiopathic

10.2.1 Primary Sclerosing Cholangitis

Primary sclerosing cholangitis (PSC) is a chronic inflammatory disorder affecting biliary epithelium which progresses to fibrosis and strictures of the intra- and extrahepatic bile ducts resulting in cholestasis and ultimately biliary cirrhosis [4].

10.2.2 Etiopathogenesis

It is a disorder of unknown aetiology. Some of the factors linked to the pathogenesis of PSC are complex immune-mediated response, genetic factors due to a strong association with HLA, environmental factors and impaired gut permeability [2, 4, 5]. PSC is a rare disease with the highest prevalence in Northern Europe and the USA, where its incidence is approximately 10/100,000, and is less common in Southern Europe and Asia [5, 6]. It occurs in adult males usually between 30 and 40 years and is twice as common in men as in women [6]. There is an association with inflammatory bowel disease, which has a prevalence of 70% in patients with PSC [5]. Of these, 87% of patients have ulcerative colitis, and 13% have Crohn's [6, 7].

10.2.3 Clinical Presentation

The onset of disease in PSC may be insidious; however, as the disease progresses, fever, jaundice, pruritus and abdominal pain may be seen due to cholestasis. With progression to biliary cirrhosis, patients can present with ascites, variceal bleed or encephalopathy. Symptoms related to ongoing ulcerative colitis such as GI bleed may be seen [4, 5].

10.3 Imaging Modality

10.3.1 Bile Duct Imaging

Large duct PSC, which accounts for 90% of cases, is diagnosed by cholangiography which is the gold standard [8]. PSC commonly affects both intrahepatic and extrahepatic ducts. Intrahepatic ducts alone are involved in about 1/4 of cases. Involvement of only the extrahepatic duct is rare, in less than 5% of cases [7, 8]. Secondary causes of PSC should always be excluded before a diagnosis of PSC is made.

10.3.2 Magnetic Resonance Cholangiopancreaticography (MRCP)

It is the imaging modality of choice for the diagnosis of PSC. MRCP is ideally performed after a 4-h period of fasting and prior to any stent placement [9]. Heavily T2-weighted sequences with gradient echo balanced steady-state free precession are used with 3D-MRCP, which provides better resolution due to thinner sections [7, 9]. However, 2D-MRCP may be utilised in the setting of inadequate breath holding or when respiratory triggering cannot be done.

10.3.3 Early Disease

Typical cholangiographic features of large duct PSC are multifocal annular short segment strictures of the extra- and intrahepatic bile ducts with only mild intervening segments of dilatation and a 'beaded appearance' of biliary radicles on MRCP [6, 10] (Fig. 10.1). Strictures occur at the bifurcation of the bile ducts.

10.3.4 Progressive Disease

With increasing fibrosis and worsening of strictures, the peripheral ducts are not visualised on cholangiogram with a 'pruned tree' appearance on MRCP. As fibrosis and strictures increase, the acute angle between the peripheral and central bile ducts becomes more obtuse [11].

Biliary diverticula or outpouchings from bile ducts and webs, which are 1–2-mm-thick, incomplete, circumferential narrowing of bile ducts, have been described with PSC, although these are not specific for this disorder [10, 12]. Pigment stones of the bile duct may be seen in 30% of cases due to bile stasis [11]. These occur as signal voids or filling defects on MRCP and can predispose to cholangitis.

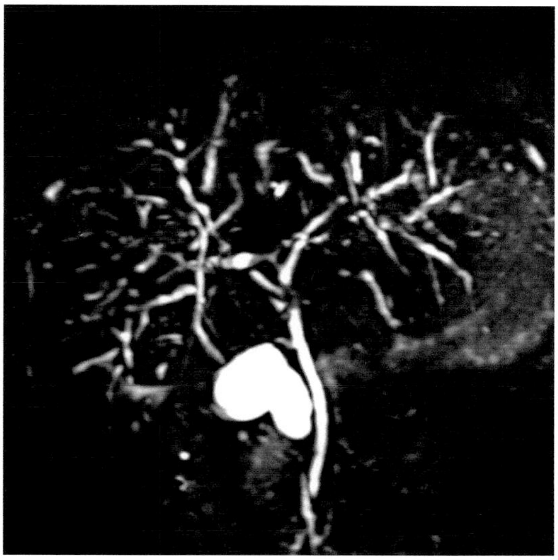

Fig. 10.1 Primary sclerosing cholangitis (PSC). MRCP images show multifocal short segment strictures and mild intervening dilatations with a beaded appearance of the biliary tree

10.3.5 Endoscopic Retrograde Cholangiopancreaticography (ERCP)

ERCP has been replaced by MRCP as the first-line modality to evaluate bile ducts, as it is less invasive, avoids radiation, is cheaper and, unlike ERCP, can provide information about bile ducts proximal to a tight stenosis [7, 11]. ERCP has a higher spatial resolution than MRCP, and thus, peripheral ductal abnormalities are better delineated on ERCP. ERCP is useful to further evaluate a tight stricture with brush cytology and also for therapeutic interventions such as dilatation of a stricture or stent placement [7].

10.3.6 Percutaneous Transhepatic Cholangiography (PTC)

This has a limited role in the evaluation of PSC. It delineates the biliary anatomy and is useful in draining obstructed systems and for stone removal.

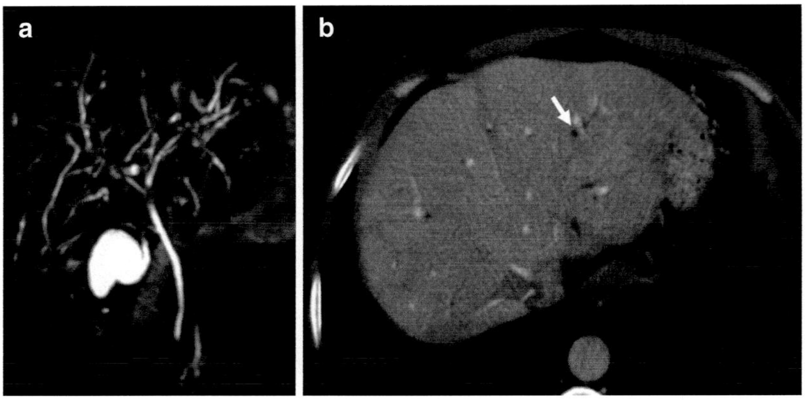

Fig. 10.2 Primary sclerosing cholangitis (PSC). MRCP (**a**) shows a beaded appearance of the biliary tree. Contrast-enhanced CT (**b**) through the upper abdomen shows mild, discontinuous and peripheral intrahepatic biliary dilatation (arrow) without an obvious mass

10.3.7 Ultrasound

Ultrasound can detect involvement of the extrahepatic bile ducts in PSC. The involved extrahepatic ducts show concentric, echogenic thickening and an echogenic portal triad. The resultant luminal narrowing usually causes only a mild proximal dilatation of intrahepatic radicles, which may or may not be visualised on ultrasound. Ultrasound has a limited role in evaluating biliary abnormality, particularly the involvement of the intrahepatic ducts in PSC [7].

10.3.8 CT

Bile duct abnormalities in PSC may be identified on CT as mild, discontinuous, segmental and peripheral intrahepatic biliary dilatation without an obvious mass (Fig. 10.2). Concentric soft tissue thickening and enhancement of the involved extrahepatic bile ducts can be seen on CT with luminal narrowing [7].

10.4 Liver Parenchymal Imaging

CT and MRI can show liver parenchymal changes that occur in advanced PSC. MRI has superior soft tissue resolution and is a better modality for evaluation of liver parenchyma [7]. MRI evaluation of liver parenchyma should include T2, T1, fat-suppressed sequences and the use of contrast medium for a complete evaluation and for the detection of mass lesions. [9].

In advanced PSC, there is an onset of secondary biliary cirrhosis with altered liver morphology which has some specific features that differentiate it from cirrhosis due to other causes. There is marked hypertrophy of the caudate lobe with atrophy of the lateral segment of the left lobe and the posterior segments of the right lobe of the liver. The relative sparing of the central portions of the liver and caudate lobe from the bile duct inflammation and cholestasis with compensatory hypertrophy leads to marked caudate lobe enlargement [7, 13] (Fig. 10.3).

On T2-weighted images, peripheral wedge-shaped areas of hyperintensity and peripheral areas of reticular, heterogenous pattern due to segmental atrophy and may be seen [14] (Fig. 10.4). Portal oedema may also be seen with periportal hyperintensity.

On contrast imaging, enhancement patterns vary. Peripheral wedge-shaped areas which show a delayed enhancement pattern may be seen [7]. In about 56% of patients, peripheral areas of arterial phase enhancement may be seen due to parenchymal inflammation and altered blood supply. In about 23% of patients, hyperintense areas on T1-weighted images can be seen [15].

Periportal lymphadenopathy is a common and nonspecific feature, seen in 77% of patients with PSC [15]. Splenomegaly, collateral vessels may be present when there is portal hypertension (Fig. 10.5).

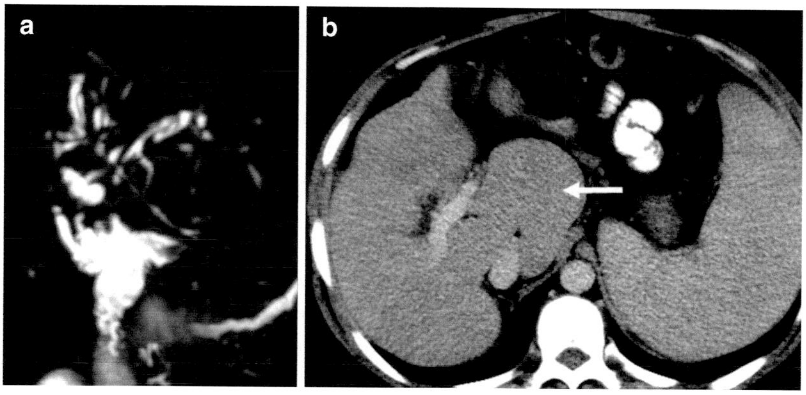

Fig. 10.3 Primary sclerosing cholangitis (PSC). MRCP (**a**) shows a beaded appearance of the biliary tree. Contrast-enhanced CT (**b**) through the upper abdomen shows the onset of secondary biliary cirrhosis with marked caudate lobe hypertrophy (arrow), classically described in secondary biliary cirrhosis due to PSC

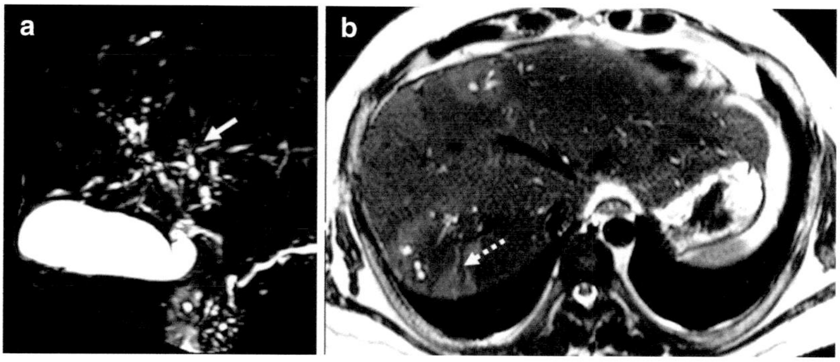

Fig. 10.4 Primary sclerosing cholangitis (PSC). MRCP (**a**) shows a beaded appearance of the biliary tree. T2-weighted axial MR images through the liver (**b**) show peripheral wedge-shaped areas of liver parenchymal hyperintensity (dashed white arrow) and mild dilatation of intrahepatic biliary radicles, described in PSC

Fig. 10.5 Primary sclerosing cholangitis (PSC). MRCP (**a**) shows a beaded appearance of the biliary tree. T2-weighted axial MR images (**b**) show cirrhotic morphology of the liver with marked splenomegaly (black arrow)

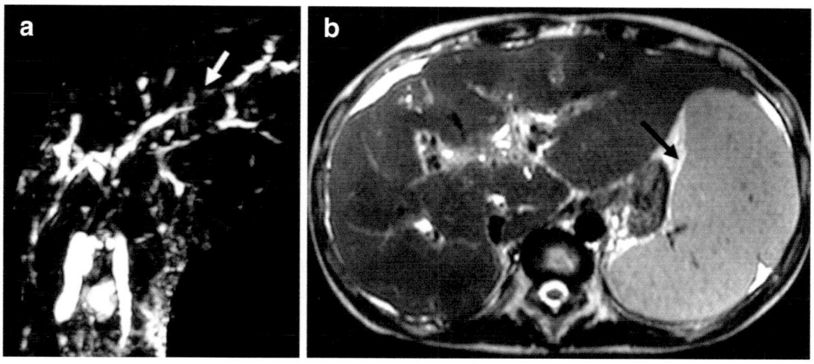

10.4.1 Complications

1. Cholangiocarcinoma

PSC is associated with the risk of hepatobiliary malignancy, the most common being cholangiocarcinoma, which occurs in 10–15% of patients with PSC [16]. The onset of cholangiocarcinoma should be suspected when a patient develops worsening jaundice, pruritus and weight loss.

10.4.2 Imaging

The most common variety of cholangiocarcinoma in PSC is the periductal infiltrating type, seen as periductal thickening with a core of fibrous tissue, in the absence of an obvious mass [7]. The lesion is hyperintense on T2-weighted images and shows delayed enhancement on contrast imaging [7, 17]. It is usually seen in common hepatic duct or its bifurcation, producing a high-grade stricture [11]. The presence of a dominant stricture, defined as narrowing of the common duct $\leq$1.5 mm and/or $\leq$ 1 mm of a hepatic duct within 2 cm of bifurcation, should arouse suspicion of cholangiocarcinoma [8]. Cholangiographic findings of new onset of cholangiocarcinoma, in the setting of PSC, include rapid progression of strictures with marked proximal biliary dilatation and intraductal polypoid mass. Screening for PSC is recommended every 6–12 months by ultrasound or MRI and Ca 19–9 [18].

10.5 Gall Bladder Calculi and Polyps

There is an increased incidence of gallstones and GB polyps in PSC. GB polyps, seen in 10–16% of patients with PSC, are largely benign with an increased risk of malignancy when they are larger than 10 mm [16]. Annual ultrasound screening of GB polyps is recommended in PSC and cholecystectomy, if the polyp size exceeds 8 mm [17].

Small Duct PSC This variant occurs in 5% of cases of PSC with a normal cholangiographic appearance of bile ducts. The diagnosis is established at histology which confirms involvement of small bile ducts with a typical periductal onion-skin fibrosis [4, 6, 17].

PSC with Autoimmune Hepatitis (AIH) Overlap This occurs in younger adults, adolescents and children [4]. An overlap of PSC with autoimmune hepatitis can occur in up to 25% of patients with PSC. In a patient with AIH, MRCP should be performed when there is cholestasis or poor response to steroids to exclude overlap syndrome. MRCP shows multifocal bile duct strictures with mild intervening dilatation, giving a beaded appearance as in PSC without overlap.

10.6 IgG4-Related Sclerosing Cholangitis

10.6.1 Introduction

IgG4-related sclerosing cholangitis (IgG4-SC) is a cholangiopathy which forms part of the spectrum of IgG4-related systemic inflammatory disease involving multiple organs [19]. It is a disorder of unknown aetiology [19]. IgG4-related sclerosing cholangitis, like other manifestations of IgG4-related disease, is associated with elevated serum IgG4 levels, infiltration of IgG4-positive plasma cells, storiform fibrosis and obliterative phlebitis in the bile duct wall with good response to treatment with steroids [20].

IgG4-related disease can involve multiple organs, the commonest being Type 1 autoimmune pancreatitis (AIP) (60%), followed by sialadenitis (34%), tubulointerstitial nephritis (23%), dacryoadenitis (23%) and periaortitis (20%) [21] (Fig. 10.6).

IgG4-SC is commonly associated with Type 1 autoimmune pancreatitis [22]. It may occasionally occur along with IgG4-related sialadenitis/dacryoadenitis and retroperitoneal fibrosis

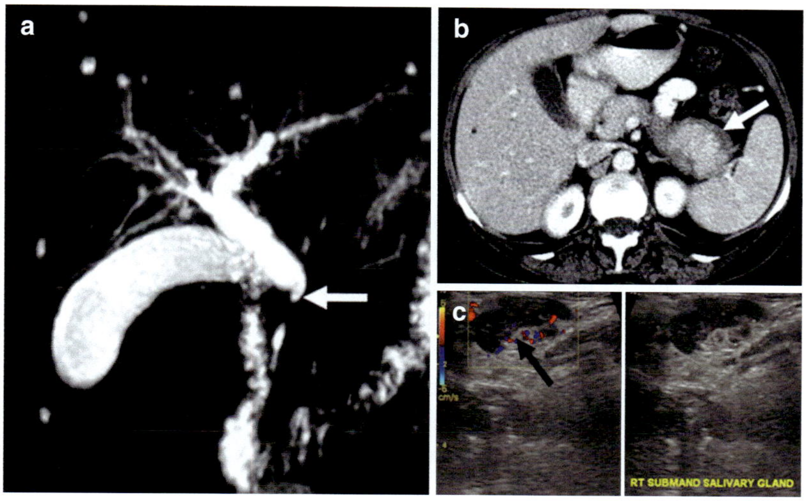

Fig. 10.6 IgG4-related sclerosing cholangitis. MRCP (**a**) shows narrowing of the lower common bile duct (white arrow). Contrast-enhanced CT (**b**) through the upper abdomen shows associated autoimmune pancreatitis with a bulky pancreatic tail with a hypodense rim (white arrow in **b**). Ultrasound images of the same patient (**c**) reveal an enlarged right submandibular gland (black arrow) with increased vascularity due to sialadenitis

[19]. IgG4-SC of the lower duct is almost always associated with Type 1 AIP and is believed to be an extension of pancreatic inflammation rather than isolated IgG4-related sclerosing cholangitis [21].

IgG4-SC involving the hilum and intrahepatic bile ducts can occur with AIP or alone. However, isolated IgG4-SC is very rare [21].

10.6.2 Pathologic Findings

Inflammatory infiltration with lymphocytes, plasma cells and also eosinophils and storiform fibrosis with an irregularly whorled pattern of collagen fibres occur around veins, leading to occlusion of veins or obliterative phlebitis. These changes occur in the submucosa of the bile duct wall with a normal epithelial layer. This helps differentiate from PSC, where inflammatory changes affect the epithelial layer [19, 23]. Cut-off values of more than 50 cells/hpf of IgG4-positive plasma cells in surgical specimens and more than 10 cells per hpf in biopsy samples with a ratio of IgG4-positive to total IgG-positive plasma cells of more than 40% are specific for IgG4-SC [21, 23].

10.6.3 Clinical Features

IgG4-SC occurs typically in elderly males. The majority of patients diagnosed with IgG4 disease are above the age of 60 years with a male-to-female ratio of 4:1. The usual presentation is with obstructive jaundice, especially when there is pancreatic involvement [21]. Occasionally, biliary involvement in IgG4-related disease may be seen as an incidental finding.

10.6.4 Investigations

High serum IgG4 levels are seen in IgG4-SC, and at a cut-off of 140 mg/dl, sensitivity was 80% for IgG4 disease [21]. However, IgG4 levels may be elevated rarely in PSC and cholangiocarcinoma, hence with lower specificity. IgG4-SC can mimic cholangiocarcinoma on imaging. At a higher cut-off of 280 mg/dl, there is a higher specificity of 90% for IgG4-SC but at a lower sensitivity of 50% [21]. When serum IgG4 elevation is four times the upper limit of normal, there is 100% specificity for IgG4-SC [24]. A ratio of IgG4/IgG >0.10 or IgG4/IgG1 > 0.24 is also specific for IgG4-SC.

10.7 Imaging

Ultrasound is often the baseline investigation in a patient with jaundice. Ultrasound shows circumferential thickening of the bile duct wall with proximal dilatation of intrahepatic ducts. However, there is low sensitivity and specificity for the diagnosis of IgG4 disease [23]. Other findings that may be seen in IgG4 disease are diffuse, hypoechoic GB wall thickening and a bulky pancreas in the setting of AIP [25].

Intraductal ultrasonography(IDUS) is useful to demonstrate the circumferential bile duct wall thickening, smooth inner and outer wall and narrow but visible lumen [21].

CT and MRI/MRCP help locate and study the extent of biliary strictures, the proximal biliary dilatation, the degree of wall thickening and the enhancement pattern of thickened bile duct wall [21].

MRCP is the best noninvasive method to delineate biliary abnormalities. CT/MRI helps delineate associated pancreatic abnormalities such as a diffusely bulky pancreas with a capsule-like rim around it and narrowing of the main pancreatic duct [21] (Fig. 10.7). Involvement of other organs such as the kidneys with cortical lesions and pelvic wall thickening may be seen.

ERCP is better than MRCP to delineate bile duct luminal abnormalities; however, it is more invasive [21, 26].

10.7.1 Bile Duct Abnormalities in IgG4-SC

Based on the location of strictures, these have been classified into four types as shown in Table 10.2.

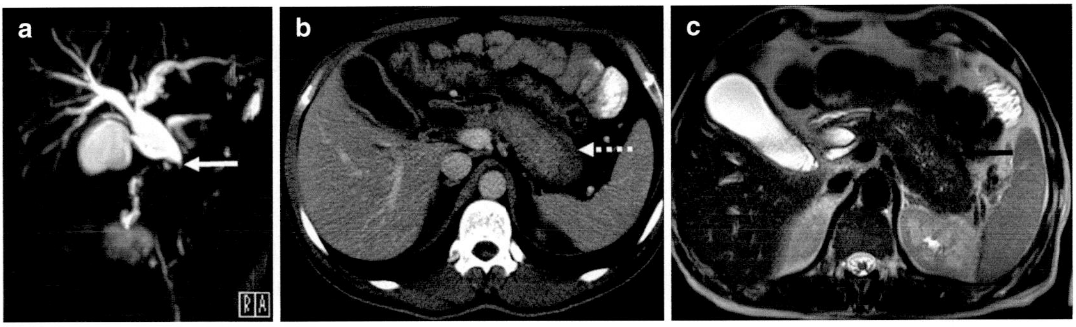

Fig. 10.7 IgG4-related sclerosing cholangitis. MRCP (**a**) shows smooth tapered narrowing of the lower common bile duct. Contrast-enhanced CT (**b**) through the upper abdomen shows associated autoimmune pancreatitis with a bulky pancreatic body and tail with a hypodense capsule-like rim around it (dashed white arrow), seen as a T2 hypointense rim (black arrow) on MRI (**c**)

Table 10.2 Classification of cholangiographic changes in IgG4-SC with AIP. (Nakazawa et al.). Adapted from Refs. 19 and 26

Types	Location of stricture	Differential diagnosis
1	Distal CBD	Pancreatic cancer, bile duct cancer, chronic pancreatitis
2	Stenosis of intrahepatic and proximal extrahepatic bile ducts	Primary sclerosing cholangitis
2a	Narrowing of intrahepatic ducts with prestenotic dilatation	
2b	Narrowing of intrahepatic bile ducts without prestenotic dilatation and reduced peripheral branches	
3	Stenosis in the lesion in the hepatic hilum and lower CBD	Cholangiocarcinoma
4	Stenosis in the lesion at the hepatic hilum	Cholangiocarcinoma

IgG4-SC IgG4-related sclerosing cholangitis, *AIP* autoimmune pancreatitis

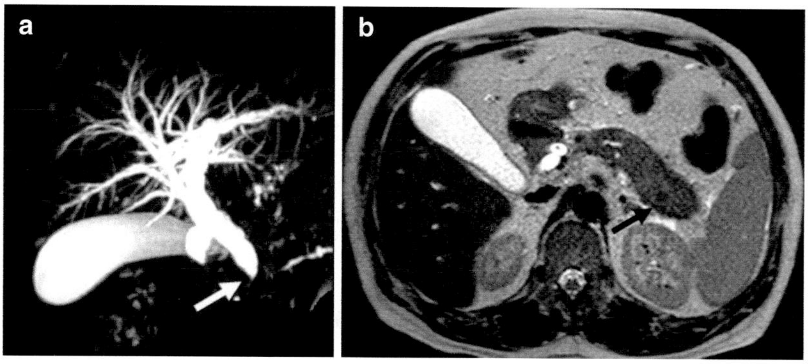

Fig. 10.8 IgG4-related sclerosing cholangitis. MRCP (**a**) shows smooth tapered narrowing of the lower common bile duct (white arrow) which represents Type 1 cholangiographic changes of sclerosing cholangitis with AIP (classification by Nakazawa et al.). T2-weighted axial MR image (**b**) shows a bulky pancreas with a T2 hypointense rim (black arrow)

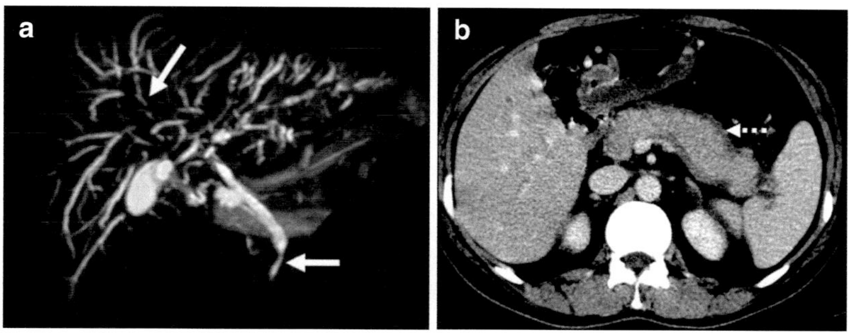

Fig. 10.9 IgG4-related sclerosing cholangitis. MRCP (**a**) shows smooth tapered narrowing of the lower common bile duct with strictures of intrahepatic bile ducts (arrows). This represents Type 2a cholangiographic changes of sclerosing cholangitis with AIP (classification by Nakazawa et al.). Contrast-enhanced CT (**b**) confirms autoimmune pancreatitis with a bulky pancreas and a hypodense rim (dashed white arrow)

Types 1 and 2 are demonstrated in Figs. 10.8 and 10.9.

Thickening of the bile duct wall in IgG4-SC is symmetrical and circular, with smooth inner and outer margins and a homogenous internal echo on ultrasound and intraductal ultrasound. These changes are also seen on CT and MRI and may be seen in nonstenotic portions of the bile duct wall as well [19, 21].

10.8 Differential Diagnosis

10.8.1 IgG4-SC versus PSC

IgG4-SC is characterised by segmental strictures; long, continuous bile duct thickening; single-layer duct wall thickness more than 2.5 mm; stricture involving the distal CBD and dilatation below the stricture at confluence. Associated diffuse GB wall thickening and absence of liver parenchymal changes are other features of IgG4-SC [19, 21, 27].

Features of PSC are band-like or short segment strictures (1–2 mm) alternating with normal or minimally dilated proximal bile ducts, giving a beaded appearance, pruned tree appearance due to decreased peripheral branches and diverticulum-like outpouchings of bile ducts [19, 27].

10.8.2 IgG4-SC versus Cholangiocarcinoma

In a study by Yata et al., a sensitivity of more than 80% for the diagnosis of IgG4-related disease was concentric thickening of the wall of the bile duct, pancreatic abnormality, unilayered contrast enhancement of the bile duct wall and homogenous attenuation on delayed scan. A specificity of more than 80% was seen in lesions involving the intrapancreatic bile duct, smooth outer margins, narrow but preserved lumen, funnel-shaped proximal bile ducts, skip lesions and pancreatic abnormality. High sensitivity and specificity for the diagnosis of IgG4 SC were seen in the presence of pancreatic abnormality [28].

10.9 Infectious Causes

10.9.1 Recurrent Pyogenic Cholangitis

10.9.1.1 Introduction

Recurrent pyogenic cholangitis (RPC) is an infectious cholangitis characterised by recurrent biliary infections, inflammatory bile duct strictures and pigmented intraductal calculi. It is prevalent in the Asian population, although increasingly seen in Western countries. It is also known by the synonyms of Oriental cholangiohepatitis and Hong Kong disease [29].

10.9.1.2 Etiopathogenesis

RPC affects men and women equally, usually in the third and fourth decades of life. There is an association with low socioeconomic status [30].

Although the exact aetiology is not known, infestations with parasites such as *Clonorchis sinensis*, *Ascaris lumbricoides*, *Fasciola hepatica* and *Opisthorchis* species are thought to be the underlying cause for RPC with superimposed bacterial infections due to reduced host immune response. Several organisms such as *Escherichia coli*, *Klebsiella*, *Pseudomonas*, *Proteus* and anaerobes have been obtained from bile cultures. Recurrent or chronic inflammation and sepsis lead to fibrosis, stricture formation and intraductal calculi due to stasis [29]. The left duct which has an acute angulation is prone to stasis, inflammation, stricture and stone formation. The stones lead to further stasis, sepsis and fibrosis with strictures [30].

10.9.1.3 Clinical Features

Patients with RPC commonly present with recurrent pain, fever and jaundice. Recurrent sepsis can cause abscesses in the liver and at distant sites. Portal vein thrombosis can occur. Cholangiocarcinoma is known to occur in 5% of patients with RPC, and this may be associated with weight loss [30].

10.9.1.4 Imaging

Ultrasound is often the initial imaging modality used for evaluation of a patient with RPC, as it is cheap and easily available. Ultrasound shows a disproportionate dilatation of the central intrahepatic and extrahepatic bile ducts with sparing of the peripheral bile ducts [30, 31]. The dilatation of central ducts is diffuse, irrespective of the presence of calculi, and has been attributed to loss of elasticity of the bile duct wall [31]. About 90% of cases will have intraductal calculi, often obscured in the presence of pneumobilia [30]. Periductal inflammation and fibrosis can cause an increase in periportal echogenicity [29].

Ultrasound can identify complications such as liver abscess and biloma. Percutaneous drainage of abscesses can be performed under ultrasound guidance.

CT is a better modality than ultrasound, particularly to detect minimal intrahepatic biliary dilatation. The disproportionate dilatation of central intrahepatic and extrahepatic ducts is well delineated on CT. On unenhanced CT, 90% of biliary calculi are hyperdense to unenhanced liver parenchyma. The presence of pneumobilia, which may be seen, can be due to varied reasons such as therapeutic procedures, passage of stones through the ampulla or cholangitis with gas-forming organisms such as *Klebsiella pneumoniae* or *Clostridium perfringens* [30, 31].

Long-standing inflammation leads to parenchymal atrophy with bile duct dilatation and crowding. These changes typically involve the lateral segment of the left lobe followed by the posterior segment of the right lobe (Fig. 10.10). These changes can be seen also on MRI, where calculi appear as signal voids and atrophic segments are iso- to mildly hyperintense on T2-weighted images [31] (Fig. 10.11).

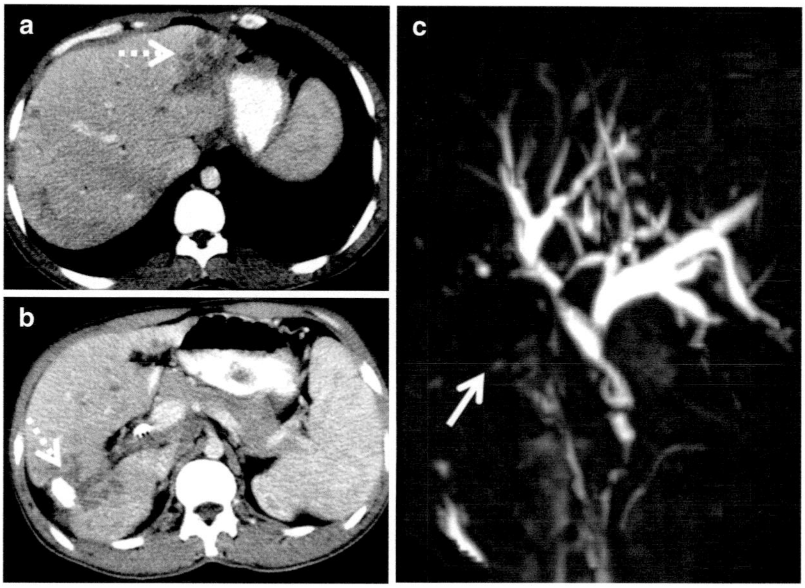

Fig. 10.10 Recurrent pyogenic cholangitis. Contrast-enhanced CT (**a**, **b**) shows crowding and dilatation of intrahepatic biliary radicles in the left lateral segment and the posterior segment of the right lobe of the liver (dashed white arrows) with atrophy of involved liver segments. A radiodense calculus is seen in the posterior segment of the right lobe. MRCP (**c**) shows poorly visualised posterior segmental duct of the right lobe due to multiple calculi in the lumen (white arrow)

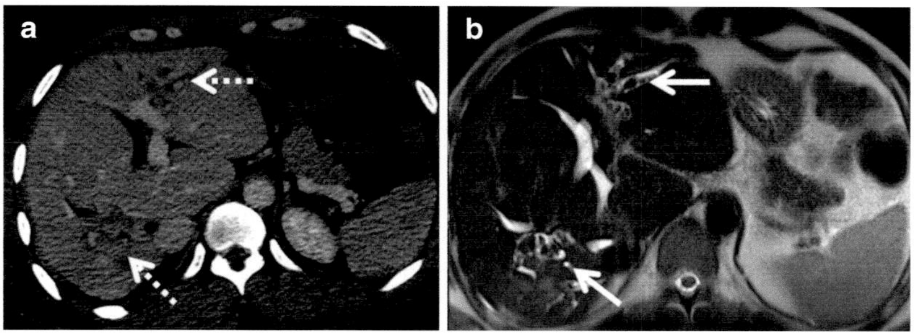

Fig. 10.11 Recurrent pyogenic cholangitis. Contrast-enhanced CT (**a**) and T2-weighted axial MRI (**b**) through the upper abdomen show crowding and dilatation of intrahepatic biliary radicles typically involving the left lateral segment and the posterior segment of the right lobe of the liver with multiple intraductal calculi (dashed white arrow in (**a**) and white arrow in (**b**))

MRCP and ERCP are useful techniques to delineate biliary anatomy. The advantages of MRCP is its ability to delineate noncalcified calculi, which are seen as signal voids, to accurately depict bile ducts proximal to tight stenosis and also the extrahepatic bile ducts (Fig. 10.12).

ERCP has better spatial resolution compared to MRCP, but it is more invasive.

Both MRCP and ERCP show disproportionate dilatation of central and extrahepatic ducts with abrupt narrowing of peripheral bile ducts [30, 31]. A cholangiogram also demonstrates strictures and the presence of calculi.

10.9.1.5 Complications

Abscess Liver abscess may be seen in 20% of patients with RPC. These occur most often in the right lobe, may be multiple, often multiseptated [30, 31]. The presence of a peripheral rim of enhancement helps differentiate from a biloma.

Portal vein thrombosis can occur.

Cholangiocarcinoma This is a rare complication, seen in 5% of patients, and affects the atrophied portions of the liver or portions of the liver with a large number of calculi. Biliary stasis, cal-

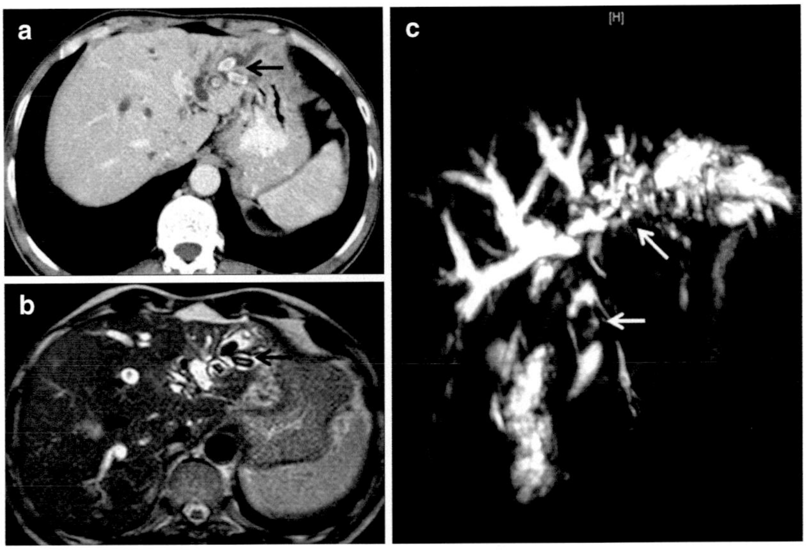

Fig. 10.12 Recurrent pyogenic cholangitis. Contrast-enhanced CT (**a**) shows multiple radiodense intraductal calculi, which appear as signal voids on T2-weighted axial MRI (black arrows in (**a**, **b**). MRCP (**c**) demonstrates multiple signal voids in the lower common bile duct and in the left hepatic ducts (white arrows)

culi and chronic infection are some of the factors thought to predispose to the formation of calculi. CT shows abrupt narrowing of the involved duct with enhancing soft tissue thickening. Lesion may show restricted diffusion on diffusion-weighted MRI [31].

10.9.1.6 Management

Treatment consists of dilatation of strictures to facilitate biliary drainage and removal of stones.

This is done by ERCP or percutaneous techniques. If these fail, surgical management includes biliary bypass procedures, segmental hepatic resection and liver transplantation.

10.10 AIDS-Related Cholangitis

Human immunodeficiency virus infection can affect the biliary tract in several ways, a spectrum known as AIDS cholangiopathy. It can cause acalculous cholecystitis, sclerosing cholangitis, papillary stenosis, lymphoma, Kaposi's sarcoma and gallstones [32]. AIDS cholangiopathy usually affects severely immunocompromised individuals with a CD4 T lymphocyte count of less than 100/mm [29, 33].

Aetiology Opportunistic infections with *Cryptosporidium* and CMV are common causes of cholangitis, but it may also occur due to ischaemia, autonomic nerve damage or direct epithelial invasion by HIV [29, 33].

Imaging There are four cholangiogram patterns which have been described: papillary stenosis with distal tapering of the CBD, sclerosing cholangitis with strictures and dilatations of intra- and extrahepatic ducts, combined papillary stenosis and sclerosing cholangitis and long strictures, more than 1 to 2 cm of the extrahepatic bile duct [33]. Thickening and enhancement of the bile duct wall may be seen on MRI [32] (Fig. 10.13).

Management HAART therapy remains the vital treatment, and antimicrobial therapy for opportunistic pathogens is often not effective [34].

Sphincterotomy, balloon dilatation and stenting of strictures may help relieve biliary obstruction [34].

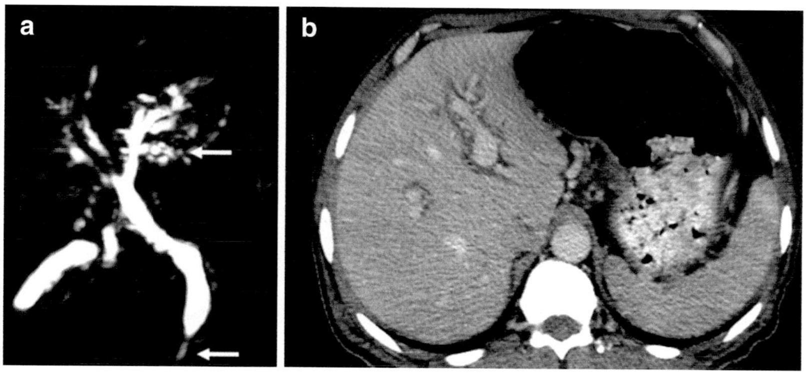

Fig. 10.13 AIDS-related cholangitis. MRCP (**a**) reveals narrowing of the terminal lower common bile duct with multiple intrahepatic bile duct strictures (white arrows) in a patient with HIV and worsening liver function tests. Contrast-enhanced CT (**b**) shows mild intrahepatic biliary dilatation

10.11 Vascular Causes

10.11.1 Portal Cavernoma Cholangiopathy

Portal cavernoma cholangiopathy (PCC) is known by various terminologies like portal biliopathy, portal hypertensive biliopathy, extrahepatic portal biliopathy, vascular biliopathy, portal ductopathy and portal cholangiopathy.

It is defined as the abnormalities caused by portal cavernoma in the extrahepatic bile duct, cystic duct and gall bladder with or without abnormalities in the first- and second-order biliary ducts. All of the following criteria need to be fulfilled for establishing the diagnosis: (a) presence of portal cavernoma, (b) typical ERCP or MRCP changes and (c) absence of other causes like bile duct injury, cholangiocarcinoma, primary sclerosing cholangitis, etc. [35].

Clinical Features PCC most commonly occurs in non-cirrhotic patients with hypercoagulable states. The majority of patients are asymptomatic with only about 21% (5–50%) demonstrating symptoms. The patients may present with chronic cholestasis and biliary colic with or without cholangitis due to biliary calculi. Choledocholithiasis is seen in 5–20% due to stasis of bile. Bleeding from collaterals leading to haemobilia is relatively rare. In the late stage, some patients may progress to secondary biliary cirrhosis [35, 36].

Pathogenesis The two main causes proposed for the biliary changes are compression by large collaterals and ischaemic injury due to chronic portal vein thrombosis (PVT) or long-standing compression. Both mechanisms can also coexist in a patient with PCC. Porto-systemic shunt surgeries can potentially reverse collateral compression [37]. The collaterals are formed by engorgement of the paracholedochal veins of Petren and the epicholedochal venous plexus of Saint. Gallstone disease is frequently associated, presumed to be contributed by (a) strictures causing stasis of bile, (b) increased lithogenicity of bile, (c) decreased gall bladder contractility due to collaterals in the wall and (d) liver parenchymal disease causing decreased bile flow [38].

10.11.2 Diagnosis

Ultrasonography with Colour Doppler This should be the initial imaging modality in suspected PCC. Attenuated or recanalised portal vein with dilated tortuous collaterals (cavernoma) at the porta hepatis can be visualised. In 95% of cases, there is extension of PVT into the SMV and splenic vein. A compensatory increase in hepatic artery flow may be seen. Pericholecystic and bile duct wall collaterals can be seen with thickened bile ducts and intrahepatic biliary dilatation [38].

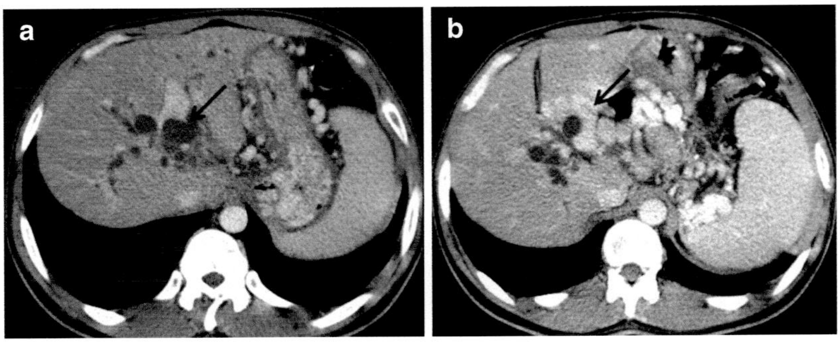

Fig. 10.14 Portal cavernoma cholangiopathy. Contrast-enhanced CT (**a**, **b**) shows a cavernoma at the porta, replacing the main portal vein. Dilated intrahepatic biliary radicles due to compression of the common bile duct at the porta by cavernoma (black arrow in (**a**, **b**))

Computed Tomography or Magnetic Resonance Imaging (MRI) CECT and MRI delineate the portal venous system well and assist in identifying the cause for portal venous thrombosis (Fig. 10.14). MR cholangiography (MRC) with MR portovenography is the modality of choice for mapping the biliary and vascular abnormalities in PCC. MRC is as accurate as ERC and clearly depicts the typical findings of biliopathy—shallow or deep extrinsic impressions/indentations, irregular duct contour, stricture, filling defects, bile duct angulation causing $\leq 145°$ angle at the site of extrinsic impression, upstream dilatation and ectasia without any downstream obstruction. Kinking or tethering of the CBD at the superior portion of the pancreatic head is also a common finding due to compression by the dilated pancreaticoduodenal veins. The angle of the CBD above the pancreatic head is more acute in the presence of PCC (averaging 110°) than in patients with portal vein thrombosis without cholangiopathy (128°) [38, 39].

MRI helps distinguish collaterals from bile duct stones. MRI also demonstrates the presence of shuntable vein and differentiates epicholedochal from paracholedochal collaterals and gall bladder varices. Epicholedochal collaterals are smaller, intramural dot-like signal voids/enhancing structures in the bile duct wall. The bile duct appears narrowed and thickened and is densely enhancing. Paracholedochal collaterals are larger, low signal intensity channels that compress and distort the bile duct [35].

Endoscopic Ultrasound (EUS) EUS is utilised when other imaging modalities are inconclusive in identifying the cause of biliary obstruction. It helps in delineating the type of choledochal collaterals (paracholedochal, epicholedochal, intracholedochal and subepithelial). This differentiation is relevant when endotherapy is being planned to avoid the risk of haemobilia [38].

Endoscopic Retrograde Cholangiography (ERC) ERC is considered the gold standard for defining the biliary changes of PCC. However, currently, it has no diagnostic role, as it is an invasive procedure. ERC is now utilised in instances where therapeutic procedures are planned. The cholangiographic abnormalities are the same as described under MR cholangiography [35, 36].

Natural Course of the Disease PCC develops early on in the event of acute PVT if recanalisation is not achieved. It is, however, a progressive condition, and symptoms may develop late in the course of portal hypertension. In addition, symptomatic patients usually have advanced or severe changes of biliopathy (Fig. 10.15). Successful endoscopic biliary drainage and shunt surgery are beneficial in patients with symptoms [35, 37].

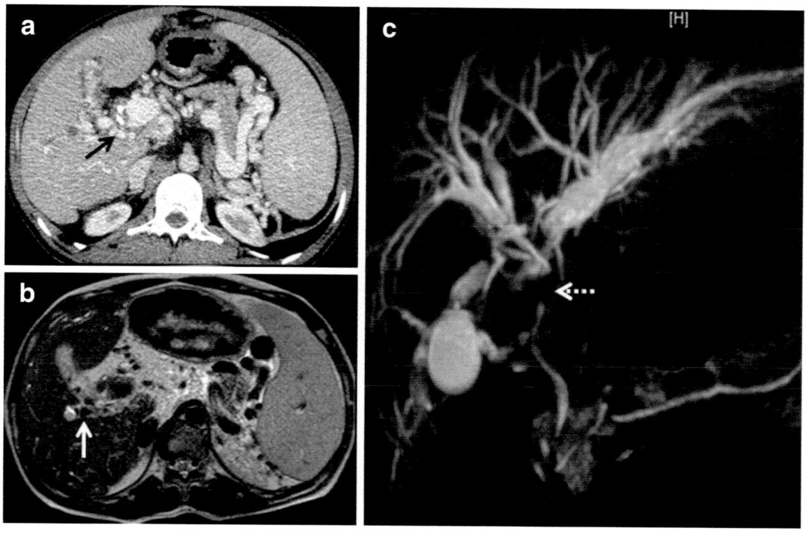

Fig. 10.15 Portal cavernoma cholangiopathy. Contrast-enhanced CT (**a**) shows collaterals at the porta (black arrow in (**a**), replacing the main portal vein and around the gall bladder with portosystemic collaterals near the splenic hilum). These are seen as multiple signal voids (white arrow) on T2-weighted MRI (**b**). MRCP (**c**) demonstrates narrowing of the proximal common hepatic duct by cavernoma and intrahepatic biliary dilatation. The common bile duct is of normal calibre

Management Relatively safe and effective procedures for PCC include biliary stent placement, sphincterotomy, stricture dilatation, lithotripsy and stone extraction. Porto-systemic decompressive surgery can cause reversal of symptoms in the presence of a shuntable vein. In persistently symptomatic patients, second-stage surgical options like hepaticojejunostomy and choledochoduodenostomy may be considered. Secondary biliary cirrhosis in complicated PCC is the only indication for liver transplantation in these patients [35].

10.12 Ischaemic Cholangiopathy

This refers to bile duct damage that results from deficient blood supply to the biliary ducts (40). These ducts receive their blood supply entirely from the hepatic artery via the rich network of peribiliary plexus surrounding the bile ducts [1, 40].

Aetiology Conditions causing ischaemic injury are thrombosis after liver transplantation, chemo-embolisation, surgical procedures, hereditary haemorrhagic telangiectasia and polyarteritis nodosa [1, 6, 40].

Imaging The most common sites of ischaemic injury are the mid-third of the bile duct followed by the hepatic confluence. Ischaemic injury to the bile ducts can present in three ways [1]. In severe injury, there is focal necrosis of the bile duct wall resulting in intrahepatic collections or biloma. In less severe injury, there is epithelial desquamation which forms biliary casts that can cause biliary obstruction [1]. Biliary casts, like calculi, may be hyperintense on T1-weighted MRI but have a linear, branching pattern [1, 6]. In chronic injury, fibrosis can cause biliary strictures which can mimic PSC or cholangiocarcinoma. The presence of peripheral areas of narrowing in PSC and a periductal mass in cholangiocarcinoma may help differentiate from ischaemic cholangiopathy [40].

Management includes several measures such as restoration of arterial flow in transplants, removal of biliary casts, drainage of biloma and biliary bypass procedures [6].

10.13 Immune-Mediated Causes

10.13.1 Primary Biliary Cholangitis

Primary biliary cholangitis (PBC) is an autoimmune-mediated, chronic inflammatory process affecting interlobular bile ducts with end-stage fibrosis, leading to cirrhosis [1]. This has a predilection for women between the fifth and seventh decades of life. The onset may be insidious. Fever and pruritus progressing to jaundice may be another presentation.

10.13.2 Etiopathogenesis

A combination of genetic and environmental factors has been implicated in the pathogenesis of PBC. Histologically, nonsuppurative inflammation of the bile ducts leads to asymmetric destruction of ducts within portal triads which ultimately leads to cirrhosis [41].

10.13.3 Imaging

Findings on imaging are mild in early stages and may not contribute to making a diagnosis of PBC. Cholangiogram in the early stage may be normal, but later, there is narrowing of ducts without post-stenotic dilatation causing ductopenia [1, 41]. The extrahepatic duct is not involved. The periportal halo sign on MRI is unique for PBC, best seen on T2-weighted MRI. This represents a ring or halo of T2 hypointensity due to fibrosis around the central portal triad [42]. In advanced stages of disease, imaging shows the onset of cirrhosis with splenomegaly and portal hypertension.

10.14 Congenital Causes

Caroli Disease This condition, also known as communicating cavernous ectasia of the intrahepatic bile ducts, is a congenital disorder characterised by nonobstructive dilatation, either saccular or fusiform, of the intrahepatic bile ducts [43].

Caroli disease results from embryonic ductal plate malformation where there is failure of remodelling and partial involution of the embryonic ductal plate. This process of remodelling of embryonic ductal plate to form bile ducts normally occurs from the hilum to the periphery of the liver with the development of the large intrahepatic bile ducts first and the smallest peripheral ductules last [44, 45]. There are two types described.

1. *Type 1 or pure type:* This is sporadic, nonhereditary and confined to one hepatic lobe. This results from arrested remodelling of the ductal plates of larger intrahepatic bile ducts. Dilatation of segmental bile ducts results in calculi and recurrent cholangitis (Fig. 10.16).
2. *Type 2 or hereditary type:* This type involves the entire liver and is usually associated with congenital hepatic fibrosis and portal hypertension. Caroli syndrome, which refers to a combination of Caroli disease and congenital hepatic fibrosis, occurs when there is arrested remodelling of the entire intrahepatic biliary tree [45]. It may be associated with other conditions such as choledochal cysts and ARPKD [43] (Fig. 10.17).

10.14.1 Imaging

Cholangiography shows the typical findings of saccular dilatation of intrahepatic bile ducts. These may contain calculi or sludge.

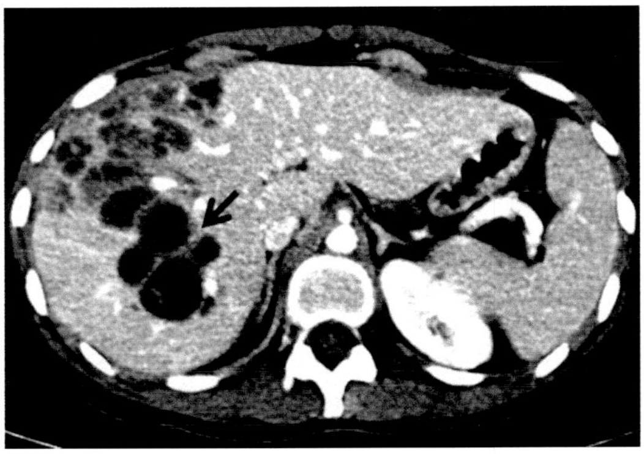

Fig. 10.16 Caroli disease Type 1. Contrast-enhanced CT shows cystic dilatation of intrahepatic biliary radicles confined to the right lobe

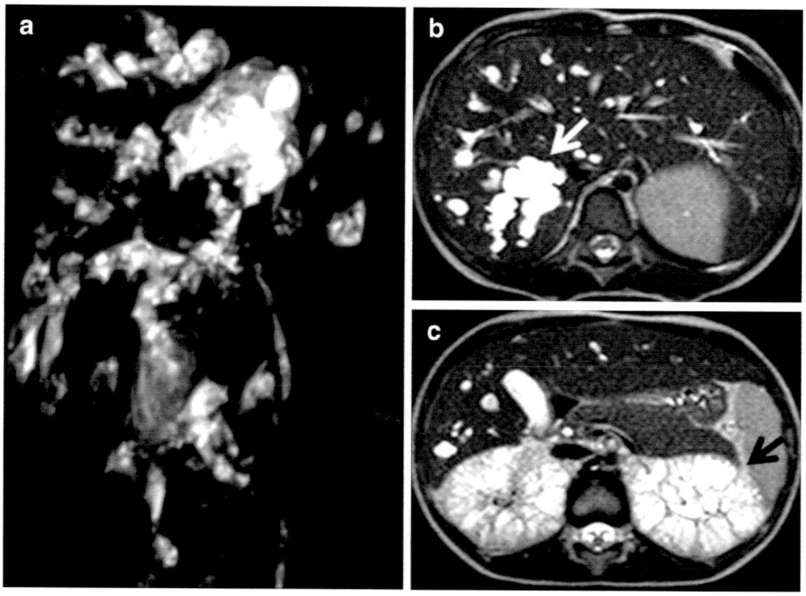

Fig. 10.17 Caroli disease Type 2. MRCP (**a**) and T2-weighted axial MR images (**b**, **c**) show cystic dilatation of biliary radicles in both lobes of the liver with normal calibre of the extrahepatic bile duct on MRCP. There is associated autosomal recessive polycystic kidney disease seen in (**c**) as marked diffuse T2 hyperintensity of both kidneys due to the presence of microcysts

Contrast-enhanced CT or MRI shows cystically dilated intrahepatic radicles communicating with the biliary tree. The central dot sign describes an enhancing fibrovascular bundle or portal vein branch within the centre of a cystically dilated radicle. The presence of communication of these cystic dilatations with the biliary tree differentiates this condition from polycystic liver disease. Complications of Caroli disease, such as stone formation and abscess due to cholangitis, are seen on imaging [44]. In the presence of these, other differential diagnoses include recurrent pyogenic cholangitis, communicating liver abscesses, choledochal cysts, PSC and obstructive biliary dilatation [45, 46]. There is also an increased risk of cholangiocarcinoma.

In Caroli syndrome, there is mild focal narrowing and only mild intervening dilatation of intrahepatic radicles. Calculi are usually absent. Associated findings of congenital hepatic fibrosis, such as shrunken liver, splenomegaly and varices, may be seen.

The association of Caroli disease with extrahepatic bile duct dilatation and choledochal cysts has also been described in the literature [45].

The salient imaging features of the cholangiopathies aforementioned are listed in Table 10.3.

Cholangiopathies, thus, represent a spectrum of disorders of varied aetiology, with often common clinical presentations such as fever and jaundice. Appropriate imaging can help in making an accurate diagnosis and also help in the follow-up of these patients.

Table 10.3 Salient imaging features of the common cholangiopathies

PSC	Short segment strictures, mild intervening dilatation, beaded appearance
	Intra- and extrahepatic ducts
	Association—IBD
IgG4-SC	Long segment strictures, symmetrical
	Smooth inner and outer margins with visible lumen
	Intra- and extrahepatic ducts
RPC	Dilated central intrahepatic ducts, sparing of peripheral bile ducts
	Intraductal calculi, lobar atrophy
	Lateral segment of the left lobe, posterior segment of the right lobe
AIDS-related cholangitis	4 patterns Papillary stenosis with narrowing of the distal CBD
	Sclerosing cholangitis with strictures and dilatations of intra- and extrahepatic ducts
	Combined papillary stenosis and sclerosing cholangitis
	Long strictures of the extrahepatic bile duct
PCC	Bile duct extrinsic indentations
	Bile duct angulation causing a $\leq 145°$ angle at the site of extrinsic impression
	Smooth strictures, upstream dilatation and ectasia, no downstream obstruction
Ischaemic cholangiopathy	3 patterns Severe injury—Necrosis of the bile duct wall, intrahepatic collections or biloma
	Less severe injury—Biliary casts by desquamated epithelium
	Chronic injury—Fibrosis causing biliary stricture
Primary biliary cholangitis	Periportal halo sign—Ring of T2 hypointensity around the central portal triad
Caroli disease	Type 1 (pure) nonhereditary, segmental cystic dilatation of intrahepatic bile ducts
	Type 2 (hereditary) entire liver, associated with congenital hepatic fibrosis
	Association—Autosomal recessive polycystic kidney disease, choledochal cysts

PSC primary sclerosing cholangitis, *IgG4-SC* IgG4-related sclerosing cholangitis, *RPC* recurrent pyogenic cholangitis, *PCC* portal cavernoma cholangiopathy

References

1. Zacarias MS, Dalla Pria HRF, Oliveira RAS, Delmonte LF, Velloni FG, D'Ippolito G. Non-neoplastic cholangiopathies: an algorithmic approach. Radiol Bras. 2020;53(4):262–72.
2. Menon S, Holt A. Large-duct cholangiopathies: aetiology, diagnosis and treatment. Frontline Gastroenterol. 2019;10(3):284–91.
3. Cheung AC, Lorenzo Pisarello MJ, LaRusso NF. Pathobiology of biliary epithelia. Biochim Biophys Acta Mol Basis Dis. 2018;1864(4 Pt B):1220–31.
4. Gidwaney NG, Pawa S, Das KM. Pathogenesis and clinical spectrum of primary sclerosing cholangitis. World J Gastroenterol. 2017;23(14):2459–69.
5. Dyson JK, Beuers U, Jones DEJ, Lohse AW, Hudson M. Primary sclerosing cholangitis. Lancet. 2018;391(10139):2547–59.
6. Seo N, Kim SY, Lee SS, Byun JH, Kim JH, Kim HJ, Lee MG. Sclerosing cholangitis: clinicopathologic features, imaging spectrum, and systemic approach to differential diagnosis. Korean J Radiol. 2016;17(1):25–38.
7. Khoshpouri P, Habibabadi RR, Hazhirkarzar B, Ameli S, Ghadimi M, Ghasabeh MA, Menias CO, Kim A, Li Z, Kamel IR. Imaging features of primary Sclerosing cholangitis: from diagnosis to liver transplant follow-up. Radiographics. 2019 Nov-Dec;39(7):1938–64.
8. Selvaraj EA, Culver EL, Bungay H, Bailey A, Chapman RW, Pavlides M. Evolving role of magnetic resonance techniques in primary sclerosing cholangitis. World J Gastroenterol. 2019;25(6):644–58.
9. Schramm C, Eaton J, Ringe KI, Venkatesh S, Yamamura J. MRI working group of the IPSCSG. Recommendations on the use of magnetic resonance imaging in PSC-A position statement from the international PSC study group. Hepatology. 2017 Nov;66(5):1675–88.
10. Elsayes KM, Oliveira EP, Narra VR, Abou El Abbass HA, Ahmed MI, Tongdee R, Brown JJ. MR and MRCP in the evaluation of primary sclerosing chol-

angitis: current applications and imaging findings. J Comput Assist Tomogr. 2006;30(3):398–404.
11. Vitellas KM, Keogan MT, Freed KS, Enns RA, Spritzer CE, Baillie JM, Nelson RC. Radiologic manifestations of sclerosing cholangitis with emphasis on MR cholangiopancreatography. Radiographics. 2000;20(4):959–75. quiz 1108–9, 1112
12. Gulliver DJ, Baker ME, Putnam W, Baillie J, Rice R, Cotton PB. Bile duct diverticula and webs: nonspecific cholangiographic features of primary sclerosing cholangitis. AJR Am J Roentgenol. 1991;157(2):281–5.
13. Düşünceli E, Erden A, Erden I, Karayalçin S. Primary sclerosing cholangitis: MR cholangiopancreatography and T2-weighted MR imaging findings. Diagn Interv Radiol. 2005 Dec;11(4):213–8.
14. Revelon G, Rashid A, Kawamoto S, Bluemke DA. Primary sclerosing cholangitis: MR imaging findings with pathologic correlation. AJR Am J Roentgenol. 1999 Oct;173(4):1037–42.
15. Ito K, Mitchell DG, Outwater EK, Blasbalg R. Primary sclerosing cholangitis: MR imaging features. AJR Am J Roentgenol. 1999 Jun;172(6):1527–33.
16. Prokopič M, Beuers U. Management of primary sclerosing cholangitis and its complications: an algorithmic approach. Hepatol Int. 2021 Feb;15(1):6–20.
17. Azizi L, Raynal M, Cazejust J, Ruiz A, Menu Y, Arrivé L. MR imaging of sclerosing cholangitis. Clin Res Hepatol Gastroenterol. 2012 Apr;36(2):130–8.
18. Lindor KD, Kowdley KV, Harrison EM. ACG clinical guideline: primary sclerosing cholangitis. Am J Gastroenterol. 2015;110(5):646–59.
19. Ohara H, Okazaki K, Tsubouchi H, Inui K, Kawa S, Kamisawa T, Tazuma S, Uchida K, Hirano K, Yoshida H, Nishino T, Ko SB, Mizuno N, Hamano H, Kanno A, Notohara K, Hasebe O, Nakazawa T, Nakanuma Y, Takikawa H. Research committee of IgG4-related diseases; research committee of intractable diseases of liver and biliary tract; Ministry of health, labor and welfare, Japan; Japan biliary association. Clinical diagnostic criteria of IgG4-related sclerosing cholangitis 2012. J Hepatobiliary Pancreat Sci. 2012 Sep;19(5):536–42.
20. Okazaki K, Uchida K, Koyabu M, Miyoshi H, Ikeura T, Takaoka M. IgG4 cholangiopathy: current concept, diagnosis, and pathogenesis. J Hepatol. 2014 Sep;61(3):690–5.
21. Zen Y, Kawakami H, Kim JH. IgG4-related sclerosing cholangitis: all we need to know. J Gastroenterol. 2016 Apr;51(4):295–312.
22. Zen Y, Nakanuma Y. IgG4 Cholangiopathy. Int J Hepatol. 2012;2012:472376.
23. Madhusudhan KS, Das P, Gunjan D, Srivastava DN, Garg PK. IgG4-related sclerosing cholangitis: a clinical and imaging review. AJR Am J Roentgenol. 2019 Dec;213(6):1221–31.
24. Oseini AM, Chaiteerakij R, Shire AM, Ghazale A, Kaiya J, Moser CD, Aderca I, Mettler TA, Therneau TM, Zhang L, Takahashi N, Chari ST, Roberts LR. Utility of serum immunoglobulin G4 in distinguishing immunoglobulin G4-associated cholangitis from cholangiocarcinoma. Hepatology. 2011;54(3):940–8.
25. Vlachou PA, Khalili K, Jang HJ, Fischer S, Hirschfield GM, Kim TK. IgG4-related sclerosing disease: autoimmune pancreatitis and extrapancreatic manifestations. Radiographics. 2011;31(5):1379–402.
26. Nakazawa T, Ohara H, Sano H, Ando T, Joh T. Schematic classification of sclerosing cholangitis with autoimmune pancreatitis by cholangiography. Pancreas. 2006 Mar;32(2):229.
27. Nakazawa T, Ohara H, Sano H, Aoki S, Kobayashi S, Okamoto T, Imai H, Nomura T, Joh T, Itoh M. Cholangiography can discriminate sclerosing cholangitis with autoimmune pancreatitis from primary sclerosing cholangitis. Gastrointest Endosc. 2004 Dec;60(6):937–44.
28. Yata M, Suzuki K, Furuhashi N, Kawakami K, Kawai Y, Naganawa S. Comparison of the multidetector-row computed tomography findings of IgG4-related sclerosing cholangitis and extrahepatic cholangiocarcinoma. Clin Radiol. 2016 Mar;71(3):203–10.
29. Catalano OA, Sahani DV, Forcione DG, Czermak B, Liu CH, Soricelli A, Arellano RS, Muller PR, Hahn PF. Biliary infections: spectrum of imaging findings and management. Radiographics. 2009 Nov;29(7):2059–80.
30. Kwan KEL, Shelat VG, Tan CH. Recurrent pyogenic cholangitis: a review of imaging findings and clinical management. Abdom Radiol (NY). 2017 Jan;42(1):46–56.
31. Heffernan EJ, Geoghegan T, Munk PL, Ho SG, Harris AC. Recurrent pyogenic cholangitis: from imaging to intervention. AJR Am J Roentgenol. 2009 Jan;192(1):W28–35.
32. Bilgin M, Balci NC, Erdogan A, Momtahen AJ, Alkaade S, Rau WS. Hepatobiliary and pancreatic MRI and MRCP findings in patients with HIV infection. AJR Am J Roentgenol. 2008 Jul;191(1):228–32.
33. Mahajani RV, Uzer MF. Cholangiopathy in HIV-infected patients. Clin Liver Dis. 1999 Aug;3(3):669–84.
34. Shanbhogue AK, Tirumani SH, Prasad SR, Fasih N, McInnes M. Benign biliary strictures: a current comprehensive clinical and imaging review. AJR Am J Roentgenol. 2011 Aug;197(2):W295–306.
35. Dhiman RK, Saraswat VA, Valla DC, Chawla Y, Behera A, Varma V, Agarwal S, Duseja A, Puri P, Kalra N, Rameshbabu CS, Bhatia V, Sharma M, Kumar M, Gupta S, Taneja S, Kaman L, Zargar SA, Nundy S, Singh SP, Acharya SK, Dilawari JB. Portal cavernoma cholangiopathy: consensus statement of a working party of the Indian National Association for study of the liver. J Clin Exp Hepatol. 2014;4(Suppl 1):S2–S14. https://doi.org/10.1016/j.jceh.2014.02.003. Epub 2014 Feb 25. PMID: 25755591; PMCID: PMC4274351
36. Ma Y, Cai R, Zhuang D, Tang Y, Cao Y, Wang X, Qiao Z. Whole clinical process in a patient with portal hypertensive biliopathy: a case report. J Int Med Res. 2020;48(3):300060520914834. https://doi.

org/10.1177/0300060520914834. PMID: 32228333; PMCID: PMC7132790
37. Dhiman RK, Puri P, Chawla Y, Minz M, Bapuraj JR, Gupta S, Nagi B, Suri S. Biliary changes in extrahepatic portal venous obstruction: compression by collaterals or ischemic? Gastrointest Endosc. 1999;50(5):646–52. https://doi.org/10.1016/s0016-5107(99)80013-3. PMID: 10536320
38. Khuroo MS, Rather AA, Khuroo NS, Khuroo MS. Portal biliopathy. World J Gastroenterol. 2016;22(35):7973–82. https://doi.org/10.3748/wjg.v22.i35.7973. PMID: 27672292; PMCID: PMC5028811
39. Walser EM, Runyan BR, Heckman MG, Bridges MD, Willingham DL, Paz-Fumagalli R, Nguyen JH. Extrahepatic portal biliopathy: proposed etiology on the basis of anatomic and clinical features. Radiology. 2011;258(1):146–53. https://doi.org/10.1148/radiol.10090923. Epub 2010 Nov 2. PMID: 21045178
40. Deltenre P, Valla DC. Ischemic cholangiopathy. Semin Liver Dis. 2008;28(3):235–46. https://doi.org/10.1055/s-0028-1085092. Epub 2008 Sep 23. PMID: 18814077
41. Yeh MJ, Kim SY, Jhaveri KS, Behr SC, Seo N, Yeh BM. Imaging of autoimmune biliary disease. Abdom Radiol (NY). 2017 Jan;42(1):3–18.
42. Meng Y, Liang Y, Liu M. The value of MRI in the diagnosis of primary biliary cirrhosis and assessment of liver fibrosis. PLoS One. 2015;10(3):e0120110.
43. Guy F, Cognet F, Dranssart M, Cercueil JP, Conciatori L, Krausé D. Caroli's disease: magnetic resonance imaging features. Eur Radiol. 2002 Nov;12(11):2730–6.
44. Brancatelli G, Federle MP, Vilgrain V, Vullierme MP, Marin D, Lagalla R. Fibropolycystic liver disease: CT and MR imaging findings. Radiographics. 2005 May-Jun;25(3):659–70.
45. Levy AD, Rohrmann CA Jr, Murakata LA, Lonergan GJ. Caroli's disease: radiologic spectrum with pathologic correlation. AJR Am J Roentgenol. 2002 Oct;179(4):1053–7.
46. Miller WJ, Sechtin AG, Campbell WL, Pieters PC. Imaging findings in Caroli's disease. AJR Am J Roentgenol. 1995 Aug;165(2):333–7.

11 Gallbladder Carcinoma Imaging and Update: Including Surgeon's Perspective

Kalpana Bansal

11.1 Introduction

Gallbladder carcinoma is the fifth most common malignancy of the gastrointestinal tract and the most common biliary tract malignancy in the world [1]. Recent advances in cross-sectional imaging techniques have increased the preoperative detection of gallbladder carcinoma. Nevertheless, an accurate imaging diagnosis of gallbladder carcinoma at early stages still remains challenging. This is due to the vague or delayed clinical presentation and non-specific appearance of early gallbladder cancer (GBCA) [2]. In advanced GBCA, the preoperative imaging for tumor recognition and non-invasive staging is essential to triage patients to appropriate care and has become more reliable due to recent advances in CT, MRI, and positron emission tomography (PET) imaging.

Ultrasonography (US) is the primary imaging modality in evaluation of biliary tract disorders [3], though conventional US is unable to distinguish benign from early malignant disease [4]. Contrast-enhanced ultrasound (CEUS) is a recent and promising technique, but its role in GBCA is not well recognized [5]. The role of endoscopic ultrasound is also limited in detecting gallbladder carcinoma [6]. Multidetector computed tomography (MDCT) is a comprehensive tool in preoperative detection as well as local staging of GBCA [7]. MDCT also allows mapping of vascular anatomy in patients being planned for resection [8]. Magnetic resonance imaging (MRI) provides excellent soft tissue contrast resolution and non-invasive imaging of the gallbladder and biliary tree [9]. It also serves as a problem-solving tool to reach a conclusive diagnosis. Recent advances in MRI including diffusion-weighted imaging (DWI) and perfusion imaging may allow greater accuracy in detection of smaller lesions [10]. Positron emission tomography is primarily employed in detection of distant metastases and post-treatment detection of residual or recurrent disease [11].

11.2 Epidemiology, Pathogenesis, and Clinical Presentation

The pathogenesis of gallbladder cancer is likely multifactorial. Risk factors for gallbladder cancer are listed as follows:

1. *Ethnicity, Gender, and Age*

Worldwide, gallbladder cancer has a low occurrence of <2 per 100,000 but has a wide variance. Gallbladder cancer is rare in developed countries. In the Unite States, it accounts for less than 5000 cases per year [12]. High rates of gall-

K. Bansal (✉)
Department of Radiodiagnosis, Govind Ballabh Pant Institute of Postgraduate Medical Education and Research Institute, New Delhi, India

© The Author(s), under exclusive license to Springer Nature Singapore Pte Ltd. 2025
B. Sureka (ed.), *Hepato-Pancreatico Biliary Imaging*, https://doi.org/10.1007/978-981-95-1699-5_11

bladder carcinoma are seen in South American countries, particularly Chile, Bolivia, and Ecuador, as well as some areas of India, Pakistan, Japan, and Korea. In Chile, mortality rates from gallbladder carcinoma are the highest in the world [13].

Sex Women are affected two to six times more often than men. Worldwide there is marked predominance of women over men, especially in northern India, in Pakistan, and in American Indian females [14].

Age Gallbladder cancer rates tend to increase with advancing age. In a Memorial Sloan-Kettering report of 435 gallbladder cancer patients, the median age at presentation was 67 years [15].

2. *Cholelithiasis*

Cholelithiasis is a well-established risk factor for the development of gallbladder carcinoma, and gallstones are present in approximately 85% of affected patients [13] (Fig. 11.1). Further, gallbladder cancer rates correlate well with the prevalence of gallstone disease. However the overall risk of gallbladder cancer in patients with cholelithiasis is low; less than 3% cases of cholelithiasis have gallbladder carcinoma [13]. The basis for this relationship likely resides in gallstones causing chronic irritation and inflammation of the gallbladder, perhaps aided by the local production of carcinogens, which leads to mucosal dysplasia and subsequent carcinoma [16]. Gallstone characteristics further influence the frequency of gallbladder cancer. Increasing stone size augments the risk of gallbladder cancer; stones >3 cm have a tenfold increased risk [17]. The stone type may also matter; cholesterol gallstone disease is found to be associated with high incidence of gallbladder cancer in American Indians and other groups [18]. In support of this association, an inverse correlation exists between cholecystectomy for cholelithiasis and gallbladder cancer rates [16].

3. *Chronic Inflammation*

Chronic inflammation is implacably linked to malignant transformation, being a major factor in carcinogenesis. Recurrent or chronic inflammatory insults are detrimental, causing deoxyribonucleic acid damage and release of inflammatory mediators and, thus, predisposing cells to oncogenic transformation [13]. Hence, cholelithiasis with its attendant repeated trauma, resulting in chronic cholecystitis, might be the mechanism for cancer development after many years. Porcelain gallbladder is an uncommon condition (<1% of gallbladder specimens) with extensive wall calcification (Fig. 11.2), which may also be the result of chronic inflammation and appears to be associated with gallbladder carcinoma in 12%–61% of patients [19].

4. *Infections*

Chronic bacterial cholangitis constitutes a clear risk for biliary tract malignancy. The organ-

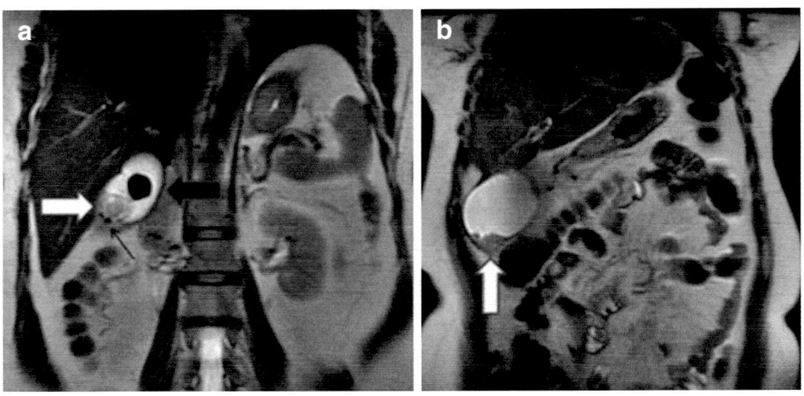

Fig. 11.1 (**a–b**): A 45-year-old female patient complaining of upper abdomen pain. Coronal T2W MR images show a large T2 hypointense (thick black arrow) and multiple small (thin black arrow) intraluminal gallbladder calculi with eccentric polypoidal soft tissue mass in the fundal region (white arrow)

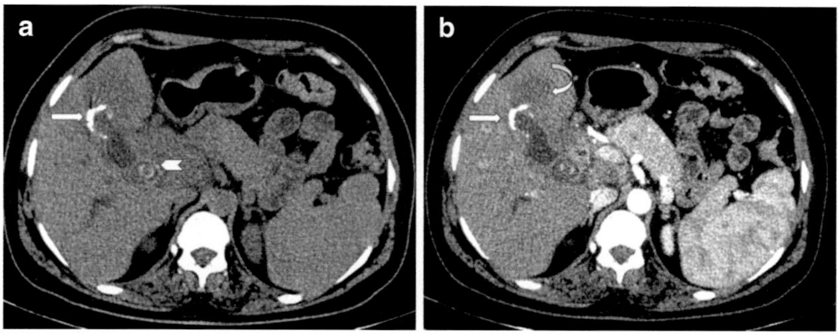

Fig. 11.2 Porcelain gallbladder with gallbladder carcinoma. (**a**) Noncontrast and (**b**) contrast-enhanced axial scans reveal a contracted gallbladder with mural calcification (white arrow), cholelithiasis (arrowhead), and hypodense mass infiltrating adjacent liver parenchyma in segment IVb (curved arrow)

isms most implicated are *Salmonella* and *Helicobacter* [20]. Some 6% of typhoid carriers develop gallbladder cancer, with a 12-fold increased risk.

5. *Primary Sclerosing Cholangitis*

There is an increased frequency of gallbladder mass lesions in patients with primary sclerosing cholangitis, presumably related to the ongoing inflammation, facilitating a metaplasia-dysplasia-carcinoma sequence [21].

6. *Exposures*

Various environmental exposures have been hypothesized to contribute to gallbladder cancer. Tobacco is a significant risk factor. Heavy metals, like nickel and cadmium, have been implicated including drugs like methyldopa and isoniazid [22]. Radon, an inhaled gas, has also been associated with cancer of the lung and gallbladder [23].

7. *Obesity*

Obese people have an increased risk of developing gallbladder cancer. For each 5-point increase in BMI, the relative risk of developing gallbladder cancer increases by 1.59 for women and 1.09 for men [24].

8. *Gallbladder Polyps*

Gallbladder polyps seen in almost 5% of adults are mostly pseudopolyps, without neoplastic potential, as cholesterol polyps (~60% of all gallbladder polyps), adenomyosis (~25%), or inflammatory polyps (~10%) (Fig. 11.3a, b).

The features of polypoidal masses that indicate malignancy include large polyps (>1 cm, 25% being malignant), a solitary polyp, a sessile polyp, polyp growth, associated gallstones, and age over 50–60 years [25] (Fig. 11.3c, d).

9. *Anomalous Pancreaticobiliary Junction*

This is a congenital malformation in which the pancreatic duct drains into the biliary tract outside the duodenal wall, potentially allowing pancreatic secretions to regurgitate into the bile ducts and gallbladder, leading to malignant changes in the mucosa [13]. Anomalous pancreaticobiliary junction malformation is found to be associated in 10% of patients with gallbladder cancer manifesting histologically as papillary carcinoma [14].

10. *Genetics*

A family history of gallbladder disease increases the risk of developing gallbladder can-

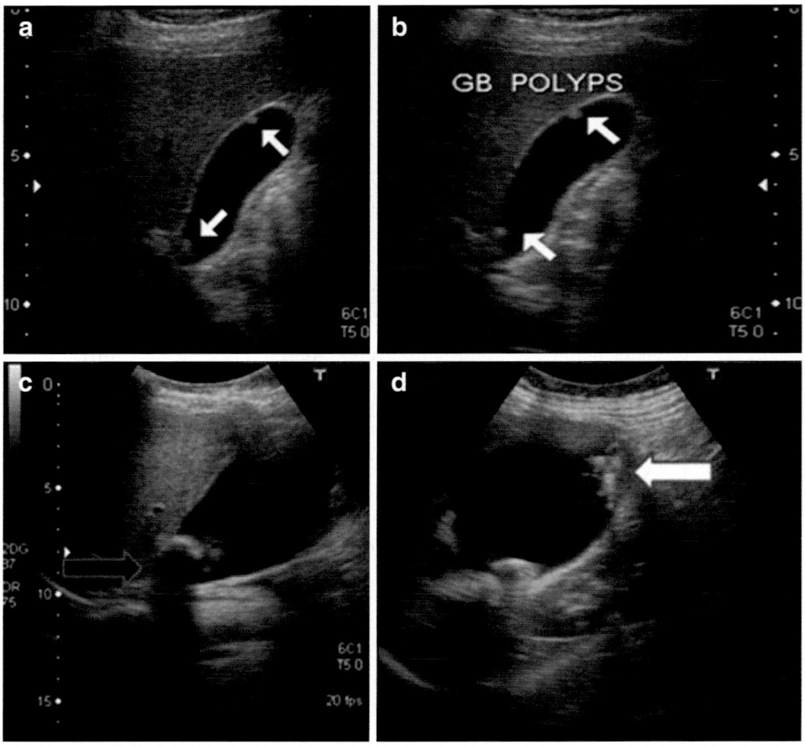

Fig. 11.3 Benign and malignant polyp. (**a**, **b**) Ultrasound depicting multiple small (<1 cm) echogenic polyps (white arrow) along the non-dependent wall of gallbladder—likely benign. (**c**, **d**) Another case displaying large irregular polypoidal soft tissue thickening in the gallbladder fundal region (white arrow) with cholelithiasis (black arrow) on US. Post-cholecystectomy histopathological examination revealed adenocarcinoma

cer, and the genetic background accounts for approximately 25% of the total gallstone disease risk [26].

11.2.1 Pathological Features

Gallbladder carcinomas are epithelial in origin and account for 98% of all gallbladder malignancies. The remainders are sarcomas, lymphomas, carcinoid, metastases, and other unusual malignancies.

Adenocarcinoma is the most common histological type (approx. 90%) of gallbladder carcinomas and is characterized by glands lined by cuboidal or columnar cells, which may contain mucin (Fig. 11.4). They may be well, moderately, or poorly differentiated. There are several recognized histologic variants of adenocarcinoma: papillary, intestinal, mucinous, signet-ring cell, and clear cell [27]. Many tumors contain more than one histologic variant.

11.2.2 Clinical Presentation

Gallbladder cancer is an incidental diagnosis in early stages, because of inflammatory symptoms related to coexistent cholelithiasis or cholecystitis. About 1% of patients undergoing cholecystectomy for cholelithiasis have an incidental gallbladder carcinoma [23]. The majority of patients with gallbladder carcinoma present with advanced disease. Chronic abdominal pain, anorexia, or weight loss are common initial symptoms [24]. Jaundice usually presents as a result of malignant obstruction of the biliary tree rather than hepatic metastasis or coexistent choledocholithiasis [25]. Physical examination may demonstrate a palpable mass, hepatomegaly, and jaundice. Elevated serum levels of alpha-fetoprotein and carcinoembryonic antigen have been reported in association with gallbladder carcinoma [28].

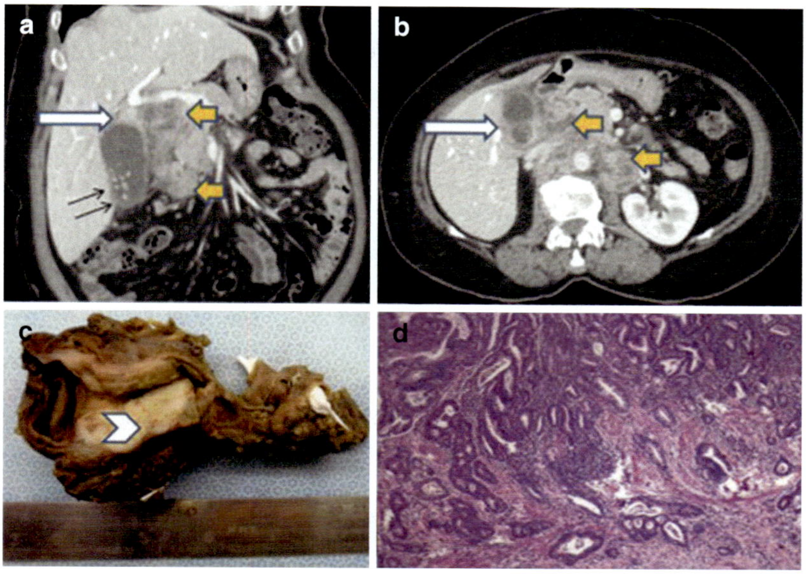

Fig. 11.4 Contrast-enhanced CT and radical cholecystectomy with lymph node dissection: (**a**, **b**) Coronal and axial CT images reveal cholelithiasis (black arrow) with annular mural thickening in the gallbladder neck region (white arrows) and periportal/peripancreatic, pre–/para-aortic lymphadenopathy (yellow arrows) (**c**). Photograph of the resected gallbladder (cut specimen) shows focal neoplastic mural thickening involving the body and neck region of the gallbladder (arrowhead) (**d**). Photomicrograph (10×; HE stain) revealed well-differentiated adenocarcinoma of the gallbladder

11.3 Imaging Modalities

11.3.1 Ultrasonography

Conventional US is the first-line modality for evaluation of the gallbladder [3]. US has limited utility in differentiation of mural thickening due to chronic cholecystitis from that of GBCA [4]. Sometimes, the biliary sludge is motionless and simulates GBCA on US [5]. It also has a limited role to provide an accurate estimate of local invasion of the gallbladder (GB) wall, adjacent liver infiltration, and nodal and peritoneal metastases [5]. GB polyps are better visualized on US (Fig. 11.3) and presence of color flow support malignancy; however, its absence does not exclude malignancy. US Doppler has a sensitivity and specificity of around 80% in diagnosis of GBCA.

High-resolution US has a higher diagnostic accuracy in distinguishing neoplastic polyps and staging GBCA compared to conventional US [29].

Contrast-enhanced US (CEUS) has been used successfully in the liver, kidney, and pancreas. However, the reports of usefulness of CEUS in GBCA have been conflicting. The pointers to malignancy are arterial tortuous tumoral vessels showing irregularly tortuous extensions [30].

11.3.1.1 Endoscopic US

Compared to conventional ultrasound and other cross-sectional imaging techniques, endoscopic US improves the characterization of local disease extent and involvement of regional lymph nodes in GBCA [31].

11.3.1.2 Multidetector Computed Tomography

MDCT is currently the work horse in investigating patients with suspected GBCA due to limitations of US including CEUS. It allows faster imaging acquisition in multiple phases following intravenous injection of contrast agent and multiplanar reconstructions (Fig. 11.4). It serves as a comprehensive tool in preoperative detection as well as local staging of GBCA [7] and allows vascular anatomy mapping in patients being planned for resection [8]. The common enhancement patterns in GBCA are strongly enhancing thick inner wall layer during the arterial phase and weakly enhancing or non-enhancing outer layer (two-layer enhancement pattern) (Fig. 11.5) or heterogeneously enhancing thick inner wall layer during both phases (one-layer enhancement pattern) [32] (Fig. 11.6). In contrast, the most common enhancement pattern of chronic cholecystitis is isoattenuation of the thin inner wall layer during both phases. Despite this MDCT still has limitations in distinguishing inflammatory disease from GBCA, particularly early-stage GBCA and low accuracy in detection of peritoneal metastases and lymph node involvement.

11.3.1.3 Magnetic Resonance Imaging

Due to a higher soft tissue, contrast resolution MRI may prove superior to MDCT in detecting

Fig. 11.5 (**a–b**): A case of a gallbladder carcinoma. Contrast-enhanced axial scans showing diffuse mural thickening in the body and fundal region with a two-layer enhancement pattern (white arrow). Note is made of ascites

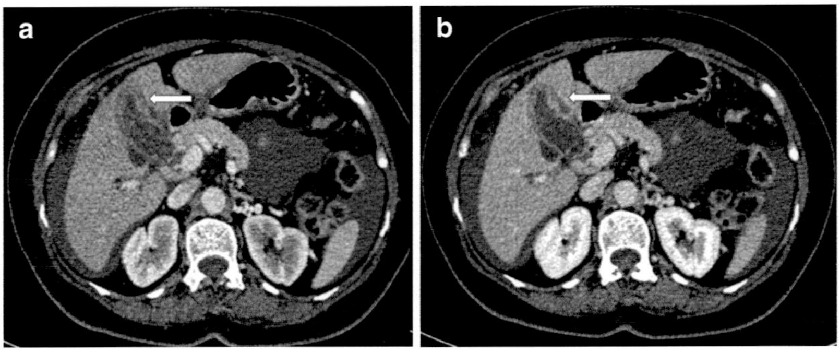

Fig. 11.6 A case of a gallbladder carcinoma: (**a**) Noncontrast and (**b–d**) triple-phase contrast-enhanced CT showing enhancing asymmetric mural thickening in the fundus and body region with a single-layer enhancement pattern (white arrow)

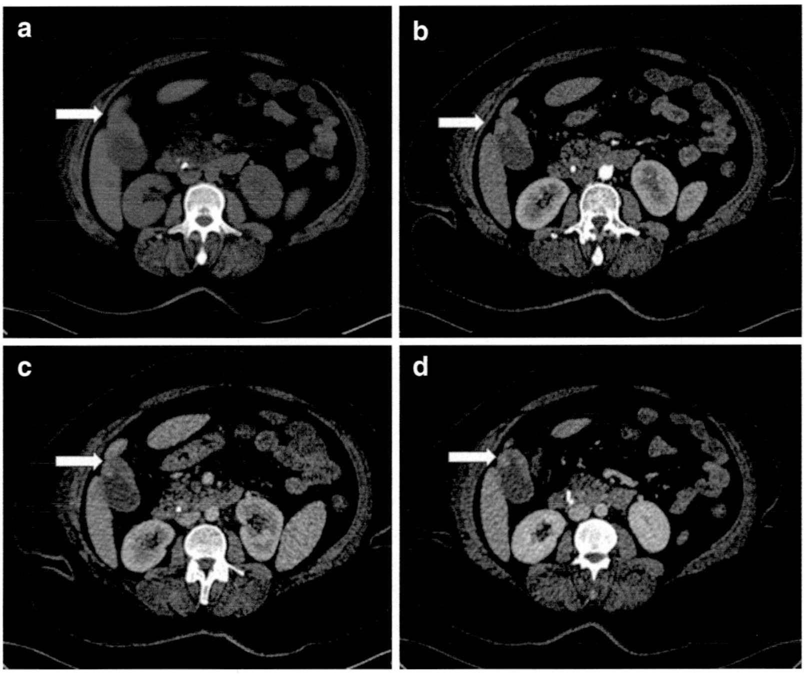

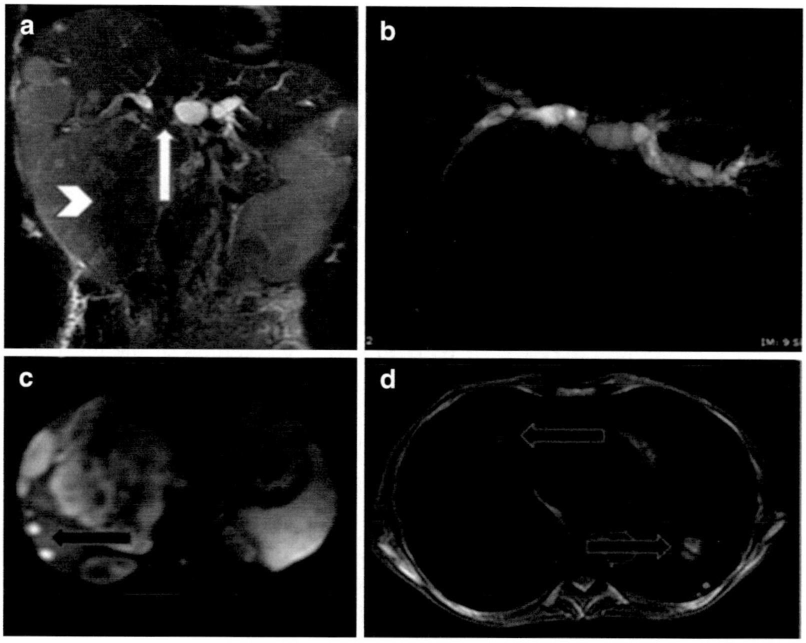

Fig. 11.7 A case of advanced carcinoma of the gallbladder: (**a**, **b**) Coronal T2WI and thick-slab 2D MRCP images reveal a large mass replacing the gallbladder with surrounding hepatic infiltration (arrowhead) and extension to the hilar region (white arrow) with resultant hilar block and attendant moderate upstream biliary dilatation. (**c**, **d**) DWI and axial T2WI reveal hepatic and pulmonary metastases (black arrows)

early gallbladder malignancy with non-specific imaging appearance. GBCA typically appears hypointense on T1W and hyperintense on T2W images (Fig. 11.7a). Associated gallstones are also better demonstrated as filling defects compared to MDCT[9]. Following gadolinium administration, GBCA shows heterogeneous arterial enhancement that persists in the venous phase. Adjacent liver invasion, bile duct invasion, lymph node metastases, and vascular invasion are better demonstrated on combining conventional MRI with magnetic resonance cholangiopancreatography (MRCP) (Fig. 11.7b) and magnetic resonance angiography. As GBCA represents a highly cellular lesion, it shows restricted diffusion [33], and apparent diffusion coefficient is a quantitative marker of diffusion restriction. DWI also has a high sensitivity in detection of liver and lymph node metastases (Fig. 11.7c). However, the specificity for nodal metastases is poor.

11.3.1.4 FDG-Pet

Fluorodeoxyglucose positron emission tomography (FDG-PET) has a high sensitivity and specificity in differentiating between benign and malignant diseases compared to conventional US, MDCT, and MRI at various sites in the body including gastrointestinal tract [34]. The efficacy of FDG-PET in diagnosing GBCA has also been reported [35] but mostly in advanced stage or bulky lesions [36]. PET is primarily employed in detection of distant metastases and post-treatment detection of residual or recurrent disease [11].

11.3.1.5 Image-Guided Fine Needle Aspiration Cytology

Several recent studies have established the efficacy of ultrasound-guided fine needle aspiration cytology to reach adequate diagnosis with high rate of sensitivity and specificity [37].

11.4 Imaging Findings

For evaluation of suspected gallbladder diseases, sonography is often the first imaging modality because of its relatively low cost and widespread availability. Although sonography has a relatively high sensitivity for the detection of advanced tumors, it has limited sensitivity and specificity in the diagnosis of early disease and is unreliable for staging. Therefore, CT and, increasingly, MRI are more widely used modalities for further characterization and preoperative evaluation of suspected malignant gallbladder lesions.

On imaging, gallbladder carcinoma may have any of the following morphological appearances: a mass completely occupying or replacing the gallbladder lumen, focal or diffuse asymmetric gallbladder wall thickening, or an intraluminal polypoid lesion [38].

11.4.1 Mass Occupying or Replacing the Gallbladder Lumen

The most common imaging appearance of GBCA is the presence of a large gallbladder mass that nearly fills or replaces the gallbladder lumen, often directly invading the surrounding liver parenchyma and may be present in 40–65% of patients at initial examination [38]. On sonography, heterogeneous, predominantly hypoechoic mass partially or completely fills the gallbladder lumen (Fig. 11.8). Anechoic foci suggestive of trapped bile or necrosis may be present, as well as echogenic foci with posterior acoustic shadowing from gallstones (Fig. 11.8a), porcelain gallbladder, or tumor calcifications [39]. GBCA usually appears hypodense on noncontrast CT (Fig. 11.9a), and MRI shows hypo-to isointense signal on T1-weighted and moderately hyperintense signal on T2-weighted images. Both CT and MRI depict intense irregular contrast enhancement at the periphery of the lesions during the early arterial phase that may be retained in fibrous stromal components of GBCA during the portal venous and delayed phases (Fig. 11.9b–d), aiding differentiating it from large central hepatocellular carcinomas, which characteristically show washout of contrast [40] (Fig. 11.10). Non-enhancing hypodense areas may represent inspissated bile or necrotic tissue, and calcific component may represent gallstones, wall calcification, or tumor calcifications. ^{18}F-FDG-PET shows an increased uptake in the region of the gallbladder mass, although it lacks specificity in distinguishing primary gallbladder carcinoma from other malignant lesions [41].

The *differential diagnosis* of a mass replacing the gallbladder lumen includes malignancies of the liver that have invaded the gallbladder fossa, such as hepatocellular carcinoma (Fig. 11.10), cholangiocarcinoma (Fig. 11.11), and metastatic disease (Fig. 11.12).

11.4.2 Focal or Diffuse Asymmetric Wall Thickening

GBCA may present as focal or diffuse asymmetric wall thickening in 20–30% of cases. Gallbladder wall thickening may be seen in many benign and inflammatory conditions, including acute and chronic cholecystitis (Fig. 11.13), xanthogranulomatous cholecystitis, and adenomyomatosis, as well as diffuse hepatic or systemic diseases such as acute hepatitis, portal hypertension, and congestive heart failure [42]. In

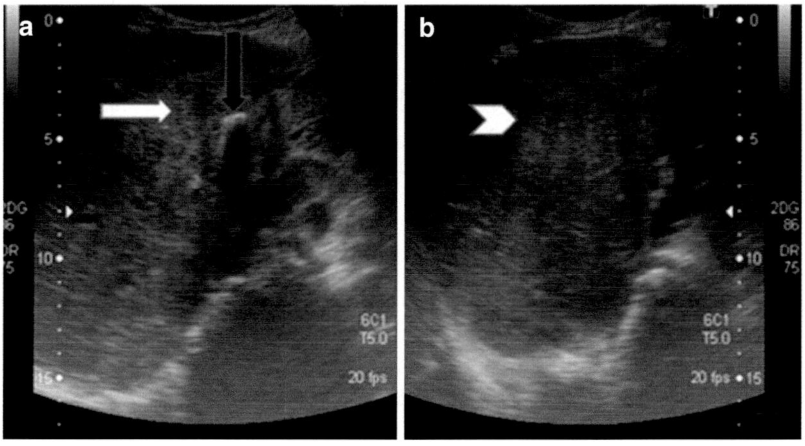

Fig. 11.8 (**a–b**): Ultrasound images showing a large poorly marginated heterogeneously hypoechoic mass lesion replacing the gallbladder (white arrow) with adjacent hepatic infiltration (arrowhead). Note echogenic focus with distal acoustic shadowing within the mass lesion suggestive of calculi (black arrow)

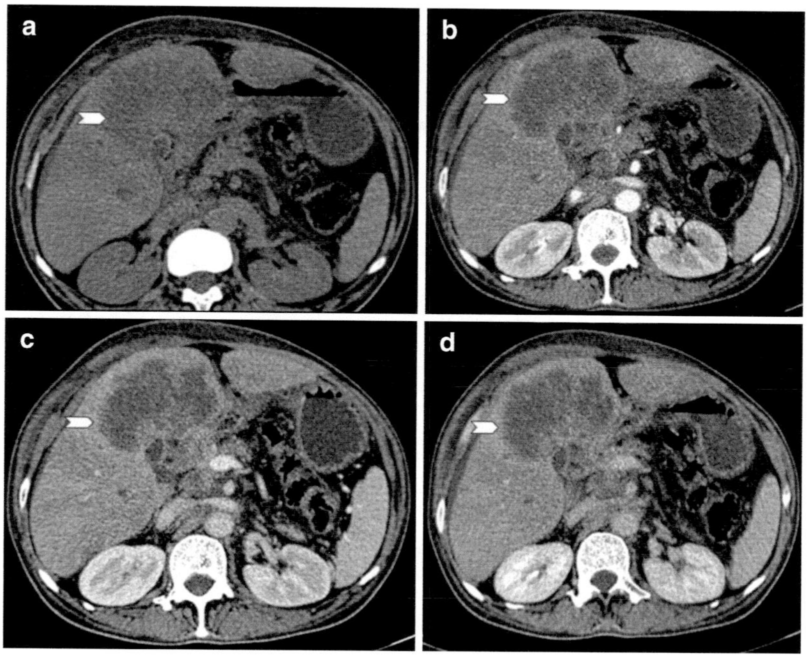

Fig. 11.9 Mass forming a gallbladder carcinoma: (**a**) Noncontrast and (**b–d**) triple-phase contrast-enhanced axial CT scan reveals a large lobulated hypodense mass in the gallbladder fossa region infiltrating into segment IVb and V of the liver (white arrow). The mass shows peripheral arterial enhancement (**b**) persisting in the portovenous (**c**) and delayed phase (**d**)

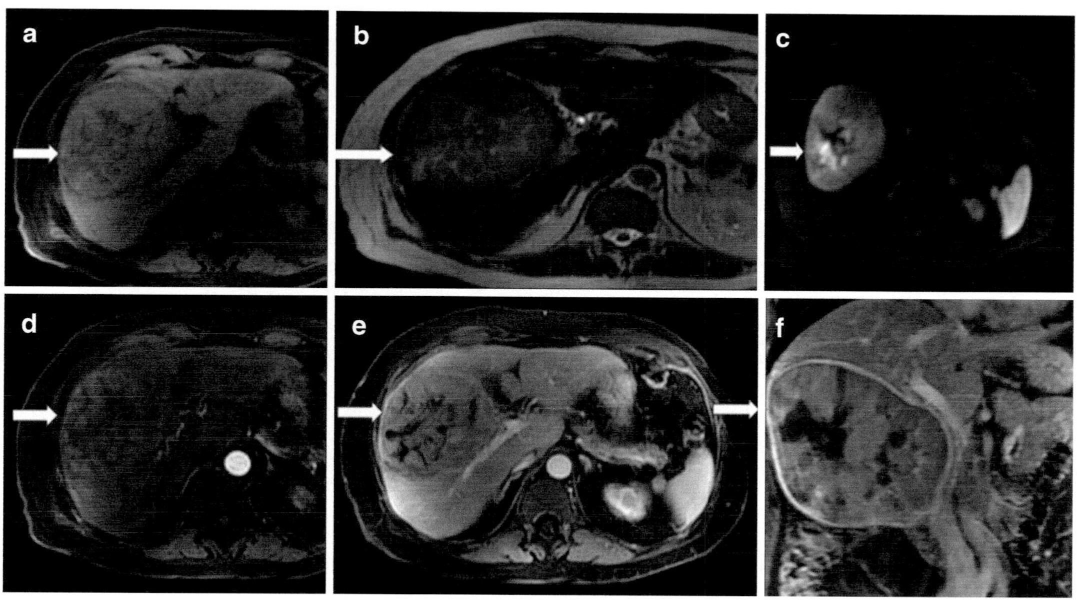

Fig. 11.10 A case of hepatocellular carcinoma: (**a–b**) Plain and (**d–f**) dynamic contrast-enhanced MR abdomen scans reveal a well-defined (**a**) T1 iso-to hypointense, (**b**) T2 hyperintense mass lesion in segment IV and V of the liver displaying (**d**) arterial enhancement and washout on (**e**) portovenous and (**f**) delayed phase images with capsule formation (white arrow)

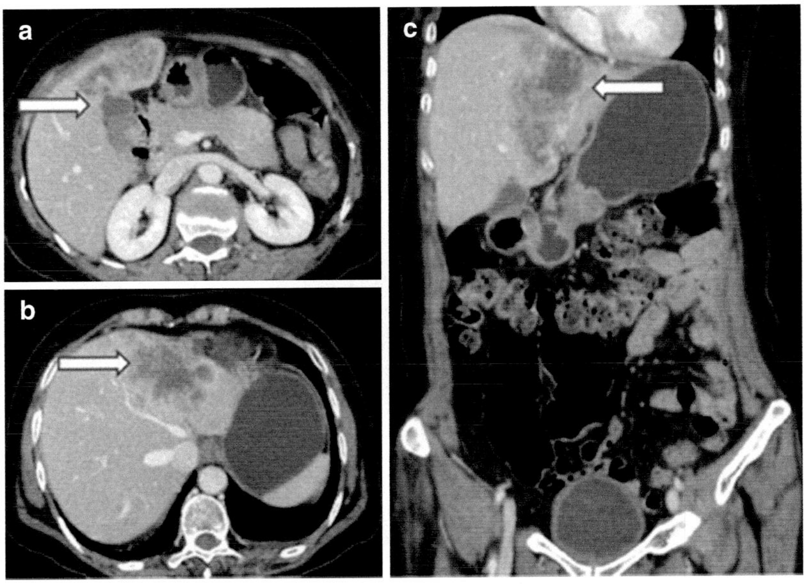

Fig. 11.11 (**a**, **b**) Axial contrast-enhanced CT and (**c**) coronal reformatted images reveal a lobulated heterogeneously enhancing mass lesion involving the left lobe of the liver (arrows) in close proximity to the gallbladder. Differentials include mass forming intrahepatic cholangiocarcinoma and gallbladder carcinoma with hepatic infiltration

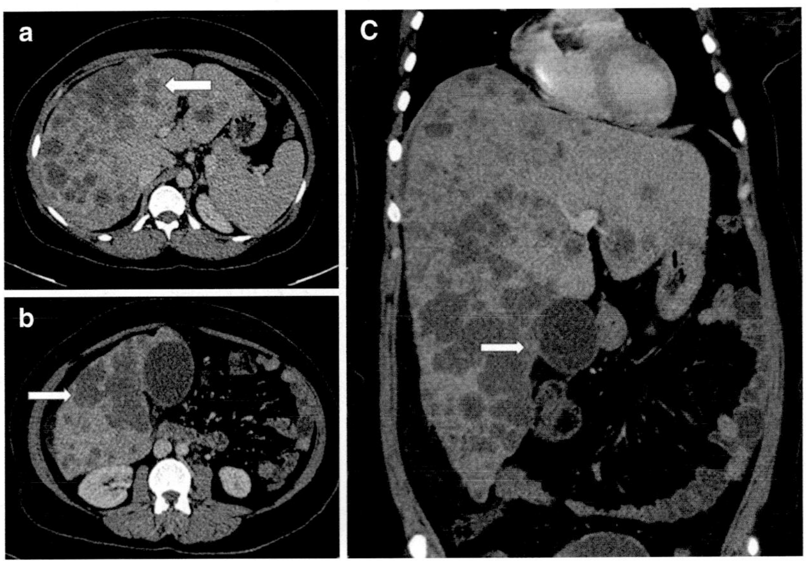

Fig. 11.12 Contrast-enhanced (**a**–**b**) axial and (**c**) coronal reformatted CT scans reveal multiple varying sizes hypoenhancing lesions in both lobes of the liver suggestive of metastases. In addition the confluent mass in segment V is showing loss of fat planes with the gallbladder with associated mild wall thickening (white arrow) in keeping with primary gallbladder carcinoma

contrast-enhanced CT and MR imaging, diffuse symmetric wall thickening suggests a nonneoplastic process, whereas asymmetric, irregular, or extensive mural thickening showing marked enhancement during the arterial phase that persists or becomes isodense or isointense to the liver during the portal venous phase favors suspicion of malignancy [40] (Fig. 11.14). Gallbladder carcinoma may also result in pre-existing background of chronic cholecystitis, which can obscure or delay the diagnosis of gallbladder cancer. FDG-PET may have a limited role because benign inflammatory lesions may also show uptake and result in false-positive results [41].

Xanthogranulomatous cholecystitis is a pseudotumoral inflammatory condition of the gallbladder that radiologically simulates gallbladder carcinoma. The CT features of xanthogranulomatous cholecystitis and gallbladder carcinoma overlap substantially (Fig. 11.15); thus, these

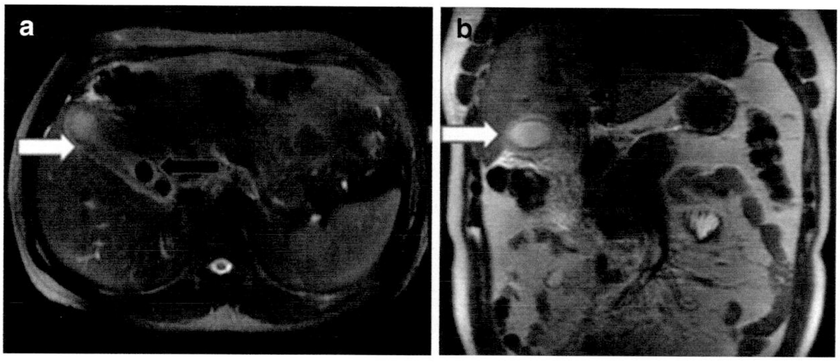

Fig. 11.13 Acute calculus cholecystitis. A 40-year-old lady complaining of severe abdominal pain: (**a**) Axial and (**b**) coronal T2W MR images reveal diffuse symmetric T2 hyperintense gallbladder wall thickening (white arrows) with T2 hypointense intraluminal calculi (black arrow) and mild pericholecystic fat stranding

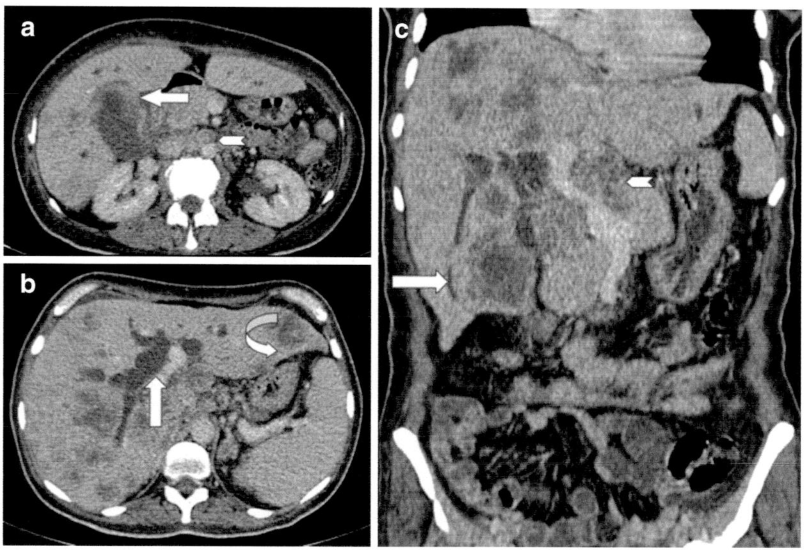

Fig. 11.14 Contrast-enhanced (**a**–**b**) axial and (**c**) coronal CT scans reveal asymmetric extensive enhancing mural thickening in the gallbladder (white arrow) with adjacent hepatic infiltration and hepatic (curved arrow) and retroperitoneal lymph node metastases (arrowhead) with resultant obstructive biliopathy (vertical arrow)

entities cannot be reliably differentiated [43]. Both diseases may demonstrate gallbladder wall thickening, infiltration of the surrounding fat, hepatic involvement, and lymphadenopathy.

Adenomyomatosis is a common tumorlike lesion of the gallbladderwith no malignant potential. It may involve the gallbladder in a focal, segmental, or diffuse form (Fig. 11.16). Its histological features include proliferation of epithelial and mural elements, and Rokitansky-Aschoff sinuses are seen as prominent infoldings of the epithelium. At US, adenomyomatosis is characterized by focal or diffuse gallbladder wall thickening and anechoic or echogenic foci in the gallbladder wall [44]. These echogenic foci may produce a ring-down reverberation artifact. Rokitansky-Aschoff sinuses are best visualized with MR imaging performed with breath-hold technique and T2-weighted pulse sequences [45]; therefore, MR imaging can be useful for distinguishing this benign entity from gallbladder carcinoma.

11.4.3 Intraluminal Polyp

Gallbladder carcinoma may present as a polypoid lesion in 15–25% of cases. Malignant lesions are usually larger than 1 cm in diameter and may have a thickened implantation base [46]

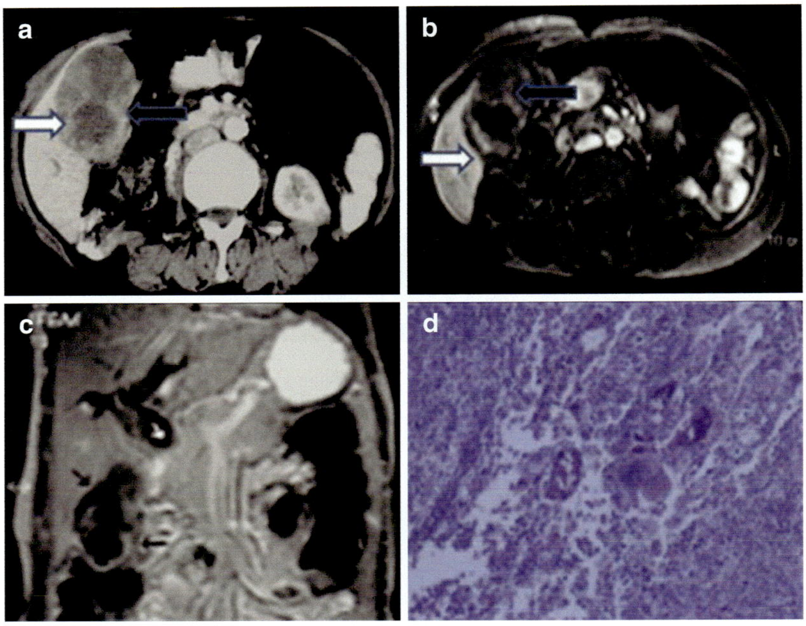

Fig. 11.15 Xanthogranulomatous cholecystitis. (**a**) Axial contrast-enhanced CT and (**b**) axial post-contrast T1W MR images reveal heterogeneously enhancing lobulated gallbladder wall thickening (white arrows) with poorly enhancing intramural areas (black arrows). (**c**) Coronal MR images reveal attendant biliary dilatation (small white arrows). (**d**) High power view showing dense inflammation comprising of foamy macrophages, lymphocytes, neutrophils, and foreign body type of giant cells

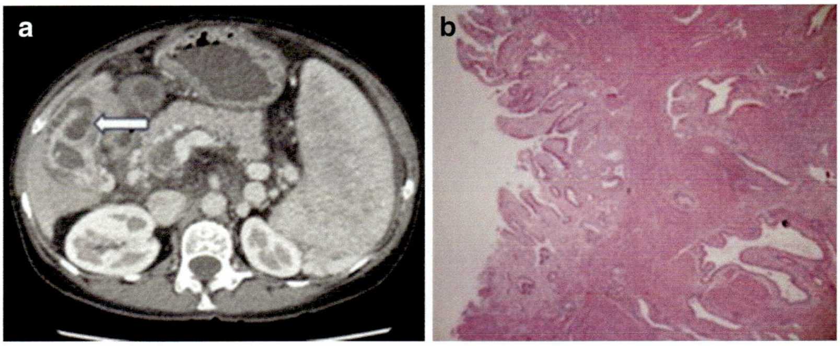

Fig. 11.16 GB adenomyomatosis. (**a**) Axial contrast-enhanced CT images reveal diffuse gallbladder wall thickening with intramural cystic spaces. Note is made of cirrhotic liver architecture with splenomegaly, multiple abdominal collaterals, and portal vein thrombosis. (**b**) Photomicrograph (40×; HE stain) shows glands in the muscle layer with stroma-adenomyomatous changes

(Figs. 11.17 and 11.18). The differential diagnosis includes adenomatous, hyperplastic, and cholesterol polyps as well as uncommon tumors such as carcinoid or melanoma metastases. At ultrasonography, movement of a polypoid lesion with a change of the patient's position suggests an alternate diagnosis of pseudotumor of biliary sludge or clot [39].

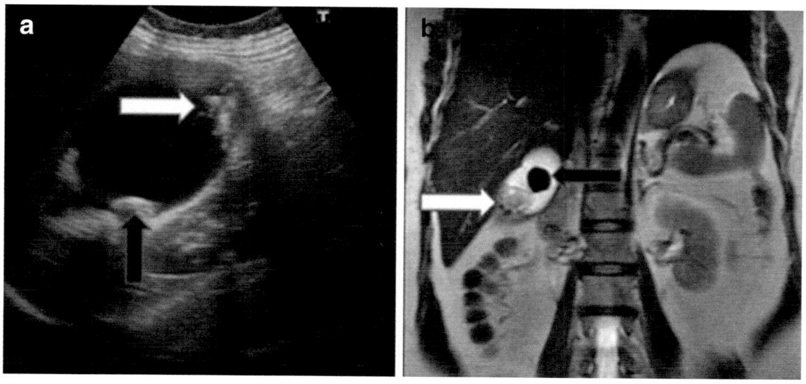

Fig. 11.17 A 56-year-old lady presented with abdominal pain: (**a**) Ultrasonography revealed cholelithiasis (black arrow) with polypoidal soft tissue thickening in the gallbladder fundal region (white arrow). Subsequently MRI confirmed a polypoidal mass in the fundus of the gallbladder displaying T2 hyperintensity on coronal T2WI (**b**). Later cholecystectomy was performed, and histopathological examination revealed mucinous adenocarcinoma

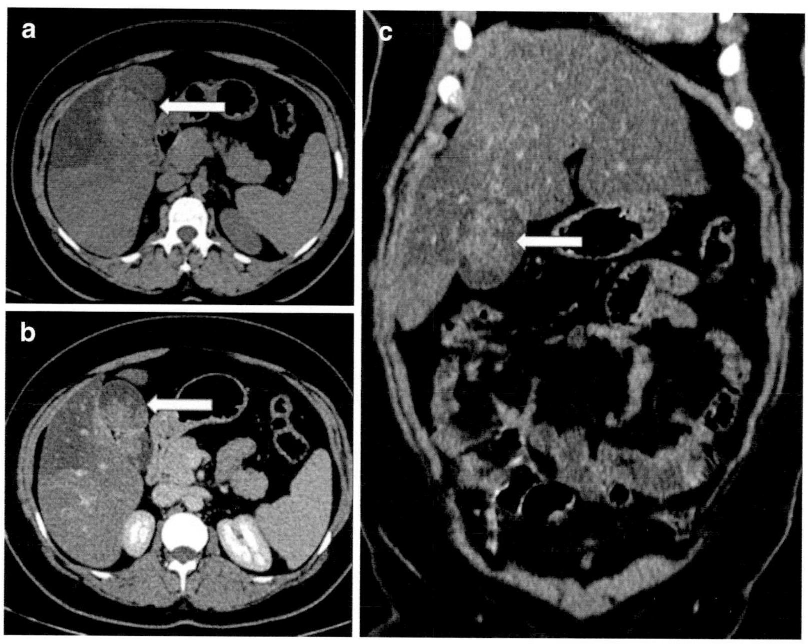

Fig. 11.18 A case of a gallbladder carcinoma: (**a**–**b**) Axial and (**c**) coronal noncontrast and contrast-enhanced CT scans reveal a large polypoidal isodense enhancing soft tissue mass in the gallbladder lumen (white arrow) with indistinct fat panes with adjacent segment V of the liver. Note is made of focal fatty infiltration in segment V

11.5 Radiologic Evaluation of Tumor Extension

The gallbladder malignancy usually presents in an advanced stage. The various modes of the spread of gallbladder carcinoma to adjacent organs are as follows:

1. *Direct extension* is the most common mode of spread as contiguous spread of tumor is facilitated by the thin gallbladder wall, which lacks a substantial lamina propria and has only a single muscular layer. In addition, the perimuscular connective tissue of the gallbladder is continuous with the interlobular connective tissue of the liver [47]. Thus, the liver is most frequently involved by direct contiguous spread (65% of cases), followed by the colon (15%) (Fig. 11.19), duodenum (15%) (Fig. 11.20a–b), and pancreas (6%) [48]. Infiltrative tumor may spread along the cystic duct to the extrahepatic bile duct, and intraductal spread of tumor results in biliary dilatation and obstruction (Fig. 11.20c–d).

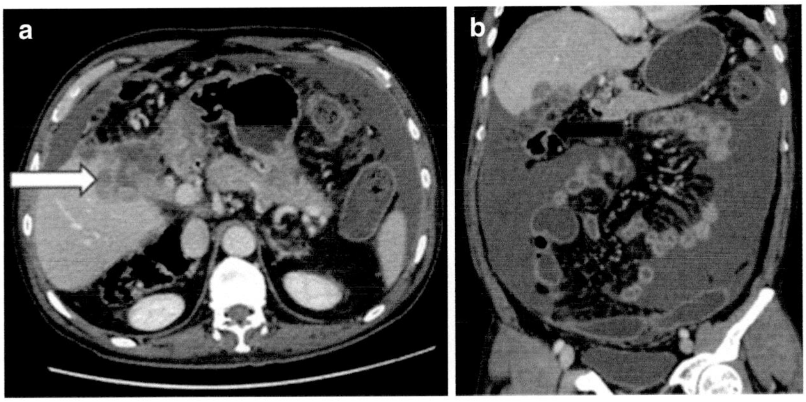

Fig. 11.19 (**a, b**): Axial and coronal contrast-enhanced CT images showing a heterogeneously enhancing lobulated soft tissue mass lesion replacing the gallbladder with adjacent hepatic (white arrow) and colonic (hepatic flexure) infiltration (black arrow). In addition, moderate ascites is also noted

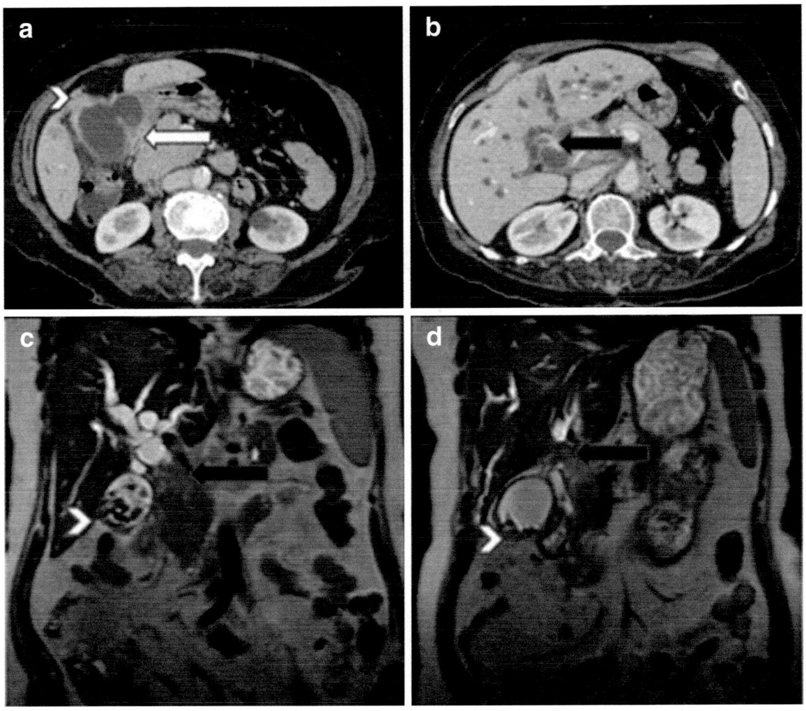

Fig. 11.20 A case of a locally advanced carcinoma of the gallbladder: (**a**, **b**) Contrast-enhanced axial CT and (**c**,**d**) coronal T2W MR images reveal diffuse asymmetric circumferential mural thickening of the gallbladder (white arrows) with adjacent hepatic (arrowhead) and duodenal infiltration (white arrow) and contiguous extension along the cystic duct to involve the proximal third of the common duct (black arrow) and resultant upstream biliary dilatation

2. *Lymphatic*—The prevalence of lymphatic spread is high in gallbladder carcinoma. Lymphatic metastases progress from the gallbladder fossa through the hepatoduodenal ligament to nodal stations near the head of the pancreas. Three pathways of lymphatic drainage have been suggested [49]: (i) cholecystoretropancreatic pathway, (ii) cholecystoceliac pathway, and (iii) cholecystomesenteric pathway.

The cystic and pericholedochal lymph nodes are the most commonly involved at surgery [50] and are a critical pathway to involvement of the celiac, superior mesenteric, and para-aortic lymph nodes (Fig. 11.21). The node of the foramen of Winslow, the superior pancreatoduodenal node, and the posterior pancreatoduodenal nodes are the most common nodes demonstrated by CT [51]. Positive lymph nodes are more likely to be greater than 10 mm in anteroposterior dimension and have ring-like or heterogeneous contrast material enhancement [52] (Fig. 11.22).

3. *Vascular*—Hematogenous metastases are most commonly seen in the liver [48] (Fig. 11.23a). Pulmonary (Fig. 11.23b), skeletal, cardiac, pancreatic, renal, adrenal, and cerebral metastases occur less frequently.
4. *Intraperitoneal*—The peritoneal spread is also common in gallbladder malignancy and may present as ascites (Fig. 11.24), enhancing omental or peritoneal nodules (Fig. 11.25) and/or "drop" metastases (Krukenberg's tumor) (Fig. 11.25).

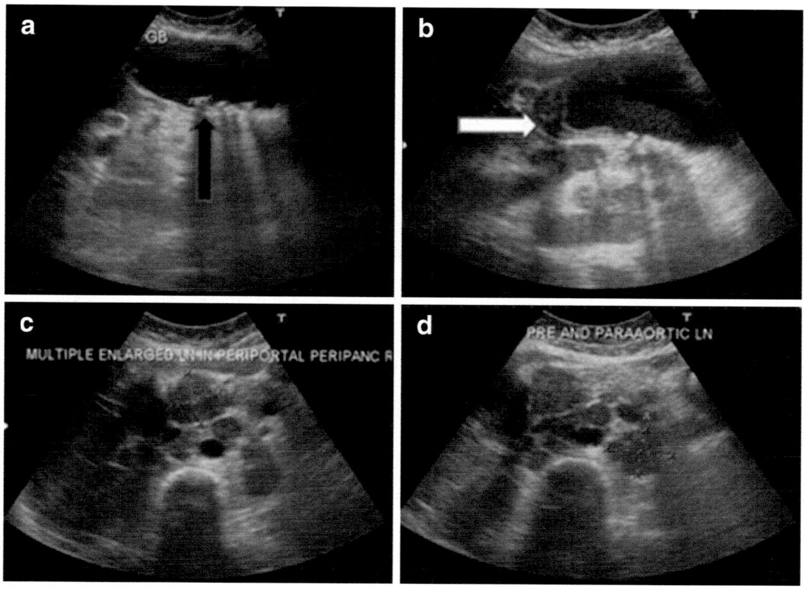

Fig. 11.21 In a known case of cholelithiasis, ultrasound images reveal (**a**) a distended gallbladder with multiple intraluminal calculi (black arrow) and layering of sludge, (**b**) annular mural thickening in the neck region of the gallbladder (white arrow) with, (**c**) periportal and peripancreatic, and (**d**) pre-and para-aortic lymphadenopathy

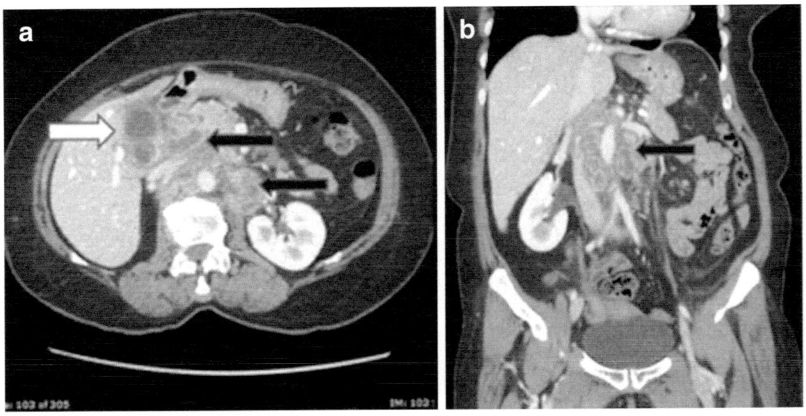

Fig. 11.22 A case of a gallbladder carcinoma: contrast-enhanced (**a**) axial and (**b**) coronal sections of the abdomen reveal annular asymmetric mural thickening of the gallbladder with adjacent hepatic infiltration (white arrow) and characteristic enlarged (>10 mm), ring-enhancing pancreatoduodenal, para-aortic, and superior mesenteric lymph nodes (black arrows)

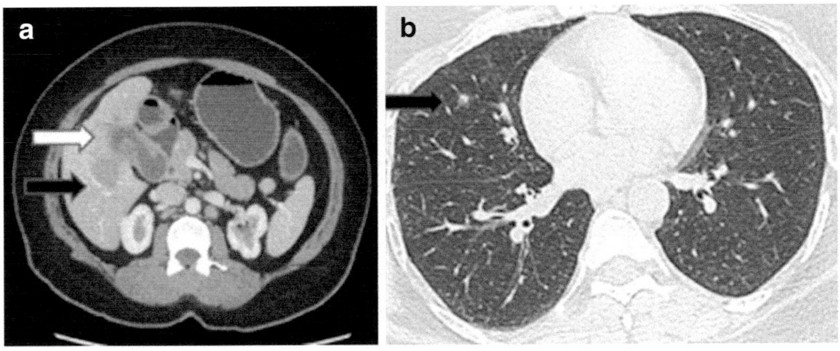

Fig. 11.23 A case of a gallbladder carcinoma; contrast-enhanced axial sections of (**a**) the abdomen and (**b**) chest reveal annular asymmetric mural thickening of the gallbladder with adjacent hepatic infiltration (white arrow) and hepatic and pulmonary metastases (black arrows)

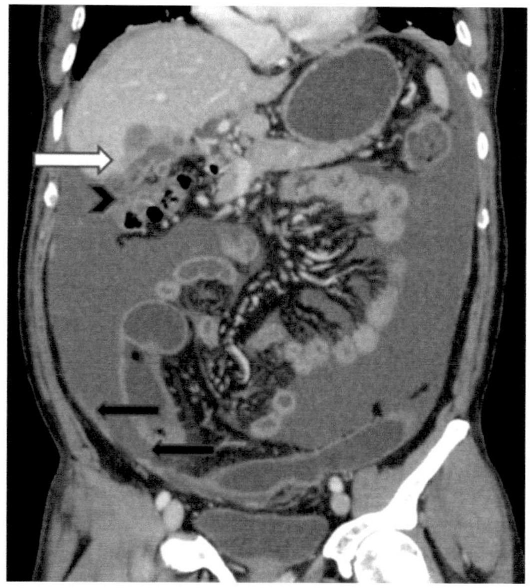

Fig. 11.24 A coronal reformatted contrast-enhanced CT image reveals a heterogeneously enhancing mass in the gallbladder fossa region (white arrow) with surrounding mesenteric fat stranding in the subhepatic region and adjacent colonic infiltration (arrowhead) with moderate ascites and nodular enhancing peritoneal thickening (black arrows) in keeping with intraperitoneal spread of gallbladder carcinoma

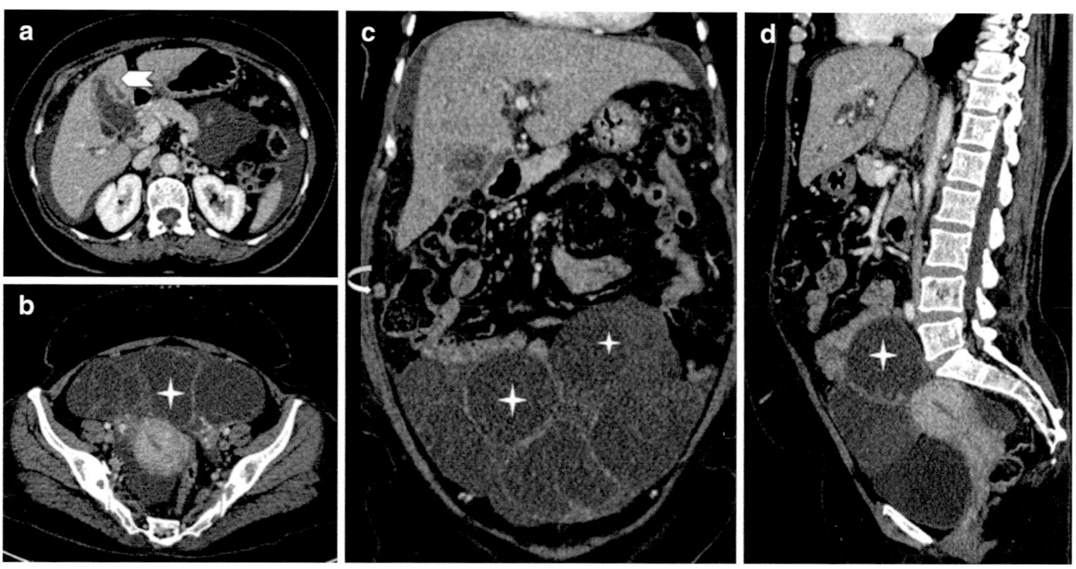

Fig. 11.25 Contrast-enhanced (**a**–**b**) axial and (**c**–**d**) coronal/sagittal reformatted CT images reveal heterogeneously enhancing asymmetric mural thickening of the gallbladder (arrow head) with ascites, omental nodule (curved arrow), and bilateral ovarian drop metastases (star)

11.6 Preoperative Evaluation and Staging

MDCT is now widely available; has robust modality to delineate hepatic and vascular invasion, lymphadenopathy, and distant metastases; and thus has a reported accuracy of up to 84% in determining the T stage and 85% in predicting resectability of primary gallbladder carcinoma [9]. It is performed as unenhanced and contrast-enhanced studies during the hepatic arterial and portal venous phases, from which multiplanar and 3D volume-rendered reconstruction images may be generated to provide a vascular road map and are useful for surgical planning [8]. Kim et al. suggest that an all-in-one protocol supplementing MRI with MRCP and contrast-enhanced arterial and portal venous phase 3D angiographic (MR angiography) images may be up to 100% sensitive for bile duct and vascular invasion; however sensitivity falls to 67% for hepatic invasion and 56% for lymph node metastases [53]. PET/CT has a promising role in the detection of distant metastases, which may alter staging and treatment [54].

The National Comprehensive Cancer Network guideline, based on the *American Joint Committee on Cancer*, eighth edition introduced in 2018, provides the following tumor, node, and metastasis (TNM) classification for gallbladder carcinoma [55].

Primary gallbladder carcinoma can be classified as T1, confined to the lamina propria or the muscle layer of the gallbladder (T1a and T1b, respectively); T2, extending to the serosa; T3, perforating the serosa and/or directly invading the liver and/or one other adjacent structure (stomach, duodenum, colon, pancreas, omentum, extrahepatic bile ducts); or T4, invading the main portal vein, the hepatic artery, or multiple extrahepatic organs (Table 11.1). Lymphatic spread is present in more than 50% of patients at the time of diagnosis and initially involves cystic, pericholedochal, hilar, periduodenal, peripancreatic, and superior mesenteric nodes, which are considered regional nodes. Portacaval, interaortocaval, and more distant nodes are considered distant or M1 disease. Gallbladder carcinoma can also disseminate via intraductal spread along the cystic duct, hematogenous and neural pathways, and intraperitoneal "drop" metastases [56].

Table 11.1 According to the eight edition of American Joint Committee on Cancer staging manual for gallbladder carcinoma; TNM staging of Gallbladder carcinoma

Stage	Definition
Note—AJCC = *American joint committee on cancer*	
Primary tumor (T)	
TX	Primary tumor cannot be assessed
T0	No evidence of primary tumor
Tis	Carcinoma in situ
T1	Tumor invades the lamina propria or muscle layer
T1a	Tumor invades the lamina propria
T1b	Tumor invades the muscle layer
T2	Tumor invades the perimuscular connective tissue on the peritoneal side without the involvement of the serosa (visceral peritoneum) OR tumor invades the perimuscular connective tissue on the hepatic side, with no extension into the liver
T2a	Tumor invades the perimuscular connective tissue on the peritoneal side without the involvement of the serosa (visceral peritoneum)
T2b	Tumor invades the perimuscular connective tissue on the hepatic side, with no extension into the liver
T3	Tumor perforates the serosa (visceral peritoneum) and/or directly invades the liver and/or one other adjacent organ or structure such as the stomach, duodenum, colon, pancreas, omentum, or extrahepatic bile ducts
T4	Tumor invades the main portal vein or hepatic artery or invades two or more extrahepatic organs or structures
Regional lymph nodes (N)	
NX	Regional lymph nodes cannot be assessed
N0	No regional lymph node metastasis
N1	Metastases to one to three regional lymph nodes
N2	Metastases to ≥4 or more regional lymph nodes
Distant metastasis (M)	
M0	No distant metastasis
M1	Distant metastasis

***American Joint Committee on Cancer* Prognostic Groups**

The following gallbladder carcinoma stages can be determined based on the TMN parameters:

- **Stage 0**: Tis; N0; M0
- **Stage I**: T1; N0; M0
- **Stage II**
  - IIA: T2a; N0; M0
  - IIB: T2b; N0; M0
- **Stage III**
  - IIIA: T3; N0; M0
  - IIIB: T1 to T3; N1; M0
- **Stage IV**
  - IVA: T4; N0 to N1; M0
  - IVB: Any T; N2; and M0 or any T; any N; and M1

11.7 Treatment and Prognosis

Because small hepatic, peritoneal, and omental tumor implants can be missed at preoperative imaging, thorough laparoscopic or open exploration should precede aggressive surgery, either at the same or at an earlier operation [56]. Patients with stage I gallbladder carcinoma who are surgical candidates may benefit from extended resection after cholecystectomy, which includes resection of hepatic margins bordering the gallbladder fossa and en bloc nodal dissection [55, 56]. Patients with stage IIA or IIB disease may also undergo exploration and subsequent resection if metastasis is confined to minimal adjacent liver or choledochal nodes. The role of radical dissection for T3 and T4 lesions is controversial [55, 56].

In patients with negative resection margins, external beam radiation therapy and systemic chemotherapy have improved survival, whereas patients with positive microscopic margins or residual disease show no added benefit from chemotherapy and are offered adjuvant radiation therapy only [57]. Although up to 60% of patients with gallbladder carcinoma who undergo extended resection may survive 5 years, the overall prognosis is only 13% [58, 59]. In patients with disseminated disease or medical contraindications to surgery, imaging-guided percutaneous biopsy for tissue confirmation can be performed before palliative therapy.

11.8 Summary

The clinical and radiologic detection of gallbladder carcinoma at an early stage remains challenging. It is imperative for radiologists to closely scrutinize the gallbladder, for subtle imaging findings that may indicate cancer, particularly in patients who are at increased risk of developing gallbladder carcinoma. MDCT is a comprehensive tool in preoperative detection as well as local staging of gallbladder carcinoma and also allows mapping of vascular anatomy in surgical candidates. MRI serves as a problem-solving tool to reach a conclusive diagnosis. PET is primarily employed in detection of distant metastases and post-treatment detection of residual or recurrent disease. Recognition of the characteristic imaging appearances of primary gallbladder carcinoma and understanding its pathways of spread and staging criteria help optimize patient triage to appropriate treatment regimens.

References

1. Roberts KW, Daugherty SF. Primary carcinoma of the gallbladder. Surg Clin North Am. 1986;66:743–9.
2. Ouchi K, Sugawara T, Ono H, et al. Diagnostic capability and rational resectional surgery for early gallbladder cancer. Hepatogastroenterology. 1999;46:1557–60.
3. Inui K, Yoshino J, Miyoshi H. Diagnosis of gallbladder tumors. Intern Med. 2011;50:1133–6.
4. Xie XH, Xu HX, Xie XY, et al. Differential diagnosis between benign and malignant gallbladder diseases with real-time contrast-enhanced ultrasound. Eur Radiol. 2010;20:239–48.
5. Liu L-N, Xu H-X, Lu M-D, et al. Contrast-enhanced ultrasound in the diagnosis of gallbladder diseases: a multi-center experience. PLoS One. 2012;10:e48371.
6. Sadamoto Y, Kubo H, Harada N, Tanaka M, Eguchi T, Nawata H. Preoperative diagnosis and staging of gallbladder carcinoma by EUS. Gastrointest Endosc. 2003;58:536–41.
7. Yoshimitsu K, Honda H, Shinozaki K, et al. Helical CT of the local spread of carcinoma of the gallbladder: evaluation according to the TNM system in patients who underwent surgical resection. AJR Am J Roentgenol. 2002;179:423–8.
8. Kalra N, Sudha S, Gupta R, et al. MDCT in the staging of gallbladder carcinoma. AJR Am J Roentgenol. 2006;186:758–62.
9. Kim SJ, Lee JM, Lee JY, et al. Accuracy of preoperative T-staging of gallbladder carcinoma using MDCT. AJR Am J Roentgenol. 2008;190:74–80.
10. Sugita R, Yamazaki T, Furuta A, Itoh K, Fujita N, Takahashi S. High b value diffusion-weighted MRI for detecting gallbladder carcinoma: preliminary study and results. Eur Radiol. 2009;19:1794–8.
11. Lee SW, Kim HJ, Park JH, et al. Clinical usefulness of 18F-FDG PET-CT for patients with gallbladder cancer and cholangiocarcinoma. J Gastroenterol. 2010;45:560–6.
12. Lazcano-Ponce EC, Miquel JF, Munoz N, et al. Epidemiology and molecular pathology of gallbladder cancer. CA Cancer J Clin. 2001;51(6):349–64.
13. Hundal R, Shaffer EA. Gallbladder cancer: epidemiology and outcome. Clin Epidemiol. 2014;6:99–109.
14. Randi G, Franceschi S, La Vecchia C. Gallbladder cancer worldwide: geographical distribution and risk factors. Int J Cancer. 2006;118(7):1591–602.

15. Duffy A, Capanu M, Abou-Alfa GK, et al. Gallbladder cancer (GBC): 10-year experience at Memorial Sloan-Kettering Cancer Centre (MSKCC). J Surg Oncol. 2008;98(7):485–9.
16. Shaffer EA. Gallbladder cancer: the basics. Gastroenterol Hepatol (NY). 2008;4(10):737–41.
17. Lowenfels AB, Walker AM, Althaus DP, Townsend G, Domellof L. Gallstone growth, size, and risk of gallbladder cancer: an interracial study. Int J Epidemiol. 1989;18(1):50–4.
18. Shaffer EA. Epidemiology of gallbladder stone disease. Best Pract Res Clin Gastroenterol. 2006;20:981–96.
19. Stephen AE, Berger DL. Carcinoma in the porcelain gallbladder: a relationship revisited. Surgery. 2001;129(6):699–703.
20. Kumar S. Infection as a risk factor for gallbladder cancer. J Surg Oncol. 2006;93(8):633–9.
21. Lewis JT, Talwalkar JA, Rosen CB, Smyrk TC. Prevalence and risk factors for gallbladder neoplasia in patients with primary sclerosing cholangitis: evidence for a metaplasia-dysplasia-carcinoma sequence. Am J Surg Pathol. 2007;31(6):907–13.
22. Pandey M. Environmental pollutants in gallbladder carcinogenesis. J Surg Oncol. 2006;93(8):640–3.
23. Darby SC, Whitley E, Howe GR, Hutchings SJ, Kusiak RA, Lubin JH, et al. Radon and cancers other than lung cancer in underground miners: a collaborative analysis of 11 studies. J Cancer Inst. 1995;87(5):378–84.
24. Wolin KY, Carson K, Colditz GA. Obesity and cancer. Oncologist. 2010;15(6):556–65.
25. Gallahan WC, Conway JD. Diagnosis and management of gallbladder polyps. Gastroenterol Hepatol. 2010;39(2):359–67.
26. Stinton LM, Shaffer EA. Epidemiology of gallbladder disease: cholelithiasis and cancer. Gut Liver. 2012;6(2):172–87.
27. Albores-Saavedra J, Henson DE, Sobin LH. WHO histological typing of tumors of the gallbladder and extrahepatic bile ducts. Berlin: Springer-Verlag; 1991.
28. Brown JA, Roberts CS. Elevated serum alphafetoprotein levels in primary gallbladder carcinoma without hepatic involvement. Cancer. 1992;70:1838–40.
29. Kim JH, Lee JY, Baek JH, et al. High-resolution sonography for distinguishing neoplastic gallbladder polyps and staging gallbladder cancer. AJR Am J Roentgenol. 2015;204:W150–9.
30. Hattori M, Inui K, Yoshino J, et al. Usefulness of contrast-enhanced ultrasonography in the differential diagnosis of polypoid gallbladder lesions. Nihon Shokakibyo Gakkai Zasshi. 2007;104:790–8. [in Japanese]
31. Fujita N, Noda Y, Kobayashi G, Kimura K, Yago A. Diagnosis of the depth of invasion of gallbladder carcinoma by EUS. Gastrointest Endosc. 1999;50:659–63.
32. Kim SJ, Lee JM, Lee JY, et al. Analysis of enhancement pattern of flat gallbladder wall thickening on MDCT to differentiate gallbladder cancer from cholecystitis. AJR Am J Roentgenol. 2008;191:765–71.
33. Le Bihan D, Breton E, Lallemand D, et al. Separation of diffusion and perfusion in intravoxel incoherent motion MR imaging. Radiology. 1988;168:497–505.
34. Rodriguez-Fernandez A, Gomez-Rio M, Llamas-Elvira JM, et al. Positron-emission tomography with fluorine-18-fluoro-2-deoxy-D-glucose for gallbladder cancer diagnosis. Am J Surg. 2004;188:171–5.
35. Ai O, Joji K, Torii K, et al. Distinguishing benign from malignant gallbladder wall thickening using FDG-PET. Ann Nucl Med. 2006;20:699–703.
36. Kim J, Ryu KJ, Kim C, Paeng JC, Kim YT. Is there any role of positron emission tomography computed tomography for predicting resectability of gallbladder cancer? J Korean Med Sci. 2014;29:680–4.
37. Iqbal M, Gondal KM, Qureshi AU, Tayyab M. Comparative study of ultrasound guided fine needle aspiration cytology with open/laparoscopic biopsy for diagnosis of carcinoma gallbladder. J Coll Physicians Surg Pak. 2009;19:17–9.
38. Levy AD, Murakata LA, Rohrmann CA. Gallbladder carcinoma: radiologic–pathologic correlation. Radiographics. 2001;21:295–314.
39. Tsuchiya Y. Early carcinoma of the gallbladder: macroscopic features and sonography findings. Radiology. 1991;179:171–5.
40. Yoshimitsu K, Honda H, Kaneko K, et al. Dynamic MRI of the gallbladder lesions: differentiation of benign from malignant. J Magn Reson Imaging. 1997;7:696–701.
41. Koh T, Taniguchi H, Yamaguchi A, Kunishima S, Yamagishi H. Differential diagnosis of gallbladder cancer using positron emission tomography with fluorine-18-labeled fluoro-deoxyglucose (FDG-PET). J Surg Oncol. 2003;84:74–81.
42. Van Breda Vriesman AC, Engelbrecht MR, Smithuis RH, Puylaert JB. Diffuse gallbladder wall thickening: differential diagnosis. AJR. 2007;188:495–501.
43. Chun KA, Ha HK, Yu ES, et al. Xanthogranulomatous cholecystitis: CT features with emphasis on differentiation from gallbladder carcinoma. Radiology. 1997;203:93–7.
44. Fowler RC, Reid WA. Ultrasound diagnosis of adenomyomatosis of the gall-bladder: ultrasonic and pathological correlation. Clin Radiol. 1988;39:402–6.
45. Yoshimitsu K, Honda H, Jimi M, et al. MR diagnosis of adenomyomatosis of the gallbladder and differentiation from gallbladder carcinoma: importance of showing Rokitansky-Aschoff sinuses. AJR Am J Roentgenol. 1999;172:1535–40.
46. Rodríguez-Fernádez A, Gómez-Río M, Medina-Benitez A, et al. Application of modern imaging methods in diagnosis of gallbladder cancer. J Surg Oncol. 2006;93:650–64.
47. Henson DE, Albores-Saavedra J, Corle D. Carcinoma of the gallbladder: histologic types, stage of disease, grade, and survival rates. Cancer. 1992;70:1493–7.

48. Sons HU, Borchard F, Joel BS. Carcinoma of the gallbladder: autopsy findings in 287 cases and review of the literature. J Surg Oncol. 1985;28:199–206.
49. Ito M, Mishima Y, Sato T. An anatomical study of the lymphatic drainage of the gallbladder. Surg Radiol Anat. 1991;13:89–104.
50. Tsukada K, Kurosaki I, Uchida K, et al. Lymph node spread from carcinoma of the gallbladder. Cancer. 1997;80:661–7.
51. Engels JT, Balfe DM, Lee JK. Biliary carcinoma: CT evaluation of extrahepatic spread. Radiology. 1989;172:35–40.
52. Ohtani T, Shirai Y, Tsukada K, Hatakeyama K, Muto T. Carcinoma of the gallbladder: CT evaluation of lymphatic spread. Radiology. 1993;189:875–80.
53. Kim JH, Kim TK, Kim BS, et al. Preoperative evaluation of gallbladder carcinoma: efficacy of combined use of MR imaging, MR cholangiography, and contrast-enhanced dual-phase three-dimensional MR angiography. J Magn Reson Imaging. 2002;16:676–84.
54. Corvera CU, Blumgart LH, Akhurst T, et al. ^{18}F-fluorodeoxyglucose positron emission tomography influences management decision in patients with biliary cancer. J Am Coll Surg. 2008;206:57–65.
55. Benson AB, D'Angelica MI, Abrams T, Abbott DE, Ahmed A, Anaya DA, Anders R, Are C, Bachini M, Binder D, Borad M, Bowlus C, Brown D, Burgoyne A, Castellanos J, Chahal P, Cloyd J, Covey AM, Glazer ES, Hawkins WG, Iyer R, Jacob R, Jennings L, Kelley RK, Kim R, Levine M, Palta M, Park JO, Raman S, Reddy S, Ronnekleiv-Kelly S, Sahai V, Singh G, Stein S, Turk A, Vauthey JN, Venook AP, Yopp A, McMillian N, Schonfeld R, Hochstetler C. NCCN guidelines® insights: biliary tract cancers, version 2.2023. J Natl Compr Cancer Netw. 2023;21(7):694–704.
56. Reid KM, Ramos-De la Medina A, Donohue JH. Diagnosis and surgical management of gallbladder cancer: a review. J Gastrointest Surg. 2007;11:671–81.
57. Mekeel KL, Hemming AW. Surgical management of gallbladder carcinoma: a review. J Gastrointest Surg. 2007;11:1188–93.
58. Kresl JJ, Schild SE, Henning GT, et al. Adjuvant external beam radiation therapy with concurrent chemotherapy in the management of gallbladder carcinoma. Int J Radiat Oncol Biol Phys. 2002;52:167–75.
59. Ito H, Matros E, Brooks DC, et al. Treatment outcomes associated with surgery for gallbladder cancer: a 20-year experience. J Gastrointest Surg. 2004;8:183–90.

Imaging in Acute Pancreatitis

12

Cristiana Boldrini, Riccardo Manfredi, Valerio Di Paola, Luca Russo, Simone Palma, Silvia De Vizio, Maria Luisa De Cicco, Angelica Marra, Silvia Amodeo, and Roberta Dattoli

12.1 Definition

Acute pancreatitis (AP) is an inflammatory disorder of the pancreas, in which the release and premature activation of the pancreatic enzymes cause tissue damage, leading to possible systemic failure. The terminology and classification scheme proposed for AP at the initial Atlanta Symposium (1992) have been reviewed, and a new consensus statement has been proposed by the Acute Pancreatitis Classification Working Group (2012).

Worldwide, AP is a common gastro-intestinal condition that is associated with substantial suffering, morbidity, and cost for the healthcare system. The mortality of acute pancreas ranges from 3% in patients with mild edematous pancreatitis to 20% in patients with pancreatic necrosis [1]. Change in habits of alcohol consumption and tobacco smoking and rising rates of obesity are contributing to increase the incidence of many diseases, including acute pancreatitis [2, 3]. Also, improving the quality of imaging modalities has modified our epidemiologic knowledge about acute pancreatitis [2–5]. The most common risk factors for AP include gallstones, alcohol, hypertriglyceridemia, drugs, post-procedural complications (endoscopic retrograde cholangiopancreatography (ERCP) or abdominal surgery), ampullary stenosis, autoimmune pancreatitis, viral infections (like coxsackie, cytomegalovirus, echovirus, Epstein-Barr virus, hepatitis A/B/C, HIV, mumps, rubella, and varicella), genetic disorders, and smoking [1].

12.2 Epidemiology

12.2.1 Incidence and Prevalence

The global incidence of acute pancreatitis in general population is estimated to be of about 34 cases per 100,000 per year [3], with no difference between men and women [6–8]. The incidence and hospitalization rates after acute pancreatitis have been increasing over the last 20 years. Although most studies have examined the Western world (North America, Europe, and Oceania), there is a paucity of research from Asian, Latin American, and African populations. The increase in incidence has been observed in both adult and pediatric populations [9]. Chronic pancreatitis (CP) occurs less frequently, reported at about 8/100,000 people per year [10]. The frequency of transition from the first episode of

C. Boldrini (✉) · R. Manfredi · V. Di Paola · L. Russo · S. Palma · S. De Vizio · M. L. De Cicco
Department of Bioimaging, Radiation Oncology and Hematology, Fondazione Policlinico Universitario A. Gemelli IRCSS, Rome, Italy
e-mail: Cristiana.boldrini@policlinicogemelli.it

A. Marra · S. Amodeo · R. Dattoli
Institute of Radiology, Catholic University of the Sacred Heart, Rome, Italy

© The Author(s), under exclusive license to Springer Nature Singapore Pte Ltd. 2025
B. Sureka (ed.), *Hepato-Pancreatico Biliary Imaging*, https://doi.org/10.1007/978-981-95-1699-5_12

acute pancreatitis to recurrent acute pancreatitis (RAP) and CP was quantified in a 2015 systematic review of cohort studies with at least 1 year of follow-up [10]. Recurrent acute pancreatitis occurs in 21% (95% Cl 17–26%) of patients after the first episode of acute pancreatitis, and CP develops in 36% (95% Cl 20–53%) of patients after recurrent acute pancreatitis [3, 10].

The mortality from an episode of acute pancreatitis evaluated in the systematic review by Xiao et al. [6] was 1.16 per 100,000 in general population per year [6]. Determinants for the increased risk for mortality in acute pancreatitis include persistent organ failure and infected pancreatic necrosis [3, 11–13].

Prevalence is more typically considered in the context of chronic diseases. Although hyperglycemia is commonly observed in patients with AP, findings of studies regarding newly diagnosed diabetes in subjects with AP are conflicting [14]. Whereas a positive relationship between pre-existing AP and development of diabetes has been observed in some studies, no association was found in others. Authors of a meta-analysis published in 2014 (Das et al.) concluded that patients treated for AP may be at higher risk of developing diabetes; however, the severity of AP had a minimal effect on the studied outcomes in this analysis [15]. The pancreatologists suggest that even patients with mild acute pancreatitis have at least twofold higher long-term risk of diabetes mellitus than the general population [3, 16, 17].

12.3 Aetiology and Clinical Presentation

AP can cause local injury, systemic inflammatory response syndrome, and multiple organ failure [18].

The two most common causes of acute pancreatitis are gallstones (30–45%) and alcohol abuse (30–35%) [5]. Less common causes include hypertriglyceridemia, hypercalcemia, viral infections (mumps, coxsackie), biliary parasites (ascaris), drugs (azathioprine, mercaptopurine, didanosine), Oddi dysfunction, tumor, trauma, surgery, ERCP, and congenital abnormalities (pancreas divisum, annular pancreas, choledochocele, duodenal duplication cyst). Acute pancreatitis is idiopathic in up to 20% of all cases, although about two-thirds of these cases are now thought to be caused by biliary sludge or microlithiasis.

According to the revised Atlanta classification (2012), diagnosis of AP requires at least two of the following three diagnostic features [3, 5]:

1. Abdominal pain consistent with acute pancreatitis
2. Serum lipase activity (or amylase activity) that are at least three times the upper limit of the normal range
3. Findings of AP on computed tomography (CT) or magnetic resonance imaging (MRI).

If the suspicion of acute pancreatitis is very strong based on the patient's clinical symptoms, imaging will be necessary for diagnosis when the serum amylase and/or lipase activity is less than three times the upper limit of normal, as may be the case with delayed presentation [5, 19, 20]. The time interval between the onset of abdominal pain (the beginning of AP) and first admission to the hospital should be noted [5].

12.3.1 Phases of AP

Acute pancreatitis is divided into *early* and *late phase* according to the Atlanta Symposium (1992). There are two overlapping phases in this dynamic disease process, with two peaks of mortality: early and late [5].

In the first week after the onset, the *early phase*, the activation of the cytokine cascade leads to systemic inflammatory response syndrome (SIRS), with an increased risk of developing organ failure, that can be "transient" if it resolves within 48 h or "persistent" if it lasts for >48 h [3, 21–24]. Patients with organ failure that resolves within 48 h of onset have been shown to have zero mortality rate. However, development of exaggerated inflammatory response (SIRS) and subsequent multiorgan failure are responsible for approximately 50% of all deaths. The *late phase* starts in the second week and can last from weeks to months; it is defined by persistent organ failure (single or multiple) and by local or systemic complications [5]. Disease progression is marked by increasing necrosis, infection, persisting systemic inflammatory response syndrome, and multiorgan failure.

12.3.2 Grading of AP

There are important reasons to stratify the severity of acute pancreatitis. First, on admission, it is important to identify patients with potentially severe acute pancreatitis who require aggressive early treatment. Second, in a secondary care setting, clinicians need to identify such patients for possible transfer to specialist care. Third, for specialists who receive such referrals, there are advantages in stratifying these patients into subgroups based on the presence of persistent organ failure and local or systemic complications [5]. According to the revised *Atlanta classification* (2008–2012), the severity of AP has been divided into three classes:

- *Mild acute pancreatitis*, with no organ failure and no local or systemic complications. Mortality is very rare [25].
- *Moderately severe AP*, characterized by the presence of transient organ failure or local or systemic complications, in the absence of persistent organ failure.
- *Severe AP*, characterized by persistent organ failure, single or multiple. These patients can have also one or more local complications, and they are at increased risk of death [22–24].

In "moderately severe AP," an example of a symptomatic local complication is a peripancreatic collection resulting in prolonged abdominal pain, leukocytosis, and fever, or that prevents the ability to maintain nutrition orally; an example of a symptomatic systemic complication is exacerbation of coronary artery disease or chronic lung disease precipitated by the acute pancreatitis [5].

Several clinical scoring systems like Marshall in 1995 or Acute Physiology and Chronic Health Disease Classification System [26, 27] aimed to predict the risk of death in AP. Balthazar et al. [28] in 1990 introduced the CT severity index for assessment of AP. In 2004, Mortele et al. [29] published the Modified CT Severity Index (MCTSI), which includes as prognostic indicators the pancreatic inflammation, the pancreatic necrosis, and extra-pancreatic complications (Table 12.1).

In 2012, the revised Atlanta classification by the "Acute Pancreatitis Classification Working Group" developed a new morphological classification based on the imaging findings, and acute pancreatitis was divided into two groups as "interstitial edematous pancreatitis" (IEP) and "necrotizing pancreatitis" (NP) [1, 3, 5, 26, 30].

Interstitial edematous pancreatitis is more common. Contrast-enhanced computed tomography (CECT) shows focal or more often diffuse enlargement of the pancreas parenchyma due to interstitial edema, with heterogeneous (patchy) enhancement; the pancreatic margins are ill-defined due to inflammation, and there are not un-enhanced (necrotic) areas (Fig. 12.1). The peripancreatic fat usually presents mild strand-

Table 12.1 Modified CT Severity Index (MCTSI)

Prognostic indicators	Points
Pancreatic inflammation:	
Normal pancreas Intrinsic pancreatic abnormalities with or without inflammatory changes in pancreatic fat Pancreatic or peripancreatic fluid collection or peripancreatic fat necrosis	**0** **2** **4**
Pancreatic necrosis:	
None ≤30% ≥30%	**0** **2** **4**
Extra-pancreatic complications:	
One or more of pleural effusion, ascites, vascular complications, parenchymal complications, or gastro-intestinal tract involvement	**2**

Total Score: Total points are given out of 10, to determine the grade of pancreatitis and aid treatment
0–2 Mild
4–6 Moderate
8–10 Severe

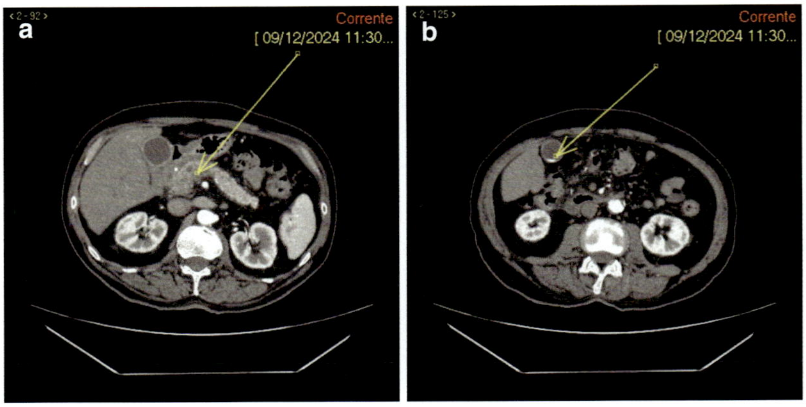

Fig. 12.1 (**a**) Interstitial acute edematous pancreatitis. Contrast-enhanced CT image, performed 3 days after the onset of acute attack, reveals increase in size and swelling of the head-isthmus of the pancreas, with evidence of dilation of the Wirsung duct in its course (maximum diameter 7 mm at the cephalic site) (arrow) (**b**) Mild ectasia and hyperemic appearance of the walls of the common bile duct are associated, in possible reactive alterations. The gallbladder is normally distended, with evidence of microlithiasis at the fundus (arrow) and no pericholecystic fluid layers

ing; there may also be peripancreatic fluid [26]. Clinical symptoms of interstitial edematous pancreatitis usually resolve within a week.

About 5–10% of patients with acute pancreatitis develop a *necrotizing pancreatitis*, usually involving both the pancreas and peripancreatic tissues (75%) and less commonly only the peripancreatic tissue or the pancreatic parenchyma alone [21]. Visualization of necrotic pancreatitis at CECT is best between 48 and 72 h after onset [30]. After the first week of the disease, a non-enhancing area of pancreatic parenchyma at CECT should be considered pathognomonic for certain pancreatic parenchymal necrosis (Fig. 12.2). CT examination should not be performed before 72 h from the onset of symptoms to grade the severity of the disease [25, 28, 31–33]. In this case, repeating CECT 5–6 days later is more accurate for a diagnosis of necrotizing pancreatitis [5].

Most of the cases, CECT imaging protocol includes an un-enhanced scan, followed by the arterial phase and the portal venous phase [3, 5]. The arterial phase on the upper abdomen is performed 35–40 s after the infusion of intravenous iodinated contrast medium or 15–20 s after the peak enhancement (the so-called pancreatic phase, with maximum contrast enhancement of the pancreatic parenchyma) and then follows the portal venous phase including the entire abdomen and pelvis [3].

12.3.3 Collections in AP

The revised Atlanta classification (2012) defines the following terms: acute peripancreatic fluid collection (APFC) occurring in the first 4 weeks in IEP, pancreatic pseudocyst as a delayed (usually >4 weeks) complication of interstitial edematous pancreatitis, and necrosis, which may be an acute necrotic collection (ANC, in the early phase and before demarcation) or walled-off necrosis (WON), which is surrounded by a radiologically identifiable capsule and rarely develops before 4 weeks from the onset of pancreatitis [5].

In IEP, APFCs can occur in the first 4 weeks; they are fluid collections in the peripancreatic region, with ill-defined walls [29, 34]. On CECT, APFCs appear as homogeneous collections, with low attenuation. On MRI, T2-weighted sequences typically demonstrate high T2 signal intensity. Most of them can be seen in the lesser sac and in the anterior pararenal space. They do not have a well-defined wall, are homogeneous, are confined by normal fascial planes in the retroperito-

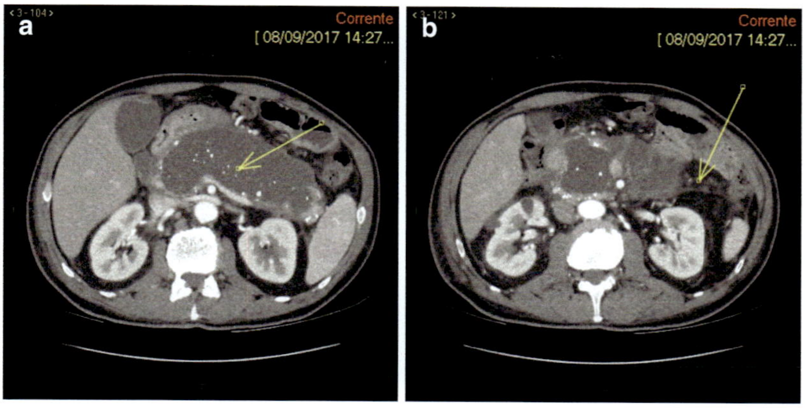

Fig. 12.2 (**a**) Necrotizing pancreatitis. The pancreas is enlarged and almost completely replaced by a voluminous fluid collection, with maximum axial dimensions of approximately 14 cm × 5.5 cm, which partially extends into the hepatogastric ligament and the root of the mesentery and which comes into contact with the stomach, the duodenum, and the first jejunal loop, the latter with moderately thickened walls. There are multiple small calcifications in the collection, due to CP (**b**) NP is associated with thickening of the right renal bands, with fluid quota in the anterior pararenal space and right perirenal space, and phenomena of steatonecrosis in the right perirenal space (arrow)

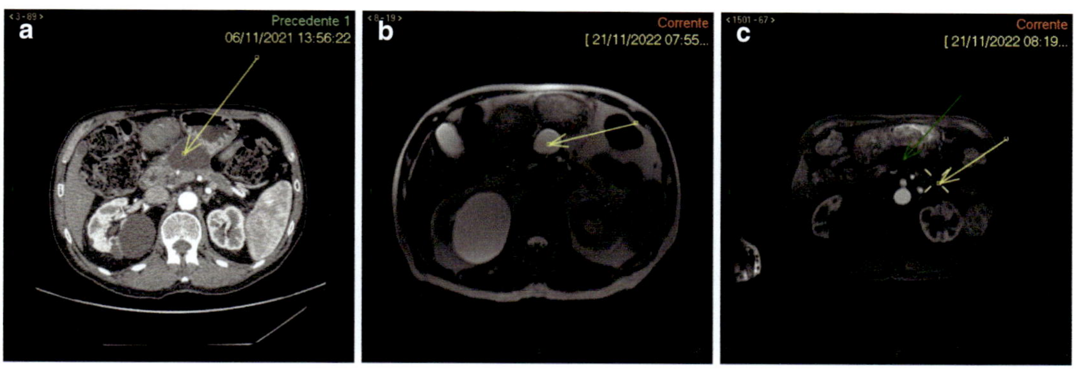

Fig. 12.3 (**a**) Pseudocyst (arrow) in a man with history of alcohol abuse and necrotizing pancreatitis. At the level of the tail, we notice ectasia of the main pancreatic duct (caliber of the main pancreatic duct of about 3 mm) and of the secondary pancreatic ducts which take on a "crown" sac-like appearance along the main pancreatic duct. At this level, the pancreatic parenchyma appears markedly thinned (**b**, **c**) At MRI, it is confirmed at the level of the body of the pancreas a well-circumscribed peripancreatic fluid collection surrounded by a well-defined enhancing capsule (yellow arrow in **b**). In the tail, the pancreatic parenchyma appears markedly thinned (yellow arrow in **c**)

neum, and may be multiple [5]. Most APFCs resolve spontaneously, without intervention, and can be followed by clinical monitoring and repeated imaging.

When a localized APFC persists beyond 4 weeks, it is likely to develop into a pancreatic pseudocyst, although this is a rare event in acute pancreatitis. A *pseudocyst* is a well-circumscribed peripancreatic fluid collection surrounded by a well-defined enhancing capsule (fibrous or granulation tissue) (Fig. 12.3), without non-liquefied components. They generally resolve spontaneously and often remain asymptomatic; only 50% of persistent pseudocysts will cause clinical symptoms or complications, such as infection [3]. Pseudocysts should be treated with endoscopic drainage or surgery if they are symptomatic, measure greater than 5 cm, or increase in size and if they persist for more than 6 weeks [35]. A pancreatic pseudocyst is thought to arise from disruption of the main pancreatic duct or its intra-pancreatic branches without any recognizable pancreatic parenchymal necrosis; this theory suggests that consequent leakage of pancreatic juice results in a persistent, localized fluid collection, usually after more than 4 weeks [5].

ANCs present within the first 4 weeks of necrotizing pancreatitis as collections of variable amounts of fluid and necrotic tissue (Figs. 12.4 and 12.5). The necrosis can involve the pancreatic parenchyma and/or the peripancreatic tissues; there is no defined wall surrounding the collection [5, 21]. Prior to 2 weeks, it may be tricky to distinguish ANCs from APFCs; however, ANCs will typically ultimately contain non-liquified debris or fat globules. On un-enhanced CT, the presence of fat attenuation within a pancreatic collection is helpful at identifying necrosis and can also help differentiate between ANCs and APFCs [3].

After 4 weeks of necrotizing pancreatitis, Acute necrotic collection (ANC) becomes WON, which resembles a pseudocyst, but can be differentiated on CECT by the presence of internal solid components (Figs. 12.6 and 12.7). As ACNs, WONs may be intra- or extra-pancreatic [5, 21]. WON is derived from necrotic pancreatic parenchyma and/or necrotic peripancreatic tissues and may be infected, multiple, and present at sites distant from the pancreas. CECT may not distinguish solid from liquid content, and for this reason, a T2-weighted MRI or ultrasound may be necessary to help identify the presence of debris in the fluid collection, in order to differentiate WON from pseudocyst [35, 36]. They can be treated conservatively if they are sterile. However, infected or symptomatic collections are usually treated with minimally invasive approaches like percutaneous or endoscopic drainage, which are demonstrated to have superior outcomes compared to open surgical debridement.

The diagnosis of infection (infected necrosis) of an ANC or of WON can be suspected by the patient's clinical course or by the presence of gas within the collection seen on CECT [5, 21]. This extraluminal gas is present in areas of necrosis and may or may not form a gas/fluid level depending on the amount of liquid content present at that stage of the disease. In cases of doubt, fine-needle aspiration (FNA) for culture may be performed, but some case series studies have shown that most patients can be managed without FNA, especially if percutaneous drainage is part of the management algorithm.

12.3.4 Complications of AP

The diagnosis of infected pancreatic necrosis is important because of the need for antibiotic treatment and likely active intervention. The presence of infection can be presumed when there is extraluminal gas in the pancreatic and/or peripancreatic tissues on CECT or when per-

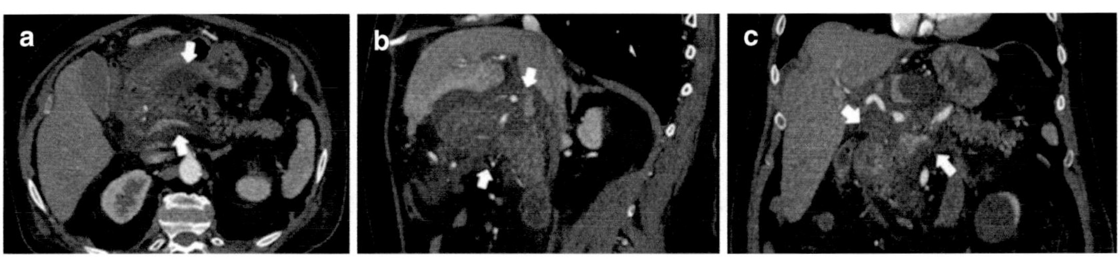

Fig. 12.4 Acute necrotic collection. The contrast-enhanced CT axial scan (**a**) shows the presence of an acute necrotic fluid collection which involves the head and the body of the pancreatic gland (white arrows). The sagittal MPR (**b**) and coronal MPR (**c**) better show the extension of the collection. (Brizi et al. [3]. Licensed under CC-BY 4.0)

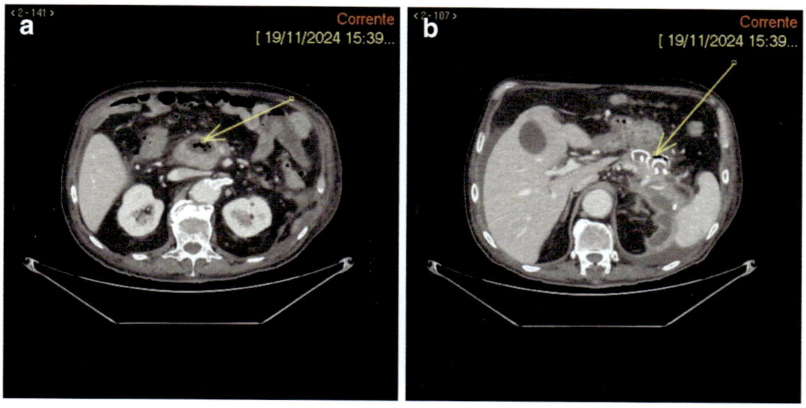

Fig. 12.5 (**a**, **b**) Necrotizing AP, 3 weeks after the onset. Results of pseudocysto-gastro-anastomosis with positioning of two Hot-Axios and two coaxial pig tails (arrow in **b**). Extensive loss of substance of the pancreatic parenchyma, which shows markedly reduced and inhomogeneous enhancement in the aftermath of acute necrotic-hemorrhagic pancreatitis. Necrotic collections coexist, with anfractuous margins delimited by thick walls and with air bubbles in the context (**a**)

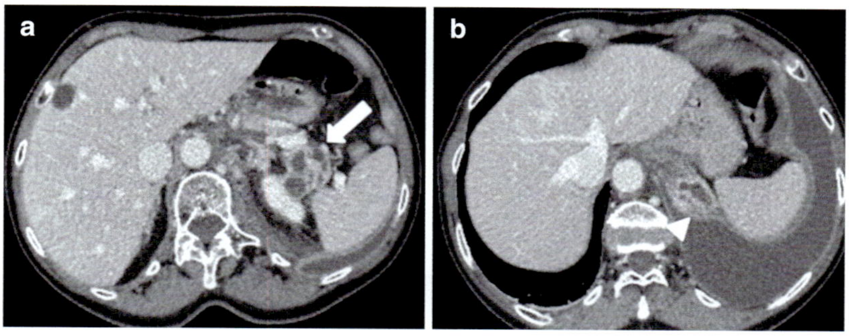

Fig. 12.6 Fistula with pleural cavity in a woman with necrotizing AP. Multiple encapsulated fluid collections in the tail of the pancreatic parenchyma (arrow in **a**) (WONs). These collections extend up to the left hemidiaphragm with pleural fistula and pleural effusion (arrow head in **b**). (Brizi et al. [3]. Licensed under CC-BY 4.0)

cutaneous, image-guided, FNA is positive for bacteria and/or fungi on Gram stain and culture. There may be a varying amount of suppuration (pus) associated with the infected pancreatic necrosis, and this suppuration tends to increase with time with liquefaction. The original Atlanta classification proposed the term "pancreatic abscess" to define a "localized collection of purulent material without significant necrotic material"; this finding is extremely uncommon, and because the term is confusing and has not been adopted widely, the term "pancreatic abscess" is not used in the current classification [5]. The development of secondary infection in pancreatic necrosis is associated with increased morbidity and mortality. The nowadays accepted management is the "step-up" approach (drainage either with a percutaneous catheter or transluminal endoscopic), with progressive escalation in case of treatment failure [3, 37, 38]. Surgical or endoscopic transluminal debridement is now only required with lack of clinical resolution and is delayed until necrosis has become WON [39]. By implementing the revised Atlanta classification, the radiologist can help the multidisciplinary team to prescribe the appropriate therapy according to the type of collection [21, 39].

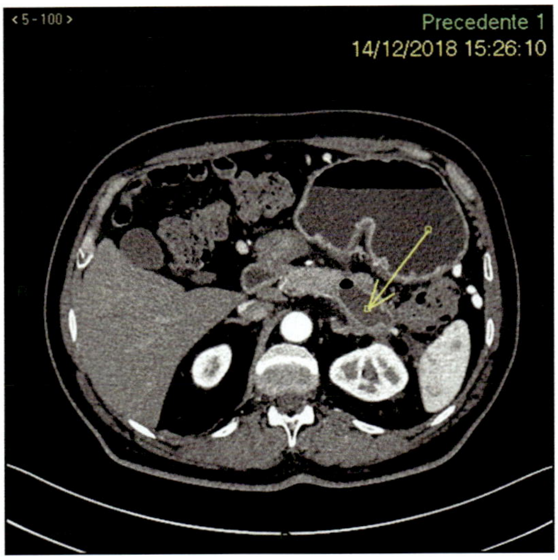

Fig. 12.7 WON evolution. Four weeks after the onset of AP, axial CECT scan shows a focal thinning of the thickness of the pancreatic parenchyma at the level of the body of the tail. The thickness and signal intensity of the pancreatic parenchyma of the head, the uncinate process, and the isthmus appear normal. A fluid collection with gas in the context is also documented in the adipose tissue of the pancreatic lodge at the level of the body and tail (arrow), with a maximum diameter of 45 mm, likely in communication with the main pancreatic duct

In addition to pancreatic and peripancreatic collections, vascular complications may occur (Fig. 12.8). The most common sources of bleeding are the splenic artery, portal vein and other peripancreatic vessels [40], due to erosion of local vasculature and pseudoaneurysm formation. However, splenic vein thrombosis represents the most common vascular complication in patients with AP, which is identifiable as either no enhancement or a filling defect of the portal vein.

Necrosis of the central pancreas results in the disruption of the main pancreatic duct in 40% of cases. This can be confirmed with pancreatic MRI and magnetic resonance cholangiopancreatography (MRCP), and later an ERCP can be executed. Another complication of necrotizing pancreatitis is pancreatic duct stricture, which may develop secondary to inflammation or healing following the successful drainage of necrotic collections [40].

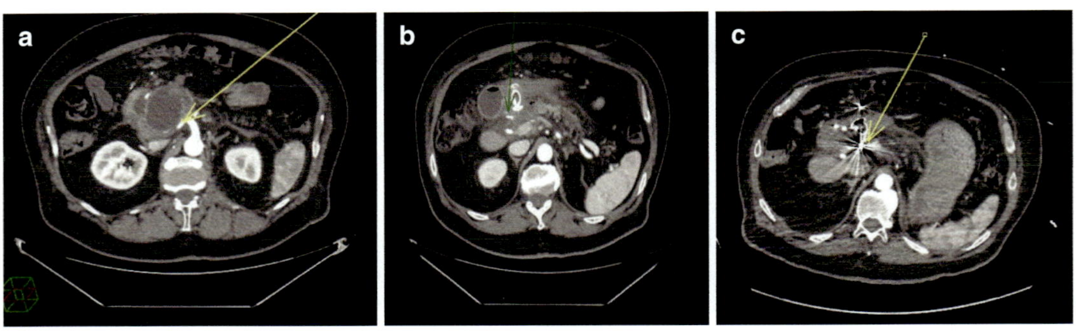

Fig. 12.8 Vascular complication of AP. Contrast-enhanced CT scan shows a collection in the retroperitoneum (pseudocyst) which contacts inferior pancreatico-duodenal artery (IPA) (yellow arrow in **a**). One month later (**b**), CECT depicts irregularity of the course of IPA, where focal dilatation of about 4 mm is appreciated—suggesting the presence of pseudoaneurysm with active bleeding (green arrow). In **c**, the CECT image after endovascular embolization procedure with evidence of metal coils in the IPA

12.4 Recurrent Acute Pancreatitis

Recurrent acute pancreatitis has been defined as a syndrome of multiple distinct acute inflammatory responses, which manifests with one or more new episodes, in individuals who experienced two or more episodes of documented AP, separated by at least 3 months [3]. The term RAP was reported in the first Marseille classification of pancreatitis, which clearly distinguished RAP from CP, and then in Toxic-metabolic, Idiopathic, Genetic, Autoimmune, Recurrent and severe acute pancreatitis and Obstructive (TIGAR-O) Pancreatitis Risk/Etiology Checklist. Toxic-metabolic, Idiopathic, Genetic, Autoimmune, Recurrent and severe acute pancreatitis and Obstructive Pancreatitis. However, the term was eliminated in the revised classifications of Marseille and Marseille-Rome, because of the difficulties of distinguishing between episodes of acute pancreatitis occurring in a normal pancreas or in CP. Pancreatitis generally recurs in a normal morpho-functional gland and is characterized by self-limited edematous changes in the pancreas. Acute episodes are generally mild to moderate; in some cases, pancreatic-like pain, with serum amylase and/or lipase elevation, lasts only a few hours, and the patient recovers without hospitalization [41, 42]. Whether recurring episodes of pancreatitis in a morphologically normal pancreas can lead to CP is still an open question, because only few, empirical data indicate whether, how often, and in which types of patients' recurrent pancreatitis progress to the chronic disease [42].

For 70–80% of patients with recurrent acute pancreatitis, a specific cause may be identified [3, 41, 42], such as gallstone disease (especially biliary microlithiasis), excessive alcohol consumption, hypertriglyceridemia, medications, intraductal papillary mucinous neoplasms, genetic disorders, and pancreato-biliary anomalies.

The investigation of RAP requires MRCP for the evaluation of ductal anatomy. MRCP can be performed also after the intravenous injection of secretin. Secretin is a hormone produced by the S cells of the duodenal mucosa in response to acid in the duodenal lumen. Its primary effect is to increase water and bicarbonate secretions by exocrine cells of the pancreas. Studies have shown that secretin increases the amount of fluid in the pancreatic ducts and may augment the sensitivity of MRCP in diagnosing pancreatic ductal disease, congenital anomalies, and CP, by leading to more conspicuous visualization of main pancreatic duct and diseased side branches; secretin is however an expensive drug [3, 43–45].

A retrospective study by Sandrasegaran et al. [44] demonstrated that secretin-enhanced MRCP is superior to conventional MRCP and T2-weighted sequences in detecting ductal abnormalities in patients with recurrent acute pancreatitis, particularly for findings related to early CP; this may obviate the need for ERCP [43]. In addition, secretin-enhanced MRCP showed a reduction in exocrine function in up to one-third of patients with recurrent acute pancreatitis. The authors believe that secretin-enhanced MRCP should be part of the MRI protocol for investigating patients with RAP, while further studies are required to determine whether patients with recurrent acute pancreatitis with impaired exocrine function on secretin-enhanced MRCP may need to be treated differently from those with normal exocrine function [43].

12.5 Imaging Modalities in AP

Imaging modalities available for the diagnosis of acute pancreatitis include US, CT, MRI, MRCP, and ERCP. The modality to be selected depends on the reason for investigation. The main purpose of the imaging in acute clinical situations is to detect the disease, to recognize the complications, and to make a differential diagnosis from other acute abdomen causes (gastro-intestinal perforation, acute cholecystitis, acute aortic dissection, and mesenteric arterial occlusion).

In the emergency setting, CT and ultrasound are the imaging modalities of choice because of accessibility and lower cost. Transabdominal ultrasound's main role in acute pancreatitis is identifying gallstones and choledocholithiasis; otherwise, ultrasound has limited use in significant measure due to difficult visualization of the pancreas [30].

In the late phase of moderately severe or severe acute pancreatitis, *MRI* has its own rule, having a superior soft tissue contrast resolution than CT (76.5%) [46] and allowing better assessment of biliary and pancreatic ducts. MRI requires patient cooperation. Because patients with pancreatitis are often young and require multiple follow-up CT examinations, substitution of MRI for CT in some patients would reduce the collective radiation dose considerably. MRI can have an important role in staging the severity of acute pancreatitis and may be superior for the characterization of peripancreatic fluid collections [47]. The use of breath-hold sequences reduces respiratory and motion artifacts, which previously limited the use of MRI. Examination times have been reduced markedly, so that the total acquisition time with a full scan is less than 30 min. The most important sequences for pancreatic evaluation are T1-weighted spoiled gradient echo with fat suppression and dynamic imaging after IV administration of gadolinium [47].

Normal pancreatic anatomy is best depicted on T1-weighted fat-suppressed images, in which the pancreas is typically hyperintense because of pancreatic acinar proteins [46–49]; on T2-weighted images, pancreatic parenchyma is typically hypointense. In interstitial edematous pancreatitis, the pancreas has diffuse or localized enlargement due to inflammatory edema, and this type of AP has no pancreatic necrosis or peripancreatic necrosis [46]. The parenchyma of the pancreas may display normal or mild hypointensity on T1-weighted images (T1WI) and hyperintensity on T2WI. Patchy-like hyperintensity on T2WI could be observed in the peripancreatic region, perirenal space, and lesser omental bursa. The pancreas shows homogeneous enhancement after an intravenous administration of a contrast agent (gadolinium). Stranding of the peripancreatic fat planes is best seen on the in-phase T1WI. In more severe cases, peripancreatic fluid collections occur because of the release of pancreatic enzymes and are best depicted on T2WI. In necrotizing pancreatitis, the necrotic areas show hypointensity on T1WI (the so-called black pancreas), hyperintensity on T2WI, and no enhancement after injection of contrast agent (gadolinium) [3, 46] (Fig. 12.9); in the necrotic zones, on MRI the presence of any gas may indicate infection [50].

APFCs usually occur in IEP within 4 weeks of the onset of symptoms; they do not have cystic walls and are homogeneously hypointense on T1WI and hyperintense on T2WI. These collections are usually sterile, and 50% of the collections can be spontaneously absorbed within 2–4 weeks [46]. They may develop into pseudocysts if acute pancreatitis lasts more than 4 weeks.

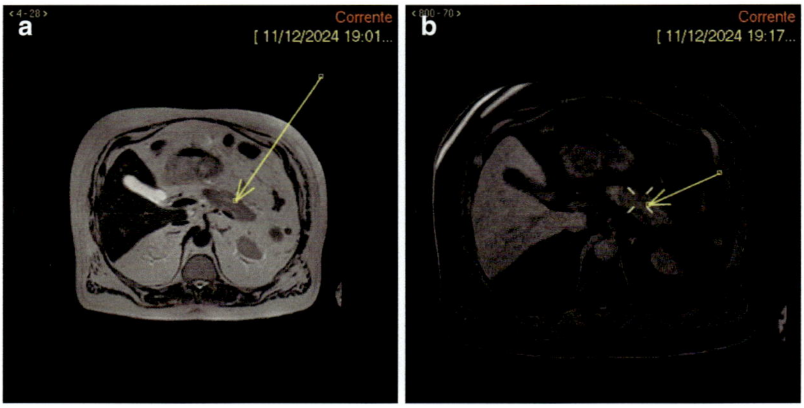

Fig. 12.9 NP at MRI. The pancreatic parenchyma of the body and tail appears uniformly increased in size, with a diffuse alteration of the signal intensity in T2 and alteration of the diffusion coefficient (**a**). In the post-contrast phase, the pancreatic parenchyma of the body-tail appears hypovascularized on T1w images (**b**)

Some researchers have found that the male sex, alcoholic pancreatitis, and ascites are risk factors for PPC formation. Pancreatic *pseudocysts* have a thin smooth wall and homogeneous intensity on T1WI and T2WI because of the liquid content with no solid component (debris) in the fluid. Pseudocysts larger than 6 cm in diameter may be associated with multiple complications, such as mass effect, infection, rupture, and bleeding [46]. T2WI, MRCP, and multiplanar reconstruction (MPR) help visualize the broken pancreatic duct and its connection with pseudocysts; from the pancreatic duct, pancreatic fluid leaks out and may cause enlargement of the pseudocysts. *ANCs* have no capsule, and they show mixed signals on T1WI and T2WI. ANCs require drainage with a catheter to prevent infection and possible sepsis [46]. A severe and persistent clinical course in acute necrotizing pancreatitis may lead to the formation of *WON* [46]. On MRI they contain multiple fragments of the tissue that are free to float, and there is no contrast enhancement on the enhanced scans [46] (Fig. 12.10). This non-liquid substance is the residue of the pancreas and extrapancreatic necrotic tissue, which is difficult to distinguish with CT. Patients with WON are commonly complicated with infection; in case of infected WON, increasing volume of WON, and vascular complications with bleeding, surgical treatment may be necessary.

When the pancreatic neck and body are totally necrotic with pancreatic duct disruption, we refer to *disconnected pancreatic duct syndrome*, which has a prevalence from 10% to 31% according to literature [46, 51–54]. Studies have reported that the diagnosis of pancreatic duct disruption should be considered if (i) peripancreatic necrosis area is at least 2 cm and (ii) MRCP shows that the main pancreatic duct of the upstream pancreatic tissue travels to the WON area of the intra- and/or extrapancreatic tissue and approaches with a right angle into the fluid or necrotic tissue [46, 54]. MRCP performed after the intravenous injection of secretin (S-MRCP) demonstrates a cut-off of the downstream pancreatic duct with enhancing upstream pancreatic parenchyma [43]; S-MRCP may show the passage of exocrine output into the collection.

MRI is also sensitive for visualizing hemorrhages. Hemorrhage can occur in patients with severe necrotizing pancreatitis or as a result of the rupture of a pseudoaneurysm and represents a life-threatening emergency. Hemorrhagic fluid collections are more evident on MRI than CT because of the following: high signal intensity methemoglobin on T1WI, low signal intensity hemosiderin on T2WI, and signal abnormalities due to hemorrhage remaining visible longer on MRI. The enzymes released by the pancreas can corrode the wall of the peripancreatic vessels, with consequent exudative damage to the pancreatic vessels: arteritis and pseudoaneurysm, phlebitis, venous thrombosis, and pancreatic portal hypertension [47, 55]. Hemorrhages on CT show a slightly high density (>35 HU) in the acute phase; the density decreases over time. Compared

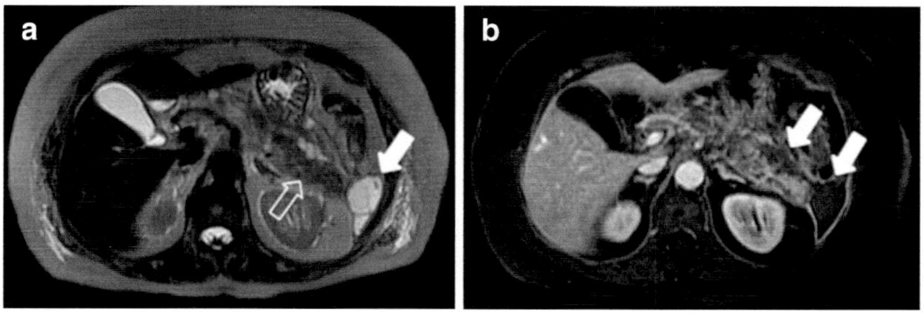

Fig. 12.10 Walled-off necrosis. T2-weighted MR image (**a**) and post-gadolinium T1w scan (**b**) show the presence of a heterogeneous encapsulated fluid collection (WON) in the pancreatic and peripancreatic area. Diffuse hyperintensity on T2w images of the pancreatic parenchyma indicates the presence of parenchymal edema (empty arrow in **a**). (Brizi et al. [3]. Licensed under CC-BY 4.0)

with CT, MRI is more sensitive for visualizing hemorrhages, which are hyperintense on T1WI during the acute phase and persist longer than on CT images [46, 55–57]. MRI findings of artery invasion consist of the loss of normal vascular flowing void effect, the blurred edge of the arterial walls, and the poor enhancement at the involving segment on contrast-enhanced arterial phase images. The splenic artery, gastroduodenal artery, and pancreaticoduodenal artery are more frequently involved [58–60].

Studies show that approximately 63% of patients with AP experience gastro-intestinal complications, characterized by dilatation, mild thickening of the gastro-intestinal wall, and stratification of the bowel wall in contrast-enhanced scans on imaging [46]. Other possible complications may involve the liver because of SIRS and bile duct obstruction, the urinary system, respiratory system, bone, and skin. Acute renal failure is an early complication of severe AP and has a high mortality rate [46, 61].

References

1. Gapp J, Tariq A, Chandra S. Acute pancreatitis. 2023 Feb 9. In: StatPearls [Internet]. Treasure Island: StatPearls Publishing; 2025.
2. Sadr-Azodi O, Orsini N, Andrén-Sandberg Å, Wolk A. Abdominal and total adiposity and the risk of acute pancreatitis: a population-based prospective cohort study. Am J Gastroenterol. 2013;108(1):133–9.
3. Brizi MG, Perillo F, Cannone F, Tuzza L, Manfredi R. The role of imaging in acute pancreatitis. Radiol Med. 2021;126(8):1017–29. Epub 2021 May 12. https://creativecommons.org/licenses/by/4.0/.
4. Kristiansen L, Grønbaek M, Becker U, Tolstrup JS. Risk of pancreatitis according to alcohol drinking habits: a population-based cohort study. Am J Epidemiol. 2008;168(8):932–7.
5. Banks PA, Bollen TL, Dervenis C, et al. Classification of acute pancreatitis—2012: revision of the Atlanta classification and definitions by international consensus. Gut. 2013;62:102–11.
6. Xiao AY, et al. Global incidence and mortality of pancreatic diseases: a systematic review, meta-analysis, and meta-regression of population-based cohort studies. Lancet Gastroenterol Hepatol. 2016;1:45–55.
7. Pendharkar SA, Mathew J, Petrov MS. Age- and sex-specific prevalence of diabetes associated with diseases of the exocrine pancreas: a population-based study. Dig Liver Dis. 2017;49:540–4.
8. Pendharkar SA, et al. Ethnic and geographic variations in the incidence of pancreatitis and post-pancreatitis diabetes mellitus in New Zealand: a nationwide population-based study. N Z Med J. 2017;130:55–68.
9. Iannuzzi JP, King JA, Leong JH, Quan J, Windsor JW, Tanyingoh D, Coward S, Forbes N, Heitman SJ, Shaheen AA, Swain M, Buie M, Underwood FE, Kaplan GG. Global incidence of acute pancreatitis is increasing over time: a systematic review and meta-analysis. Gastroenterology. 2022;162(1):122–34. Epub 2021 Sep 25.
10. Petrov MS, Yadav D. Global epidemiology and holistic prevention of pancreatitis. Nat Rev Gastroenterol Hepatol. 2019;16(3):175–84.
11. Frey C, Zhou H, Harvey D, White RH. Co-morbidity is a strong predictor of early death and multi-organ system failure among patients with acute pancreatitis. J Gastrointest Surg. 2007;11:733–42.
12. Wang SQ, Li SJ, Feng QX, Feng XY, Xu L, Zhao QC. Overweight is an additional prognostic factor in acute pancreatitis: a meta-analysis. Pancreatology. 2011;11(2):92–8.
13. Petrov MS, Shanbhag S, Chakraborty M, Phillips AR, Windsor JA. Organ failure and infection of pancreatic necrosis as determinants of mortality in patients with acute pancreatitis. Gastroenterology. 2010;139:813–20.
14. Lee YK, Huang MY, Hsu CY, Su YC. Bidirectional relationship between diabetes and acute pancreatitis: a population-based cohort study in Taiwan. Medicine (Baltimore). 2016;95(2):e2448.
15. Das SL, Singh PP, Phillips AR, et al. Newly diagnosed diabetes mellitus after acute pancreatitis: a systematic review and metaanalysis. Gut. 2014;63:818–31.
16. Shen HN, Chang YH, Chen HF, Lu CL, Li CY. Increased risk of severe acute pancreatitis in patients with diabetes. Diabet Med. 2012;29(11):1419–24.
17. Lai SW, Muo CH, Liao KF, Sung FC, Chen PC. Risk of acute pancreatitis in type 2 diabetes and risk reduction on anti-diabetic drugs: a population-based cohort study in Taiwan. Am J Gastroenterol. 2011;106(9):1697–704.
18. Crockett SD, et al. American Gastroenterological Association Institute guideline on initial management of acute pancreatitis. Gastroenterology. 2018;154:1096–101.
19. Bollen TL, van Santvoort HC, Besselink MG, et al. Update on acute pancreatitis: ultrasound, computed tomography, and magnetic resonance imaging features. Semin Ultrasound CT MR. 2007;28:371–83.
20. Morgan DE. Imaging of acute pancreatitis and its complications. Clin Gastroenterol Hepatol. 2008;6:1077–85.
21. Fung C, Svystun O, Fouladi DF, Kawamoto S. CT imaging, classification, and complications of acute pancreatitis. Abdom Radiol. 2020;45(5):1243–52.

22. Lytras D, Manes K, Triantopoulou C, Paraskeva C, Delis S, Avgerinos C, Dervenis C. Persistent early organ failure: defining the high-risk group of patients with severe acute pancreatitis? Pancreas. 2008;36(3):249–54.
23. Du W, Wang H, Zhang SW, Wang BE. Investigation on the relation between systemic inflammatory response syndrome and severity of acute pancreatitis. Zhongguo Wei Zhong Bing Ji Jiu Yi Xue. 2005;17(5):279–81.
24. Carnovale A, Rabitti PG, Manes G, Esposito P, Pacelli L, Uomo G. Mortality in acute pancreatitis: is it an early or a late event? JOP. 2005;6(5):438–44.
25. Singh VK, Bollen TL, Wu BU, et al. An assessment of the severity of interstitial pancreatitis. Clin Gastroenterol Hepatol. 2011;9:1098–103.
26. Marshall JC, Cook DJ, Christou NV, Bernard GR, Sprung CL, Sibbald WJ. Multiple organ dysfunction score: a reliable descriptor of a complex clinical outcome. Crit Care Med. 1995;23(10):1638–52.
27. Mederos MA, Reber HA, Girgis MD. Acute pancreatitis: a review. JAMA. 2021;325(4):382–90.
28. Balthazar EJ, Robinson DL, Megibow AJ, Ranson JH. Acute pancreatitis: value of CT in establishing prognosis. Radiology. 1990;174(2):331–6.
29. Mortele KJ, et al. A modified CT severity index for evaluating acute pancreatitis: improved correlation with patient outcome. AJR Am J Roentgenol. 2004;183:1261–5.
30. Stevens KJ, Lisanti C. Pancreas imaging. 2023 Mar 6. In: StatPearls [Internet]. Treasure Island: StatPearls Publishing; 2025.
31. Spanier BWM, Nio Y, van der Hulst RWN, et al. Practice and yield of early CT scan in acute pancreatitis: a Dutch observational multicenter study. Pancreatology. 2010;10:222–8.
32. Bollen TL, Singh VK, Maurer R, et al. A comparative evaluation of radiologic and clinical scoring systems in the early prediction of severity of acute pancreatitis. Am J Gastroenterol. 2012;107:612–9.
33. Isenmann R, Buechler M, Uhl W, et al. Pancreatic necrosis: an early finding in severe acute pancreatitis. Pancreas. 1993;8:358–61.
34. Lenhart DK, Balthazar EJ. MDCT of acute mild (nonnecrotizing) pancreatitis: abdominal complications and fate of fluid collections. AJR Am J Roentgenol. 2008;190:643–9.
35. Thoeni RF. The revised Atlanta classification of acute pancreatitis: its importance for the radiologist and its effect on treatment. Radiology. 2012;262(3):751–64.
36. Zhao K, Adam SZ, Keswani RN, et al. Acute pancreatitis: revised Atlanta classification and the role of cross-sectional imaging. AJR. 2015;205:W32–41.
37. Rerknimitr R, Lakananurak N, Prueksapanich P, Sallapant S, Angsuwatcharakon P, Kongkam P, Kullavanijaya P. A fatal case of a colonic fistula communicating with a walled-off area of pancreatic necrosis. Endoscopy. 2014;46(Suppl 1 UCTN):E30–1.
38. Van Santvoort HC, Besselink MG, Bakker OJ, et al. A step-up approach or open necrosectomy for necrotizing pancreatitis. N Engl J Med. 2010;362:1491–502.
39. Da Costa DW, Boerma D, van Santvoort HC, et al. Staged multidisciplinary step-up management for necrotizing pancreatitis. Br J Surg. 2014;101:e65–79.
40. Shyu JY, Saianani NI, Sahni VA, et al. Necrotizing pancreatitis: diagnosis, imaging and intervention. Radiographics. 2014;34:1218–39.
41. Guda NM, Trikudanathan G, Freeman ML. Idiopathic recurrent acute pancreatitis. Lancet Gastroenterol Hepatol. 2018;3(10):720–8.
42. Testoni PA. Acute recurrent pancreatitis: etiopathogenesis, diagnosis and treatment. World J Gastroenterol. 2014;20:16891–901.
43. Tirkes T, Sandrasegaran K, Sanyal R, et al. Secretin enhanced MR cholangiopancreatography: spectrum of findings. Radiographics. 2013;33(7):1889–906.
44. Sandrasegaran K, Tahir B, Barad U, Fogel E, Akisik F, Tirkes T, Sherman S. The value of secretin-enhanced MRCP in patients with recurrent acute pancreatitis. AJR Am J Roentgenol. 2017;208(2):315–21.
45. Borak GD, Romagnuolo J, Alsolaiman M, Holt EW, Cotton PB. Long-term clinical outcomes after endoscopic minor papilla therapy in symptomatic patients with pancreas divisum. Pancreas. 2009;38(8):903–6.
46. Sun H, Zuo HD, Lin Q, Yang DD, Zhou T, Tang MY, Wáng YX, Zhang XM. MR imaging for acute pancreatitis: the current status of clinical applications. Ann Transl Med. 2019;7(12):269.
47. Miller FH, Keppke AL, Dalal K, Ly JN, Kamler VA, Sica GT. MRI of pancreatitis and its complications: part 1, acute pancreatitis. AJR Am J Roentgenol. 2004;183:1637–44.
48. Testoni PA, Mariani A, Curioni S, et al. MRCP-secretin test-guided management of idiopathic recurrent pancreatitis: long-term outcomes. Gastrointest Endosc. 2008;67:1028–34.
49. Ditkofsky NG, Singh A, Avery L, Novelline RA. The role of emergency MRI in the setting of acute abdominal pain. Emerg Radiol. 2014;21:615–24.
50. Türkvatan A, Erden A, Seçil M, Türkoğlu MA. Fluid collections associated with acute pancreatitis: a pictorial essay. Can Assoc Radiol J. 2014;65(3):260–6.
51. Sandrasegaran K, Tann M, Jennings SG, et al. Disconnection of the pancreatic duct: an important but overlooked complication of severe acute pancreatitis. Radiographics. 2007;27:1389–400.
52. Tyberg A, Karia K, Gabr M, Desai A, Doshi R, Gaidhane M, Sharaiha RZ, Kahaleh M. Management of pancreatic fluid collections: a comprehensive review of the literature. World J Gastroenterol. 2016;22(7):2256–70.
53. Uomo G, Molino D, Visconti M, et al. The incidence of main pancreatic duct disruption in severe biliary pancreatitis. Am J Surg. 1998;176:49–52.
54. Balci NC, Bieneman BK, Bilgin M, Akduman IE, Fattahi R, Burton FR. Magnetic resonance imag-

ing in pancreatitis. Top Magn Reson Imaging. 2009;20(1):25–30.
55. Tang MY, Chen TW, Bollen TL, et al. MR imaging of hemorrhage associated with acute pancreatitis. Pancreatology. 2018;18:363–9.
56. Yang R, Jing ZL, Zhang XM, Tang W, Xiao B, Huang XH, Yang L, Feng ZS. MR imaging of acute pancreatitis: correlation of abdominal wall edema with severity scores. Eur J Radiol. 2012;81(11):3041–7.
57. Domagk D, Wessling J, Reimer P, Hertel L, Poremba C, Senninger N, Heinecke A, Domschke W, Menzel J. Endoscopic retrograde cholangiopancreatography, intraductal ultrasonography, and magnetic resonance cholangiopancreatography in bile duct strictures: a prospective comparison of imaging diagnostics with histopathological correlation. Am J Gastroenterol. 2004;99(9):1684–9.
58. Bates DD, LeBedis CA, Soto JA, et al. Use of magnetic resonance in pancreaticobiliary emergencies. Magn Reson Imaging Clin N Am. 2016;24(2):433–48.
59. Kim MJ, Han SJ, Yoon CS, Kim JH, Oh JT, Chung KS, Yoo HS. Using MR cholangiopancreatography to reveal anomalous pancreaticobiliary ductal union in infants and children with choledochal cysts. AJR Am J Roentgenol. 2002;179(1):209–14.
60. Chen CC. The efficacy of endoscopic ultrasound for the diagnosis of common bile duct stones as compared to CT, MRCP, and ERCP. J Chin Med Assoc. 2012;75(7):301–2.
61. Naqvi R. Acute kidney injury in association with acute pancreatitis. Pak J Med Sci. 2018;34:606–9.

Chronic Pancreatitis: Differentiation from Pancreatic Adenocarcinoma

13

Cristiana Boldrini, Valerio Di Paola, Luca Russo, Simone Palma, Maria Luisa De Cicco, Silvia De Vizio, Angelica Marra, Silvia Amodeo, Roberta Dattoli, and Riccardo Manfredi

13.1 Introduction

Pancreatic cancer is the 5th leading cause of death from cancer, and the 11th most common cancer in the United States. The incidence of chronic pancreatitis (CP) varies between 4 and 14/100000 worldwide; additionally, patients with CP carry a 13.3-fold higher risk for developing pancreatic ductal adenocarcinoma. The most common symptom of CP is abdominal pain, with other symptoms such as exocrine pancreatic insufficiency and diabetes developing at highly variable rates. CP is most caused by toxins such as alcohol or tobacco, genetic polymorphisms, and recurrent attacks of acute pancreatitis, although no history of acute pancreatitis is seen in many affected patients. On the other hand, CP sometimes may present as a solid mass, mimicking ductal adenocarcinoma of the pancreas (PDAC). Misdiagnosis of MF-CP as focal pancreatic malignancy results in unnecessary surgical treatment, and misdiagnosis of PC as focal pancreatitis may delay necessary surgical intervention. The imaging diagnosis is not always simple and immediate, so in addition to CT and MRI, endosonography or invasive procedures may help make the correct approach.

13.2 Chronic Pancreatitis: Definition

Chronic pancreatitis is historically defined as an irreversible inflammatory condition of the pancreas leading to various degrees of exocrine and endocrine dysfunction [1, 2, 3, 4]. Before 2016, CP was defined using a traditional clinico-pathologic approach with typical signs and symptoms—i.e., chronic inflammation and irreversible fibrosis without infection. Obtaining the pancreatic tissue was thought to be the "gold standard" for a pathologic diagnosis; three consensus conferences in Marseille, France, between 1963 and 1989 defined CP on the basis of clinical, functional, and histologic evidence [5]. In 1984, the "Cambridge definition" was proposed as a clinically useful alternative to biopsy by using an endoscopic retrograde cholangiopancreatography

The original version of the chapter has been revised. A correction to this chapter can be found at https://doi.org/10.1007/978-981-95-1699-5_22

C. Boldrini (✉)
Department of Bioimaging, Radiation Oncology and Hematology, Fondazione Policlinico Universitario A. Gemelli IRCSS, Rome, Italy
e-mail: Cristiana.boldrini@policlinicogemelli.it

V. Di Paola · L. Russo · S. Palma · M. L. De Cicco · S. De Vizio · A. Marra · S. Amodeo · R. Dattoli · R. Manfredi
Department of Diagnostic Imaging, Oncological Radiotherapy, and Hematology - Diagnostic Imaging Area, Rome, Italy

Fondazione Policlinico Universitario Agostino Gemelli IRCCS, Rome, Italy

© The Author(s), under exclusive license to Springer Nature Singapore Pte Ltd. 2025, corrected publication 2026

B. Sureka (ed.), *Hepato-Pancreatico Biliary Imaging*, https://doi.org/10.1007/978-981-95-1699-5_13

(ERCP) scoring system as a surrogate for the tissue [6]. An international group of doctors interested in pancreatic disease met in Cambridge under the auspices of the Pancreatic Society of Great Britain and Ireland, to discuss the classification of pancreatitis in the light of developments that had taken place in 20 years since the crucial conference in Marseille. *CP was defined as a continuing inflammatory disease of the pancreas, characterized by irreversible morphological change, and typically causing pain and/or permanent loss of function.* This definition served as the basis for imaging approaches to the diagnosis of CP (in the context of typical symptoms and loss of function) and for the foundation for most consensus statements and clinical guidelines for the next three decades.

13.3 Epidemiology and Risk Factors

The development of CP is multifactorial, with numerous risk factors playing significant contributory roles. In western countries, the incidence and prevalence of clinical CP range from 4.03 to 14 per 100,000 person-years and from 13.5 to 143 per 100,000 at risk [7]. Recently, the incidence of CP has increased, indicating a growing burden of this disease. Beyond the clinical presentation, 26%–29% of patients without lifestyle risk factors for CP versus 42%–47% of smokers and alcoholics have pancreatic fibrosis on autopsy [7–9]. Compared to the general population, CP patients have a 35.8% increase in death rate over a 20-year observation period; moreover, CP patients are predisposed to pain, bile duct strictures, pseudocysts, ascites, pancreatic exocrine, and endocrine insufficiencies leading to type 3C diabetes mellitus [10, 11]. *Most importantly, CP is a risk factor for PDAC, with a relative risk of PDAC of 13.3 compared to the general population* [12]. Like CP, the incidence of PDAC has increased in the USA from 11 to 13.1 per 100,000 person-years between 2002 and 2017. Despite modest incidence, PDAC is the third leading cause of cancer-related mortality, accounting for about 47,050 cancer-related deaths in 2020 only in the USA [12, 13], and due to increasing incidence and poor prognosis, PDAC is projected to be the second leading cause of cancer-related mortality by 2030.

The TIGAR-O system, used to help categorize an etiology to explain CP, has proven useful in multiple international studies, and was recently revised to include new insights from the past 20 years; the acronym stands for T (toxic-metabolic), I (idiopathic), G (genetic), A (autoimmune), R (recurrent acute or severe pancreatitis), and O (obstructive) [5]. The Toxic-metabolic, Idiopathic, Genetic, Autoimmune, Recurrent and severe acute pancreatitis and Obstructive (TIGAR-O) Pancreatitis Risk/Etiology Checklist (TIGAR-O_V1) is a broad classification system that lists the major risk factors and etiologies of recurrent acute pancreatitis, chronic pancreatitis, and overlapping pancreatic disorders with or without genetic, immunologic, metabolic, nutritional, neurological, metaplastic, or other features. Toxic-metabolic causes include: alcohol, tobacco smoking, hypercalcemia and hyperparathyroidism, hyperlipidemia (rare and controversial), chronic renal failure, medications, phenacetin abuse (possibly from chronic renal insufficiency), toxins, organotin compounds (e.g., DBTC). Idiopathic causes include early onset and late onset, tropical pancreatitis and fibrocalculous pancreatic diabetes. Genetic causes can be autosomal dominant or autosomal recessive. Autoimmune factors include isolated autoimmune chronic pancreatitis and syndromic autoimmune chronic pancreatitis. Recurrent and severe acute pancreatitis may be postnecrotic, due to vascular diseases/ischemic, or post-irradiation. Obstructive factors include pancreas divisum, sphincter of Oddi disorders (controversial), and duct obstruction (e.g., tumor). The pancreatitis with multiple risk factors such as alcohol consumption, nicotine consumption, nutritional factors, hereditary factors, efferent duct factors, immunological factors, miscellaneous and rare metabolic factors (M-ANNHEIM) system is a similar multirisk factor classification system that attempts to add information on disease activity and stage and has been used to evaluate the impact and interaction of various risk factors on the course of CP [5].

13.4 Risk of Pancreatic Cancer in CP

Lowenfels et al. in 1993 were the first to describe a significantly increased risk of developing pancreatic cancer in patients with CP [14]. They undertook a multicenter historical cohort study of 2015 subjects; a total of 56 cancers were identified among these patients during a mean (±SD) follow-up of 7.4 ± 6.2 years. The expected number of cases of cancer calculated from country-specific incidence data and adjusted for age and sex was 2.13, yielding a standardized incidence ratio (the ratio of observed to expected cases) of 26.3 (95 percent confidence interval, 19.9 to 34.2). For subjects with a minimum of two or five years of follow-up, the respective standardized incidence ratios were 16.5 (95 percent confidence interval, 11.1 to 23.7) and 14.4 (95 percent confidence interval, 8.5 to 22.8) [14]. Talamini et al. in 1999 analyzed 715 cases of chronic pancreatitis with a median follow-up of 10 years; during this observation period, they recorded 61 neoplasms, 14 of which were pancreatic cancers. They found a standardized incidence ratio of pancreatic cancer in CP patients of 13.3 [15]. According to the authors, there does not appear to be an increased risk of pancreatic cancer in non-smokers, while in smokers the risk increases 15.6 times [15]. Other studies in literature have reported that the risk of pancreatic cancer diminishes with long-term follow-up, and that although a first episode of acute pancreatitis may be related to pancreatic cancer, this risk is mainly present in patients who progress to chronic pancreatitis [16, 17, 18].

13.5 Diagnosis

CP represents a later stage of progressive disorders resulting in irreversible morphologic damage of the pancreas. The diagnosis is made using a combination of modalities, including exposure risk, underlying predisposition, cross-sectional imaging (CT and MRI), and direct and/or indirect pancreatic function tests. It is critical to assess the patient's risk factors for CP, including family and exposure history, the nature and character of the patient's pain, whether or not they have had previous episodes of acute pancreatitis, and whether they have related conditions such as steatorrhea and/or symptoms of vitamin deficiency. In patients with clinical symptoms of an inflammatory disorder of the pancreas (previous episode of acute pancreatitis, characteristic pain, and/or maldigestion) and/or a suggestive gene-environment risk assessment, imaging should be the first test used to establish the diagnosis of CP because it is universally available, reproducible, and valid when compared with other modalities. The best evidence comparing modalities is from a systematic review and meta-analysis (published in 2017 by Issa et al.) of 43 studies and 3460 patients with suspected CP, in which the sensitivity estimates of endoscopic ultrasonography (EUS), magnetic resonance imaging (MRI), and computed tomography (CT) were 81% (95% confidence interval [CI]: 70%–89%), 78% (95% CI: 69%–85%), and 75% (95% CI: 66%–83%), respectively, and did not differ significantly from each other [19]. Estimates of specificity were comparable for EUS (90%; 95% CI: 82%–95%), ERCP (94%; 95% CI: 87%–98%), CT (91%; 95% CI: 81%–96%), MRI (96%; 95% CI: 90%–98%), and ultrasound (US) (98%; 95% CI: 89%–100%). A limitation of this meta-analysis, however, was that not all the studies included a histologic gold standard to establish the type of inflammation for comparison. *Given the vast discrepancy in cost, availability, invasiveness, and objectivity, cross-sectional imaging is nowadays considered the first-line test for the diagnosis of CP.* Owing to its invasiveness and issues about availability, intra-rate reproducibility, and discrepancy, EUS should be used to diagnose CP alone if there is uncertainty following cross-sectional imaging [20]. Multiple other imaging modalities and scoring systems have been used to establish the diagnosis of CP, including contrast enhanced EUS, ERCP, trans-cutaneous ultrasonography, and pancreatic elastography [21]. However, high-quality randomized clinical trial evidence is not available to warrant their inclusion as first-line diagnostic tests for CP in place of cross-sectional imaging (CT, MRI) or EUS.

13.6 Pancreatic Ductal Adenocarcinoma as an Incidental Finding in Chronic Pancreatitis

Prospective cohort studies have reported at least 20 possible risk factors for PDAC, including smoking, heavy alcohol drinking, adiposity, diabetes, and pancreatitis, but population attributable fractions of individual risk factors are small (mostly <10%). The association of CP and PDAC is well established. The study of Birgin et al. in 2018 [18] found that about 30% of patients with CP who underwent surgery also had concomitant PDAC. Malinka et al. in 2018 in a large retrospective study [20] defined the prevalence of incidental PDAC found at pancreatic resections for CP; PDAC was found in the surgical specimen of 7.1%. Evaluation of mean overall survival demonstrated a clear disadvantage for patients with CP and incidental carcinoma (11.7 vs. 216.1 months) [20]. Numerous studies have found a strong link between CP and pancreatic cancer. Patients with hereditary pancreatitis and an early onset have a markedly increased risk at least 50-fold greater than the general population [21]. Furthermore, a meta-analysis evidenced a relative risk of 13.3 for developing PDAC in patients with CP, with a 10-to 20-year lag between pancreatitis and development of pancreatic malignancy [22].

13.7 Mass-Forming Chronic Pancreatitis: Imaging Features

At transabdominal US (ultrasound), it is difficult to distinguish mass-forming chronic pancreatitis (MF-CP) from PDAC because the imaging features overlap, and masses may be obscured by overlying bowel gas or the patient's body habitus. Endoscopic US offers improved visualization of masses and is used routinely to perform targeted biopsies. Cross-sectional imaging represents the most available mean to obtain information for the radiologist. The typical appearance of MF-CP is a hypoattenuating mass at unenhanced CT, which is hypovascular on CT contrast-enhanced scans (Fig. 13.1) [1]. These masses are most often located in the pancreatic head. The masses in MF-CP are usually hypointense at T1-weighted gradient-recalled echo (GRE) magnetic resonance (MR) imaging and iso- to hyperintense at T2-weighted MRI; they are hypointense at arterial phase enhanced MRI, with moderate enhancement at venous phase scans, showing moderate hypointensity to isointensity in later phases (Fig. 13.2) [1]. ADC (apparent diffusion coefficient) values in MF-CP are higher than in PDAC. There are some imaging features which help make a differential diagnosis. None of the secondary signs of PDAC and

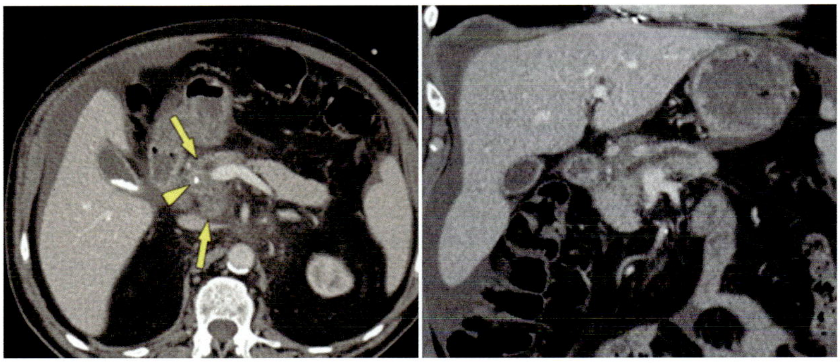

Fig. 13.1 MF-CP in a 52-year-old male patient [1]. Axial and coronal multidetector CT images demonstrate a hypoattenuating mass in the pancreatic head (arrows). There is a single small parenchymal calcification (arrowhead), which isn't intraductally located. The differential diagnosis from PDAC in this case was very difficult only on the basis of CT imaging. (Schima et al. [1]. Licensed under CC-BY 4.0)

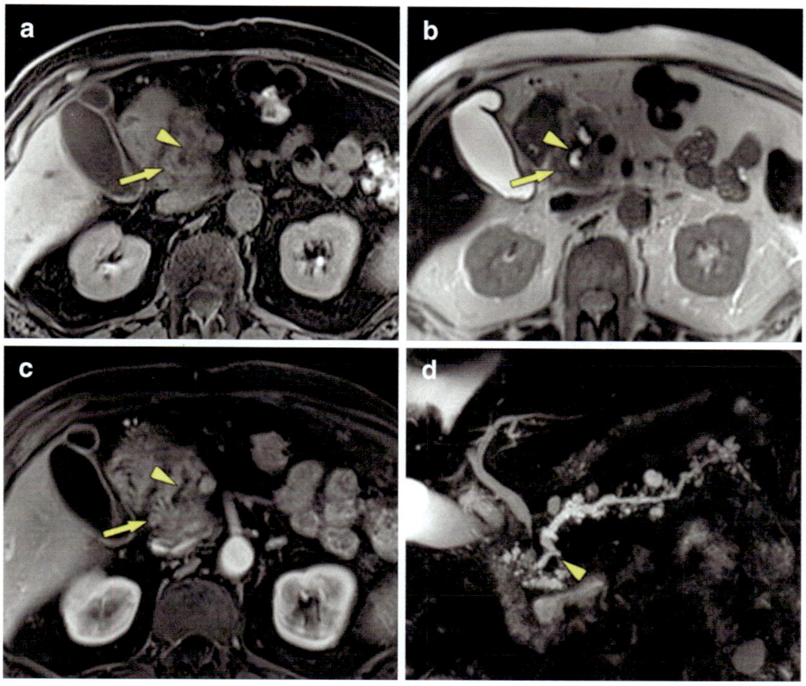

Fig. 13.2 T1w GRE fatsat, T2w TSE, and gadolinium-enhanced T1w GRE images (**a–c**) [1] show a solid mass in the head of the pancreas (arrows). The pancreatic duct traverses the mass (arrowheads) (duct-penetrating sign), which is typical for an inflammatory mass. In **d**, MRCP shows duct-penetrating sign (arrowhead) in a better way. Other typical signs of CP include ductal irregularities and dilated side branches. (Schima et al. [1]. Licensed under CC-BY 4.0)

mass-forming pancreatitis have 100% sensitivity or specificity. A diagnosis can be favored if more secondary imaging signs are present to support either a benign inflammatory process or a neoplastic process.

Parenchymal calcifications are seen in about 60% of CP patients; in particular, the combination of diffused parenchymal calcifications with ductal calcifications, atrophy, and cystic lesions is quite specific for the diagnosis of CP [23] (Fig. 13.3). Campisi et al. examined the imaging of patients who had chronic pancreatitis ($n = 70$), neuroendocrine tumors ($n = 14$), intraductal papillary mucinous neoplasm (IPMN) ($n = 11$), pancreatic adenocarcinoma ($n = 4$), and serous cystadenoma ($n = 4$). Four CT findings had a specificity of over 60% for the diagnosis of chronic pancreatitis: parenchymal calcifications, intraductal calcifications, parenchymal atrophy, and cystic lesions. Also, pancreatic neuroendocrine tumors, IPMN, and PDAC may show spotted calcifications, with the principal difference that in these neoplasms the calcifications do not tend to be diffuse or intraductally located [1]. It is well established that the development of a new tissue mass displacing calcifications or the presence of a soft tissue mass in a diffusely calcified chronic pancreatitis at imaging raises the suspicion of the onset of PDAC in CP [1].

The presence of a narrowing of the main pancreatic duct in the context of a pancreatic mass (***duct-penetrating sign***) without abrupt or complete obstruction leans for the diagnosis of an inflammatory pseudotumor and pancreatitis [24] (Fig. 13.4). PDAC, as a densely fibrotic tumor, usually causes abrupt narrowing or even complete obstruction of the pancreatic duct, while a chronic inflammatory mass most often results in gradual stenosis, with visualization of the pancreatic duct that traverses the mass. This sign, described by Ichikawa et al. in 2001 [24], was found to be accurate in about 94% of patients with MF-CP or PDAC. In this study, MRCP, CT, and MR images were compared by means of receiver operating characteristic analysis for 11 inflammatory pancreatic mass (IPMs) and 43 conventional pancreatic carcinoma (CPCs). With the MRCP images, a morphologic classification of the main pancreatic duct was attempted for all lesions. On the basis of this classification and the enhancement patterns of a lesion, all readers graded the presence of IPM or CPC on a scale for

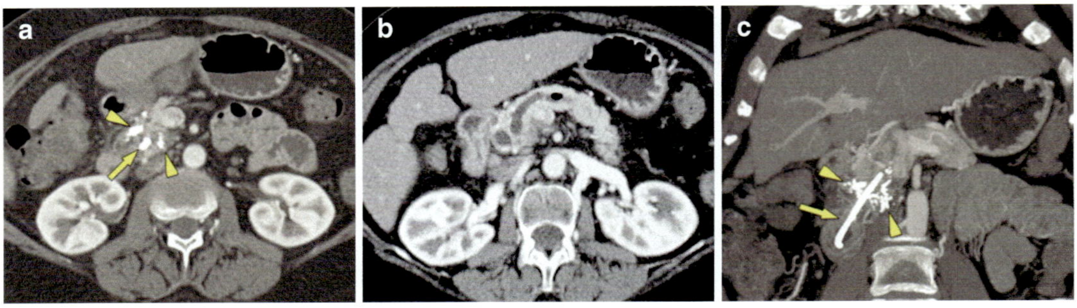

Fig. 13.3 Axial contrast-enhanced CT shows a hypoattenuating mass of the head with coarse calcifications (arrowheads) and a pancreatic plastic stent in place (arrow) (**a**, **b**). There are no signs of CP in the rest of the pancreas. Paracoronal reformation image demonstrates the stent (arrow) in the pancreatic head and the parenchymal calcifications (**c**) [1]. (Schima et al. [1]. Licensed under CC-BY 4.0)

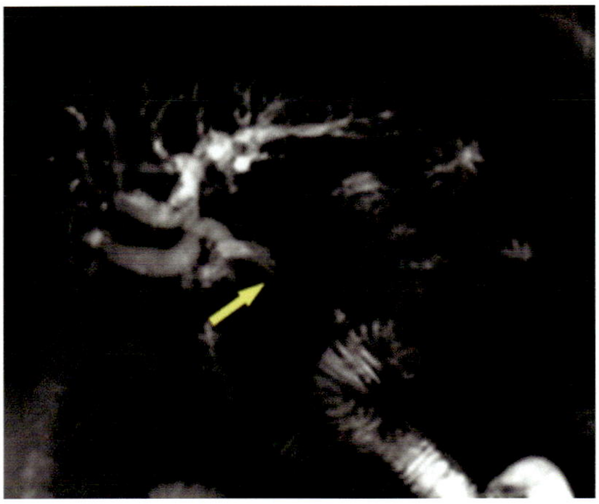

Fig. 13.4 MRCP shows abrupt stenosis of the CBD (arrow) with dilatation. Surgical histology revealed PDAC in CP [1]. (Schima et al. [1]. Licensed under CC-BY 4.0)

all images. Duct-penetrating sign is best seen on magnetic resonance cholangiopancreatography (MRCP), with visualization of the duct sometimes improved by secretin administration. With MRCP it is possible to study also side branches penetrating an inflammatory mass [1]. It is important to remember that the duct-penetrating sign on MRCP images sometimes is considered more helpful to distinguish an inflammatory pancreatic mass from CPC than the enhancement patterns on CT and MR images [1, 24].

The common bile duct (CBD) and the main pancreatic duct form a junction at a level of the major papilla; an obstruction at the papilla or in the periampullary region (pancreatic head) may cause stenosis of both ductal systems, with subsequent pre-stenotic ductal dilatation. This imaging feature of dilatation of both ductal systems is known as ***double-duct sign*** (Fig. 13.5) [1, 25], and is more often seen in PDAC than in any inflammatory condition, with a reported incidence of 80%. Double-duct sign may occur as well in mass forming chronic pancreatitis (MF-CP) or autoimmune pancreatitis (AIP), but is usually defined by a more smooth narrowing of the common bile duct and main pancreatic duct, with less severe pre-stenotic dilatation.

Both chronic pancreatitis and pancreatic adenocarcinoma share the modification in the morphology of pancreatic duct and side branches. The main pancreatic duct is usually visible at CT or MRI from the papilla to the tail. A duct diameter of more than 3.5 mm in the head is considered abnormal. In case of advanced stage CP, not only focal strictures, but also contour irregularities of the duct upstream are present. Pancreatic duct dilatation upstream to PDAC is usually severe, but quite smooth, and also includes severe parenchymal atrophy [26]. The results of the study by Kim et al. show that several CT findings (i.e., non-head location, long transition of the PD ($\geq$ 6.1 mm), abrupt transition of the PD, absence of duct penetrating sign, PD or CBD enhancement at the transition area, and presence of attenuation difference in upstream pancreatic parenchyma) are significant predictors of malig-

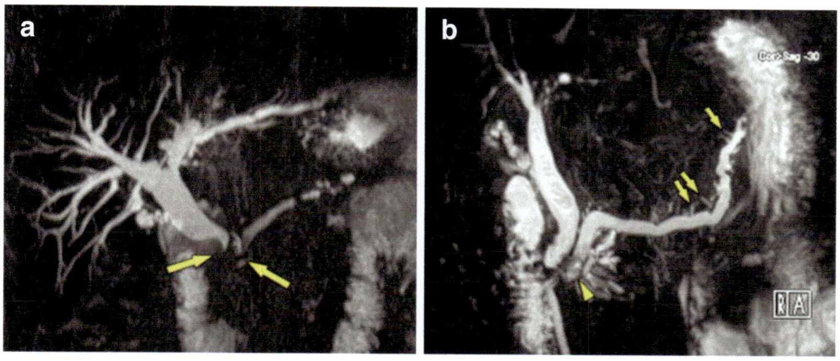

Fig. 13.5 (**a**) Double-duct sign in PDAC: MRCP shows abrupt cut-off of the common bile duct and main pancreatic duct in the pancreatic head (arrows), very suggestive of neoplasm. Histology confirmed PDAC in this patient. (**b**) Lack of double-duct sign in CP: MRCP shows duct dilatation without abrupt cut-off and contour irregularities of the main duct with dilated side branches (small arrows), typical for CP. There are also irregular filling defects in the main duct, suggestive of stones (arrowhead) [1]. (Schima et al. [1]. Licensed under CC-BY 4.0)

nant MPD dilatation in the differentiation of benign and malignant MPD dilatation [1, 26].

Vessel encasement The extension of a pancreatic mass toward the celiac trunk or the superior mesenteric artery with the presence of the soft tissue that surrounds the vessels is called "vessel encasement" and is strongly suggestive of PDAC. The "SMV teardrop sign," a teardrop-shaped deformity of the SMV, is highly indicative of SMV encasement; although uncommon, inflammatory conditions may result in loss of fat planes with peripancreatic vessels. Rarely the vessel encasement can be observed in patients with chronic inflammation of the pancreatic gland; venous deformation of the confluence, superior mesenteric vein, or splenic vein is more likely in PDAC than in MF-CP, but unfortunately is not specific [1]. Occlusion of the splenic vein with extensive venous collaterals formation is a typical feature in patients with recurrent pancreatitis of the body and tail, while the presence of soft tissue encasement of the peripancreatic arteries is quite specific for a developing neoplasm and usually indicates already locally advanced (and most likely unresectable) PDAC (Fig. 13.6).

Studies on *perfusion CT* revealed promising results concerning the differentiation between MF-CP and PDAC. Perfusion CT not only allowed differentiation between normal parenchyma and MF-CP and PDAC but also between the latter two [1, 27]. The mean blood flow (BF), blood volume (BV), and permeability surface area product (PS) were significantly higher in MF-CP than in adenocarcinoma. There was no significant difference in mean transit time between MF-CP and adenocarcinoma. The combination of threshold values for BV, BF, and PS yielded excellent sensitivity and specificity for differentiation between MF-CP and PDAC [1, 27]. However, these results have to be corroborated by other studies with perfusion software of different vendors.

A preliminary study evaluated the role of *gadolinium-enhanced perfusion MRI* for differentiation between MF-CP and PDAC. Although it showed differences in perfusion curves between MFCP and PDAC, this feature alone did not allow reliable diagnosis [1, 28]. The combination of perfusion MRI and diffusion-weighted imaging (DWI) achieved better results, because the mean ADC value of PDAC was significantly lower than that of MF-CP ($1.17 \pm 0.23 <$ vs. 1.47 ± 0.18, $p < 0.01$, obtained at 3.0 T MRI) [28]. The time-signal intensity curve of dynamic contrast-enhanced MRI (DCE-MRI) and ADC value of DWI for pancreatic mass were found to provide reliable information in differentiating pancreatic carcinoma from mass-forming focal pancreatitis; the combination of DCE-MRI and DWI achieved a higher sensitivity, specificity, and diagnostic accuracy.

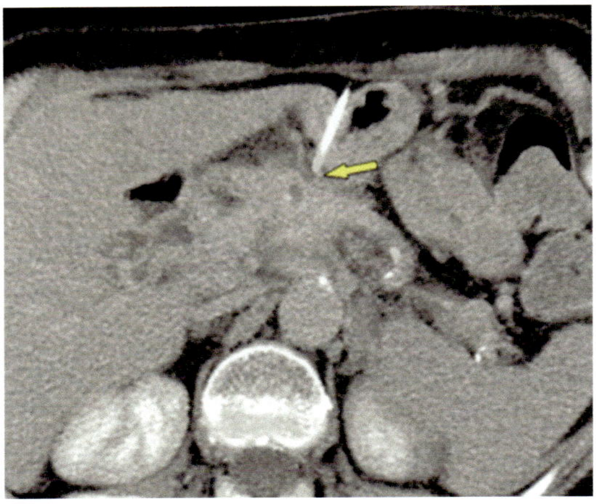

Fig. 13.6 Soft tissue mass with vessel encasement in calcified CP and locally advanced PDAC at CT imaging. Diagnosis of PDAC was confirmed by percutaneous CT-guided transgastric biopsy (arrow) [1]. (Schima et al. [1]. Licensed under CC-BY 4.0)

13.8 Multi-modal imaging and biopsy to distinguish pancreatic cancer from mass-forming chronic pancreatitis

There is no single imaging feature that alone allows differentiation between MF-CP and PDAC. In a retrospective study in 2018, Ruan et al. [29] analyzed computerized tomography (CT), magnetic resonance imaging (MRI) and positron emission tomography - computerized tomography (PET/CT) data to identify features that may distinguish pancreatic carcinoma (PC) from mass-forming chronic pancreatitis (MF-CP) of the pancreatic head; the found that at FDG-PET/CT, the standardized uptake value (SUV) of MF-CP was usually lower (cut-off value 4.90) than in PC. Complete obstruction of the main pancreatic duct by the mass with disappearance of the "duct penetration sign", the "double duct sign" due to periampullary obstruction, vessel encasement by a soft tissue mass, and displacement of previously observed calcifications by newly appearing tissue are all highly suspicious features of PDAC development in inflammatory CP, which should prompt further diagnostic procedures. Endoscopic ultra-sound (EUS) and Endoscopic US-guided fine-needle aspiration/biopsy is generally very sensitive in characterizing focal pancreatic masses, but in CP it may be unfortunately burdened by low sensitivity. In the study by Fritscher-Ravens et al., sensitivity for the detection of PDAC with endoscopic US-guided fine-needle aspiration was markedly lower when a mass was present in patients with chronic pancreatitis (sensitivity, 54%; specificity, 100%; accuracy, 91%) [30]. In this work, its sensitivity in patients with CP was shown to be unacceptably low, and tumor resection using standard surgical techniques was still usually necessary to confirm the correct diagnosis. Evaluation of a focal pancreatic mass in the setting of chronic pancreatitis is a diagnostic challenge. A study conducted by Varadarajulu et al. in 2005 aimed to compare the diagnostic yield and accuracy of EUS-guided FNA in the evaluation of pancreatic mass lesions, in the presence or the absence of CP [31]. A lower sensitivity for EUS-FNA was observed in patients with CP than in those without CP (73.9% vs. 91.3%; $p = 0.02$). False-negative cytology was encountered in 24 cases: 6/71 (8%) with CP vs. 18/222 (8%) without CP. Patients with CP required more EUS-FNA passes to establish a diagnosis vs. those without CP (median, 5 vs. 2; $p < 0.001$) [31].

Bibliography

1. Schima W, Böhm G, Rösch CS, Klaus A, Függer R, Kopf H. Mass-forming pancreatitis versus pancreatic ductal adenocarcinoma: CT and MR imaging for differentiation. Cancer Imaging. 2020;20(1):52.
2. Petrov MS, Yadav D. Global epidemiology and holistic prevention of pancreatitis. Nat Rev Gastroenterol Hepatol. 2019;16(3):175–84.
3. Elsherif SB, Virarkar M, Javadi S, Ibarra-Rovira JJ, Tamm EP, Bhosale PR. Pancreatitis and PDAC: association and differentiation. Abdom Radiol. 2019;45:1324.
4. Cannon A, Thompson CM, Bhatia R, Armstrong KA, Solheim JC, Kumar S, Batra SK. Molecular mechanisms of pancreatic myofibroblast activation in chronic pancreatitis and pancreatic ductal adenocarcinoma. J Gastroenterol. 2021;56(8):689–703.

https://doi.org/10.1007/s00535-021-01800-4. Epub 2021 Jul 19.
5. Gardner TB, Adler DG, Forsmark CE, Sauer BG, Taylor JR, Whitcomb DC. ACG clinical guideline: chronic pancreatitis. Am J Gastroenterol. 2020;115(3):322–39.
6. Sarner M, Cotton PB. Classification of pancreatitis. Gut. 1984;25(7):756–9. https://doi.org/10.1136/gut.25.7.756.
7. Beyer G, Habtezion A, Werner J, et al. Chronic pancreatitis. Lancet. 2020;396:499–512.
8. Levy P, Dominguez-Munoz E, Imrie C, et al. Epidemiology of chronic pancreatitis: burden of the disease and consequences. United Eur Gastroenterol J. 2014;2:345–54.
9. Yadav D, Lowenfels AB. The epidemiology of pancreatitis and pancreatic cancer. Gastroenterology. 2013;144:1252–61. [PubMed: 23622135].
10. Yadav D, Timmons L, Benson JT, et al. Incidence, prevalence, and survival of chronic pancreatitis: a population-based study. Am J Gastroenterol. 2011;106:2192–9.
11. Hirota M, Shimosegawa T, Masamune A, et al. The seventh nationwide epidemiological survey for chronic pancreatitis in Japan: clinical significance of smoking habit in Japanese patients. Pancreatology. 2014;14:490–6.
12. Machicado JD, Dudekula A, Tang G, et al. Period prevalence of chronic pancreatitis diagnosis from 2001–2013 in the commercially insured population of the United States. Pancreatology. 2019;19:813–8.
13. Capurso G, Archibugi L, Pasquali P, et al. Prevalence of chronic pancreatitis: results of a primary care physician-based population study. Dig Liver Dis. 2017;49:535–9.
14. Lowenfels AB, Maisonneuve P, Cavallini G, Ammann RW, Lankisch PG, Andersen JR, et al. Pancreatitis and the risk of pancreatic cancer. International pancreatitis study group. N Engl J Med. 1993;328:1433–7.
15. Talamini G, Falconi M, Bassi C, Sartori N, Salvia R, Caldiron E, et al. Incidence of cancer in the course of chronic pancreatitis. Am J Gastroenterol. 1999;94:1253–60.
16. Kirkegård J, Mortensen FV, Cronin-Fenton D. Chronic pancreatitis and pancreatic cancer risk: a systematic review and meta-analysis. Am J Gastroenterol. 2017;112:1366–72.
17. Syed A, Babich O, Thakkar P, Patel A, Abdul-Baki H, Farah K, et al. Defining pancreatitis as a risk factor for pancreatic cancer: the role, incidence, and timeline of development. Pancreas. 2019;48:1098–101.
18. Birgin E, Hablawetz P, Téoule P, Rückert F, Wilhelm TJ. Chronic pancreatitis and resectable synchronous pancreatic carcinoma: a survival analysis. Pancreatology. 2018;18:394–8.
19. Issa Y, Kempeneers MA, van Santvoort HC, et al. Diagnostic performance of imaging modalities in chronic pancreatitis: a systematic review and meta-analysis. Eur Radiol. 2017;27(9):3820–44.
20. Malinka T, Klein F, Le Thu T, Rösch CS, Wundsam H, Biebl M, et al. A binational analysis of 252 pancreatic resections for chronic pancreatitis with regard to incidental carcinoma sequence and overall postoperative outcome. Anticancer Res. 2018;38:4947–52.
21. Becker AE, Hernandez YG, Frucht H, Lucas AL. Pancreatic ductal adenocarcinoma: risk factors, screening, and early detection. World J Gastroenterol. 2014;20(32):11182–98.
22. Raimondi S, Lowenfels AB, Morselli-Labate AM, Maisonneuve P, Pezzilli R. Pancreatic cancer in chronic pancreatitis; aetiology, incidence, and early detection. Best Pract Res Clin Gastroenterol. 2010;24(3):349–58.
23. Campisi A, Brancatelli G, Vullierme MP, Levy P, Ruszniewski P, Vilgrain V. Are pancreatic calcifications specific for the diagnosis of chronic pancreatitis? A multidetector-row CT analysis. Clin Radiol. 2009;64:903–11.
24. Ichikawa T, Sou H, Araki T, Arbab AS, Yoshikawa T, Ishigame K, et al. Duct-penetrating sign at MRCP: usefulness for differentiating inflammatory pancreatic mass from pancreatic carcinomas. Radiology. 2001;221:107–16.
25. Tirkes T. Chronic pancreatitis: what the clinician wants to know from MR imaging. Magn Reson Imaging Clin N Am. 2018;26:451–61.
26. Kim SW, Kim SH, Lee DH, Lee SM, Kim YS, Jang JY, Han JK. Isolated Main Pancreatic Duct Dilatation: CT Differentiation Between Benign and Malignant Causes. AJR Am J Roentgenol. 2017;209(5):1046–55
27. Yadav AK, Sharma R, Kandasamy D, Pradhan RK, Garg PK, Bhalla AS, et al. Perfusion CT–can it resolve the pancreatic carcinoma versus mass forming chronic pancreatitis conundrum? Pancreatology. 2016;16:979–87.
28. Zhang TT, Wang L, Liu HH, Zhang CY, Li XM, Lu JP, Wang DB. Differentiation of pancreatic carcinoma and mass-forming focal pancreatitis: qualitative and quantitative assessment by dynamic contrast-enhanced MRI combined with diffusion-weighted imaging. Oncotarget. 2017 Jan 3;8(1):1744–59. https://doi.org/10.18632/oncotarget.12120.
29. Ruan Z, Jiao J, Min D, Qu J, Li J, Chen J, et al. Multimodality imaging features distinguish pancreatic carcinoma from mass-forming chronic pancreatitis of the pancreatic head. Oncol Lett. 2018;15:9735–44.
30. Fritscher-Ravens A, Brand L, Knöfel WT, et al. Comparison of endoscopic ultrasound-guided fine needle aspiration for focal pancreatic lesions in patients with normal parenchyma and chronic pancreatitis. Am J Gastroenterol. 2002;97(11):2768–75.
31. Varadarajulu S, Tamhane A, Eloubeidi MA. Yield of EUS-guided FNA of pancreatic masses in the presence or the absence of chronic pancreatitis. Gastrointest Endosc. 2005;62(5):728–36; quiz 751, 753.

Approach to Solid Pancreatic Tumors

14

Smily Sharma and Taruna Yadav

14.1 Introduction

Solid pancreatic lesions encompass a myriad of neoplastic and non-neoplastic lesions affecting the pancreas. Imaging plays a pivotal role in their diagnosis, staging, determining the management protocol, and assessing the post-treatment outcome. This chapter provides a comprehensive discussion of key imaging features and approach to common solid pancreatic masses.

14.2 Classification

Solid pancreatic masses can be broadly classified into neoplastic or non-neoplastic lesions as detailed in Table 14.1 [1].

Table 14.1 Classification of solid pancreatic lesions [1]

Neoplastic lesions	Non-neoplastic lesions
Pancreatic ductal adenocarcinoma (PDAC)	Focal pancreatitis
Solid pseudopapillary tumor (SPT)	Focal autoimmune pancreatitis
Pancreatic lymphoma	Intrapancreatic splenule
Pancreatoblastoma	Focal fatty infiltration
Pancreatic metastasis Miscellaneous neoplasms: 1. Epithelial tumors: acinar cell carcinoma, giant cell tumor, colloid carcinoma 2. Mesenchymal tumors: granular cell tumor, fibrous histiocytoma, juvenile hemangioendothelioma, fibroma, inflammatory myoblastic tumor, sarcoma 3. Mixed tumors: squamous cell carcinoma, mixed endocrine-exocrine tumor	Miscellaneous lesions: Pancreatic sarcoidosis Pancreatic tuberculosis Castleman disease affecting the pancreas

S. Sharma · T. Yadav (✉)
Department of Diagnostic and Interventional Radiology, AIIMS Jodhpur, Jodhpur, Rajasthan, India

© The Author(s), under exclusive license to Springer Nature Singapore Pte Ltd. 2025
B. Sureka (ed.), *Hepato-Pancreatico Biliary Imaging*, https://doi.org/10.1007/978-981-95-1699-5_14

14.3 Pancreatic Ductal Adenocarcinoma

PDAC is the most common malignant pancreatic tumor, accounting for 85%–95% of the masses. Patients usually present at the seventh or eighth decade of life, with nonresectability in 75% of cases and metastasis in 85% cases at presentation with male-to-female ratio of 2:1 [1, 2]. Patients present late with complaints of abdominal pain, jaundice, and weight loss. Precursor lesions include pancreatic intraepithelial neoplasm and intraductal papillary mucinous neoplasm (IPMN). KRAS mutation is the most common oncogene mutation associated with PDAC and is associated with poor prognosis. CA-19-9 is a sensitive but non-specific tumor marker and is rarely positive in tumors measuring <1 cm in diameter [3].

14.3.1 Imaging Features

The most common location of the PDAC is in the pancreatic head (60%–70%) followed by body (10%–20%) and tail (5%–10%). Few cases (5%) show diffuse involvement of the pancreas [1]. The average size of PDAC in the head is 3 cm, while the average size of PDAC in the body and tail is 5–7 cm, as pancreatic head tumors become symptomatic earlier due to common bile duct (CBD) and main pancreatic duct (MPD) obstruction secondary to their intense desmoplastic reaction [1–3].

PDAC can show extensive infiltration of retroperitoneum and invasion of surrounding anatomic structures including the vessels and neural structures. Regional lymph node metastasis (incidence: 80%) is common and is associated with a poor prognosis. The usual sites of distant metastasis include liver and peritoneum [3].

Imaging aims to detect and characterize the pancreatic tumors and screen high-risk patients, aids in their staging, and helps decide their surgical resectability, thereby guiding the management of the tumor [3]. The candidates for screening include patients with first-degree relative affected with pancreatic cancer (two to six times increased relative risk for developing pancreatic cancer), members of families with a history of hereditary cancer syndromes such as Peutz-Jeghers syndrome, and patients with hereditary pancreatitis [3, 4].

Abdominal ultrasound is the first-line investigation. *Dual-phase (pancreatic parenchymal and portal venous) contrast-enhanced CT (CECT)* of the abdomen with neutral oral contrast has an accuracy of 85%–95% for detection of PDAC and forms the mainstay for evaluation of pancreatic tumors [1, 3, 5, 6].

Pancreatic parenchymal phase aims to accurately detect the tumor and assess the involvement of peripancreatic arteries. The maximum pancreatic parenchymal enhancement and maximum attenuation difference between tumor and parenchyma are found in this phase. PDAC is hypodense on CT with irregular margins. Being a hypovascular tumor, it shows relative *hypo-enhancement* as compared to the rest of the pancreas on the pancreatic phase. *Portal venous phase* allows for adequate evaluation of hepatic metastasis and status of the peripancreatic veins [1, 3, 6].

In 10% of the cases, the tumor is isoattenuating and thus may not be visualized on CECT [5]. However, certain *secondary effects* like mass effect, loss of pancreatic lobulations, deformity of the contours of the pancreas, obstruction of the upstream duct with parenchymal atrophy, and invasion of the surrounding vasculature can suggest its presence and location. Pancreatic head tumors can cause obstruction and dilatation of both CBD and MPD leading to "double-duct sign" (Fig. 14.1). Pancreatic body tumors on the other hand lead to dilatation of only the upstream MPD [1–3, 5].

Vascular involvement is seen as a soft tissue surrounding the peripancreatic vessels accompanied by loss of perivascular fat planes. Deformity in the contour of the vessel, thrombosis, and collateral formation are other signs of vascular invasion [1, 7]. "Tear drop" sign is the change in contour of superior mesenteric vein from the round shape on axial CT images to a shape of teardrop caused by the tumor infiltration or peritumoral fibrosis [1, 8].

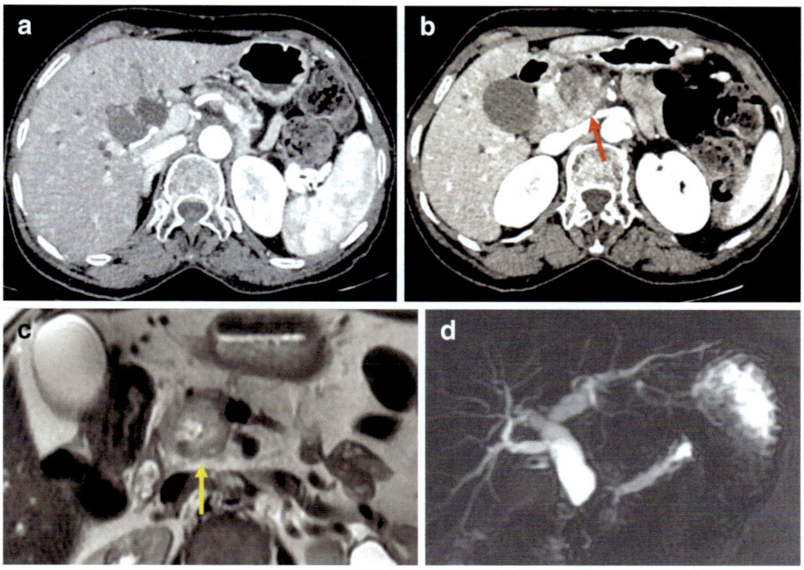

Fig. 14.1 Pancreatic ductal adenocarcinoma in two different patients with abdominal pain and jaundice. Patient 1, a 62-year-old, CT (**a**, **b**): pancreatic head mass (red arrow) with upstream pancreatic and common bile ductal dilation and pancreatic parenchymal atrophy. Patient 2, a 71-year-old, MRI (**c**, **d**): A T2 hyperintense mass is evident in the head of the pancreas (yellow arrow) with a double-duct sign with dilated CBD and MPD on the MRCP image

Extrapancreatic perineural invasion is one of the characteristic modes of the spread of PDAC due to infiltration of the tumor along the neural fascicles. It is a very poor prognostic marker and is the cause of recurrence even after complete resection. It has been reported to occur in 53%–100% of cases of PDAC. Its incidence is not related to the size of the tumor and can even occur in tumors <2 cm in size. On CT, it is seen as a confluent soft tissue mass spreading along the peripancreatic neural plexus which is contiguous with and having an attenuation similar to that of the primary tumor [9–11].

Dual-energy CT (DECT) is especially useful to improve detection of isoattenuating pancreatic lesions. The tumor becomes more conspicuous at lower x-ray energy virtual monochromatic images (50–60 keV) due to better tissue contrast. Qualitative (iodine overlay maps) and quantitative information of iodine distribution with MDI (material density iodine) images help evaluate the correct extent of the lesion. DECT helps in staging of PDAC by improved assessment of vascular invasion, peripancreatic fat stranding, and distant metastasis. It helps in post-operative imaging by improving differentiation between the post-surgical changes and local recurrences.

CT perfusion can be used to detect isoattenuating PDAC and differentiate PDAC from mass-forming chronic pancreatitis (MFCP). Blood flow (BF) and Blood Volume (BV) are reduced in both PDAC and MFCP, but the extent of reduction is greater in PDAC than in MFCP [6, 12].

Magnetic resonance imaging (MRI) is found to be 90%–100% accurate in detection of PDAC due to its superior contrast resolution [1, 13]. It mainly serves as a problem-solving tool in indeterminate CT findings. 2D and 3D MRCP help in accurate ductal evaluation. PDAC is hypointense on T1 and shows variable signal on T2-weighted (T2W) sequences depending on the extent of fibrosis [14]. Tumor enhances less than pancreatic parenchyma in pancreatic parenchymal phase with a thin rim of greater enhancement around the tumor with progressive enhancement of tumor in the subsequent phases.

Diffusion-weighted imaging (DWI) may be instrumental in detection of smaller tumors (Fig. 14.2). Liver and peritoneal metastases from PDAC are best visualized on T2W image and DWI [3]. It can aid in screening of patients with a high risk of pancreatic malignancy, in differentiating PDAC from mass-forming pancreatitis [15]. ADC values can be used for prognostication and also serve as a marker of response to chemotherapy [16, 17].

Endoscopic ultrasound (EUS) is complimentary to CECT and is especially useful for detec-

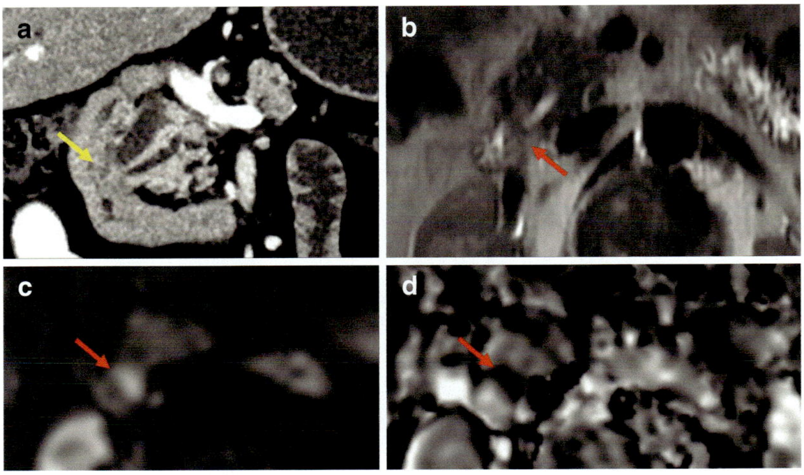

Fig. 14.2 A 55-year-old male with jaundice. (**a**) Oblique coronal image of CT shows slightly bulky ampulla with a small equivocal isoenhancing mass in the periampullary region due to inadequate duodenal distension. MRI (**b**) T2W image depicts a hyperintense mass (red arrows) which is best delineated on diffusion-weighted image (**c**) with diffusion restriction on ADC map (**d**)

tion of small tumors (as small as 2–3 mm) [1, 18]. EUS has the highest accuracy for assessment of regional lymphadenopathy associated with the tumor with EUS-guided fine-needle aspiration for sampling [3]. PDAC appears as a heterogeneously hypoechoic lesion on EUS with an ill-defined margin. However, EUS is limited by operator dependence and longer learning curve, and it cannot be used for evaluation of distant metastasis due to its narrow field of view.

Fluorodeoxyglucose positron emission tomography (FDG-PET) CT or MR can also be used to detect PDAC as it shows an intense uptake of FDG along with detection of small metastasis. However, false positives due to inflammation and false negatives due to physiological uptake in the bowel in periampullary carcinoma may occur [1].

14.3.2 Staging of Pancreatic Ductal Adenocarcinoma

Staging of PDAC is aimed to identify candidates of surgical resection as only R0 (complete) resection can improve survival. Pancreatic protocol CT is ideal for assessment of resectability of PDAC. Staging should be performed <4 weeks before surgery and prior to CBD stenting. MRI with DWI can be useful for isoattenuating lesions on CT and for assessing indeterminate liver and peritoneal metastasis. Biopsy is usually not required in resectable disease but is necessary in cases requiring neoadjuvant therapy [19, 20].

The two commonly used staging systems of PDAC include tumor, node, and metastasis (TNM) staging based on "American Joint Committee on Cancer (AJCC)" and "National Comprehensive Cancer Network (NCCN)" staging systems. AJCC staging is mainly used to determine prognosis and long-term survival of the patients, whereas NCCN staging is used for planning of treatment [3, 19, 20].

In TNM staging, the locoregional peripancreatic lymph nodes which are resected during surgery are included under N stage, whereas involvement of para-aortic lymph nodes and the nodes outside the lymphatic drainage pathway are considered under M stage [3, 19].

The NCCN staging is based on the "American Hepato-Pancreatico-Biliary Association" consensus report. Resectability of PDAC mainly depends on:

1. Distant metastases: Presence renders the tumor unresectable.
2. Major vascular involvement like superior mesenteric artery, celiac axis with/without aortic involvement, superior mesenteric vein, and portal vein.

In the absence of metastasis, NCCN classifies PDAC into three main categories: resectable, borderline resectable, or unresectable/locally advanced stages based on vascular (arterial and venous contact) involvement (Figs. 14.3 and 14.4) and location of tumor. The extension of the tumor to adjacent visceral structures is not an absolute contraindication for resection of the tumor as they can be removed along with the primary tumor (Fig. 14.5) [20–23].

A structured reporting template for evaluation of PDAC can help improve the accuracy of staging by imaging. It should include morphological evaluation, evaluation of arterial and venous involvement along with mention of arterial vari-

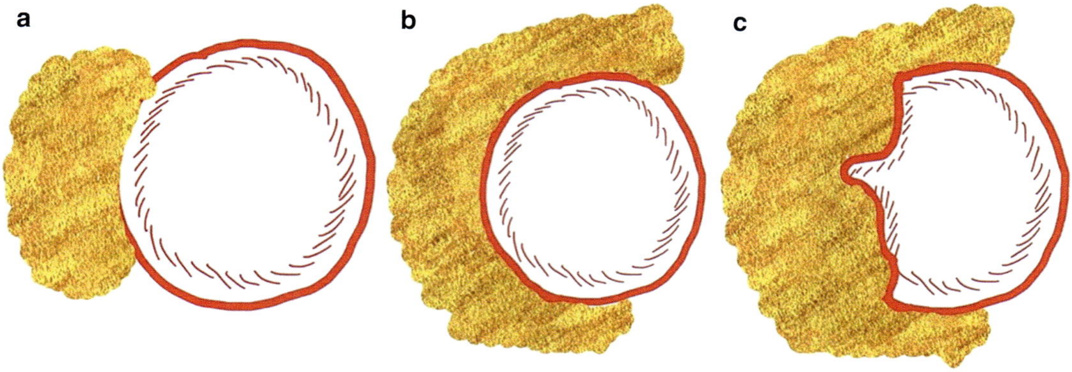

Fig. 14.3 Image showing arterial tumor contact: (**a**) ≤180-degree contact without deformity: vessel abutment. (**b**) >180-degree contact without deformity: vessel encasement. (**c**) Tumor contact with deformity

Fig. 14.4 Image showing vein tumor contact: (**a**) ≤180-degree contact without deformity. (**b**) >180-degree contact without deformity. (**c**) ≤180-degree contact with deformity. (**d**) Teardrop deformity

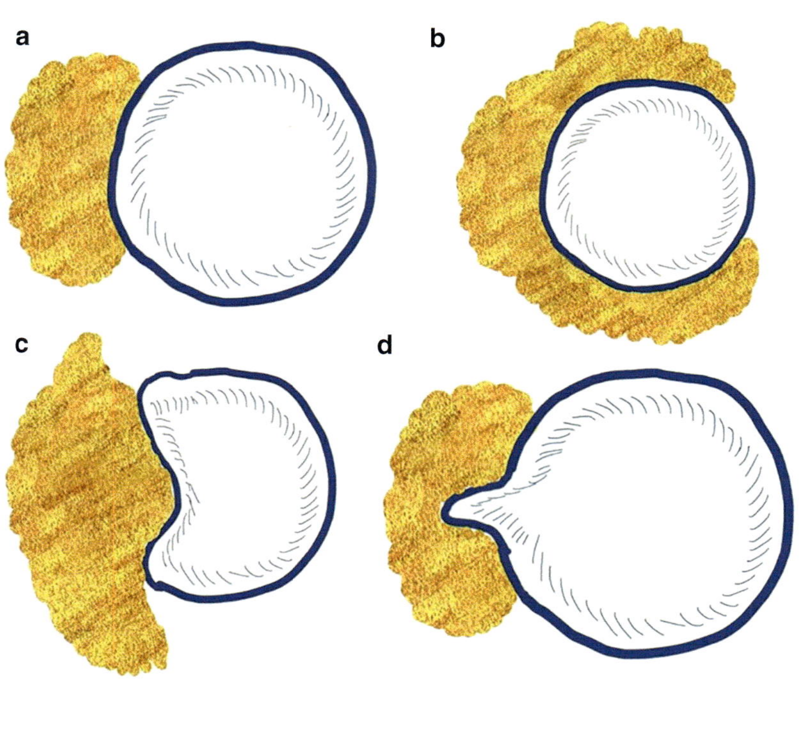

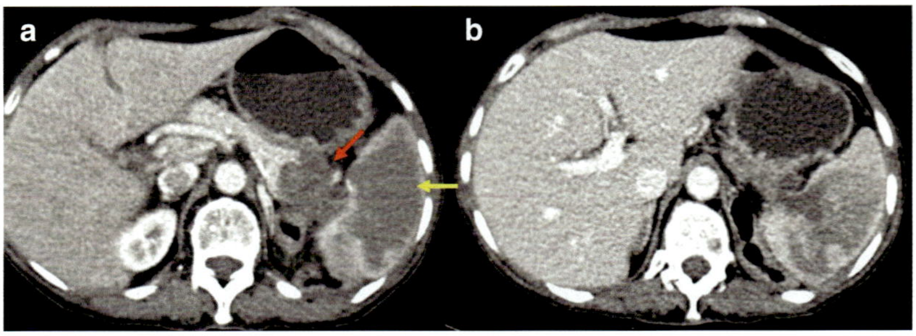

Fig. 14.5 A 59-year-old male with adenocarcinoma in the tail of the pancreas on CT (**a**, **b**). Hypoenhancing mass (red arrow) is causing splenic hilar involvement with invasion of splenic vessels leading to splenic infarcts (yellow arrow) and infiltrating posterior wall of the stomach

ants, and extrapancreatic involvement including liver and peritoneal metastasis, ascites, locoregional invasion, and involvement of lymph nodes [19, 22–24]. Reader should refer to NCCN criteria for detailed discussion on resectability of PDAC [21, 22].

14.3.3 Differential Diagnosis

Imaging mimics of PDAC include other pancreatic pathologies with solid morphology. Features favoring a diagnosis other than adenocarcinoma include hyperenhancement, lack of significant duct dilatation, large size (>5 cm), and intralesional ducts or cysts [25].

14.3.3.1 Mass-Forming Chronic Pancreatitis

Focal chronic pancreatitis may have a mass-like appearance and is associated with dilatation of MPD. However, the dilated duct in chronic pancreatitis is irregular with strictures in contrast to smoothly dilated obstructed duct in PDAC. Other features like pancreatic calcifications and pancreatic ductal calculi are common in MFCP than PDAC. Differences between MFCP and PDAC are outlined in Table 14.2. Pancreatic "duct width to total gland ratio" of >0.5 is suggestive of PDAC [3]. Nevertheless, PDAC may be associated with chronic pancreatitis where the distinction further becomes difficult. The most specific sign for differentiating MFCP from PDAC is "duct-penetrating sign" on MRCP [26]. It refers to a stenotic or normal MPD penetrating the mass and is seen in MFCP rather than PDAC. If the pancreatic mass completely obstructs and causes dilatation of the upstream duct, it is referred to as "duct-interruption sign" and is seen in PDAC. "Corona sign" is also positive in PDAC and refers to the absence of any dilated side branches of the

Table 14.2 Differences between MFCP and PDAC

	MFCP	PDAC
Duct dilatation	+, Irregularly dilated MPD with strictures	+++, Smooth dilatation of the obstructed MPD
Pancreatic calcification, pancreatic ductal calculi	Common	Rare
Pancreatic duct width to total gland ratio	<0.5	>0.5
Duct-penetrating sign	+	–
Duct interruption sign	–	+
Corona sign	–	+
Duct attraction sign	+	–
CT perfusion	Low BV and BF	BV and BF even lower value than MFCP
DWI	No diffusion restriction	Diffusion restriction +
IVIM	D and D* lower F value higher	D and D* higher F value lower

obstructed MPD within the mass. "Duct-interrupted" sign and "corona sign" are highly specific for PDAC [27]. "Attraction" sign is positive in MFCP, refers to the presence of dilated CBD near the pancreatic mass, and is relatively specific for MFCP (Fig. 14.6).

14.3.3.2 Autoimmune Pancreatitis

Focal forms of autoimmune pancreatitis (AIP) are difficult to differentiate from PDAC. However, few imaging features of AIP are absent in PDAC, as detailed in Table 14.3. AIP causes long segment irregular narrowing of the pancreatic duct rather than cut-off and upstream dilatation. Serum markers like IgG4 and antibodies like ALA, ACA II, ASMA, and ANA are elevated in AIP. Fine-needle aspiration may be useful, but the patchy nature of AIP may make pathological evaluation inadequate. A trial of corticosteroid therapy serves as a diagnostic and therapeutic tool as AIP shows excellent response to steroids [3, 4, 25, 28, 29].

14.3.3.3 Miscellaneous

Groove pancreatitis appears as a sheet-like mass in pancreaticoduodenal groove. However, in contrast to PDAC, it does not show dilatation of MPD and has other features like small intralesional ducts or cysts and cystic dystrophy in the duodenal wall (Fig. 14.7) [3].

Rarely pancreatic ductal adenocarcinoma may arise in IPMN (more frequently in the main duct than in branch duct IPMN) and pose a diagnostic dilemma on imaging. The concerning features of malignancy in IPMN include obstructive jaundice in cystic neoplasm, enhancing mural nodule $\geq$5 mm, and main pancreatic duct diameter $\geq$10 mm [25].

14.3.4 Treatment and Prognosis

Complete surgical resection with adjuvant therapy is the best cure. However, less than 20% of the tumors are resectable on diagnosis. Whipple procedure (pancreaticoduodenectomy) is the surgery of choice for curative resection. Chemotherapy and/or radiotherapy can be used in locally advanced tumors which are not amenable to surgery or tumors with distant metastasis [3].

PDAC is the fourth leading cause of cancer-related deaths. It has a very poor prognosis with 1-year survival rate of <20% and 5-year survival rate of <5%. The post-surgical 5-year survival rate is only 20% [1]. Patients with distant metas-

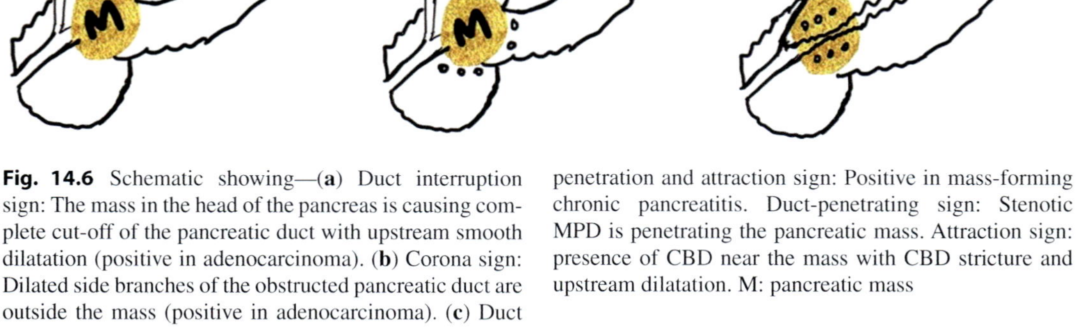

Fig. 14.6 Schematic showing—(**a**) Duct interruption sign: The mass in the head of the pancreas is causing complete cut-off of the pancreatic duct with upstream smooth dilatation (positive in adenocarcinoma). (**b**) Corona sign: Dilated side branches of the obstructed pancreatic duct are outside the mass (positive in adenocarcinoma). (**c**) Duct penetration and attraction sign: Positive in mass-forming chronic pancreatitis. Duct-penetrating sign: Stenotic MPD is penetrating the pancreatic mass. Attraction sign: presence of CBD near the mass with CBD stricture and upstream dilatation. M: pancreatic mass

Table 14.3 Differences between autoimmune pancreatitis and PDAC

	Autoimmune pancreatitis	PDAC
Types	Focal, diffuse	Focal mass
Appearance: Sausage-shaped enlargement of the pancreas	Present	Absent
Hypodense/T2 hypointense rim (halo)	Present	Absent
Enhancement pattern	Hypo-enhancing but shows prolonged enhancement on the delayed phase	Hypo-enhancing, no delayed enhancement
Duct involvement	Diffuse/long segment irregular narrowing of the MPD and compression or narrowing of distal CBD secondary to swelling of the pancreas	Cut-off of the duct with dilatation of the upstream duct
Serum/tumor marker	Elevated IgG4	Elevated CA-19-9
Extrapancreatic manifestations-inflammatory pseudotumors	Present	Absent
Treatment	Steroids	Surgery: only curative treatment, chemoradiotherapy in unresectable cases
Response to steroids (serial imaging 2–4 weeks after initiation of steroid therapy)	Complete resolution: diagnostic	Partial or no resolution

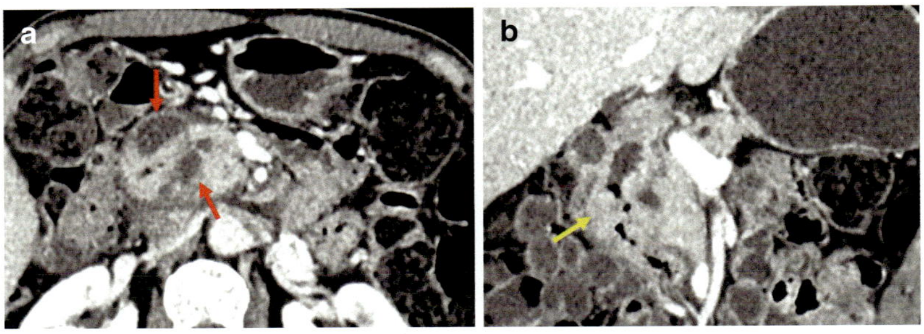

Fig. 14.7 A 39-year-old male with abdominal pain and vomiting depicting features of groove pancreatitis on CT. (**a**) Axial image shows few cystic areas in pancreaticoduodenal groove (red arrows) with (**b**) inflammatory changes extending into the duodenal wall causing its stenosis (yellow arrow)

tasis do not show significant improvement in survival or quality of life even with chemotherapy [3].

14.4 Pancreatic Neuroendocrine Tumors

Pancreatic neuroendocrine tumors (PNETs) account for 1%–5% of all pancreatic tumors. They are classified under gastroenteropancreatic NETs according to the World Health Organization. They originate from pluripotential stem cells in ductal epithelium [1, 30]. Pathologically these tumors show uniform nuclei, clear cytoplasm, and secretory granules which stain positive for chromogranin A and neuron-specific enolase. Most cases are sporadic, but syndromic association with multiple endocrine neoplasia type 1 (MEN 1), neurofibromatosis type 1, von Hippel-Lindau syndrome (VHL), and tuberous sclerosis is seen [1].

PNETs can be functioning or non-functioning based on the presence of hormone overproduction [3]. They are further divided according to their specific hormone production and differ in location and clinical features as detailed in Table 14.4.

Table 14.4 Specific features of neuroendocrine tumors

Functioning tumors (15%–52%)	Clinical features	Location	Size	Malignancy rate	Any specific feature	Survival
Insulinoma (50%): most common functioning NET	Hypoglycemia, atypical seizures No gender predilection Age: 30–60 years	90% in the pancreas Equal distribution in head, body, and tail	<2 cm, 90% cases; <1.5 cm, 66% cases; <1 cm, 40% cases	10%	Usually solitary (90%) Association with MEN 1	100% after resection
Gastrinoma (20%)	Zollinger-Ellison syndrome with peptic ulceration and diarrhea Male predilection Age: fifth decade	25%–60% in the pancreas 90% in the gastrinoma triangle	Mean size: 4 cm	60%, metastasis in up to 60%	Usually multiple (20%–40%) Most common pancreatic NET associated with MEN 1 (~30% associated)	10-year survival rate of 90% following complete resection
Vipoma (3%)	WDHA/Werner- Morrison syndrome (watery diarrhea, hypokalemia, achlorhydria-hypochlorhydria) Female predilection (3:1)	90% pancreas: most commonly in the tail 10%–20% extrapancreatic: Most commonly in adrenal glands and retroperitoneal sympathetic chain	Mean 5 cm	50%–75%, metastasis in up to 70%	WDHA syndrome	5-year survival rate of 95% following complete resection; 60% in metastatic tumors
Glucagonoma (1%)	Necrolytic migratory erythema, weight loss, diabetes, diarrhea, and mild hyperglycemia may occur	>90% in the pancreas: location is in the pancreatic body and tail	2–6 cm	70%, metastasis in up to 60%	Associated with 4D syndrome	More favorable with complete resection, prolonged even with liver metastasis
Somatostatinoma (<1%)	Cholelithiasis, weight loss, steatorrhea, diarrhea, diabetes Mean age: 51 years Female predilection	50% pancreas, 50% duodenum	>5 cm	50%, metastasis in up to 50%	Associated with neurofibromatosis type 1 in 50% cases, inhibitory syndrome	5-year survival rate of 95% following complete resection; 60% in metastatic tumors
Non-functioning tumors (15%–50%)	Clinical features due to mass effect Age: fourth or fifth decade	Pancreatic head	>10 cm in 30% cases Range: 3–24 cm (large size at presentation)	90%, metastasis in up to 50%	Higher resectability rate and better chemotherapy response than pancreatic adenocarcinoma	5-year survival >50% following complete resection

Adapted from Refs. [1, 3, 29]

14.4.1 Imaging Features

NETs associated with syndromes like MEN 1 and VHL tend to be multiple in number. Functioning tumors (15%–52%) manifest at a small size as they become symptomatic earlier, whereas non-functioning tumors present when they become large in size and cause symptoms mainly related to their mass effect [1, 3].

Dual-phase CT and MRI form the principal imaging modalities for detection and staging of PNETs. Small tumors are usually homogeneous, solid, and hyperenhancing on CT, whereas larger ones may show necrosis and cystic degeneration with calcification seen in up to 20% of PNETs [1, 31].

The diagnostic feature of NETs is their avid arterial enhancement due to the presence of rich vascular supply which is homogeneous in small tumors (<2 cm), whereas larger tumors show a heterogeneous pattern of enhancement which may be more pronounced peripherally, thereby appearing as a ring-like pattern. On the portal venous phase, the tumors may remain hyperenhancing or show iso- or hypoattenuation compared to the rest of the pancreas (Figs. 14.8, 14.9, and 14.10) [1, 3]. Metastasis to regional lymph nodes and liver can occur.

PNETs may be well-differentiated tumors (grade 1–3) or poorly differentiated neuroendocrine carcinoma (small or large cell type) or mixed endocrine non-endocrine neoplasms. Poorly differentiated carcinomas show features like local spread, retroperitoneal invasion, vascular infiltration with tumor thrombosis, significant lymphadenopathy, and distant metastasis with more prevalence of central necrosis and calcifications (Fig. 14.11). Lymph nodes and metastases show similar hyperenhancement pattern as the primary PNET [6, 32].

Indium 111 octreotide SPECT/CT: Indium 111-radiolabeled octreotide is a somatostatin analogue and is taken up by somatostatin receptors 2 and 5 which are found in most of the PNETs except for insulinoma. Therefore, it is very useful for detection of PNETs (except insulinoma) with a sensitivity of 90% and specificity of 80% [1, 33]. Another advantage is scanning of the whole body for detection of metastasis and other small tumors.

Gallium 68 DOTATATE PET/CT: Gallium 68 is a somatostatin receptor analogue like indium 111. Gallium 68 has a shorter half-life and therefore results in lesser radiation dose to the patient. In addition, PET/CT helps provide better speed and resolution compared with gamma camera of SPECT/CT. Owing to its superior accuracy, it has become a new reference standard for evaluation of PNETs and their metastases [34].

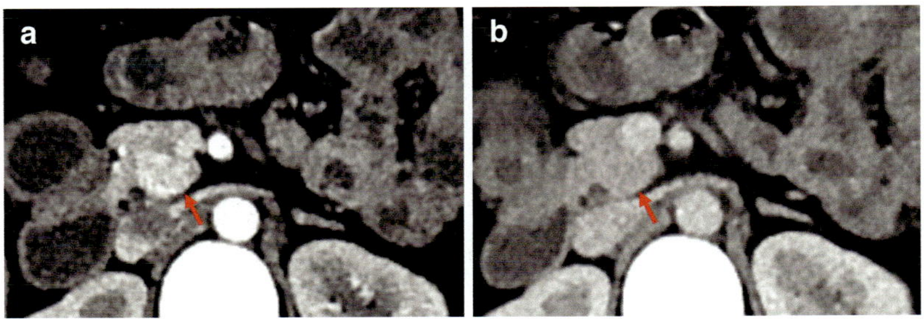

Fig. 14.8 Dual-phase contrast-enhanced CT in a 25-year-old female with recurrent episodes of hypoglycemia and pancreatic insulinoma. (**a**) Arterial phase shows an avidly enhancing mass lesion in the uncinate process of the pancreas (red arrows). (**b**) In the venous phase, the mass becomes isodense without any contour bulge and has the potential to be missed, if only venous phase imaging is done

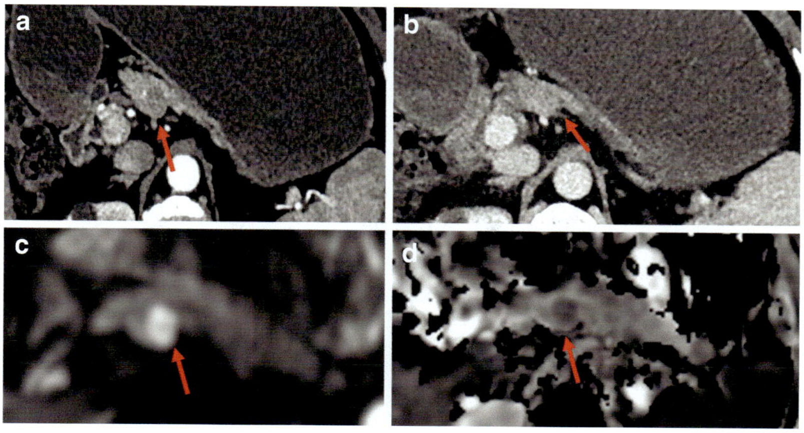

Fig. 14.9 A 35-year-old male with suspected insulinoma. (**a**) A small hypoenhancing mass lesion is seen in the arterial phase (red arrows) which demonstrates progressive enhancement on venous phase (**b**). Diffusion-weighted imaging (**c**) delineates the lesion well with diffusion restriction on ADC map (**d**) and increases the diagnostic confidence in lesions with atypical enhancement patterns. Enucleation was done, and histopathology confirmed insulinoma

Fig. 14.10 Multiphasic CT in a 45-year-old female with upper abdominal pain and multiple gastrinomas. Arterial phase: (**a**) axial and (**b**) sagittal images showing multiple avidly enhancing nodular masses along the pylorus and proximal duodenum in Passaro's triangle. Venous phase: (**c**) axial and (**d**) sagittal images showing progressive enhancement of masses (yellow arrows) along with multiple arterially enhancing liver metastases (red arrows)

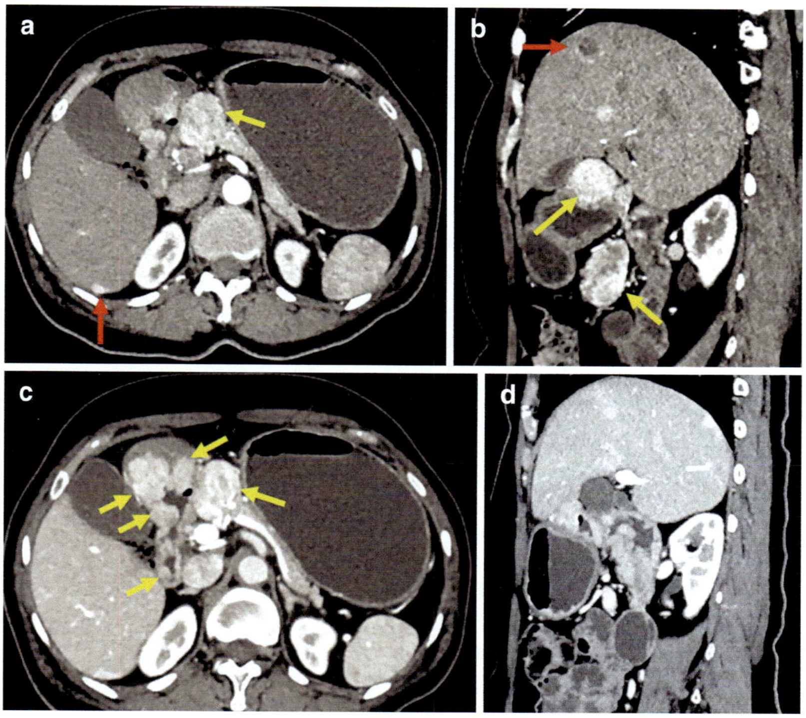

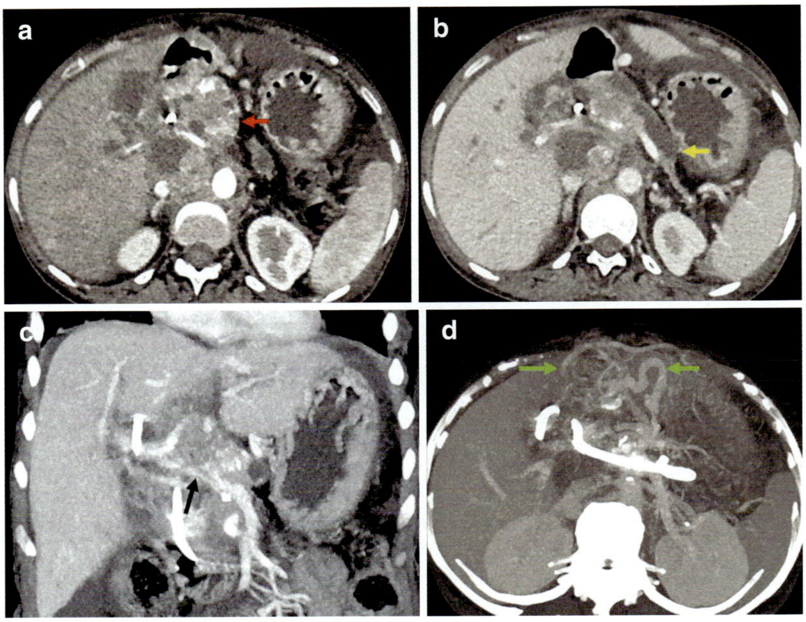

Fig. 14.11 A 58-year-old female with abdominal pain and jaundice for 2 months. (**a**) Axial section, arterial phase demonstrates a large infiltrating tumor depicting arterial enhancement with few cystic areas, encasing common hepatic artery, invading main portal vein (MPV), extending into the retroperitoneum in the aortocaval region. (**b**) Venous phase, axial image shows a dilated main pancreatic duct (yellow arrow) with distal pancreatic atrophy and lipomatosis. (**c**) Coronal image confirming MPV invasion (black arrow) with CBD stent in situ. (**d**) Axial maximum intensity projection image depicts multiple gastroepiploic collaterals (green arrows). Biopsy was suggestive of neuroendocrine carcinoma

FDG PET/CT: It is useful for evaluation of poorly differentiated NETs which are usually negative on octreotide scan. These tumors have a high proliferation rate and therefore show the increased uptake of FDG PET. Well-differentiated NETs on the other hand usually do not show avid uptake due to their low cellular proliferation [1].

14.4.2 Differential Diagnosis

NETs should be differentiated from the rest of the pancreatic tumors with the main differential being metastasis from renal cell carcinoma (RCC), intrapancreatic accessory spleen (Fig. 14.12), or PDAC as detailed in Table 14.5 [3].

14.4.3 Treatment and Prognosis

Treatment is based on the type of NET and involves surgical resection. Chemotherapy may be required in non-functioning NETs. Prognosis is better than pancreatic ductal carcinoma with good post-operative and post-chemotherapy response.

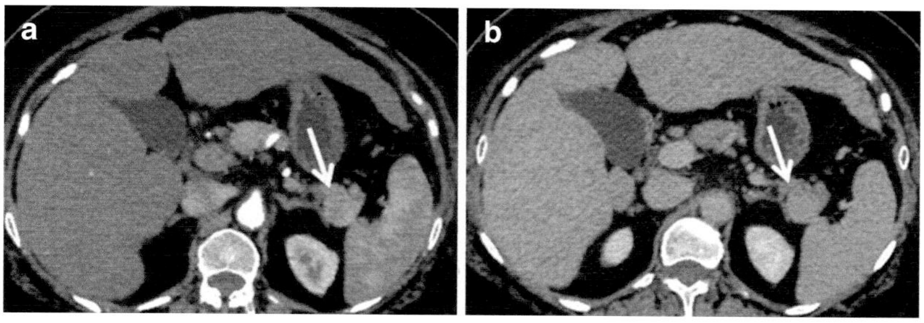

Fig. 14.12 Incidental intrapancreatic spleen in the tail of the pancreas on CT. (**a**) Arterial and (**b**) venous phases showing an enhancing lesion in the tail of the pancreas (white arrows). Lesion shows enhancement similar to the spleen in both phases. Note the patient had chronic liver disease

Table 14.5 Differences between pancreatic NET and pancreatic ductal adenocarcinoma [1]

	Pancreatic NET	Pancreatic ductal adenocarcinoma
Post-contrast enhancement	Hyperenhancing	Hypoenhancing compared to rest of the pancreas
Calcification	Common (20%)	Rare (2%)
Vessel involvement	Vascular infiltration with tumor thrombosis in cases of malignant NET	Vessel encasement
Obstruction of MPD ± CBD	Less common	Common
Cystic/necrotic degeneration	Common	Rare

14.5 Pancreatoblastoma

Pancreatoblastoma is the most common primary pancreatic neoplasm of childhood and accounts for 0.2% of all pancreatic neoplasms [1]. Young children (mean age: 5 years) are usually affected with a male predisposition. One third of the cases have elevated alpha-fetoprotein levels. Syndromic association with Beckwith-Wiedemann syndrome has been described [1, 35, 36].

14.5.1 Imaging Features

Pancreatoblastomas are slow growing and present as large solitary abdominal masses with most tumors located in the head (50%). On ultrasound, they appear as hetero-echoic masses with multiseptated hypoechoic cystic areas secondary to hemorrhagic changes and cystic degeneration. Pancreatoblastomas associated with Beckwith-Wiedemann have predominant cystic appearance. On CT, they appear as heterogenous multiloculated mass with enhancing internal septations. Calcifications may be present in a rim-like or clustered pattern.

Despite being large in size, they rarely cause obstruction of the duodenum or biliary tree because of their gelatinous consistency. Complications include vascular encasement and local lymphadenopathy. The liver is the most common site of distant metastasis followed by the lymph nodes, lung, bone, posterior mediastinum, peritoneum, and omentum [1, 35, 36].

14.5.2 Differential Diagnosis

Large tumors with a suspicious organ of origin call for consideration of other embryonal tumors such as hepatoblastoma, nephroblastoma, and neuroblastoma. Biopsy is often necessary to make a definitive diagnosis.

14.5.3 Treatment and Prognosis

Complete surgical resection forms the mainstay of management. Follow-up imaging and long-term surveillance are required as 14% tumors progress even after resection. Pancreatic body and tail tumors are difficult to excise completely and therefore carry a poor prognosis [1].

14.6 Pancreatic Lymphoma

Pancreatic lymphoma can be primary or secondary (more common). It is a B-cell non-Hodgkin lymphoma in most cases. Secondary lymphoma is usually the result of direct extension from involved peripancreatic lymph nodes. Primary pancreatic lymphoma (PPL) is rare accounting for 0.5% of pancreatic neoplasms and <2% of extranodal lymphomas. It is defined when pancreatic lymphoma is associated with only locoregional lymphadenopathy, absence of other lymphadenopathy, normal leukocyte count, and no hepatic or splenic involvement [37]. Secondary lymphoma is associated with extensive locoregional and systemic lymphadenopathy.

Mid-aged patients between 35 and 75 years of age (mean age: 55 years) and immunocompromised patients are more commonly affected with male predilection (male/female: 7:1). Patients present with non-specific clinical features like abdominal pain, mass, and weight loss [1, 3].

14.6.1 Imaging Features

Pancreatic lymphoma may manifest in two forms: [1] Focal well-circumscribed mass/masses and [2] diffuse form. The focal form usually affects the pancreatic head and has a large size at presentation (mean: 8 cm). It often extends to extrapancreatic regions and does not respect any anatomic boundaries. It appears hypodense on CT. Calcifications and necrosis are not present and can be used to exclude the diagnosis. Differences between pancreatic lymphoma and PDAC are detailed in Table 14.6. It causes no or only mild dilatation of upstream MPD and affects CBD more than MPD (Fig. 14.13). These are hypointense on T1W and intermediate/hyperintense on T2W images, hypoenhancing with significant diffusion restriction indicating high cellularity.

Diffuse Involvement occurs as poorly defined infiltrative mass causing enlargement of the pancreas and needs to be differentiated from AIP. It appears hypointense on both T1W and T2W sequences with near homogeneous post-contrast enhancement. Histopathological evaluation is usually required for a definitive diagnosis.

14.6.2 Differential Diagnosis

PDAC and PNET are the main differentials of pancreatic lymphoma. Faint post-contrast enhancement, absence of necrosis, and calcification are features differentiating it from PNET.

Table 14.6 Differences between pancreatic lymphoma and PDAC

	Pancreatic lymphoma	PDAC
Age, size	Mean age: 55 years, large size (mean: 8 cm)	Usually >60 years (rare before 30 years), mean size (3 cm)
Duct cut-off with dilatation of MPD	Non-significant	Marked
Lymphadenopathy	Bulky, non-locoregional, common below the level of the renal vein	Locoregional lymphadenopathy present
Respect for anatomic boundaries	Absent, infiltrates retroperitoneum, upper abdominal organs, and the gastrointestinal tract	Present
Vascular invasion	Less common	More common
Necrosis	Absent	May be present
Calcification	Absent	May be present

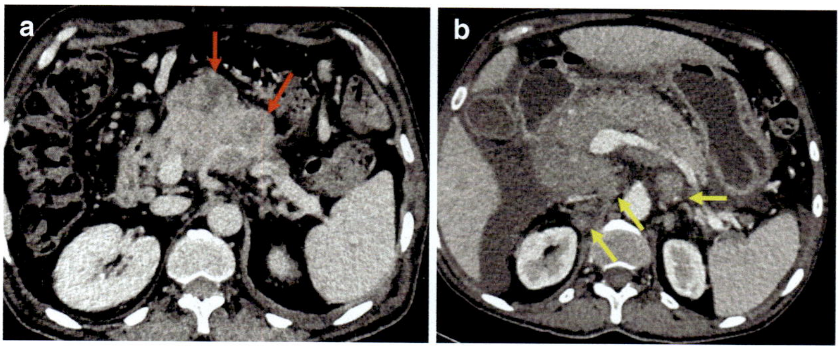

Fig. 14.13 Pancreatic lymphoma on CT in two different patients. (**a**) A 57-year-old male with PPL with multifocal hypodense masses (red arrows) encasing splenic artery without narrowing with the absence of other systemic involvement and mild peripancreatic lymphadenopathy. (**b**) Secondary pancreatic lymphoma with diffuse involvement of the pancreas with retroperitoneal lymphadenopathy (yellow arrow) with ascites. Note the absence of pancreatic duct dilatation in both cases

14.6.3 Treatment and Prognosis

Treatment includes chemotherapy, and surgery is often not required. Prognosis is better than PDAC because of its good response to chemotherapy.

14.7 Metastases to the Pancreas

Metastases to the pancreas account for 2%–5% of the malignant tumors of the pancreas. The most common primary sites include RCC and carcinoma lung followed by breast carcinoma, colorectal carcinoma, and melanoma. The patients present with non-specific clinical features with 50%–83% of the patients being asymptomatic at presentation [1, 3, 38]. The time interval between the diagnosis of primary tumor and detection of metastasis in the pancreas is generally <3 years. RCC metastasis, however, usually presents 6–12 years after nephrectomy [39].

14.7.1 Imaging Features

Pancreatic metastasis can occur in solitary (50%–70% cases), multifocal (5%–10%), and diffuse (15%–44%) patterns. The average size at diagnosis is 4.6 cm [3]. They may show varied appearances on ultrasound or CT and are usually T1W hypointense and T2W hyperintense. The enhancement characteristics of the metastases resemble those of the primary tumor (Fig. 14.14). Metastases from RCC are well defined and show hyperenhancement with the central necrotic core [1, 3, 39, 40].

14.7.2 Differential Diagnosis

Pancreatic metastasis from RCC may mimic PNETs as both show hyperenhancement with central necrotic degeneration. Hypovascular metastasis from the lung, colon, and breast needs to be differentiated from PDAC especially if they are solitary. The past medical history of malignancy may help [1, 39].

14.7.3 Treatment and Prognosis

Surgical resection of pancreatic metastasis can be carried out in patients with long disease-free interval between resection of primary tumor and development of metastasis or in those where metastasis is confined only in the pancreas. About 80% of the patients with RCC do not show any other organ involvement. The prognosis is favorable than PDAC [1, 39].

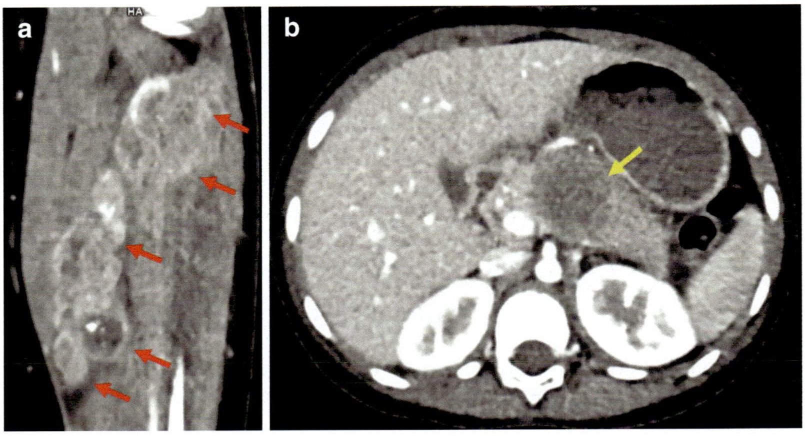

Fig. 14.14 Contrast-enhanced CT in a 6-year-old female with an asymptomatic solitary pancreatic metastasis that developed 3 years after the treatment of primary rhabdomyosarcoma (RMS) in leg. (**a**) Coronal image depicting the primary RMS in the leg (red arrows). (**b**) Axial image of follow-up CT showing pancreatic metastasis (yellow arrow). Note the absence of ductal dilatation despite the significant size of the mass

14.8 Solid Pseudopapillary Tumor

Solid pseudopapillary tumor (SPT) accounts for 1%–2% of all pancreatic tumors. It is a benign exocrine tumor of the pancreas occurring in young adults. It most commonly affects females with female-to-male predilection of 9:1. Gradually enlarging abdominal mass and vague abdominal pain are the usual clinical complaints or are asymptomatic (15%) [1, 3].

14.8.1 Imaging Features

The most common location of tumor is in the pancreatic tail followed by the head; the tumor is typically large in size (mean size −9 cm) and slow growing [1, 41]. Metastases are uncommon (7%–9%). The most common site of metastasis is the liver followed by the omentum and peritoneum [1].

Smaller SPTs (<3 cm) appear completely solid, whereas larger lesions are mixed solid-cystic [42]. Hallmark feature of SPT is internal hemorrhage and cystic degeneration, owing to the presence of fragile vascular network, best seen on MRI where subacute hemorrhage in the tumor is T1 hyperintense with variable signal on T2WI (Fig. 14.15). Chronic hemorrhage appears hypointense on both T1- and T2-weighted sequences. Few cases (10%–18%) may show fluid-fluid levels due to the hematocrit effect [1, 43].

SPTs have a thick fibrous pseudocapsule which appears hypodense on CT and hypointense on T1W and T2W sequences [3]. Peripheral calcification may be present in 30% cases [43]. SPTs show heterogeneous post-contrast enhancement with enhancing solid areas predominantly located in the periphery and cystic spaces located in the center [3]. There is a progressive increase in enhancement on the portal venous phase, but it usually remains less than the normal pancreas [1, 44].

14.8.2 Differential Diagnosis

Cystic PNETs are the main differential diagnosis of SPTs with differences outlined in Table 14.7.

14.8.3 Treatment and Prognosis

Complete surgical resection is usually curative with excellent prognosis [1]. Tumors undergoing malignant degeneration are called "solid pseudopapillary carcinomas" and may occur in older patients with male predilection [3].

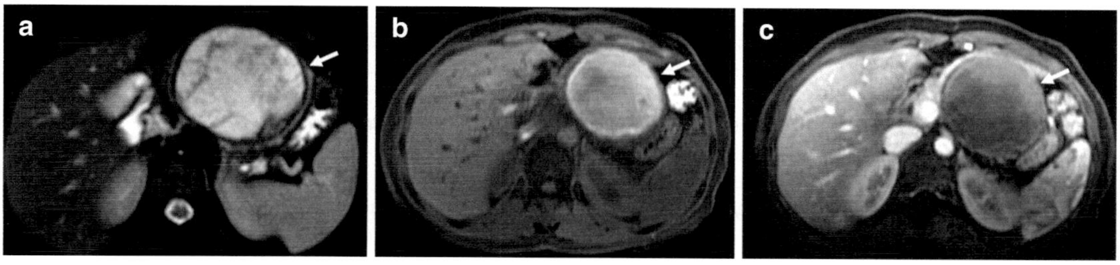

Fig. 14.15 MRI in a 19-year-old female with abdominal pain and a cystic lesion detected on ultrasound. (**a**) Axial T2-weighted image shows a T2 hyperintense cystic lesion (arrow) with multiple T2 hypointense septations. (**b**) Axial pre-contrast T1W image shows internal T1 hyperintensity in the lesion due to hemorrhage. (**c**) Post-contrast T1WI in the venous phase showing no enhancement of septations with minimal peripheral enhancement. Surgical resection followed by histopathology confirmed solid pseudopapillary tumor

Table 14.7 Differences between SPT and cystic NET of the pancreas [1, 3]

	SPT	Pancreatic NET
Age at presentation	Mean age: 25 years	Rare before 30 years
MRI signal intensity	Hyperintense on T1-weighted sequence owing to the presence of hemorrhage	Hypointense on T1-weighted imaging
Post-contrast enhancement	Progressive heterogenous post-contrast enhancement of the peripheral solid areas; enhancement usually remains less than that of the surrounding pancreatic parenchyma	Diffuse or ring hyperenhancement

14.9 Miscellaneous Neoplasms

One of the rare neoplasms (1%) of the pancreas is acinar cell carcinoma (ACC). Excess production of lipase by the tumor can lead to "lipid hypersecretion syndrome" which manifests as "subcutaneous fat necrosis, bone infarcts and polyarthritis." It predominantly involves uncinate process and head of the pancreas with a mean size of 7 cm. Calcification in ACCs (50%) may be either in peripheral or central stellate patterns. A well-defined enhancing capsule is present around the tumor in 60% of the cases with discontinuation or infiltration at places, a feature lacking in PDAC and PNET. Central necrosis is present in 80% of the cases, a feature rare in PDAC and present in 18% of the functional PNETs. Macroscopic hemorrhage has not been reported in ACC, a feature distinguishing it from SPT [1, 3].

14.10 Summary

Imaging plays a fundamental role in the management of solid pancreatic tumors with newer advances like dual-energy CT and CT perfusion further helping in improved detection, staging, post-operative evaluation, and prognostication. Adequate dual-phase pancreatic protocol and structured reporting format are important for optimal evaluation of resectability. CT forms the work horse for assessment, but multimodality imaging approach is of paramount importance in indeterminate cases.

References

1. Low G, Panu A, Millo N, Leen E. Multimodality imaging of neoplastic and non-neoplastic solid lesions of the pancreas. Radiographics. 2011;31(4):993–1015.
2. Ros PR, Mortele KJ. Imaging features of pancreatic neoplasms. J Belg Radiol. 2001;84(6):239–49.
3. Haaga J, Boll D. CT and MRI of the whole body. 6th ed. Philadelphia: Elsevier; 2017. Pancreas. p. 1406–78.

4. Gore R, Levine M. Texbook of gastrointestinal radiology. 4th ed. Philadelphia: Elsevier; 2015. Pancreatic neoplasms. p. 1838–55.
5. Brennan DD, Zamboni GA, Raptopoulos VD, Kruskal JB. Comprehensive preoperative assessment of pancreatic adenocarcinoma with 64-section volumetric CT. Radiographics. 2007;27(6):1653–66.
6. Almeida RR, Lo GC, Patino M, Bizzo B, Canellas R, Sahani DV. Advances in pancreatic CT imaging. Am J Roentgenol. 2018;211(1):52–66.
7. DSK L, Reber HA, Krasny RM, Kadell BM, Sayre J. Local staging of pancreatic cancer: criteria for unresectability of major vessels as revealed by pancreatic-phase, thin-section helical CT. AJR Am J Roentgenol. 1997;168:1439–43.
8. Hough T, Raptopoulos V, Siewert B, Matthews B. Teardrop-shaped superior mesenteric vein. AJR Am J Roentgenol. 1999;173:1509–12.
9. Deshmukh SD, Willmann JK, Jeffrey RB. Pathways of extrapancreatic perineural invasion by pancreatic adenocarcinoma: evaluation with 3D volume-rendered MDCT imaging. Am J Roentgenol. 2010;194(3):668–74.
10. Patel BN, Olcott E, Jeffrey RB. Extrapancreatic perineural invasion in pancreatic adenocarcinoma. Abdom Radiol. 2018;43(2):323–31.
11. Khristenko E, Shrainer I, Setdikova G, Palkina O, Sinitsyn V, Lyadov V. Preoperative CT-based detection of extrapancreatic perineural invasion in pancreatic cancer. Sci Rep. 2021;11(1):1–11. Available from: https://doi.org/10.1038/s41598-021-81322-4.
12. Yadav AK, Sharma R, Kandasamy D, Pradhan RK, Garg PK, Bhalla AS, et al. Perfusion CT–can it resolve the pancreatic carcinoma versus mass forming chronic pancreatitis conundrum? Pancreatology. 2016;16(6):979–87. Available from: https://doi.org/10.1016/j.pan.2016.08.011.
13. Hanbidge AE. Cancer of the pancreas: the best image for early detection–CT, MRI, PET or US? Can J Gastroenterol. 2002;16(2):101–5.
14. Winston C, Mitchell DG, Outwater EK, Ehrlich SM. Pancreatic signal intensity on T1- clinical correlation. JMRI. 1995;5(3):267–71.
15. Ichikawa T, Erturk SM, Motosugi U, Sou H, Iino H, Araki T, et al. High-b value diffusion-weighted MRI for detecting pancreatic adenocarcinoma: preliminary results. Am J Roentgenol. 2007;188(2):409–14.
16. Tang M-Y, Zhang X-M, Chen T-W, Huang X-H. Various diffusion magnetic resonance imaging techniques for pancreatic cancer. World J Radiol. 2015;7(12):424.
17. Kang KM, Lee JM, Yoon JH, Kiefer B, Han JK, Choi BI. Intravoxel incoherent motion diffusion-weighted MR imaging for characterization of focal pancreatic lesions. Radiology. 2014;270(2):444–53.
18. DeWitt J, Devereaux B, Chriswell M, McGreevy K, Howard T, Imperiale TF, et al. Comparison of endoscopic ultrasonography and multidetector computed tomography for detecting and staging pancreatic cancer. Ann Intern Med. 2004;141(10):753–64.
19. Al-Hawary MM, Francis IR, Chari ST, Fishman EK, Hough DM, Lu DS, et al. Pancreatic ductal adenocarcinoma radiology reporting template: consensus statement of the society of abdominal radiology and the american pancreatic association. Radiology. 2014;270(1):248–60.
20. Hong SB, Lee SS, Kim JH, Kim HJ, Ho J. Pancreatic cancer CT: prediction of resectability according to NCCN Criteria. Radiology. 2018;289:710–8.
21. Tempero M, Malafa M, Al-Hawary M, et al. Clinical practice guidelines in oncology: pancreatic adenocarcinoma. National Comprehensive Cancer Network. 2021; version 2. Available at: http://www.nccn.org/. Accessed June 2021.
22. Zins M, Matos C, Cassinotto C. Pancreatic adenocarcinoma staging in the era of preoperative chemotherapy and radiation therapy. Radiology. 2018;287(2):374–90.
23. Fowler KJ. CT assessment of pancreatic cancer: what are the gaps in predicting surgical outcomes? Radiology. 2018;289:719–20.
24. Brook OR, Brook A, Vollmer CM, Kent TS, et al. Structured reporting of multiphasic CT for pancreatic cancer brook. Radiology. 2015;274:464–72.
25. Coakley FV, Hanley-Knutson K, Mongan J, Barajas R, Bucknor M, Qayyum A. Pancreatic imaging mimics: part 1, imaging mimics of pancreatic adenocarcinoma. Am J Roentgenol. 2012;199(2):301–8.
26. Ichikawa T, Sou H, Araki T, Arbab AS, Yoshikawa T, Ishigame K, et al. Duct-penetrating sign at MRCP: usefulness for differentiating inflammatory pancreatic mass from pancreatic carcinomas. Radiology. 2001;221(1):107–16.
27. Beker K, Lee KS, Tsai LL, Hegazi T, Garces-Descovich A, Brook A, et al. Differentiation of pancreatic head ductal adenocarcinoma from inflammatory pancreatic pseudomass by MR cholangiopancreatography: utility of the duct-interrupted, corona, and attraction signs. Abdom Radiol. 2019;44(12):4048–56. Available from: https://doi.org/10.1007/s00261-019-02155-4.
28. Zaheer A, Singh VK, Akshintala VS, Kawamoto S, Tsai SD, Gage KL, Fishman EK. Differentiating autoimmune pancreatitis from pancreatic adenocarcinoma using dual-phase computed tomography: an inter-observer study. J Comput Assist Tomogr. 2015;38(1):146–52.
29. Lewis RB, Lattin GE, Paal E. Pancreatic endocrine tumors: radiologic-clinicopathologic correlation. Radiographics. 2010;30(6):1445–64.
30. Oberg K, Eriksson B. Endocrine tumours of the pancreas. Best Pract Res Clin Gastroenterol. 2005;19(5 SPEC. ISS):753–81.
31. Noone TC, Hosey J, Zeynep F, Semelka RC. Imaging and localization of islet-cell tumours of the pancreas on CT and MRI. Best Pract Res Clin Endocrinol Metab. 2005;19(2):195–211.
32. Gouya H, Vignaux O, Augui J, Dousset B, Palazzo L, Louvel A, et al. CT, endoscopic sonography, and a combined protocol for preoperative evalua-

tion of pancreatic insulinomas. Am J Roentgenol. 2003;181(4):987–92.
33. Wiedenmann B, Ricke J, Mignon M. Standardisation of imaging in neuroendocrine tumours: results of a European delphi process. Eur J Radiol. 2001;37:8–17.
34. Hofman MS, Eddie Lau WF, Hicks RJ. Somatostatin receptor imaging with 68Ga DOTATATE PET/CT: clinical utility, normal patterns, pearls, and pitfalls in interpretation. Radiographics. 2015;35(2):500–16.
35. Montemarano H, Lonergan GJ, Bulas DI, Selby DM. Pancreatoblastoma: imaging findings in 10 patients and review of the literature. Radiology. 2000;214(2):476–82.
36. Chung EM, Travis MD, Conran RM. From the archives of the AFIP pancreatic tumors in children: objectives. Radiographics. 2006;26(4):1211–39. Available from: http://radiographics.rsnajnls.org/cgi/doi/10.1148/rg.264065012.
37. Fujinaga Y, Lall C, Patel A, Matsushita T, Sanyal R, Kadoya M. MR features of primary and secondary malignant lymphoma of the pancreas: a pictorial review. Insights Imaging. 2013;4(3):321–9.
38. Tsitouridis I, Diamantopoulou A, Michaelides M, Arvanity M, Papaioannou S. Pancreatic metastases: CT and MRI findings. Diagn Interv Radiol. 2010;16(1):45–51.
39. Merkle EM, Boaz T, Kolokythas O, Haaga JR, Lewin JS, Brambs HJ. Metastases to the pancreas. Br J Radiol. 1998;71:1208–14.
40. Klein KA, Stephens DH, Welch TJ. CT characteristics of metastatic disease of the pancreas. Radiographics. 1998;18:369–78.
41. Xiuzhong Y, Yuan J, Mengsu Z, Rao Shengxiang BY. Solid pseudopapillary tumor of the pancreas: cross-sectional imaging and pathologic correlation. Pancreas. 2010;39(4):486–91.
42. Gandhi D, Sharma P, Parashar K, Kochar PS, Ahuja K, Sawhney H, et al. Solid pseudopapillary tumor of the pancreas: radiological and surgical review. Clin Imaging. 2020;67:101–7. Available from: https://doi.org/10.1016/j.clinimag.2020.06.008.
43. Buetow PC, Buck JL, Ros PR. Solid and papillary epithelial neoplasm of the pancreas: imaging-pathologic correlation in 56 cases. Radiology. 1996;199:707–11.
44. Cantisani V, Mortele KJ, Levy A, Glickman JN, Ricci P, Passariello R, et al. MR imaging features of solid pseudopapillary tumor of the pancreas in adult and pediatric patients. Am J Roentgenol. 2003;181(2):395–401.

Approach to Cystic Pancreatic Lesions

15

Martina Borzi, Clizia Gasparini, Maria Chiara Ambrosetti, and Giulia A. Zamboni

15.1 Introduction

Pancreatic cystic lesions (PCLs) are a large group of pancreatic lesions with different demographical, morphological, histological, and clinical characteristics.

The prevalence of PCLs is about 2.6% and increases with aging: the reported prevalence is 25% in the eighth decade and 37% in the ninth decade.

They are increasingly common incidental findings in asymptomatic patients undergoing imaging examinations for diseases unrelated to the pancreas.

PCLs are found in 2.6–3% of patients undergoing abdominal computed tomography (CT) [1] and in up to 49% of patients undergoing abdominal magnetic resonance imaging (MRI) for non-pancreatic indications.

Up to 50% of the patients may report mild or vague symptoms like abdominal pain or bloating, but generally they are unlikely to be directly related to the PCL [2].

PCLs represent a heterogeneous group of lesions that include two of the three known precursors of pancreatic cancer: intraductal papillary mucinous neoplasms (IPMN) and mucinous cystic neoplasms (MCNs). Approximately 8% of pancreatic cancers arise from these lesions, so careful surveillance and timely surgery represent an opportunity for early curative resection [3].

The standard workup of newly diagnosed PCLs starts from evaluating symptoms suggestive of malignancy, e.g., jaundice or significant weight loss. It continues with imaging evaluation with gadolinium-enhanced MRI with magnetic resonance cholangiopancreatography (MRCP) or pancreatic protocol CT.

After detecting a cystic lesion, it is essential to differentiate between a non-neoplastic cyst, most commonly a pseudocyst, and a neoplasm. Knowing the clinical history of the patient is vital because pseudocysts are most common in patients with a previous history of acute or chronic pancreatitis, abdominal trauma, or stone disease. With no history of pancreatitis, trauma, or stone

M. Borzi · C. Gasparini · G. A. Zamboni (✉)
Institute of Radiology, University of Verona, Policlinico GB Rossi, Verona, Italy
e-mail: giulia.zamboni@univr.it

M. C. Ambrosetti
Radiology Unit, Department of Pathology and Diagnostics, Azienda Ospedaliera Universitaria Integrata of Verona, Verona, Italy

© The Author(s), under exclusive license to Springer Nature Singapore Pte Ltd. 2025
B. Sureka (ed.), *Hepato-Pancreatico Biliary Imaging*, https://doi.org/10.1007/978-981-95-1699-5_15

Table 15.1 Classification of pancreatic cystic lesions [9, 10]

Epithelial non-neoplastic	*Epithelial neoplastic*
Mucinous non-neoplastic cyst	Intraductal papillary mucinous neoplasm
Lymphoepithelial cyst	Serous cystic adenoma (microcystic oligocystic/macrocystic)
Paraampullary duodenal wall cyst	VHL-associated serous cystic adenoma
Retention cyst	Mucinous cystic neoplasm
Congenital cyst (in malformation syndromes)	Cystic neuroendocrine tumor G1–G2
Endometrial cyst	Serous cystadenocarcinoma
	Acinar cell cystadenoma
	Cystic acinar cell carcinoma
	Cystic metastatic epithelial neoplasm
	Solid pseudopapillary neoplasm
	Accessory-splenic epidermoid cyst
	Cystic hamartoma
	Cystic teratoma (dermoid cyst)
	Cystic ductal adenocarcinoma
	Cystic pancreatoblastoma
	Others
Non-epithelial non-neoplastic	*Non-epithelial neoplastic*
Pancreatitis-associated pseudocyst	Benign non-epithelial neoplasm (e.g., lymphangioma)
Parasitic cyst	Malignant non-epithelial neoplasms (e.g., sarcomas)

disease, the most probable option is neoplasm. After the clinical evaluation, diagnostic imaging is fundamental to identify and characterize these lesions and perform a differential diagnosis. Regarding the imaging modalities used in the workup of PCLs, MRI is more accurate than CT in defining the nature and the internal structure of the cyst and the relationship with the ductal system. Endoscopic ultrasound (EUS) plays an important role in this diagnostic process because it allows for a detailed morphological study and fluid sampling for analysis.

Imaging features most often allow a correct classification and diagnosis of PCL. This is enhanced by the analysis of serum tumor markers, which can be used to diagnose IPMN and MCN and to differentiate them from other PCLs or malignant transformation [4, 5].

A correct diagnosis of IPMNs and MCNs is especially important because these are possible precursor lesions to pancreatic cancer [6], and they can be easily identified on cross-sectional imaging [7]. Given that approximately 8% of all pancreatic cancers are believed to arise from these lesions, radiological surveillance offers an opportunity for early cancer detection [8].

Correct identification and characterization of PCLs are fundamental because the prognosis of these lesions is good, and the interventions are curative if the diagnosis is timely.

The World Health Organization (WHO) classification divides PCLs into two main classes of tumors based on the presence of epithelial tissue (Table 15.1).

A more clinically oriented classification differentiates non-neoplastic and neoplastic cysts, more commonly defined as pancreatic cystic neoplasms (PCNs) (Table 15.2).

Table 15.2 Main characteristics of PCLs [11]

	BD-IPMN and MD-IPMN	MCN	SCN	Pseudocyst
Epidemiology	Most common PCL Mostly >50 years Low male prevalence	F >> M Fifth–sixth decade	F>M Seventh decade	History of pancreatitis, middle-aged men
Location	Often in the head, multifocal	Body and tail Single lesion	No prevalent location	No prevalent location
Morphology	MD: diffuse or segmental MPD dilatation without obstruction BD: cysts connected to the MPD	Single cyst, sometimes with septa, mural nodules, or calcifications	Most frequently microcystic 20–30% have a central stellate scar	Unilocular with clear content, inside or close to the pancreas
Cytology	Epithelial mucinous cells with variable atypia Mucin stain +	Ovarian-type stroma, mucinous cells with variable atypia Mucin stain +	Cubic cells Glycogen stain +	Inflammatory cells, histiocytes, no epithelial cells
Fluid content	High amylase, CEA >192 ng/mL	Amylase generally low CEA >192 ng/mL	Low amylase CEA <5 ng/mL	Amylase >250 U/L, CEA <5 ng/mL

MPD main pancreatic duct, *BD* branch duct, *MD* main duct, *IPMN* intraductal papillary mucinous cystic neoplasm, *SCN* serous cystic neoplasm, *MCN* mucinous cystic neoplasm, *CEA* carcinoembryonic antigen

15.2 Mucinous Cystic Lesions

According to the WHO classification, mucinous cystic lesions are divided into IPMN and MCN. Mucinous cystic lesions are especially significant for their malignant potential: imaging is important in detecting features suggestive of degeneration.

15.2.1 IPMN

The WHO has defined IPMNs as intraductal papillary mucinous neoplasms with tall, columnar, mucin-containing epithelium, with or without papillary projections, involving the main pancreatic duct (MPD) and/or branch ducts [12]. The prevalence of IPMNs increases with aging. The true prevalence of IPMN is unknown, ranging from 20% to 50% [13]. The most common location is the head of the pancreas, and in 20–30% of cases, they are multifocal. IPMNs are most commonly asymptomatic and generally discovered incidentally in the fifth decade of life with a low male dominance. However, some patients may present with recurrent non-specific or pancreatitis-like symptoms such as abdominal discomfort, abdominal pain, nausea, and vomiting. In patients with associated invasive carcinoma, symptoms such as weight loss, diabetes, and jaundice can be present.

IPMNs are divided into two main types: main duct IPMN (MD-IPMN) and branch duct IPMN (BD-IPMN). When both sites are involved, they are defined as mixed type IPMN (MT-IPMN).

15.2.2 Pathology

Depending on the microscopic morphological features, four types of IPMNs can be identified: gastric, intestinal, pancreaticobiliary, and oncocytic. The gastric type derives from the branch ducts, while the other three types derive from the main duct. There is a correlation between the histological background and type and the possibility of developing carcinoma of epithelial type.

IPMNs can be non-invasive or invasive neoplasms.

Non-invasive IPMNs are classified into low-/moderate-/high-grade dysplasia, and high-grade dysplasia is already considered carcinoma in situ.

The epithelial background plays an important role in defining the biology and prognosis of invasive IPMNs.

Tubular, colloid, and oncocytic invasive IPMNs have varying prognoses and arise from different epithelial subtypes. Colloid and oncocytic types have improved biology, whereas the tubular type has a course similar to pancreatic ductal adenocarcinoma (PDAC) [14]. Invasive IPMNs are classified as IPMNs associated with invasive carcinoma.

Most MD-IPMNs belong to the intestinal type and can evolve into invasive carcinoma, typically of the colloid type [15]. They are generally unifocal, but recent studies have demonstrated the possibility of potential synchronous or metachronous lesions [16].

The majority of BD-IPMNs are of gastric type. Gastric type is typically low grade, with a small percentage evolving to carcinoma. When it evolves into carcinoma, it is usually of tubular type and behaves like a PDAC [15]. The oncocytic type is characterized by complex arborizing papillae with delicate cores, oncocytic cells, and intraepithelial luminal formation. This type tends to form large lesions, relatively uncommon and with limited invasiveness. It has an excellent prognosis and a tendency for recurrence in the remnant pancreas years after the initial resection [17]. The pancreaticobiliary type is the least common, and it is considered the high-grade version of the gastric type. Invasive carcinoma associated with this type is usually tubular and aggressive [14].

15.2.3 MD-IPMN

Main duct IPMNs involve the main pancreatic duct and are most often observed in the proximal part of the gland (75%).

They are characterized by a dilatation of the duct of 1 centimeter or more because of the presence of mucus that can be found extruding from the ampulla.

Imaging has a central role in the detection and characterization of these lesions. The mucosal layer of IPMNs is generally thin, and when a nodule or a thickened portion is found, they are suggestive of malignant transformation, especially if enhancing after contrast administration. EUS can be used for the identification and definition of malignant characteristics, such as intracystic structures [18]. After contrast administration, the accuracy in detecting mural nodules is 98%. Another benefit of EUS is allowing cyst fluid collection with FNA, which is indicated in the case of indefinite imaging findings [14]. Cytological cyst fluid analysis has a high specificity (91%) but low sensitivity (65%) in differentiating benign and malignant IPMN. The sensitivity may be increased when the cyst wall and solid components are sampled [19].

15.2.4 Diagnostic Imaging

At US a dilated and hypoechoic main pancreatic duct without a cause of obstruction is usually visible. A differential diagnosis with chronic pancreatitis at US may be difficult.

At CT the main duct is dilated with hypodense content. Solid mural nodules isodense to the rest of the pancreatic parenchyma and with enhancement after contrast administration can be identified inside the main pancreatic duct (Fig. 15.1).

In invasive IPMNs CT can promptly assess lesion resectability, vessel infiltration, or presence of distant metastases.

MRI and in particular MCRP have replaced CT for studying and following up IPMNs.

The duct can be entirely or segmentally dilated, surrounded by pancreatic parenchyma that can be atrophic.

The duct content is hyperintense on T2-weighted images, while nodes and thickened components are hypointense and characterized by contrast enhancement, concerning for degeneration of IPMN (Fig. 15.2).

Even if endoscopic retrograde cholangiopancreatography (ERCP) can show with high sensitivity dilatation and filling defects of the pancreatic ducts due to possible solid nodules, signs suggestive of malignancy, it is no longer used for imaging and is used preferentially to confirm the presence of mucus in the main pan-

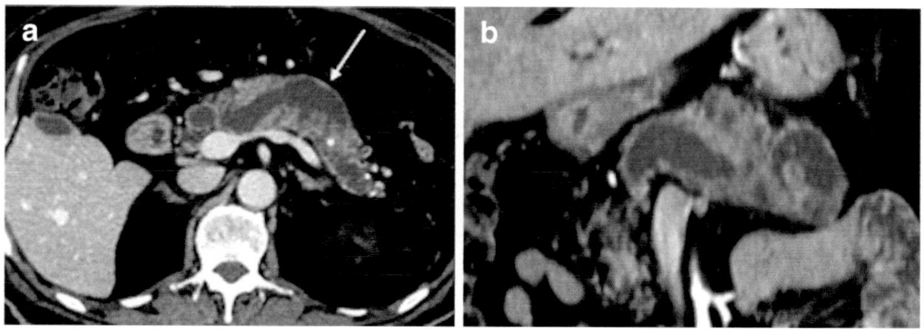

Fig. 15.1 A 77-year-old man with a MD-IPMN without signs of degeneration. Postcontrast CT axial (**a**) and coronal (**b**) images in the arterial phase show dilatation of the whole main pancreatic duct (arrow)

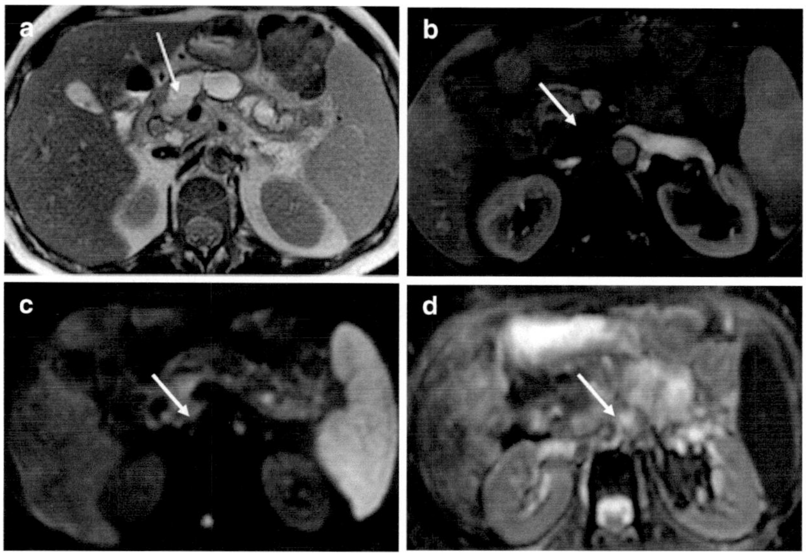

Fig. 15.2 A 67-year-old woman with MD-IPMN with signs of degeneration. (**a**) T2-weighted image shows a hypointense solid tissue (arrow) inside the dilated main pancreatic duct. (**b**) In the arterial phase, enhancing the solid tissue is visualized (arrow). On DWI (**c**) the solid tissue is hyperintense (arrow) with restricted diffusion in the Apparent Diffusion Coefficient map (**d**) (arrow)

creatic duct or at the papilla and to perform biopsies.

The presence of mucus is considered a confirmatory finding of IPMN.

15.2.5 BD-IPMN

BD-IPMNs are defined as a grape-like cyst (>5 mm) that communicates with the MPD [20]. BD-IPMNs account for 41–64% of IPMNs and can be multifocal, with a predilection for the uncinate process. They have a lower risk of malignant progression (7–42%), but their multifocality (40%) and high post-surgical recurrence rate (7–8%) are insidious elements in the choice of management. Multifocality has not been proven to increase the risk of malignancy [20] (Fig. 15.3).

Macroscopically the lesion is surrounded by a thin layer of pancreatic parenchyma and can consist of a single cyst or conglomerated communicating cysts separated by multiple septa. Dilatation of the main pancreatic duct can be associated because mucus obstructs the drainage of pancreatic juice from the upstream pancreatic duct. Atrophy of the pancreas may be severe. Similar to MD-IPMN, imaging is the first choice for diagnosis. At CT, US, and MRI with MRCP, the tumor appears as clustered small cysts with a lobulated margin with septa or as a single unilocular cyst. When a tumor is present, it is frequently hardly seen because it is generally flat. At ERCP branch ducts are cystically dilated with mucin appearing as elongated bandlike strings and sometimes as nodular filling defects. Duodenal endoscopy can show thick mucus oozing through the duodenal papilla. The duodenal

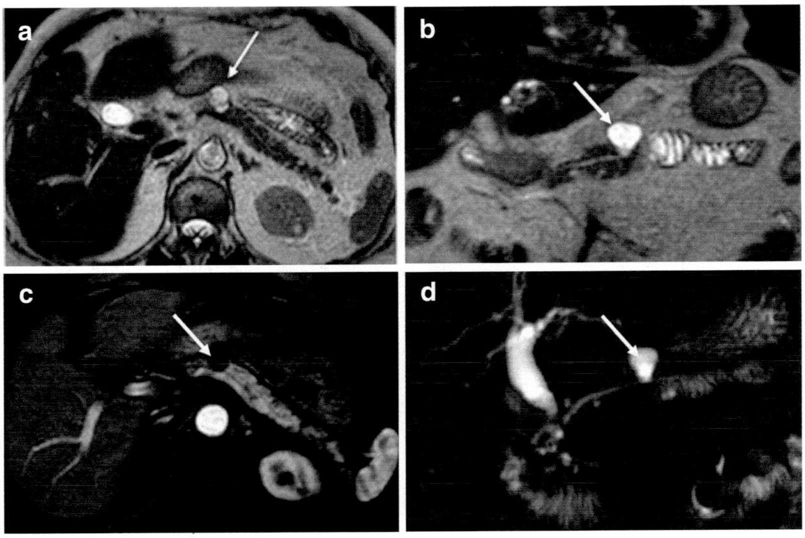

Fig. 15.3 A 76-year-old woman with multiple BD-IPMNs without signs of degeneration. (**a**) T2-weighted axial and (**b**) coronal images with hyperintense dilatations of BD (arrow). (**c**) In the arterial phase, no enhancing solid tissue is seen inside the BD-IPMN (arrow). (**d**) On MRCP multiple BD dilatations without filling defects are visualized (arrow)

papilla protrudes into the lumen of the duodenum, easily visible at CT or MR. A bulging duodenal papilla and a severe dilatation of the main pancreatic duct are frequent in the malignant form.

15.2.6 Diagnostic Imaging

The main characteristic of these tumors, such as MD-IPMN, is the communication with branch pancreatic ducts.

At US small thin-walled pancreatic cysts or hypoechoic ducts are visible. Polypoid mural nodes or mucinous luminal filling defects can be found, suggestive for malignancy. Mural nodes or mucin globules can be hyperechoic and therefore difficult to distinguish from the adjacent pancreatic parenchyma.

CT typically shows multiple hypodense pancreatic cystic lesions. Communication with pancreatic branch ducts can be difficult to demonstrate.

MRI most commonly shows normal parenchyma, with marked dilatation of the side branches, that appear like multiple cystic masses. These aspects make IPMN similar to serous cystic neoplasm (SCN), and once again the communication with the main duct is discriminatory of BD-IPMNs (Fig. 15.4).

Solid mural nodes or wall thickenings are concerning for degeneration of IPMN, especially if enhancing after contrast administration (Figs. 15.5 and 15.6).

Also, in this case, ERCP can be useful to show mucus slowly flowing within the ducts.

15.2.7 Differential Diagnosis

The differential diagnosis of IPMNs is based on the age of the patient, the clinical presentation, and the radiological findings [21, 22]. The most likely differentials include chronic pancreatitis, mucinous cystadenoma, serous cystadenoma (SCA), simple cysts, and pseudocysts [22]. Side branch dilatation is usually found in the head and uncinate process, and it is the pattern that causes most diagnostic difficulties [20]. This pattern is similar to pseudocyst, simple cyst, or serous cystadenoma. EUS performed to demonstrate the presence of mural nodules and communication with the MPD and analysis of the cyst fluid for cytology, extracellular mucin, and carcinoembryonic antigen (CEA) levels may help in establishing the diagnosis [23]. BD-IPMNs also enter into differential diagnosis with SCNs of the small olygocystic type. EUS-FNA is sometimes necessary to evaluate the CEA level. If a very low CEA level and acellular fluid

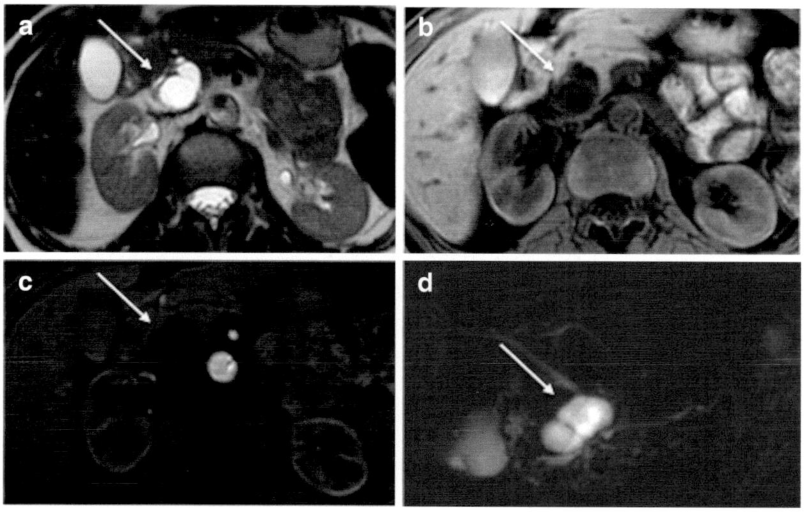

Fig. 15.4 A 64-year-old woman with BD-IPMN without signs of degeneration. (**a**) The T2-weighted image shows a hyperintense mass in the head of the pancreas (arrow). (**b**) On the T1-weighted fat-suppressed image, the lesion is completely hypointense (arrow). (**c**) Postcontrast T1-weighted fat-suppressed image, in the arterial phase, shows no enhancement. (**d**) On MRCP the communication between BD-IPMN and the main pancreatic duct is visible (arrow)

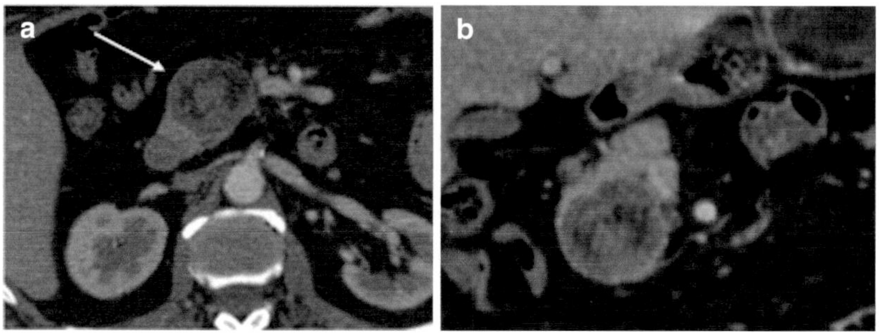

Fig. 15.5 A 66-year-old man with a degenerated BD-IPMN of the body of the pancreas. Axial- (**a**) and coronal (**b**) arterial-phase CT images show an enhancing solid component inside the lesion (arrow)

are found, these favor the diagnosis of SCN. In the presence of ductal dilatation, calcifications, and parenchymal atrophy, differentiating IPMN from chronic pancreatitis becomes important [24]. Sex, age, and lifestyle habits such as alcohol consumption and smoking suggest chronic pancreatitis, while jaundice and diabetes are suggestive of malignancy. It is difficult to differentiate IPMNs (MD and BD) from MCNs because tumor cells of MCN have the same cytology as IPMN [25]. MCNs are more common in young asymptomatic women, while patients with the malignant variant may be a few years older. On the other side, MD-IPMN, which occurs commonly in the pancreatic head, can be single or multifocal and is more common in men [16]. Another point that differentiates BD-IPMN from MCNs is that BD-IPMNs are mainly found in the uncinate process.

15.2.8 Prognosis, Treatment, and Follow-Up Strategies

The management of MD-IPMN and BD-IPMN is currently based on clinical and imaging features, to detect promptly malignant degeneration. The most used guidelines for managing IPMNs are the Fukuoka guidelines, which recognize two layers of criteria to assess the possible malignant

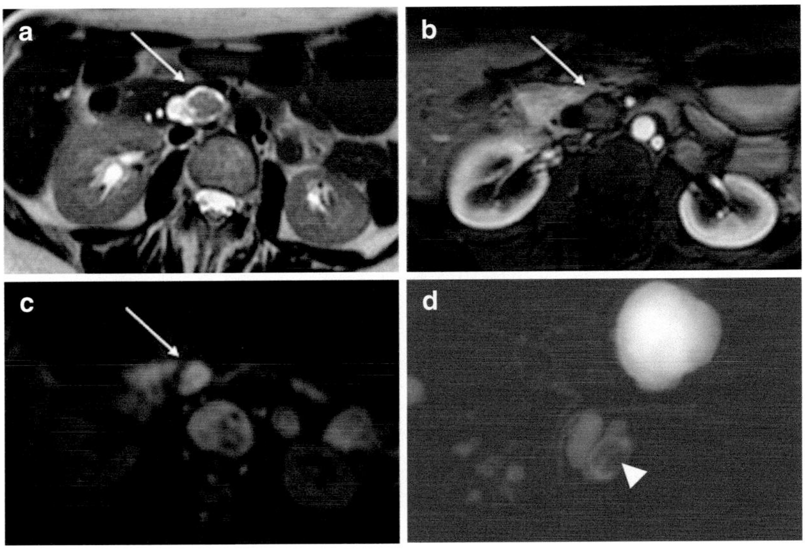

Fig. 15.6 A 57-year-old woman with degenerated BD-IPMN in the pancreatic head. (**a**) T2-weighted image shows a hyperintense lesion with internal hypointense solid tissue (arrow). (**b**) The arterial phase shows enhancement of the solid tissue (arrow). (**c**) On DWI the solid tissue is hyperintense. (**d**) MRCP demonstrates filling defects inside the BD-IPMN (arrow) and the communication of the lesion with the main pancreatic duct (arrowhead)

behavior of IPMNs: "high-risk stigmata" and "worrisome features." *High-risk stigmata* are indicative of malignancy and include obstructive jaundice, enhancing solid component, and main pancreatic duct >10 mm.

Worrisome features are indications pointing toward malignancy and include cyst size ≥3 cm, enhancing mural nodule <5 mm, thickened enhanced cyst walls, MPD caliber of 5–9 mm, abrupt change in the MPD caliber with distal pancreatic atrophy, lymphadenopathy, elevated serum levels of carbohydrate antigen (CA)19-9 and a rapid rate of cyst growth >5 mm/2 years [26].

Over the years, the treatment of MD-IPMN has not changed: most patients with MD-IPMNs undergo tumor resection if they are fit for surgery at the time of diagnosis. In patients fit for surgery, the presence of one or more high-risk stigmata makes surgery mandatory. After resection, patients undergo radiological surveillance every 6 months in case of family history of PDAC, surgical margins with high-grade dysplasia, and non-intestinal type IPMN. Patients without these risk factors undergo surveillance every 6–12 months.

Regarding BD-IPMN, their management is controversial and evolved over the years. After the Sendai consensus guidelines, the strategy has become more conservative in terms of surveillance. Once a patient is diagnosed with a BD-IPMN, surveillance is recommended, with timing based mainly on the size of the cyst and its growth. MRI is the first choice to reduce radiation exposure. When the size is <1 cm, patients should undergo surveillance every 6 months for the first 2 years and then every 2 years, in case of no pathological findings; between 1 and 2 cm every 6 months for the first year, yearly for the second year, and every 2 years after the third year; between 2 and 3 cm every 3–6 months, then yearly lifelong; and when the size is >3 cm every 3–6 months [9]. When one of the elements cited above is found, then surgery becomes the first choice for patients who are fit for surgery. The guidelines recommend surgery only in case of one or more high-risk stigmata or one or more worrisome features or one of the following findings: mural nodule ≥5 mm, suspicious MPD, and suspicious cytology. In case of suspected malignancy, oncologically sound surgery should be performed. In multifocal IPMNs the most suspicious lesions must be all removed. A total pancreatectomy is only recommended in the case of multiple worrisome features throughout the pancreas or post-surgical recurrence in the remnant pancreas. After surgery, surveillance follows the same timelines as MD-IPMN, basing the decision on the presence or not of risk factors. Around 40% of BD-IPMNs are multifocal, and this increases the rate of early recurrence of IPMN in the remnant pancreas. This is the reason why lifelong surveillance should be performed. A large observational study by Marchegiani et al. found a 5-year survival after resection of 77% for all IPMNs, in particular 69% for MD-IPMN and 82% for BD-IPMN, with a median survival of 17 months. In the case of postoperative pathological diagnosis of invasive IPMN, the overall survival decreases significantly from 77% to 30–42%. All patients with IPMN-associated adenocarcinoma have a poor survival rate because at the time of diagnosis 53% of cases have lymph node metastases, 58% peri-neural invasion, and 33% vascular invasion [27].

15.2.9 Mucinous Cystic Neoplasms

Mucinous cystic neoplasms represent about 4% of all PCNs. These neoplasms are mostly diagnosed at the age of 40–60 years, with a very strong female prevalence [28].

MCNs are most often located in the body-tail of the pancreas.

The discovery of many MCNs is incidental, if not the patient may present with non-specific symptoms such as abdominal discomfort or pain. Patients may suffer also from anorexia, obstructive jaundice, or weight loss, suggestive of malignancy.

15.2.10 Pathology

The pathogenesis of MCNs is uncertain, and these lesions share clinical and pathological characteristics with biliary and ovarian tumors.

MCNs are defined as mucin-producing cysts that are surrounded by ovarian-type stroma [29]. Macroscopically these neoplasms can have unilocular or multilocular cystic architecture, with large cystic spaces ranging in size from one to several centimeters. The presence of septa is also common. The masses show well-defined margins and contain mucin or mucin with hemorrhagic material. The macrocystic multilocular pattern is the most typical, while a unilocular pattern is common with other cystic lesions. These tumors do not communicate with the pancreatic ductal system and have thick fibrotic walls that may show calcifications. The presence of mural nodules or papillary projections and septa is suggestive of malignancy [30].

According to the Mayo Clinic classification, these tumors are divided into *mucinous cystadenomas* (65% of MCNs) which contain a uniform single layer of benign columnar mucinous cells, *non-invasive, proliferative* MCNs (30% of MCNs) composed of various degrees of atypia, dysplasia but without tissue invasion, and *mucinous cystadenocarcinomas* characterized by stromal invasion beyond the epithelium [31].

Large tumor size (>4 cm), associated with mural nodules, mass, eggshell calcification, asymmetric thickened wall, and age are risk factors for malignancy of MCNs [32].

15.2.11 Diagnostic Imaging

Given the potential for progressing to malignancy, a correct diagnosis is mandatory. Cross-sectional imaging is unable to distinguish MCNs with malignant epithelium from benign ones, unless in case of vascular invasion, adjacent organ infiltration, or metastatic disease, but may identify signs of malignancy.

At US macrocystic multilocular lesions appear as defined masses, hypoechoic, with variably thin septa, thickened wall, and rim calcifications. On CT, the density of MCNs depends on their content, from mucoid to hemorrhagic fluid. The precontrast scan can easily show rim calcifications. After contrast administration, solid components and septa may have delayed enhancement due to

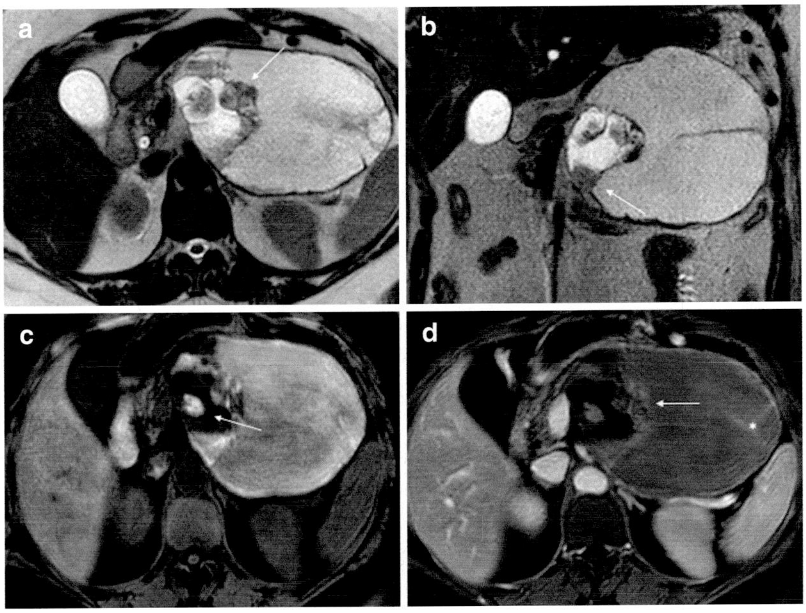

Fig. 15.7 A 58-year-old woman with mucinous cystadenocarcinoma in the pancreatic tail. (**a**, **b**) Axial (**a**) and coronal (**b**) T2-weighted fat-suppressed images show a large multilocular cystic lesion with hypointense solid elements (arrow) (**c**). T1-weighted fat-suppressed image demonstrates hypertense portions due to the presence of mucin or blood (arrow). (**d**) Portal venous T1-weighted image shows enhancing soft tissue elements and septa (*)

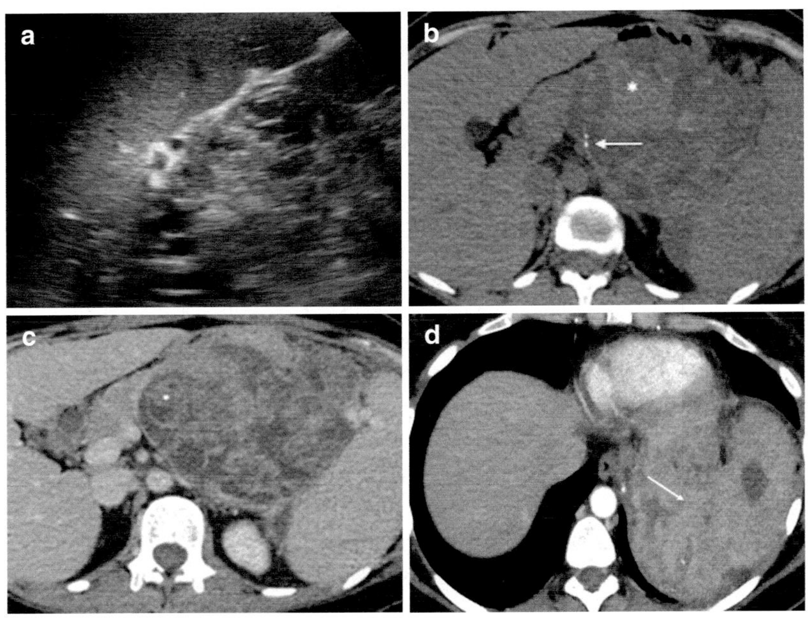

Fig. 15.8 A 35-year-old woman with mucinous cystadenocarcinoma. (**a**) US shows a large mass of the pancreas adjacent to the spleen with a heterogeneous structure. (**b**) Precontrast CT scan demonstrates lamellar calcifications (arrow) and hyperdense portions due to recent bleeding (*). (**c**) Portal venous phase CT better demonstrates enhancing soft tissue elements (arrow). (**d**) The tumor invades the splenic parenchyma (arrow)

their fibrous composition [10]. Malignancy signs that can be identified on CT are walls thickened more than 1–2 mm, septa, rim calcifications, and mural nodules, which have a 95% probability of malignancy [30]. CT also is useful in assessing local invasion and metastatic disease (Figs. 15.7 and 15.8).

MRI provides a better morphological characterization of MCNs. On T1-weighted unenhanced images, the signal is variable, depending on the lesion content. On T2-weighed sequences, the content is hyperintense and septa hypointense. After contrast administration, especially in the portal venous phase, similar to CT, septa, mural

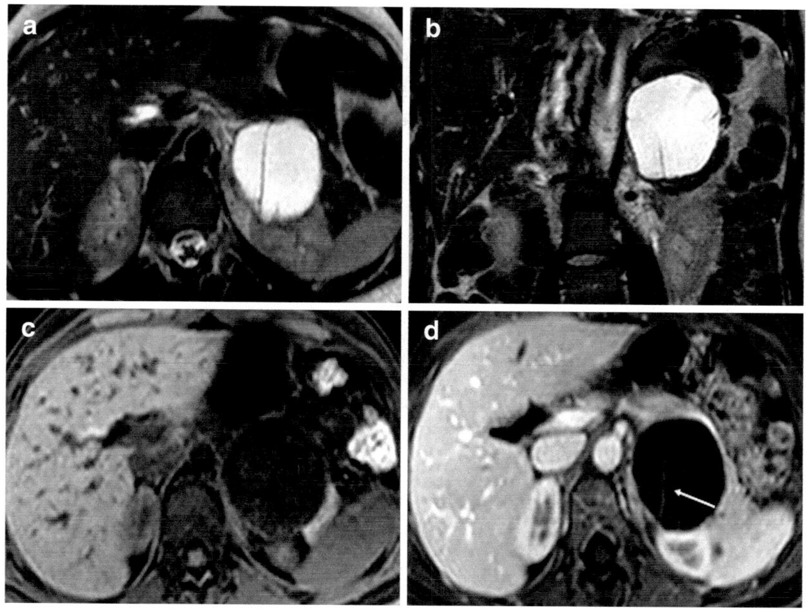

Fig. 15.9 A 31-year-old woman with mucinous cystadenoma in the pancreatic tail. (**a**, **b**) Axial (**a**) and coronal (**b**) T2-weighted images show a rounded multilocular cystic mass with hypointense septa. (**c**) On the T1-weighted fat-suppressed image, the mass is homogeneously hypointense. (**d**) Portal venous T1-weighted image demonstrates enhancement of thin septa (arrow) and the absence of enhancing soft tissue elements

nodules, and solid components can be better visualized [33] (Fig. 15.9). ERCP is useful for the visualization of the communication between the lesion and the pancreatic duct, important in the differentiation between IPMN and MCNs [22]. ERCP also may reveal the deformity of pancreatic and/or biliary ducts, a suggestive sign of malignancy. However, this imaging modality is not routinely part of the assessment of MCNs, because MRCP, in a non-invasive way and with fewer risks, can demonstrate the lack of communication with the pancreatic ductal system. EUS is often employed in the assessment of MCNs since lesion architecture and the remaining pancreatic parenchyma can easily be examined [34]. EUS findings must be correlated with clinical history, laboratory findings, and cross-sectional imaging studies to best define the tumor type. Furthermore, EUS allows cyst content aspiration and wall biopsy. MCNs' cystic fluid aspirates typically show increased CEA titers and low amylase levels [35].

15.2.12 Differential Diagnosis

The differential diagnosis of macrocystic unilocular MCNs includes pseudocysts, oligocystic serous neoplasms, IPMNs, solid pseudopapillary, and cystic endocrine tumors. In the case of pseudocysts, a clinical history of pancreatitis and laboratory data is essential for a correct differential diagnosis [36]. Macrocystic MCNs can be indistinguishable from oligocystic SNCs, so in most cases, it is impossible to make a preoperative accurate diagnosis (Fig. 15.10). Branch-duct IPMNs may mimic MCNs, and the differential diagnosis is based on the demonstration of communication with the pancreatic ductal system. In neuroendocrine and pseudopapillary tumors, the cystic component is a sign of tumor degeneration.

15.2.13 Prognosis, Treatment, and Follow-Up Strategies

All MCNs should be considered as premalignant conditions. As defined by the Fukuoka guidelines, surgical resection is recommended for all surgically fit patients, and the first-line surgical approach is typically a distal pancreatectomy, given the preferential MCN localization in the pancreatic body or tail. Parenchyma-sparing resections (central pancreatectomy) and distal pancreatectomy with spleen preservation can be

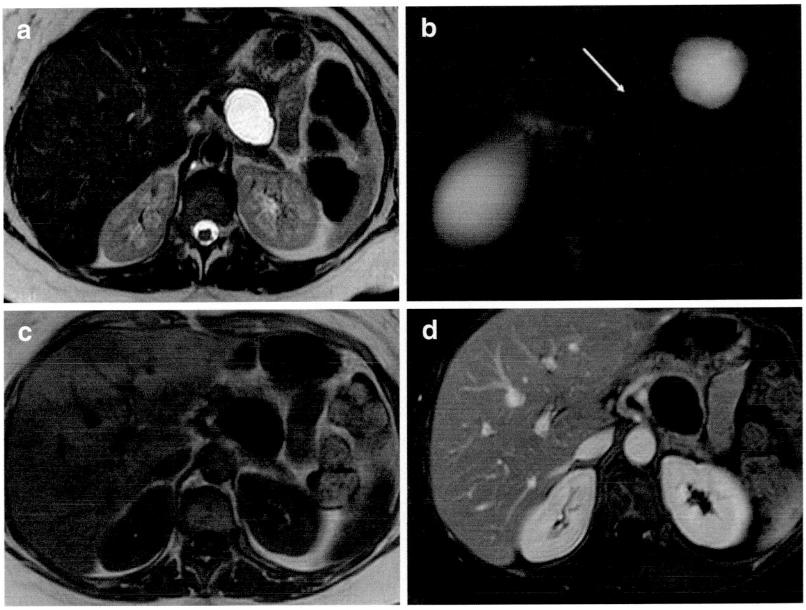

Fig. 15.10 A 55-year-old woman with unilocular mucinous cystadenoma in the pancreatic tail. (**a**) T2-weighted image shows a rounded thick-walled cyst. (**b**) On MR cholangiopancreatographic image, the main pancreatic duct is not dilated (*arrow*). (**c**) On the T1-weighted fat-suppressed image, the lesion is homogeneously hypointense, and soft tissue elements are not visualized. (**d**) Portal venous T1-weighted image demonstrates faint wall enhancement

considered in patients with MCNs smaller than 4 cm without mural nodules [21]. However, a more conservative approach has been established over time. According to European guidelines, MCNs larger than 4 cm should undergo resection. Also, symptomatic MCNs or those with mural nodules should be resected, regardless of their size. MCNs smaller than 4 cm, in the absence of risk features, can undergo surveillance [25].

Post-resection follow-up is not strictly necessary in patients with non-invasive MCNs, since these neoplasms usually do not recur locally or at a distance after complete surgical resection. On the other hand, patients with invasive MCN should be followed up with CT or MRI every 6 months after resection, to detect local recurrence or metastases [37]. Five-year disease survival rate of patients with invasive MCNs is 57% [32].

15.2.14 Serous Cystic Neoplasm

SCNs represent about 30% of all cystic neoplasms of the pancreas. The mean age at diagnosis is 62 years, with a female predilection (65%) [38].

In most cases SCNs are asymptomatic, and the diagnosis is incidental, these lesions being identified at cross-sectional imaging done for unrelated symptoms. Whenever present, the most common symptoms are abdominal discomfort and weight loss.

SCNs can arise in any portion of the pancreas but are mostly located in the head [33].

15.2.15 Pathology

The pathogenesis of SCNs is uncertain; however, these lesions share ultrastructural characteristics with normal centro-acinar cells.

According to the WHO classification, serous cystic neoplasms are divided into SCA and serous cystadenocarcinoma, but reported cases of malignancy are extremely rare, the reason why SNCs should be considered benign [10].

SCA may be associated with von Hippel-Lindau syndrome, a rare autosomal dominantly inherited disease caused by mutation of the tumor suppressor gene VHL and characterized by multi-organ involvement [39]. Also in sporadic SCAs, VHL loss of function mutations may play a role in tumor development [40].

SCNs are variable in size between 1 and 25 cm [38]. The lesions are well demarcated from the surrounding parenchyma and have no communication with the pancreatic ducts. These tumors usually are unifocal, but in von Hippel-Lindau disease can be multifocal and can involve the entire pancreatic parenchyma. Macroscopically SCNs may have the following patterns: microcystic, macrocystic, mixed micro-macrocystic, and solid. The most frequent is the microcystic pattern (70%) characterized by a solitary multicystic mass with a honeycombing architecture. The lesion presents a thin wall and thin multiple septa, in some cases oriented toward a central scar which is considered pathognomonic for SCA [41]. The central scar can present a stellate pattern of calcifications. In the macrocystic pattern, previously also called oligocystic, the mass is characterized by a small number of cysts >2 cm, sometimes only one. In the solid variant, the tumor is a well-demarcated nodule with very small cysts and multiple thick fibrous septa. The mixed pattern has the characteristics of both microcystic and macrocystic types.

Histologically, all patterns of SNCs present cystic spaces lined by a cubic flat epithelium with clear cytoplasm glycogen-rich cells.

15.2.16 Diagnostic Imaging

The majority of SNCs are initially diagnosed incidentally on cross-sectional abdominal imaging.

In most cases, US shows a multilobulated mass with a honeycombing architecture due to the presence of multiple septa lining cystic spaces [35].

However, on US a microcystic pattern lesion, due to the proximity of septa, may simulate a solid pancreatic lesion. Also, sometimes, the unilocular macrocystic pattern could be confused with mucinous cystadenoma [42].

In the diagnostic evaluation of SCNs, CT is useful for spatial resolution, availability, and low cost. On unenhanced CT images, lesions with a microcystic pattern show lobulated margins and are homogeneously hypodense or isodense to the adjacent parenchyma with well recognizable, whenever present, central calcifications [42]. After contrast media administration, the internal septa exhibit contrast uptake, and the central scar is hypodense due to its fibrous nature, with retention of contrast in the portal and delayed phases. The solid variant, after contrast injection, has the appearance of an enhancing solid pancreatic mass due to its prevalence of vascularized septa over the cystic component; these features may make difficult the differentiation from neuroendocrine neoplasms. The macrocystic pattern when unilocular can be indistinguishable from MCNs. MRI plays a key role in the diagnosis of SCNs thanks to the fact that the multiplanar sequences and the use of contrast medium allow to better investigate the morphology and the constitution of the lesion. In addition, the use of MRCP is essential to prove the lack of communication with the main pancreatic duct. Microcystic SCNs show a typical honeycombing architecture with a thin wall (less than 2 mm). The T2-weighted multiplanar images allow evaluating the cystic nature of the lesion showing a hyperintense mass with hypointense septa. Sometimes a hypointense central scar is visualized [42] (Fig. 15.11). After contrast administration, MRI provides the same information as CT, with enhancement of septa and walls. The main limit of MRI is the low sensitivity for calcifications, which are better detected with CT. Macrocystic types are lobulated cystic-like masses, hyperintense on T2-weighted sequences (Fig. 15.12). These aspects are non-specific, and MRI does not allow to differentiate them from MCN [43]. EUS can supply additional information when CT or MRI

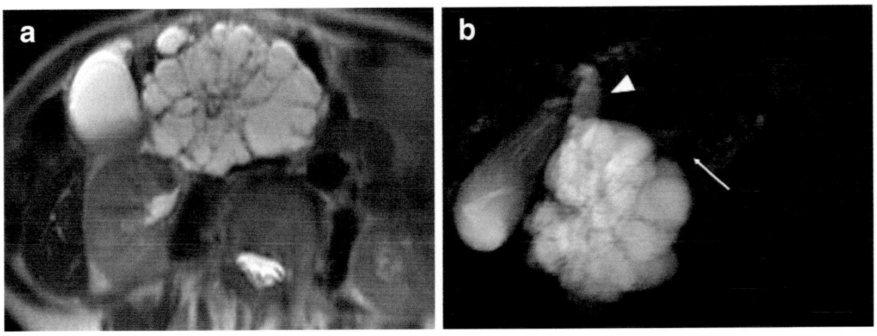

Fig. 15.11 A 75-year-old woman with a microcystic serous cystadenoma in the pancreatic head. (**a**) Axial T2-weighted image shows a lobulated cystic lesion with multiple hypointense septa oriented toward a central scar. (**b**) MR cholangiopancreatographic image demonstrates the dilation of the common bile duct (*arrowhead*) and the main pancreatic duct due to the large size of the lesion (*arrow*)

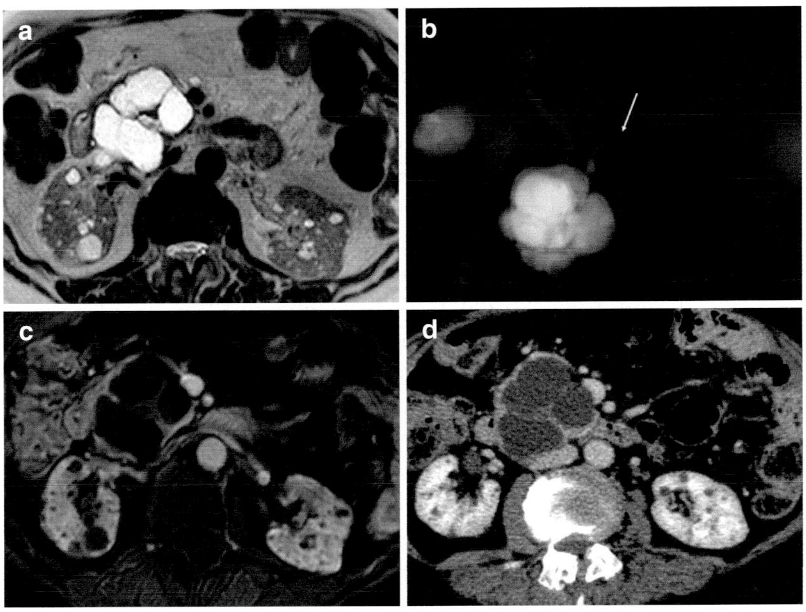

Fig. 15.12 A 74-year-old woman with macrocystic serous cystadenoma. (**a**) T2-weighted image shows a hyperintense mass with cystic spaces >2 cm and thin hypointense septa. (**b**) MRCP image demonstrates a regular and not-dilated main pancreatic duct (arrow). (**c**, **d**) After contrast injection on T1-weighted fat-suppressed image (**c**) and on CT (**d**), enhancement of the septa is visualized

does not allow a definitive diagnosis. EUS, with its high resolution, accurately shows every cystic element such as margins, wall, internal architecture, and the lack of communication between the cyst and the main pancreatic duct. In addition, it is possible to perform EUS-guided FNA for cytological and biochemical analyses of cystic fluid. The fluid content of SCAs is colorless and watery (non-viscous) and shows low levels of tumor markers such as CEA [44].

15.2.17 Differential Diagnosis

The differential diagnosis of SCNs includes other cystic pancreatic lesions such as pseudocysts, IPMNs, and MCNs. Solid variants of SCNs may simulate solid neoplasms such as neuroendocrine tumors, pancreatic ductal adenocarcinomas, and solid pseudopapillary neoplasms. For unilocular serous cysts, the main differential diagnosis is represented by pseudocysts: for the correct diagnosis,

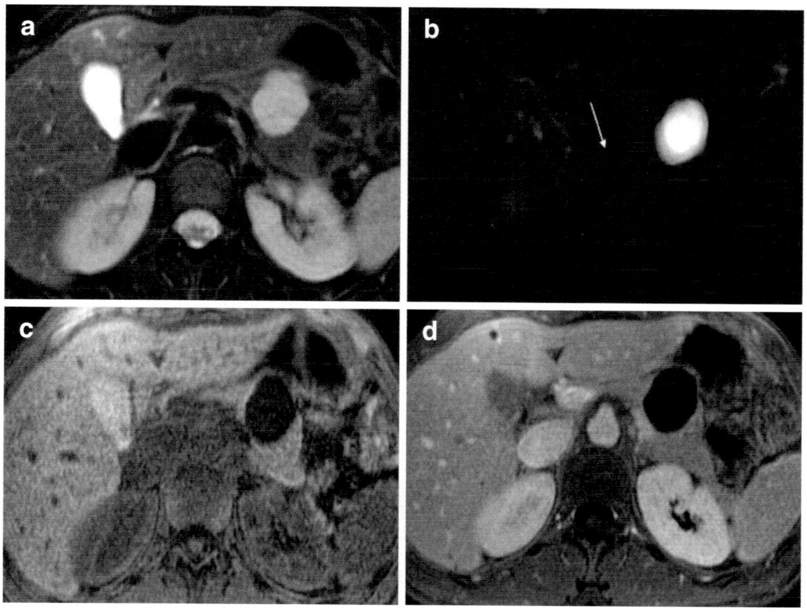

Fig. 15.13 A 33-year-old woman with unilocular serous cystadenoma. (**a**) T2-weighted fat-suppressed image shows a smoothly marginated cyst with clear fluid content. (**b**) On MRCP the main pancreatic duct is regular and is not dilated (*arrow*). (**c**, **d**) On the T1-weighted fat-suppressed images before (**c**), and after contrast injection (**d**) the tumor is hypointense without septa or thickening of the cyst wall. Imaging features of this lesion overlap with those of unilocular mucinous cystadenoma

it is fundamental to investigate a clinical history of pancreatitis [45]. In addition, pseudocysts affect more often the body or the tail of the pancreas and on T1-weighted images may have mixed signal, not completely fluid. Another differential diagnosis of oligocystic SCNs is MCNs, but in most cases, these cannot be pre-operatively differentiated because both can have a unilocular structure (Fig. 15.13). For the differential diagnosis of IPMNs, it is fundamental to evaluate the communication with the pancreatic duct system [46].

15.2.18 Prognosis, Treatment, and Follow-Up Strategies

SCNs are generally considered benign with slow growth and a small risk of malignancy (<3%) [47] so surveillance is recommended. According to the European guidelines, asymptomatic patients should be followed up for 1 year. After 1 year a follow-up based on symptoms is recommended [25]. In symptomatic patients, or when the differentiation from MCNs is not certain, surgical resection is recommended.

The prognosis of all variants of SCN is excellent, and the overall 5-year survival is almost 100%. In the literature, the reported cases of cystadenocarcinoma are exceedingly rare, and its biological behavior is still not clear [48].

15.2.19 Solid Pseudopapillary Neoplasm

Solid pseudopapillary tumors (SPNs) represent about 4% of pancreatic cystic lesions. A neoplasm with pseudopapillary characteristics was reported for the first time in 1959 by Franz, but only in 1996 WHO renamed this tumor SPN. In most cases, SPN affects young women and is located in the pancreatic body or tail. Although the disease is generally asymptomatic, sometimes patients present compressive symptoms, due to lesion size, such as nausea and epigastric pain.

15.2.20 Pathology

The pathogenesis of this lesion is unclear. Many authors have suggested that SPNs originate from multipotent primordial cells, whereas others suggest an extra-pancreatic origin, from genital ridge angle-related cells [49]. SPNs typically show benign behavior but in some cases can present malignant degeneration [50]. WHO classification defines an SPN as a solid-pseudopapillary carcinoma when this neoplasm presents the following criteria of malignancy: vascular and nerve invasion or lymph node and liver metastases.

Macroscopically, SPN is a large, well-encapsulated mass that can contain necrosis, hemorrhage, and cystic changes, due to tumor degeneration. Microscopically, SPN is characterized by two histological patterns: solid and papillary. Solid areas are formed by a single layer of neoplastic cells, while the papillary component is characterized by a fibrovascular stalk surrounded by several layers of epithelial cells [51].

15.2.21 Diagnostic Imaging

CT shows a well-encapsulated mass with a variable solid and cystic component. After contrast media administration, peripheral enhancing solid areas are emphasized while cystic spaces, usually central, do not enhance [52]. On MRI, SPTs present a heterogeneous signal on T1- and T2-weighted images due to their complex nature. On T1-weighted sequences, it is possible to well recognize hemorrhage, whenever present, because it shows high signal intensity and a fluid-debris level [53] (Figs. 15.14 and 15.15). EUS with FNA can be useful in a pre-operative evaluation to distinguish SPT from other pancreatic cystic lesions.

15.2.22 Differential Diagnosis

The differential diagnosis of SPNs includes pseudocysts, neuroendocrine tumors, and ductal adenocarcinomas.

For pseudocysts, clinical history and laboratory data must be considered. Suggestive criteria of SPNs are a mass found in a young woman, the lack of a clinical history of pancreatitis, and a lesion characterized by variable solid and cystic components. In the case of neuroendocrine tumors, the main feature is the strong hypervascularity after contrast injection on the arterial phase. Ductal adenocarcinoma is most typical in elderly men, and it has infiltrative growth.

15.2.23 Prognosis, Treatment, and Follow-Up Strategies

A surgical approach is the treatment of choice for SPN, based on the potential malignancy of these tumors. Complete resection is usually curative, with a 97% 5-year overall survival rate [54].

15.2.24 Cystic Degeneration of Solid Tumor

Ductal adenocarcinoma is in most cases a solid tumor; however, it may exhibit cystic degeneration, due to central tumor necrosis or an obstruction of secondary ducts with the generation of small retention cysts. It is important to consider, especially in the differential diagnosis with other cystic lesions, that ductal adenocarcinoma is a hypovascular infiltrative neoplasm with possible infiltration and obstruction of main pancreatic or common bile ducts [55].

Endocrine neoplasms may present cystic formation due to tumor degeneration too. They can show a unilocular or a multilocular cyst pattern. Typically these neoplasms are asymptomatic and non-functional [56]. On CT, after contrast media administration, cystic portions do not present contrast enhancement with only a rim of the enhancing tissue in the arterial phase [57] (Fig. 15.16). These masses may be indistinguishable on imaging from other cystic lesions, but a correct diagnosis can be achieved with Fine Needle Aspiration Cytology and with the demonstration of endocrine markers such as synaptophysin and chromogranin A.

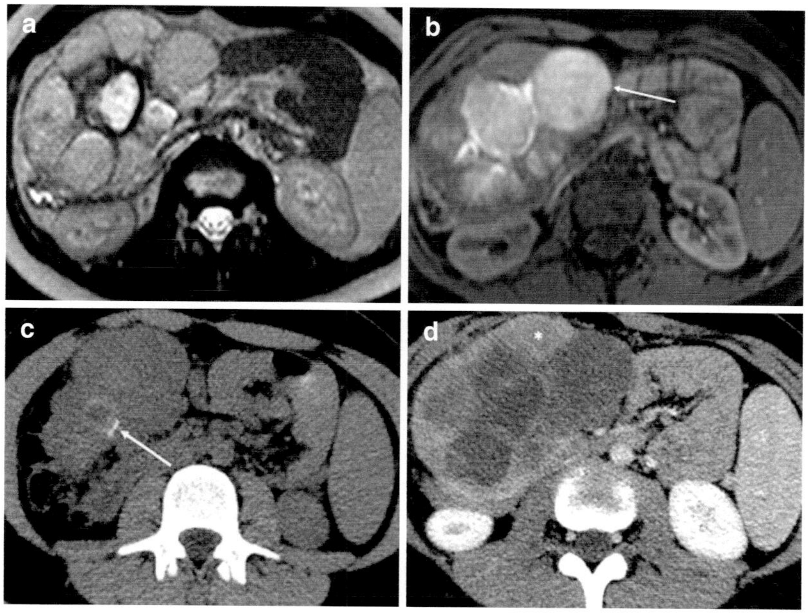

Fig. 15.14 A 14-year-old girl with a solid pseudopapillary tumor in the pancreatic head. (**a**) T2-weighted image shows a large encapsulated and multilocular mass characterized by cystic portions. (**b**) On T1-weighted fat-suppressed image, the hemorrhagic component appears hyperintense (*arrow*). (**c**) Precontrast CT scan demonstrates some calcifications (*arrow*). (**d**) Portal venous CT scan better depicts central cystic spaces with enhancing peripherical solid areas (*)

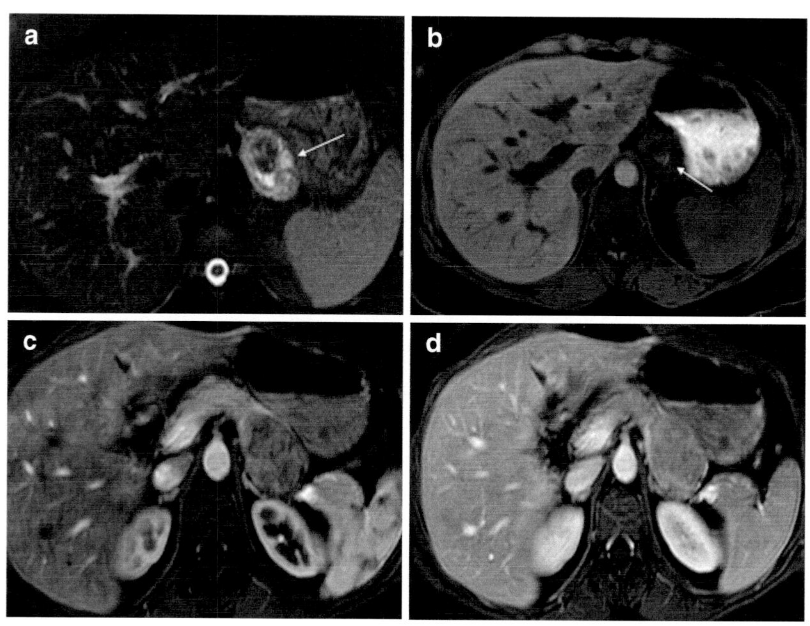

Fig. 15.15 A 31-year-old woman with a solid pseudopapillary tumor in the pancreatic body. (**a**) A T2-weighted fat-suppressed image demonstrates a solid lesion with cystic component (arrow). (**b**) A T1-weighted fat-suppressed image depicts a focal hemorrhage (arrow). (**c**, **d**) Arterial (**c**) and portal venous (**d**) phase T1-weighted images show a gradual accumulation of contrast material in the tumor

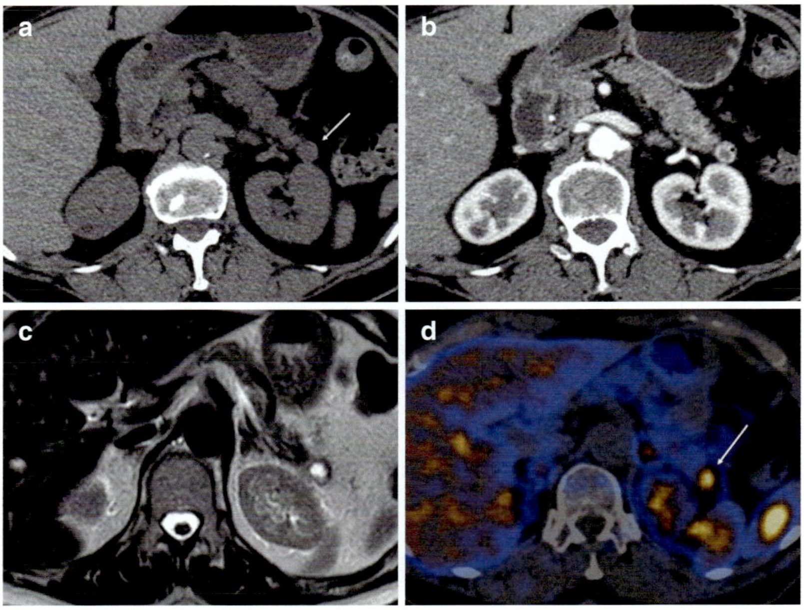

Fig. 15.16 A 64-year-old woman with cystic pancreatic neuroendocrine tumor (PNET). (**a**) Precontrast CT shows a slightly hypodense lesion in the pancreatic tail (*arrow*). (**b**) Arterial phase CT demonstrates a well-defined hypodense fluid lesion with a rim of well-vascularized enhancing tissue. (**c**) T2-weighted image shows better the cystic nature of the lesion. (**d**) The mass is hypermetabolic on GA-68 DOTA-TOC PET (*arrow*)

15.3 Pseudocyst

Pseudocysts are collections containing fluid [58], rich in amylase and pancreatic enzymes. They are not only one of the possible consequences of episodes of acute or chronic interstitial edematous pancreatitis but also of abdominal trauma or surgery [59]. According to the revised Atlanta classification, they develop after at least 4 weeks after the acute episode, as the evolution of acute peripancreatic fluid collections [58]. They account for 10% of all pancreatic cystic lesions [58]. The incidence of pseudocysts is 1.6–4.5 per 100,000 adults each year [60], and the prevalence ranges from 10% to 20% in acute pancreatitis and from 20% to 40% in chronic pancreatitis.

The age of presentation is between 35 and 60 years with a male predilection. Most of these lesions are asymptomatic. In general, the size and duration of the clinical course of the pseudocyst are the most important predictors of symptoms [61]. When patients present symptoms, these are usually mild or poor, due to the mass effect with biliary or gastric obstruction. The common ones are abdominal pain, early satiety, nausea, and vomiting. Weight loss is observed in 20% of patients with mass effects to the stomach. Jaundice due to compression of bile ducts, with dark urine, pruritus, and acholic stools, may be noted in 10% of patients. Fever is unusual in uncomplicated lesions; when present it can be a sign of superinfection [62].

15.3.1 Pathology

Pseudocysts originate from the disruption of pancreatic ducts with consequent leakage and accumulation of pancreatic juice usually in the peripancreatic fat; it can be intrapancreatic in cases of prior necrosectomy with a persistent pancreatic duct leak. Since there is no necrosis, it contains only fluid without non-liquefied components. Pseudocysts have no epithelial lining; walls are made of fibrosis and inflammatory tissue. Content is rich in pancreatic enzymes and usually sterile. In 10% of patients, pseudocysts can be multiple.

They are round or oval, multilocular, and irregular in shape, ranging in size from 2 to 20 cm, without solid components, central scars, or wall calcifications.

15.3.2 Diagnostic Imaging

At US pseudocysts appear as hypoechoic or anechoic fluid collections, with a well-defined wall, sometimes with fluid-fluid levels. On CT these lesions have round morphology and fluid density (<15 Hounsfield units) and are surrounded by a well-defined wall. The wall is smooth and symmetric and thin or thick and shows contrast enhancement. CT gives detailed information about the surrounding anatomy and can highlight additional pathologies, including pancreatic duct dilatation and calcifications and common bile duct dilatation. However, it can be challenging to differentiate between a pseudocyst and a cystic neoplasm on CT.

At MRI, pseudocysts are homogeneously hyperintense on T2-weighted images without debris or solid components. On T1-weighted images, the lesions are hypointense with an early enhancement of the wall that becomes progressively more intense.

At MR cholangiopancreatography, a connection between the pseudocyst and the pancreatic ductal system can be seen (Fig. 15.17).

15.3.3 Differential Diagnosis

Differential diagnosis of pseudocysts includes PCNs such as SCNs and MCNs, BD-IPMNs, and other solid neoplasms with cystic degeneration. Imaging features and history of acute or chronic pancreatitis can help make a diagnosis of pseudocyst.

The most challenging differential diagnosis is with the unilocular serous or mucinous cysts; for the correct diagnosis, it is mandatory to investigate a clinical history of pancreatitis.

15.3.4 Prognosis, Treatment, and Follow-Up Strategies

Pseudocyst can be stable in dimension, increase, or decrease in size over time. In selected cases treatment is required because of mass effect or infection. Treatment options include open surgery or cistoenterostomy, percutaneous or endoscopic drainage, and octreotide infusion.

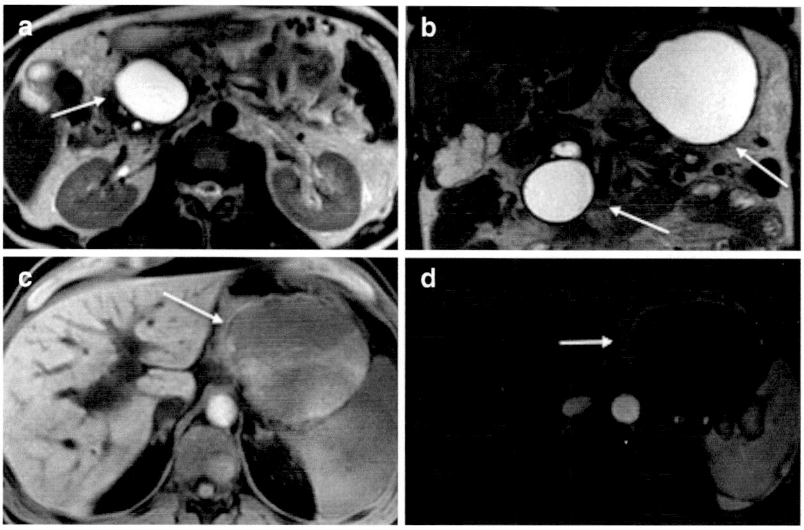

Fig. 15.17 A 41-year-old man with two pseudocysts in the head and tail of the pancreas. (**a**) A T2-weighted axial image shows a homogeneous hyperintense fluid collection in the pancreatic head (arrow). (**b**) A T2-weighted coronal image demonstrates both pseudocysts (arrows). (**c**) On the non-enhanced T1-weighted fat-suppressed image, the lesion in the pancreatic tail is hypointense (arrow). (**d**) After contrast administration, a slight enhancement of the wall is visible (arrow)

References

1. Laffan TA, Horton KM, Klein AP, Berlanstein B, Siegelman SS, Kawamoto S, et al. Prevalence of unsuspected pancreatic cysts on MDCT. Am J Roentgenol. 2008;191(3):802–7.
2. Fernández-Del Castillo C, Targarona J, Thayer SP, Rattner DW, Brugge WR, Warshaw AL, et al. Incidental pancreatic cysts: clinicopathologic characteristics and comparison with symptomatic patients. Arch Surg. 2003;138:427–34.
3. Keane MG, Afghani E. A review of the diagnosis and management of premalignant pancreatic cystic lesions. J Clin Med. 2021;10(6):1284.
4. Bassi C, Salvia R, Gumbs AA, Butturini G, Falconi M, Pederzoli P. The value of standard serum tumor markers in differentiating mucinous from serous cystic tumors of the pancreas: CEA, Ca 19-9, Ca 125, Ca 15-3. Langenbeck's Arch Surg. 2002;387(7–8):281–5.
5. Maire F, Hammel P, Terris B, Paye F, Scoazec JY, Cellier C, et al. Prognosis of malignant intraductal papillary mucinous tumours of the pancreas after surgical resection. Comparison with pancreatic ductal adenocarcinoma. Gut. 2002;51(5):717–22.
6. Pergolini I, Sahora K, Ferrone CR, Morales-Oyarvide V, Wolpin BM, Mucci LA, et al. Long-term risk of pancreatic malignancy in patients with branch duct Intraductal papillary mucinous neoplasm in a referral center. Gastroenterology. 2017;153(5):1284–94.e1.
7. Nara S, Onaya H, Hiraoka N, Shimada K, Sano T, Sakamoto Y, et al. Preoperative evaluation of invasive and noninvasive intraductal papillary-mucinous neoplasms of the pancreas: clinical, radiological, and pathological analysis of 123 cases. Pancreas. 2009;38(1):8–16.
8. Le H, Ziogas A, Rhee JM, Lee JG, Lipkin SM, Zell JA. A population-based, descriptive analysis of malignant intraductal papillary mucinous neoplasms of the pancreas. Cancer Epidemiol Biomarkers Prev. 2008;17(10):2737–41.
9. del Chiaro M, Verbeke C, Salvia R, Klöppel G, Werner J, McKay C, et al. European experts consensus statement on cystic tumours of the pancreas. Dig Liver Dis. 2013;45(9):703–11.
10. Brugge WR. Diagnosis and management of cystic lesions of the pancreas. J Gastrointest Oncol. 2015;6:375–88. Pioneer Bioscience Publishing.
11. Herranz Pérez R, de la Morena LF, Santander VC. Neoplasias quísticas pancreáticas, enfoque diagnóstico. Rev Colomb Gastroenterol. 2019;34(1):52.
12. Farrell RJ, Agarwal B, Brandwein SL, Underhill J, Chuttani R, Pleskow DK. Intraductal US is a useful adjunct to ERCP for distinguishing malignant from benign biliary strictures. Gastrointest Endosc. 2002;56(5):681–7.
13. Sahani DV, Lin DJ, Venkatesan AM, Sainani N, Mino-Kenudson M, Brugge WR, et al. Multidisciplinary approach to diagnosis and management of intraductal papillary mucinous neoplasms of the pancreas. Clin Gastroenterol Hepatol. 2009;7:259–69.
14. Mino-Kenudson M, Fernández-del Castillo C, Baba Y, Valsangkar NP, Liss AS, Hsu M, et al. Prognosis of invasive intraductal papillary mucinous neoplasm depends on histological and precursor epithelial subtypes. Gut. 2011;60(12):1712–20.
15. Volkan AN. Cystic lesions of the pancreas. Mod Pathol. 2007;20(S1):S71–93.
16. Hirono S, Yamaue H. Surgical strategy for intraductal papillary mucinous neoplasms of the pancreas. Surgery Today. 2020;50:50–5. Springer.
17. Andrejevic-Blant S, Kosmahl M, Sipos B, Klöppel G. Pancreatic intraductal papillary-mucinous neoplasms: a new and evolving entity. Virchows Arch. 2007;451:863–9.
18. Kamata K, Kitano M, Kudo M, Sakamoto H, Kadosaka K, Miyata T, et al. Value of EUS in early detection of pancreatic ductal adenocarcinomas in patients with intraductal papillary mucinous neoplasms. Endoscopy. 2014;46(1):22–9.
19. Rodríguez-D'Jesús A, Fernández-Esparrach G, Boadas J, Busquets J, Fernández-Cruz L, Ferrer J, et al. Impact of endoscopic ultrasonography (EUS) and EUS-guided fine-needle aspiration on the management of pancreatic cystic lesions. Eur J Gastroenterol Hepatol. 2016;28(9):1094–9.
20. Stark A, Donahue TR, Reber HA, Joe HO. Pancreatic cyst disease a review. JAMA. 2016;315:1882–93.
21. Tanaka M, Fernández-Del Castillo C, Adsay V, Chari S, Falconi M, Jang JY, et al. International consensus guidelines 2012 for the management of IPMN and MCN of the pancreas. In: Pancreatology. Elsevier B.V; 2012. p. 183–97.
22. Gourgiotis S, Germanos S, Ridolfini MP. Presentation and management of pancreatic cystic neoplasms. J Clin Gastroenterol. 2007;41(6):599–608.
23. Matthaei H, Schulick RD, Hruban RH, Maitra A. Cystic precursors to invasive pancreatic cancer. Nat Rev Gastroenterol Hepatol. 2011;8:141–50.
24. Sakorafas GH, Smyrniotis V, Reid-Lombardo KM, Sarr MG. Primary pancreatic cystic neoplasms revisited: part II.Mucinous cystic neoplasms. Surg Oncol. 2011;20(2):e93–101.
25. Del Chiaro M, Besselink MG, Scholten L, Bruno MJ, Cahen DL, Gress TM, et al. European evidence-based guidelines on pancreatic cystic neoplasms. Gut. 2018;67:789–804. BMJ Publishing Group.
26. Tanaka M, Fernández-del Castillo C, Kamisawa T, Jang JY, Levy P, Ohtsuka T, et al. Revisions of international consensus Fukuoka guidelines for the man-

agement of IPMN of the pancreas. Pancreatology. 2017;17(5):738–53.
27. Turrini O, Waters JA, Schnelldorfer T, Lillemoe KD, Yiannoutsos CT, Farnell MB, et al. Invasive intraductal papillary mucinous neoplasm: predictors of survival and role of adjuvant therapy. HPB. 2010;12(7):447–55.
28. Nilsson LN, Keane MG, Shamali A, Millastre Bocos J, Marijinissen van Zanten M, Antila A, et al. Nature and management of pancreatic mucinous cystic neoplasm (MCN): a systematic review of the literature. Pancreatology. 2016;16(6):1028–36.
29. Elmer P, Naveed S, Qari H, Banday T, Altaf A, Para M. Mucinous cystic neoplasms of pancreas. Gastroenterol Res. 2014;7(2):44–50.
30. Procacci C, Carbognin G, Accordini S, Biasiutti C, Guarise A, Lombardo F, et al. CT features of malignant mucinous cystic tumors of the pancreas. Eur Radiol. 2001;11(9):1626–30.
31. Sarr MG, Carpenter HA, Prabhakar LP, Orchard TF, Hughes S, van Heerden JA, et al. Clinical and pathologic correlation of 84 mucinous cystic neoplasms of the pancreas. Ann Surg. 2000;231(2):205–12.
32. Crippa S, Salvia R, Warshaw AL, Domínguez I, Bassi C, Falconi M, et al. Mucinous cystic neoplasm of the pancreas is not an aggressive entity: lessons from 163 resected patients. Ann Surg. 2008;247(4):571–9.
33. Sidden CR, Mortele KJ. Cystic tumors of the pancreas: ultrasound, computed tomography, and magnetic resonance imaging features. Semin Ultrasound CT MR. 2007;28(5):339–56.
34. Karoumpalis I, Christodoulou DK. Cystic lesions of the pancreas. Ann Gastroenterol. 2016;29(2):155–61.
35. Al-Haddad M, Schmidt MC, Sandrasegaran K, Dewitt J. Diagnosis and treatment of cystic pancreatic tumors. Clin Gastroenterol Hepatol. 2011;9(8):635–48.
36. Buetow PC, Rao P, Thompson LDR. From the archives of the AFIP: mucinous cystic neoplasms of the pancreas: radiologic-pathologic correlation. Radiographics. 1998;18(2):433–49.
37. Sahani DV, Kambadakone A, Macari M, Takahashi N, Chari S, Castillo CF. Diagnosis and management of cystic pancreatic lesions. Am J Roentgenol. 2013;200:343–54.
38. Sarr MG, Kendrick ML, Nagorney DM, Thompson GB, Farley DR, Farnell MB. Cystic neoplasms of the pancreas benign to malignant epithelial neoplasms. Surg Clin North Am. 2001;81:497–509.
39. Lonser RR, Glenn GM, Walther M, Chew EY, Libutti SK, Linehan WM, et al. von Hippel-Lindau disease. Lancet. 2003;361(9374):2059–67.
40. Mohr VH, Vortmeyer AO, Zhuang Z, Libutti SK, Walther MM, Choyke PL, et al. Histopathology and molecular genetics of multiple cysts and microcystic (serous) adenomas of the pancreas in von Hippel-Lindau patients. Am J Pathol. 2000;157(5):1615–21.
41. Antonini F, Fuccio L, Fabbri C, Macarri G, Palazzo L. Management of serous cystic neoplasms of the pancreas. Expert Rev Gastroenterol Hepatol. 2015;9(1):115–25.
42. Sarno A, Tedesco G, de Robertis R, Marchegiani G, Salvia R, D'Onofrio M. Pancreatic cystic neoplasm diagnosis: role of imaging. Endosc Ultrasound. 2018;7(5):297–300.
43. Kalb B, Sarmiento JM, Kooby DA, Adsay NV, Martin DR. MR imaging of cystic lesions of the pancreas. Radiographics. 2009;29(6):1749–65.
44. Levy MJ, Clain JE. Evaluation and management of cystic pancreatic tumors: emphasis on the role of EUS FNA. Clin Gastroenterol Hepatol. 2004;2(8):639–53.
45. Ishigami K. Imaging pitfalls of pancreatic serous cystic neoplasm and its potential mimickers. World J Radiol. 2014;6(3):36.
46. Dietrich CF, Dong Y, Jenssen C, Ciaravino V, Hocke M, Wang WP, et al. Serous pancreatic neoplasia, data and review. World J Gastroenterol. 2017;23:5567–78. Baishideng Publishing Group Co.
47. Strobel O, Z'graggen K, Schmitz-Winnenthal FH, Friess H, Kappeler A, Zimmermann A, et al. Risk of malignancy in serous cystic neoplasms of the pancreas. Digestion. 2003;68(1):24–33.
48. Reid MD, Choi HJ, Memis B, Krasinskas AM, Jang KT, Akkas G, et al. Serous neoplasms of the pancreas: a clinicopathologic analysis of 193 cases and literature review with new insights on macrocystic and solid variants and critical reappraisal of so-called serous cystadenocarcinoma. Am J Surg Pathol. 2015;39(12):1597–610. https://pubmed.ncbi.nlm.nih.gov/26559376/.
49. Zuriarrain A, Nir I, Bocklage T, Rajput A. Pseudopapillary tumor of the pancreas in a 17-year-old girl. J Clin Oncol. 2011;29(14):e395–6.
50. Coleman KM, Doherty MC, Bigler SA. Solid-pseudopapillary tumor of the pancreas. Radiographics. 2003;23(6):1644–8.
51. Lam KY, Lo CY, Fan ST. Pancreatic solid-cystic-papillary tumor: clinicopathologic features in eight patients from Hong Kong and review of the literature. World J Surg. 1999;23:1045–50.
52. Kehagias D, Smyrniotis V, Gouliamos A, Vlahos L. Cystic pancreatic neoplasms: computed tomography and magnetic resonance imaging findings. Int J Gastrointest Cancer. 2000;28(3):223–30.
53. Buetow PC, Buck JL, Pantongrag-Brown L, Beck KG, Ros PR, Adair CF. Solid and papillary epithelial neoplasm of the pancreas: imaging-pathologic correlation on 56 cases. Radiology. 1996;199(3):707–11.
54. Eder F, Schulz H-U, Röcken C, Lippert H. Solid-pseudopapillary tumor of the pancreatic tail. World J Gastroenterol. 2005;11(26):4117–9. Elsevier.
55. Kucera JN, Kucera S, Perrin SD, Caracciolo JT, Schmulewitz N, Kedar RP. Cystic lesions of the

pancreas: radiologic-endosonographic correlation. Radiographics. 2012;32(7):E283–301.
56. Horton KM, Hruban RH, Yeo C, Fishman EK. Multi–detector row CT of pancreatic islet cell tumors. Radiographics. 2006;26(2):453–64.
57. Bordeianou L, Vagefi PA, Sahani D, Deshpande V, Rakhlin E, Warshaw AL, et al. Cystic pancreatic endocrine neoplasms: a distinct tumor type? J Am Coll Surg. 2008;206(6):1154–8.
58. Foster BR, Jensen KK, Bakis G, Shaaban AM, Coakley FV. Revised Atlanta classification for acute pancreatitis: a pictorial essay. Radiographics. 2016;36:675–87. Radiological Society of North America Inc.
59. Tan JH, Chin W, Shaikh AL, Zheng S. Pancreatic pseudocyst: dilemma of its recent management (review). Exp Ther Med. 2020;21(2):159.
60. Kim HS, Jang J-Y. Management algorithms for pancreatic cystic neoplasms: the surgeon's perspective. Archives of Pathology & Laboratory Medicine; 2021.
61. Cannon JW, Callery MP, Vollmer CM. Diagnosis and management of pancreatic pseudocysts: what is the evidence? J Am Coll Surg. 2009;209:385–93.
62. Brugge WR, Lauwers GY, Sahani D, Fernandez-Del Castillo C, Warshaw AL. Cystic neoplasms of the pancreas. N Engl J Med. 2004;351(12):1218–26.

Approach to Periampullary Pathologies

16

Binit Sureka and Satya Jha

16.1 Introduction

Periampullary pathologies create various challenges to radiologists, pathologists, and the treating physicians and surgeons, owing to the complex anatomy and plethora of pathologies possible in this location.

The common bile duct (CBD) and main pancreatic duct unite with each other to form a small dilated common channel of ~3 mm, known as the ampulla of Vater, which opens in the medial wall of the second part of the duodenum. This opening in the duodenal wall is called the papilla. It measures ~1 mm in diameter. However, not all cases show a classic ampulla [1].

In other individuals, these two ducts may join with each other to form a common channel without the classically described dilatation. Sometimes, the two ducts may open separately into a single opening in the duodenal papilla (giving it a double-barrel appearance). In rare cases, two openings at the duodenal papilla may be seen adjacent to each other (Fig. 16.1).

The distal-most part of the common bile duct and main pancreatic duct, along with the ampulla, is surrounded by the sphincter of Oddi. Circular and longitudinal smooth muscles form the sphincter of Oddi. It covers the distal bile duct and distal pancreatic duct for varied lengths and is composed of three smaller sphincters, namely, the sphincter pancreaticus (around pancreatic duct), sphincter choledochus (around the common bile duct), and sphincter papilla (around the duodenal papillae) (Fig. 16.2) [2]. Various benign and malignant periampullary pathologies are listed in Table 16.1.

B. Sureka (✉) · S. Jha
Department of Diagnostic & Interventional Radiology, AIIMS Jodhpur, Jodhpur, India

© The Author(s), under exclusive license to Springer Nature Singapore Pte Ltd. 2025

B. Sureka (ed.), *Hepato-Pancreatico Biliary Imaging*, https://doi.org/10.1007/978-981-95-1699-5_16

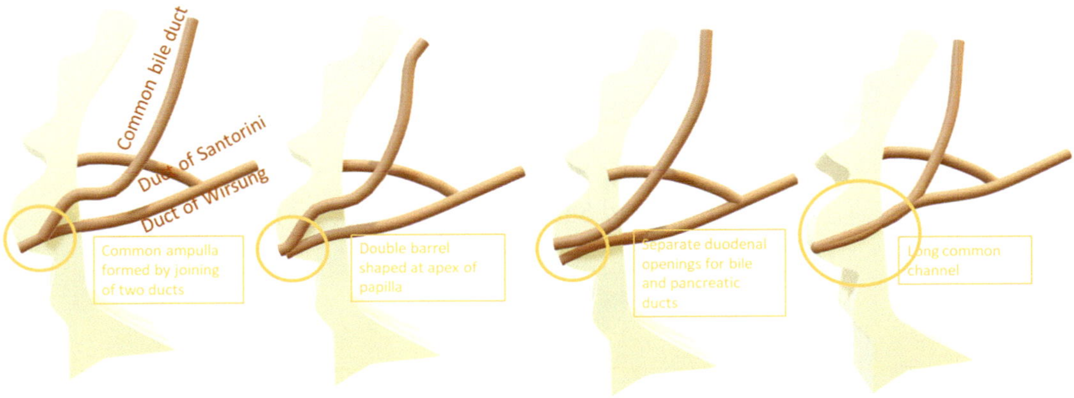

Fig. 16.1 Line diagram showing various morphologies of pancreaticobiliary union

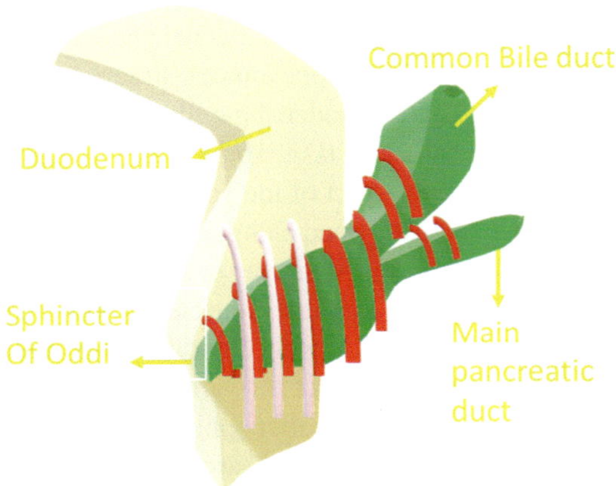

Fig. 16.2 Line diagram depicting the ampullary anatomy

Table 16.1 Differential diagnosis of periampullary lesions

Malignant	Benign
Ampullary cancer	Ampullary adenoma
Pancreatic adenocarcinoma	Lipoma
Distal CBD cholangiocarcinoma	Hematoma
Duodenal adenocarcinoma	Diverticulum (Lemmel syndrome)
Neuroendocrine tumors	Papillitis
	Choledocholithiasis
	Inflammatory stricture
	Groove pancreatitis
	Autoimmune pancreatitis
	Duodenitis
	Pseudoaneurysm

16.2 Goals of Imaging

Delineation of the tumor epicenter Determination of the site of origin of tumor plays a vital role in affecting patient outcome. Ampullary tumors and distal bile duct cholangiocarcinoma are found to be detected in the resectable stage more often than the pancreatic cancer. Ampullary (39%) and duodenal periampullary carcinomas (59%) offers a better 5-year survival rate than pancreatic (15%) and distal CBD periampullary carcinoma (27%) [3].

Evaluation of extent, prediction of resectability, and staging Even in the presence of lymphadenopathy, aggressive removal of all the tumor components may yield better results in cases of ampullary and duodenal carcinoma [4]. Hence locating the metastatic lymph node is very important in deciding the type of surgery.

16.3 Stepwise Approach to Cross-Sectional Imaging

When it comes to imaging, the foremost part is to get a hold of the normal cross-sectional anatomy of the periampullary region, surrounding arterial and venous structures, knowledge of draining lymph nodes, along with ductal anatomy. When one comes across a CT scan in the suspected case of periampullary malignancy for interpretation, it is important to ask yourself, "Are there visibly dilated common bile duct and pancreatic duct?"

The next step in such a case is to trace the course of dilated CBD, by scrolling through subsequent slices of data, until its distal point where it is not dilated anymore. Look carefully at and around this point to find any abnormally attenuating lesion or mass. The mass may be present at ampulla, medial wall of the second part of the duodenum, distal portion of the bile duct, pancreatic head, or more than one of these locations.

The mass lesion may be nodular, irregular, or ill-defined. At this point, it would be wise to remember that, in general, polypoidal and nodular tumors have a better outcome than infiltrating tumors. Polypoidal morphology is more common in ampullary and duodenal variants than in periampullary and pancreatic variants. If a mass lesion is not seen, look for linear, abnormal enhancing wall thickening at the ampulla, in the distal bile duct, or along the duodenum wall. Look for any alteration in the outline or contour of the shape of the duodenum.

Atrophic pancreatic parenchyma with a disproportionately dilated pancreatic duct points toward a periampullary involving the pancreatic head. Irrespective of whether one finds a periampullary tumor on CT or not, it is vital to assess the surrounding nodal stations, including para-aortic and inter aortocaval nodes.

It is essential to look at the fat planes around the abdominal aorta's major branches and define encased or distortion of vessels by the mass, especially of the celiac axis and its branches, superior mesenteric artery and vein, and portal vein. It is also a must to note for variant anatomies such as replaced right hepatic artery arising from the superior mesenteric artery or a left hepatic artery arising from the left gastric artery. Other important areas to look at the solid organs, omentum, peritoneum, mesocolon, and mesentery for the presence of any nodular deposits or abnormal suspicious thickening, suggesting carcinomatosis.

16.4 Significance of Histological Sub-classification

Even on histopathology, the exact origin of a periampullary carcinoma may be difficult to conclude, particularly in larger tumors that involve more than one site. Kimura et al. [5] first subclassified the ampullary adenocarcinomas into "intestinal" and "pancreatobiliary" type of differentiation. The pancreatobiliary types are associated with an overall poor prognosis. This classification is now applied to other periampullary adenocarcinomas as well.

Ivanovic et al. [6] demonstrated MDCT features that could accurately differentiate between the pancreatobiliary and intestinal subtypes. On imaging, intestinal subtypes are more likely to be nodular in morphology. On the other hand, pancreatobiliary subtypes can have either an infiltrative or nodular morphology. Differentiating features between the two is highlighted in Table 16.2.

16.5 Implication of Nodal Evaluation on CT Scan

Staging laparoscopy is often used to evaluate locoregional lymph nodal metastases. However, a preoperative CT scan has a clear advantage of being fast and noninvasive in identifying regional

Table 16.2 Differentiating features between pancreaticobiliary and intestinal subtype

Imaging features	Pancreaticobiliary subtype	Intestinal subtype
CT morphology	Infiltrative	Nodular
Papilla	Retracted	Bulging
Common bile duct	Dilated with abrupt cut-off	Stricture or tapering
Main pancreatic duct	Dilated with abrupt cut-off	Stricture or tapering
Pancreaticoduodenal groove	Involved	Free
Enhancement	Hypoenhancing	Iso or hyperenhancing

lymph nodes. On CT scan, the CBD node, which is located behind and lateral to suprapancreatic CBD, is found to be highly correlating with staging laparoscopy. Another such nodal group is the gastroduodenal artery (GDA) node, which is located anterior and medial to the origin of the gastroduodenal artery [7].

Maithel et al. [7] found that tumor metastasis to the GDA node was associated with reduced survival in the postoperative period. So, the GDA node impacted the patient outcome, similar to that of liver metastases. However, metastasis to the CBD node did not show any such significant association.

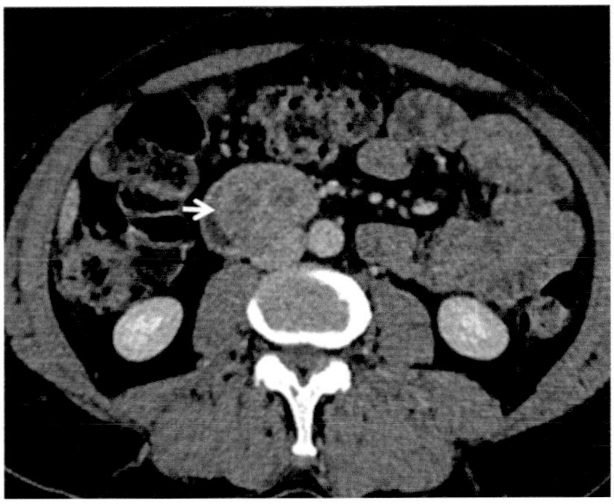

Fig. 16.3 Axial contrast-enhanced CT showing polypoidal heterogeneously enhancing lesion centered at the ampulla (arrow) bulging into the duodenum in a case of ampullary carcinoma

16.6 Ampullary Carcinoma

Adenocarcinoma epicentered in the ampulla is relatively uncommon among other gastrointestinal malignancies. A tiny tumor can obstruct the distal common bile duct due to its location, obstructing the entire biliary tree and a prominent central pancreatic duct leading to hampered drainage of pancreatic juices. Thus these tumors are more likely to be detected early in the resectable stage, as the patient becomes symptomatic early. Jaundice occurs before abdominal pain, nausea, and vomiting in these cases.

On imaging, very often, a solid nodular mass is seen at the ampulla. It is frequently picked up on ultrasound by tracing the dilated duct up to the point of cut-off. On non-contrast CT, one can see a solid lesion at the ampulla, isoattenuating to the pancreas. On post-contrast imaging, the tumor may enhance gradually on arterial and portal venous phases. It is seen as a well-circumscribed lesion or an infiltrating mass at the ampulla (Fig. 16.3). On magnetic resonance imaging (MRI), the smaller masses can be hypointense on T2. They show restricted diffusion. They may cause an irregular nodular filling defect (nodular type) or periductal thickening at the ampulla or the pancreaticobiliary junction on magnetic resonance cholangiopancreatography (MRCP). Many cases may show bulging of the papilla into the duodenal lumen. Some instances can show only common bile duct dilated, without pancreatic duct dilatation. On MRCP, the pancreaticobiliary junction/ampulla usually shows an abrupt blunted cut-off but, in some cases, may display a meniscus-shaped cut-off. Pancreatic side branch dilatation is an uncommon finding.

However, in many cases, double-duct sign is the only manifestation that makes the suspicion of ampullary malignancy. Localizing the mass may not always be feasible, not even on endoscopic ultrasound or ERCP.

16.7 Distal CBD (Extrahepatic) Cholangiocarcinoma

Grossly, these can be either polypoidal or infiltrating type. On cross-sectional imaging, the infiltrating type is seen as enhancing ductal walls with narrowed or obliterated lumen in the involved segment [8]. A polypoidal mass, on the other hand, is seen as polyp-like growth occupying the ductal lumen, causing partial obliteration of the lumen, and upstream dilatation (Fig. 16.4).

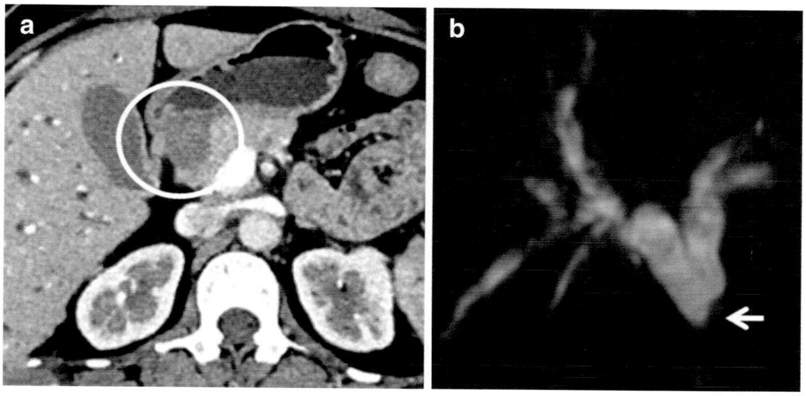

Fig. 16.4 (**a**) Axial contrast-enhanced CT showing infiltrative hypoenhancing lesion (circle) centered on the suprapancreatic CBD. (**b**) Thick-slab MRCP showing abrupt cut-off (arrow) in a case of extrahepatic cholangiocarcinoma

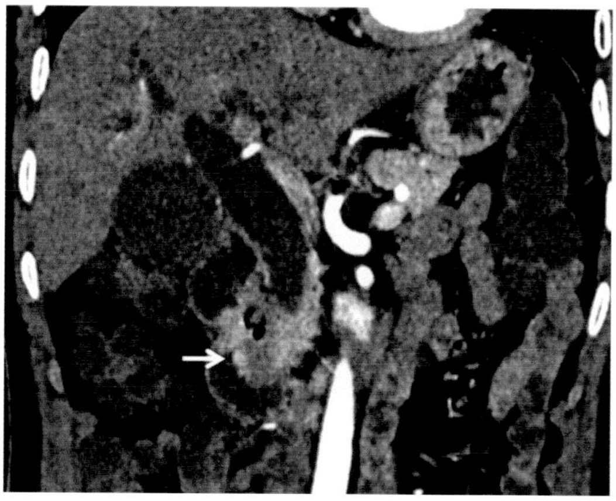

Fig. 16.5 Coronal contrast-enhanced CT image showing an intraluminal enhancing mass (arrow) in the duodenum causing ampullary invasion and dilatation of the CBD in a proven case of duodenal adenocarcinoma

16.8 Duodenal Adenocarcinoma

A periampullary duodenal adenocarcinoma arises from the duodenal wall. When large enough, it invades the major duodenal papilla, leading to upstream biliary dilatation. It may have varying morphology, the common ones being a polypoidal, intraluminal mass, eccentric duodenal wall thickening, or concentric thickening with annular stricture formation (Fig. 16.5). This may lead to gastric outlet obstruction.

These arise from the intestinal epithelium of the duodenum and are histologically found to be similar to ampullary carcinoma. On contrast-enhanced CT studies, these are usually hypovascular. Similar features are seen on contrast-enhanced MRI, along with diffusion restriction.

16.9 Pancreatic Adenocarcinoma

Adenocarcinoma of the head of the pancreas may be periampullary if its epicenter is close enough to the ampulla. In such cases, there is ampullary invasion and resultant obstructive jaundice. It is, in fact, the most frequent type of periampullary malignancy encountered [8].

These are classically hypovascular tumors, thus appearing hypoenhancing on CT and MRI. The signal intensity on the T2-weighted image may vary from hypointense to hyperintense, depending on the amount of internal necrosis or desmoplastic within the tumor. On MRCP, the classic double-duct sign with an abrupt cut-off at the periampullary location may be seen. The shape of cut-off may be rat tail shaped, beaked, or abruptly blunted. In some cases, pancreatic duct thickening may be the only abnormality seen, instead of a mass. A four-segment sign may be seen in many cases [1]. This means, in addition to the classic doubt duct sign, a short

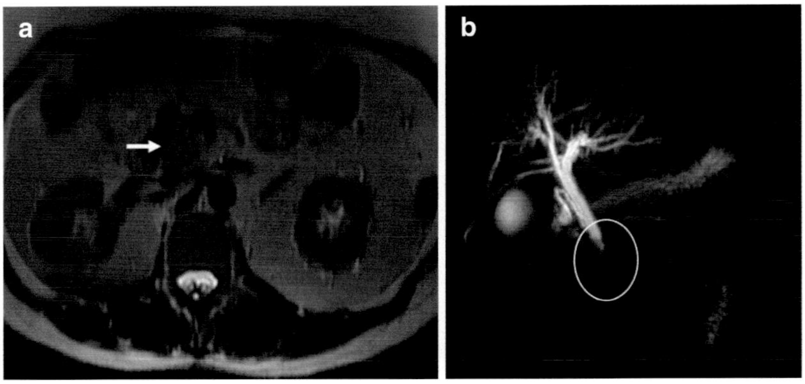

Fig. 16.6 (**a**) Axial T2-weighted MR image showing a mass (arrow) in the head-uncinate process of the pancreas which is mildly hyperintense. (**b**) 3D-coronal MRCP MIP images showing four-duct sign (circle) in a case of pancreatic adenocarcinoma

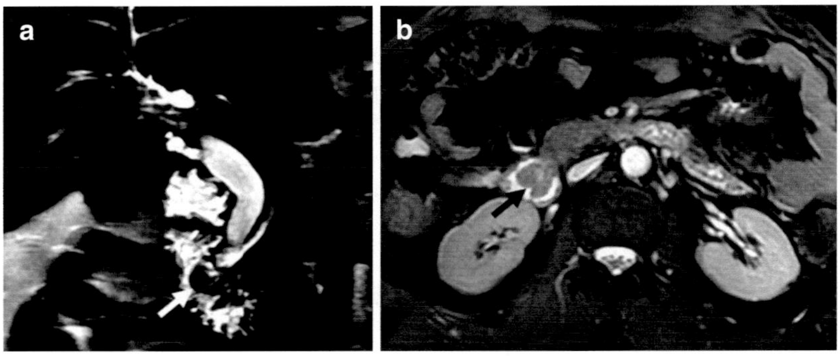

Fig. 16.7 (**a**) 3D-MRCP image showing polypoidal well-marginated lesion (arrow) at the ampulla causing dilatation of the bile duct and pancreatic duct. (**b**) Axial T2-weighted MR image showing a mildly hyperintense lesion (black arrow) bulging into the duodenum in a case of ampullary adenoma

segment of the common bile duct and pancreatic duct may also be visualized, distal to the cut-off by the mass (Fig. 16.6). Very often, dilated side branches of the main pancreatic duct are also seen adjacent to the narrowed/cut-off segment. This finding is said to be very specific for the pancreatic type of periampullary carcinoma.

16.10 Benign Periampullary Pathologies

16.10.1 Ampullary Adenoma

Ampullary adenomas need special mention, as they are benign and nevertheless premalignant and may transform into adenocarcinoma. These may be sporadic or familial. On imaging, they are seen as well-defined lesion of soft tissue density, may cause irregularity of the ampulla, and upstream ductal dilatation (Fig. 16.7) [8, 9].

16.10.2 Groove Pancreatitis

Groove pancreatitis is a rare form of pancreatitis that affects the pancreaticoduodenal groove. It often poses a diagnostic challenge to radiologists and pathologists. It is seen as a pure type that solely affects the pancreaticoduodenal groove or a segmental type that affects the head of the pancreas. Both these forms show inflammatory sheet-like thickening in the median paraduodenal location, with associated thickened walls of the second part of the duodenum (Fig. 16.8). A particular feature identified in this disease is cysts in the duodenal wall and the groove [10].

16.10.3 Periampullary Lipoma

A periampullary duodenal lipoma is a rare lesion and may be seen incidentally in CT scans of elderly patients, being scanned for other indications. These are typically as well marginated lesions of fat attenuation [11]. On MR, these are hyperintense of T1 and T2 and show loss of signal on fat-suppressed sequences. In rare cases, an unusually large lipoma may cause ampullary obstruction and obstructive jaundice.

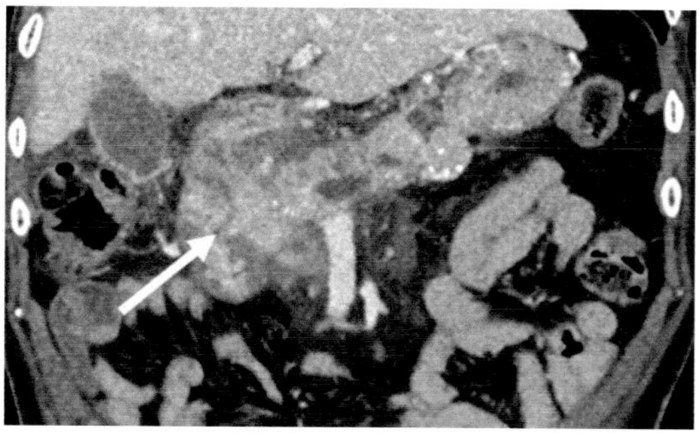

Fig. 16.8 Coronal multiplanar reconstruction contrast-enhanced CT showing inflammatory wall thickening (arrow) centered on the pancreaticoduodenal groove region with changes of peripancreatic inflammation in a case of groove pancreatitis

16.10.4 Lemmel Syndrome

This is a rather rare abnormality. A large duodenal diverticulum (air or air fluid-filled structure) arising from the medial duodenal wall, at the second part of the duodenum, may cause obstructive jaundice similar to a periampullary neoplasm [12].

In conclusion, there are various other pathologies in the periampullary region like duodenitis, papillitis, and hematoma which needs clinic-radiological correlation as these entities can be mislabeled as malignancy. Figure 16.9 highlights an algorithmic approach in differentiating the origin of these malignancies.

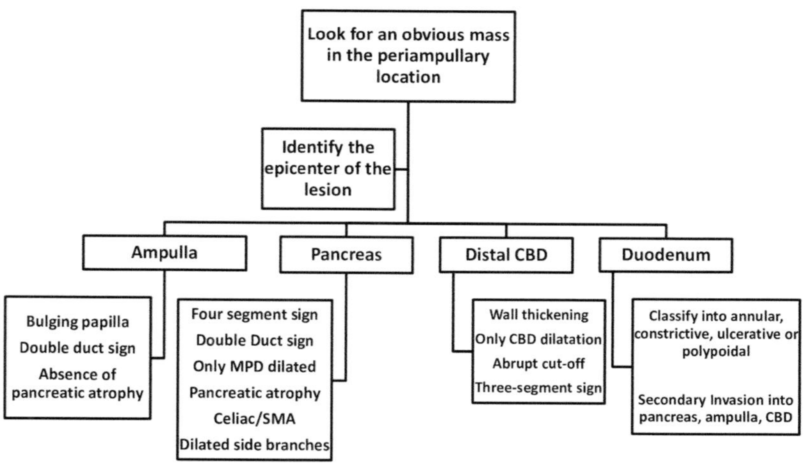

Fig. 16.9 Algorithmic approach in differentiating periampullary malignancies

References

1. Kim JH, Kim M-J, Chung J-J, Lee WJ, Yoo HS, Lee JT. Differential diagnosis of periampullary carcinomas at MR imaging. RadioGraphics. 2002;22:1335–52.
2. Seetharam P, Rodrigues G. Sphincter of oddi and its dysfunction. Saudi J Gastroenterol. 2008;14:1–6.
3. Riall TS, Cameron JL, Lillemoe KD, Winter JM, Campbell KA, Hruban RH, et al. Resected periampullary adenocarcinoma: 5-year survivors and their 6- to 10-year follow-up. Surgery. 2006;140:764–72.
4. Panzeri F. Management of ampullary neoplasms: a tailored approach between endoscopy and surgery. World J Gastroenterol. 2015;21:7970.
5. Kimura W, Futakawa N, Zhao B. Neoplastic diseases of the papilla of Vater. J Hepato-Biliary-Pancreat Surg. 2004;11(4):223–31.
6. Ivanovic AM, Alessandrino F, Maksimovic R, Micev M, Ostojic S, Gore RM, et al. Pathologic subtypes of ampullary adenocarcinoma: value of ampullary MDCT for noninvasive preoperative differentiation. AJR Am J Roentgenol. 2017;208:W71–8.
7. Maithel SK, Khalili K, Dixon E, Guindi M, Callery MP, Cattral MS, et al. Impact of regional lymph node evaluation in staging patients with periampullary tumors. Ann Surg Oncol. 2007;14:202–10.
8. Nikolaidis P, Hammond NA, Day K, Yaghmai V, Wood CG, Mosbach DS, et al. Imaging features of benign and malignant ampullary and periampullary lesions. RadioGraphics. 2014;34:624–41.
9. Lee M, Kim M-J, Park M-S, Choi J-Y, Chung YE. Using multi-detector-row CT to diagnose ampullary adenoma or adenocarcinoma in situ. Eur J Radiol. 2011;80:e340–5.
10. Addeo G, Beccani D, Cozzi D, Ferrari R, Lanzetta MM, Paolantonio P, et al. Groove pancreatitis: a challenging imaging diagnosis. Gland Surg. 2019;8:S178–87.
11. Fang S-H, Dong D-J, Chen F-H, Jin M, Zhong B-S. Small intestinal lipomas: diagnostic value of multi-slice CT enterography. World J Gastroenterol. 2010;16:2677–81.
12. Carmona Agúndez M, López Guerra D, Fernández Pérez J, Blanco Fernández G. Lemmel's syndrome: obstructive jaundice secondary to a duodenal diverticulum. Cir Esp (English Edition). 2017;95:550–1.

17 Imaging in Hepatobiliary-Pancreatic Trauma

Atin Kumar and Ankit Sangwan

17.1 Introduction

Trauma is one of the leading causes of death and causes substantial morbidity in the productive age group [1]. Road traffic accidents constitute the bulk of causes of severe physical trauma. Abdominal trauma accounts for 5% of mortality in isolation and contributes about 15% to mortality as part of polytrauma [2]. Excessive bleeding accounts for 80–90% of acute deaths from abdominal injury out of which the liver and spleen form the major component.

Blunt abdominal trauma is much more common than penetrating abdominal trauma with road traffic accidents being the dominant cause. And with conservative non-surgical management becoming the preferred treatment for most blunt injury patients, computed tomography (CT) examination findings are of utmost importance to describe the extent of injury and guide the trauma management team towards a non-surgical trial of treatment.

Penetrating abdominal trauma is usually caused to firearm injury or stab wounds. These injuries may have only subtle findings on the outside but can be very complex and damaging once inside the peritoneum. Knowledge of the projectile kinetics and the mechanism of assault can help the radiologist in diagnosing subtle and overt traumatic injuries which can guide prompt operative management and decrease the omission of life-threatening findings intraoperatively.

The hepatobiliary system consists of the liver, the intrahepatic bile ducts (IHBDs) and extrahepatic bile ducts including the gall bladder (GB). The liver is the most commonly injured organ in blunt abdominal trauma and the second most commonly injured organ in penetrating abdominal trauma [3]. While liver injuries represent one of the most frequent life-threatening injuries in trauma patients [4], the incidence of biliary injury following trauma has not been studied and characterised extensively [5]. The incidence of biliary complications after blunt hepatic trauma has been reported to be 2.8–7.4% [6]. Extrahepatic biliary trauma is even rarer, accounting for less than 1% of all blunt abdominal injuries according to most series [7]. Gall bladder injury is also an uncommon occurrence following trauma. Majority (89%) of gall bladder injuries result from penetrating trauma [8]. In recent years, advances in cross-sectional imaging coupled with image-guided interventional therapy have enabled increased detection, recognition and non-surgical management of hepatobiliary injuries in blunt abdominal trauma.

A. Kumar (✉) · A. Sangwan
Radiodiagnosis and Interventional Radiology, All India Institute of Medical Sciences, New Delhi, New Delhi, India

© The Author(s), under exclusive license to Springer Nature Singapore Pte Ltd. 2025

B. Sureka (ed.), *Hepato-Pancreatico Biliary Imaging*, https://doi.org/10.1007/978-981-95-1699-5_17

Pancreatic injuries are uncommon, incidence has been reported as 0.2–2% in patients with blunt trauma and 1–12% in patients with penetrating trauma [9]. Retroperitoneal location of the pancreas has been stated as one of the reasons for low incidence of pancreatic injuries in abdominal trauma. However, its location also means that pancreatic injury is a marker of severe abdominal trauma and is usually associated with significant injuries to other abdominal visceral and vascular structures with significant morbidity as well as mortality due to complications—including but not limited to pancreatitis, pseudocyst and pancreatic fistula [10]. The major determinant in the management of pancreatic trauma is the integrity of pancreatic duct as well as associated injuries, both of which can be detected with high sensitivity using modern imaging tools like contrast-enhanced CT, magnetic resonance cholangiopancreatography (MRCP) and endoscopic retrograde cholangiopancreatography (ERCP).

A radiologist must have an understanding of the patterns of injury associated with the many mechanisms of trauma, assessment of hemodynamic status and need for any prompt operative management as well as common imaging artefacts. Injuries in the abdomen if accurately and quickly diagnosed can be treated with very good results, and the radiologist plays an important role in the evaluation of all polytrauma patients. In a background of systematic and orderly resuscitation and support, imaging evaluation enables optimal management of the severely injured patients.

17.2 Role of Imaging/Imaging Modalities

Various imaging modalities used and their current role in evaluation of hepatobiliary and pancreatic trauma are:

Plain radiography It is not routinely done in a case of trauma to the abdomen since it is not very sensitive in detecting the site of injury or presence of mild to moderate hemoperitoneum. As part of adjunct to primary survey and resuscitation, chest radiograph and pelvic radiographs are recommended. They can help in detecting the various chest injuries like rib fractures, pneumothorax and hemothorax and thus may give a clue to underlying liver injury. In cases of penetrating trauma, radiographs can help in direct visualisation and localisation of foreign bodies like bullet fragments or shrapnel.

Ultrasonography (US) Focused abdominal sonography for trauma (FAST) is the primary modality for determination of hemoperitoneum in an unstable patient. Its advantages are wide availability, rapid evaluation and a fast learning curve. In severe or high-grade liver injuries, detection of free fluid in the subphrenic space (as a lenticular collection), Morrison's pouch (triangular collection) and pelvis (ovoid collection) helps in detection of hemoperitoneum and guide further management (Fig. 17.1). The FAST scan should be completed in a few minutes without focusing upon the solid organs despite the ability of sonography to visualise solid parenchymal organ injuries in some cases.

FAST has a high sensitivity for detection of intraperitoneal fluid, ranging from 64% to 98% and specificity 86% to 100% [11]. Positive FAST scan should direct the need for a tailored imaging protocol to detect any active extravasation or vascular injury along with the solid parenchymal organ injuries. Negative FAST scan should be interpreted as the absence of hemoperitoneum and not the absence of intraparenchymal injury.

Ultrasound can help in direct visualisation of high-grade injuries to the liver as well as continuity of the gall bladder. The presence of isolated fluid around the porta and in the GB fossa can suggest biliary injuries. In thin patients, the pancreas can also be evaluated, and the presence of peripancreatic fluid and complications like pseudocyst and vascular injuries is also seen occasionally. Doppler US can help in detection of vascular injury (pseudoaneurysm with the typical appearance of Yin-Yang sign). Contrast-enhanced ultrasound (CEUS) can help in the detection of vascular injuries (pseudoaneurysm and active

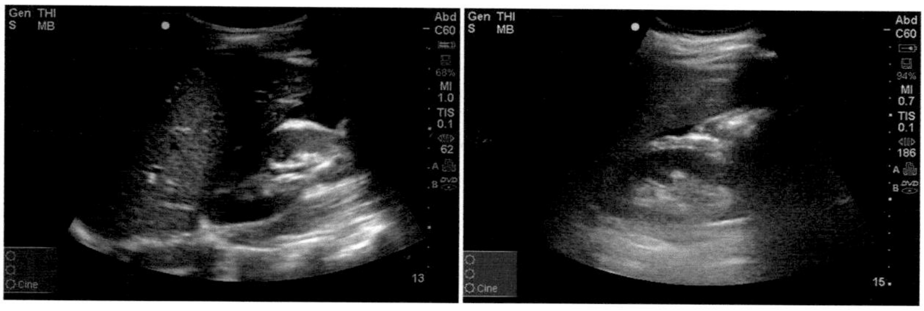

Fig. 17.1 Two different cases of road traffic accident. FAST reveals free fluid in the hepatorenal space suggesting the presence of hemoperitoneum. Liver injury was seen in both cases

extravasation) with higher sensitivity than Doppler US. CEUS can also help in the detection of solid parenchymal injuries like contusions and lacerations with a higher sensitivity than grey scale US.

Ultrasound is also useful for follow-up imaging of previously diagnosed injuries in the liver which underwent conservative management. Complications in case of pancreatic injury can be picked up early using ultrasound and help in prompt management. Protocol ultrasound which involves ruling out any vascular injury in the solid organs is frequently done in our institute before discharging a patient who has undergone conservative treatment for a high-grade solid organ injury.

Ultrasound has certain limitations in evaluation of hepatobiliary and pancreatic injuries. Operator dependence, suboptimal visualisation in the presence of excessive bowel gas (post-traumatic paralytic ileus) and wounds on the abdomen and lack of direct visualisation of biliary injuries make it an insensitive investigation for hepatobiliary and pancreatic trauma.

CT Contrast-enhanced computed tomography (CECT) is the most important imaging modality in the evaluation of trauma to the abdomen in general and hepatobiliary injuries specifically. It not only helps in the detection of occult injuries but also helps in grading the severity of injury and determines treatment approach. It is an objective imaging technique that helps in visualisation of both the parenchymal injuries and vascular injuries distinctly. A hemodynamically stable patient who has sustained significant trauma to the abdomen should undergo a CECT of the chest and abdomen to detect and rule out any injuries to the internal structures. This is important because if the initial abdominal CT of a stable patient is negative, the patient can be safely discharged from the trauma emergency without a period of observation.

An optimised CT imaging protocol should be employed which should consider the type and amount of contrast material, number and timing of phases to be acquired. At our institution (a tertiary care apex trauma centre), all patients who have sustained significant trauma undergo CECT chest and abdomen with 80–100 mL of non-ionic low osmolar iodinated (350 mg iodine per millilitre) contrast injected with a power injector at the rate of 3–5 mL/s through a 18 or 20 gauge cannula in a peripheral vein. The number and timing of phase acquired are determined by the result of FAST scan. All FAST-positive patients undergo CECT with acquisition of both arterial and portal venous phases to detect vascular injury along with parenchymal injury leading to hemoperitoneum. Both the chest and the abdomen are included in the arterial phase which is acquired using bolus tracking by keeping the threshold marker at the descending thoracic aorta. The portal venous phase is acquired after approximately 60 s of injection of contrast, and coverage is confined to the abdomen. The isolated portal venous phase is acquired in FAST-negative patients, and both the chest and the abdomen are acquired in the single phase. Delayed scans (1–2-minute delay) can be taken for suspected active contrast extravasation or pseudoaneurysm. Some centres have started using a split bolus technique which achieves both arterial and venous phase images using two separate contrast boluses [12]. When the suspicion of pancreatic injury is high, a repeat contrast-enhanced CT acquired in the pancreatic phase (35–45 seconds after start of contrast injection) done within 24–48 hours of trauma depicts injuries that were not evident on the initial CT (done in the portal venous phase according to routine trauma protocol) [13]. Image quality improvement with minimisation of artifacts is achieved using adequate patient positioning—arms raised above the head (if possible) for imaging of the torso, transient displacement of metallic monitoring devices like electrocardiogram leads, wires, etc.

Dual-energy CT is being increasingly used in the evaluation of trauma to the abdomen. By using different attenuation properties of different materials at low and high-energy spectra, it offers improved material characterisation and visualisation of hepatic injuries [14, 15]. Low-energy virtual monoenergetic images increase contrast-to-noise ratio and help in the detection of liver injuries [15]. Iodine selective images also increase the sensitivity of detection of lacerations, haematomas and vascular injuries [14]. Given that dual-energy CT help in better visualisation and characterisation of pancreatic duct and hypovascular masses, there is a potential in its use to improve the detection of lacerations and contusions in the pancreas [16].

17.3 CT Signs in Hepatobiliary and Pancreatic Trauma

Hemoperitoneum The presence of free blood in the peritoneum may not be the most sensitive sign, but it is usually the first sign to be seen in a case of hepatobiliary trauma. The appearance on imaging depends upon the time that has elapsed from the onset of trauma. Hyperacute free intraperitoneal bleed shows an attenuation similar to a patient's haematocrit, that is, 30–40 HU (Fig. 17.2). In anaemic patients, the attenuation may be even lesser and confuse with that of ascites or biliary leak. After few minutes to a couple of hours, the coagulation of free blood starts, and attenuation increases to 45–70 HU [17]. As time progresses, blood product degradation starts, and attenuation reduces to that of water in a couple of weeks. Detection of fluid in a suspected case of

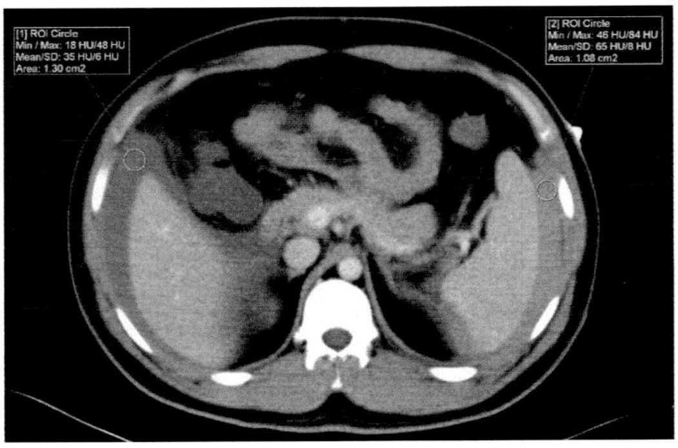

Fig. 17.2 Hemoperitoneum as seen on CECT. Fluid seen in the perihepatic region with high attenuation (35 HU) suggesting hyperacute haemorrhage

abdominal trauma is considered hemoperitoneum unless proven otherwise. It can also be seen as a physiological finding when a small amount of free fluid is seen in the pouch of Douglas or pelvis in women of reproductive age group.

Haemorrhage arising from an injured liver which is associated with capsular rupture appears as a perihepatic haemorrhage. If larger in amount, it extends below into the paracolic gutter. Accumulation of blood in the abdomen and pelvis suggests an amount of haemorrhage being at least 500 mL. Sometimes, following injury to the hepatobiliary system, the haemorrhage may appear in remote location like the pelvis or pouch of Douglas in women. The location of high-density blood in a case of trauma is an important clue to the site of injury. Focal accumulation of clotted blood (>60 HU) compared to haemorrhage of decreased attenuation elsewhere is described as the 'sentinel clot' sign and suggests the source of haemorrhage [18]. In coagulopathic states (when the patient is on anticoagulation treatment), there is layering of higher attenuating content dependently within a collection of free peritoneal blood [19]. This appearance may also be seen in recent haemorrhage in individuals with normal clotting profiles.

Lacerations Lacerations appear as linear or curvilinear hypoattenuating observations in the background of homogeneously enhancing parenchyma during the portal venous phase. They may show variable appearance (irregular or branch-

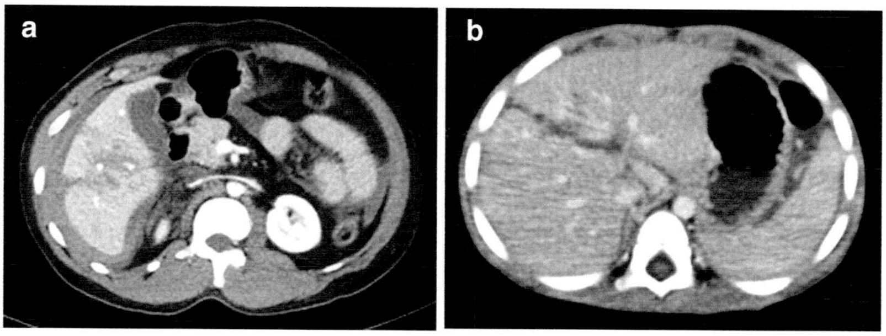

Fig. 17.3 Lacerations in the liver. Multiple lacerations with hemoperitoneum seen in (**a**). Deep laceration reaching up to the juxtacaval region in (**b**)

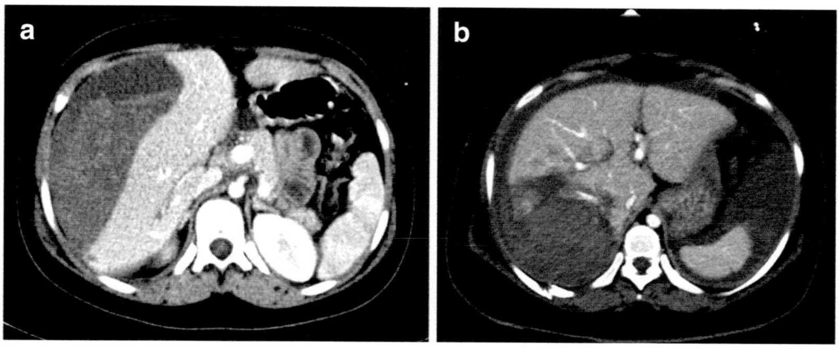

Fig. 17.4 Large subcapsular haematoma causing indentation of the liver surface in (**a**). Differential densities of blood seen in the subcapsular haematoma. Large intraparenchymal haematoma with laceration as well as hemoperitoneum seen in (**b**). No deformation of the liver surface seen in case of intraparenchymal haematoma

ing) and number as well as site in different cases depending upon the mechanism and severity of trauma (Fig. 17.3). Lower rib fractures are associated with a high incidence of hepatic lacerations and loss of capsular integrity with hemoperitoneum. They can be differentiated from contusions on the basis of linear (one-dimensional) morphology, and delayed filling is seen from the margins if additional phases are acquired. It is important to describe both the length (largest dimension) and depth of laceration (perpendicular distance from the capsule) to grade the liver injury accordingly. Multiple large and deep lacerations may lead to disruption of major part of a lobe or entire parenchyma and give rise to the appearance known as the shattered liver (usually seen operatively). Deep lacerations extending up to the porta hepatis can lead to biliary duct injuries with complications. The gall bladder may also be injured in deep lacerations especially in penetrating trauma. Pancreatic lacerations tend to occur at the junction of the body and tail due to shearing injuries with compression against the spine. They are much more likely to be associated with ductal injury (which is the major prognostic indicator) than contusions. Disruption of the pancreatic duct is inferred by visualisation of laceration involving more than 50% of pancreatic thickness. Laceration extending through the entire thickness of the pancreas can lead to pancreatic fracture with two separate ends seen on imaging.

Haematoma Haematoma can be subcapsular or intraparenchymal, meaning collections of blood contained by the liver capsule or parenchyma, respectively. Subcapsular haematomas are crescentic in shape and located peripherally, whereas intraparenchymal haematomas are usually elliptical in shape. Both subcapsular and intraparenchymal haematomas displace the hepatic parenchyma, which helps in differentiating it from contusions or perihepatic haemorrhage (Fig. 17.4). They appear as hypodense areas in and around the higher and more uniformly attenuating liver parenchyma. In the setting of hepatic steatosis, they may appear hyperattenuating. For grading according to American Association for the Surgery of Trauma (AAST) classification, the area of a subcapsular haematoma should be estimated and compared relative to the surface area of the organ.

Vascular injury CECT when acquired in both arterial and portal venous phases helps in direct visualisation of vascular injury as well as indirect signs of vascular injury [20]. Uncontained vascular injury in the form of active contrast extravasation is seen as a focus or amorphous area of high attenuation that increases in volume on the repeat phase (arterial and venous phases or venous and delayed phases as per acquisition) (Fig. 17.5). The arterial phase when acquired is more sensitive for the detection of active contrast extravasation. The extravasated contrast is usually within 10 HU of the vessel of origin and may help in localising the source of bleed [21]. Active visceral arterial bleeding usually requires immediate endovascular or surgical intervention. Non-bleeding vascular injury can be pseudoaneurysm or arteriovenous fistula (AVF) which appear as focal rounded or tubular areas of high-density contrast pooling which mirrors the attenuation of surrounding vessels. Early filling of the venous structure helps in differentiating the arteriovenous fistula from pseudoaneurysm. The arterial phase helps in the detection of non-bleeding vascular injuries better than the portal venous phase alone. Both pseudoaneurysm and AVF are usually treated by embolisation. Another type of vascular injury seen in the liver is arterioportal venous fistula (APF), usually following penetrating trauma or interventional procedure. It is seen in association with a hypoattenuating wedge-shaped area in the liver (called as transient hepatic attenuation difference). Other manifestations include early filling of peripheral or central intrahepatic portal vein. Simultaneous enhancement of portal vein as well as hepatic artery branch is seen as double barrel or rail track appearance [22]. It is important to embolise larger APF as they can cause portal hypertension and high-output cardiac failure. In a case of pancreatic injury, sudden drop in haemoglobin should alert to a possibility of pseudoaneurysm in the splenic artery (or its branches) against a backdrop of trauma-induced pancreatitis.

Contusion Contusion is an irregular hypodense area in an organ with interstitial blood suffusion. Unlike haematoma, it does not cause a mass effect, and blood vessels can be seen coursing through the contusion. Isolated contusion without laceration or haematoma is uncommon in the liver. However, pancreatic trauma (due to compression against the vertebra posteriorly) does frequently lead to contusions which are also evaluated in grading the pancreatic injury.

Organ infarct Segmental liver infarct is rare in the liver as there is dual blood supply from hepatic artery and portal venous system. When it happens, some degree of hepatic artery and portal venous occlusion is expected. It appears as a geographical or triangular hypoattenuating area with the apex directed towards the hilum. It can be complicated by secondary abscess.

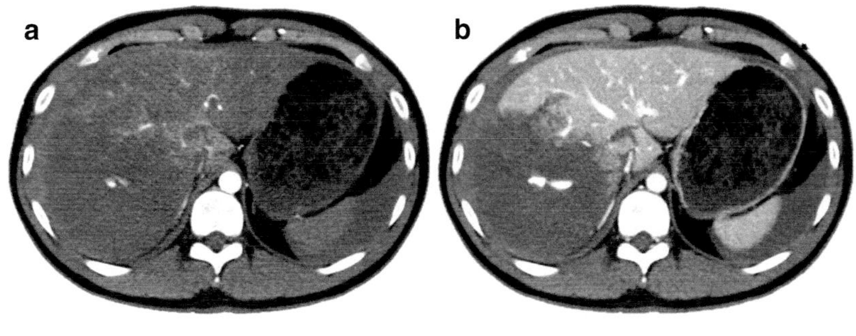

Fig. 17.5 Active extravasation seen in a large intraparenchymal haematoma in the liver. CT acquired in the early arterial phase (**a**) shows a blob of contrast that increases in size on the portal venous phase (**b**) suggesting active extravasation

Hypoperfusion In cases of severe trauma leading to major haemorrhage, signs of hypoperfusion are seen in abdominal CECT like hyperenhancement of adrenals, increased bowel wall enhancement and renal cortical enhancement [23]. The inferior vena cava (IVC) and aortic diameter are reduced.

17.4 Classification of Hepatic and Extrahepatic Biliary Injuries

The AAST Organ Injury Scale (OIS) is the most widely used traumatic organ injury classification system and was most recently updated in 2018 [24]. It classified various hepatic injuries according to extent and severity as well as included vascular injury.

17.5 Liver

The liver is said to be the most commonly injured organ in abdominal trauma. The right lobe is injured more commonly than the left, and the posterior segment is injured more commonly. Lacerations are the most common hepatic injuries [25]. It is important to note that lacerations in the bare area of liver extending to the posterior and superior aspect of segment VII can lead to significant haemorrhage in retroperitoneum as this part communicates directly with retroperitoneum. Other injuries seen commonly are haematomas (both intraparenchymal and subcapsular), active haemorrhage and pseudoaneurysms. Arterioportal venous fistulas and infarction may also be seen rarely. Intrahepatic or subcapsular air is seen rarely up to 2 days after trauma and is attributed to necrosis. Haemobilia is seen sometimes due to increased intrahepatic pressure following trauma leading to parenchymal necrosis and blood spilling into the biliary tree and gall bladder.

According to the AAST-OIS, the liver injuries are classified as *Grade 1*, subcapsular haematoma of <10% surface area or laceration <1 cm depth; *Grade 2*, subcapsular haematoma of 10–50% surface area or parenchymal haematoma of <10 cm or laceration 1–3 cm depth and <10 cm length; *Grade 3*, subcapsular haematoma of >50% surface area, ruptured subcapsular or parenchymal haematoma or parenchymal haematoma of >10 cm or laceration >3 cm depth and >10 cm length or hepatic vascular injury or active contrast extravasation contained within liver parenchyma; *Grade 4*, parenchymal disruption involving 25–75% of a hepatic lobe or active contrast extravasation extending beyond liver parenchyma into the peritoneum; *Grade 5*, parenchymal disruption involving >75% of a hepatic lobe or juxtahepatic venous injury involving IVC or hepatic veins.

Few important points to note are:

- If multiple injuries are present, advance one grade up to Grade 3.
- Vascular injuries refer to pseudoaneurysm or arteriovenous fistula.
- Most common hepatic injuries are Grade II followed by Grade 1.
- The final AAST class is ultimately based upon the highest grade obtained on imaging, at time of operation or pathology.

Major venous injury is an important scenario to detect and manage in hepatobiliary trauma. It occurs when hepatic laceration extends into the IVC and/or hepatic veins (Fig. 17.6). CT shows active extravasation, contour abnormality and associated hepatic injury [26]. It is graded as AAST Grade 4 injury and requires operative management mostly as the mortality rates are up to 100%, 78% and 33% for suprahepatic, retrohepatic and suprarenal injuries, respectively [26].

With the increasing tendency and approach towards NOM (non-operative management) in most of patients with liver trauma, there is an increased frequency of delayed complications which are recognised on follow-up investigations. These include:

- Delayed haemorrhage: usually secondary to a pseudoaneurysm, expanding biloma or an initial minimal injury expanding in size to include the vessels secondarily. It can also

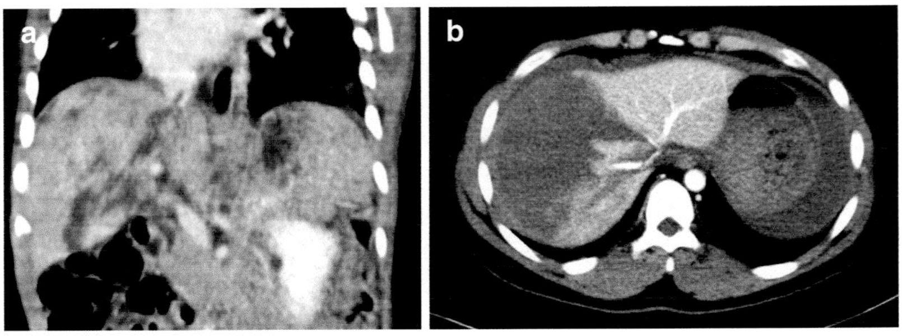

Fig. 17.6 Coronal CT image shows multiple lacerations in the liver and spleen (**a**). One of the lacerations seen extending up to intrahepatic IVC. An axial CT image (**b**) of a different patient with a large haematoma in the right lobe of the liver and lacerations extending along the hepatic veins into the intrahepatic IVC

present as haemobilia if the pseudoaneurysm ruptures into the biliary tree.

Abscess: seen as a hypodense lesion showing fluid density with air foci or air-fluid levels. Should be managed by percutaneous drainage.

Biliary complications: Biloma, biliary extravasation and biliary peritonitis can occur secondary to high-grade hepatic trauma.

Follow-up investigations are usually not required in most cases of low-grade hepatic trauma. However, in cases of high-grade trauma or if any complication is suspected, investigations like ultrasound or contrast-enhanced ultrasound (if high suspicion of vascular injury) can be performed as alternative to CT before discharging the patient or after 7–10 days of initial trauma.

Digital subtraction angiography (DSA) is usually performed with a therapeutic intent to treat any vascular injury or simply reduce the hepatic perfusion pressure in cases of high-grade liver injury in combination with surgical packing. Superselective catheterisation of the arteries and their distal branches helps in reducing ischemia when coupled with portal venous supply of liver, making angioembolisation a safe approach in patients of liver trauma. In a hemodynamically stable patient post severe trauma, if there is the presence of active contrast extravasation/pseudoaneurysm as seen on CT, or there is a drop in haemoglobin during NOM, angioembolisation is done to identify the offending vessel and embolise it using gelfoam or coils [27]. Traumatic pseudoaneurysms occur in 15% of patients with liver trauma. Delayed rupture of pseudoaneurysms can have devastating consequences, so all pseudoaneurysms are treated with embolisation as soon as possible. Coil embolisation is preferred over gelfoam embolisation in case of pseudoaneurysm(s). Arteriovenous or arterioportal shunting is a rare vascular injury subset that occurs secondary to trauma. It can be assessed on multiphase CT; however definitive diagnosis is made on DSA. These patients are also treated with coil embolisation of the feeding artery.

17.6 Biliary Tract Injuries

Biliary tract injuries are rarely seen (2–3%) due to the protective effect of the liver [28]. Gall bladder injuries are more frequent as compared to extrahepatic biliary tract and IHBD. Isolated biliary tract injuries are extremely uncommon, and they are usually associated with additional injuries to the liver, spleen and duodenum [28]. Traumatic bile leaks are increasing in prevalence due to the trend of NOM of hepatic injuries [29]. It is important to diagnose them early to reduce the morbidity in patients with hepatic trauma managed conservatively.

CT findings Various injuries occurring in the gall bladder are contusions (most common), lacerations, perforations and avulsions. Contusions

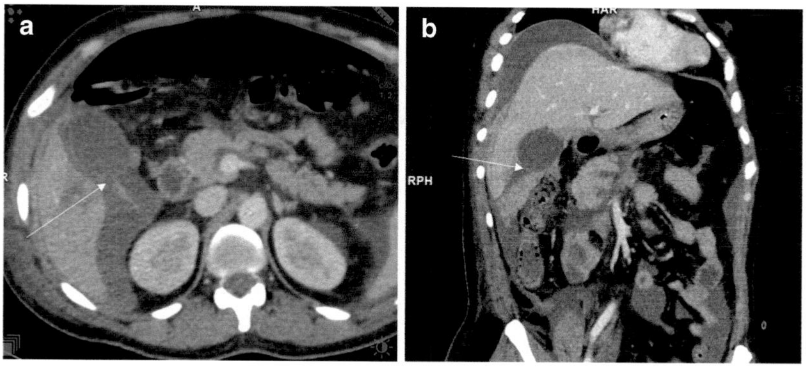

Fig. 17.7 CECT axial (**a**) and coronal (**b**) images in a man after road traffic accident show a thin discontinuous wall (arrow) of the gall bladder with extensive perihepatic and intraperitoneal free fluid (hemoperitoneum)

may present with subtle wall thickening (due to intramural haematoma) and are the mildest form of injuries to the gall bladder. Lacerations or perforations may present as the collapsed gall bladder lumen with pericholecystic fluid and discontinuous gall bladder wall enhancement (Fig. 17.7). Avulsions are the most severe injuries and may reveal gall bladder displaced from the fossa with or without associated injury to the cystic duct and cystic artery with significant haemorrhage [30]. Gall bladder may be filled with hyperdense contents suggesting haemobilia in cases of trauma.

Bile leak is usually associated with significant trauma to the biliary tree. It may present as either contained fluid around GB fossa or liver parenchyma called as bilomas or may freely leak into the peritoneum making it indistinguishable from ascites and hemoperitoneum in many cases. Intrahepatic bilomas are usually well-defined circumscribed lobular hypodense collections, while intraperitoneal bile leak is suspected when there are signs of biliary peritonitis [31]. Biliary peritonitis can be seen as persistent or increase in the amount of intraperitoneal fluid and thickening and enhancement of the peritoneum.

Imaging risk factors for biliary tract injuries include high-grade hepatic injuries, lacerations extending to the porta, gall bladder fossa, or near IVC and low-density perihepatic fluid. Factors that predispose the gall bladder to injury are distension and increased sphincter of Oddi tone. If there is high index of suspicion of trauma to the biliary tract, other investigations can be used to confirm the diagnosis.

Hepatobiliary scintigraphy It demonstrates physiologic biliary excretion and has the ability to demonstrate active bile leaks. Progressive accumulation of a radiotracer in the abdomen not conforming to the appearance of the bowel is diagnostic of bile leak [32]. It can also help in determining the severity and rapidity of bile leak with the use of dynamic imaging. However, it is limited by poor spatial resolution and anatomical details which necessitates the use of MRCP in conjunction.

Magnetic resonance cholangiopancreatography A non-contrast MRCP can be performed to assess the biliary tract and look for any irregularity or discontinuity. MRCP with a hepatobiliary contrast is a powerful alternative to hepatobiliary scintigraphy in the dynamic evaluation of the biliary system as it has the unique ability to reveal the exact location of a bile leak [33]. It is limited in the trauma setting by its long acquisition times as well as signal noise by injury to surrounding tissues and inadequate patient preparation.

Percutaneous transhepatic cholangiography (PTC) During the need of an intervention such as percutaneous transhepatic biliary drain (PTBD) placement to decompress an obstructed biliary system and control bile leakage, it is combined with PTC to detect and localise the site of injury and leak. PTC is superior to ERCP for the evaluation of proximal bile duct injuries, common duct ligation or transection. It is an invasive procedure with a major complication rate of 2%, hence not used routinely when non-invasive diagnosis of biliary tract injury suffices [34].

Biliary tract injury management requires a skilled multidisciplinary team including interventional radiology, gastroenterology and hepatobiliary surgery. Percutaneous and endoscopic interventions provide definitive treatment for several types of bile duct injuries. Cholecystectomy is usually the treatment for severe gall bladder injuries.

17.7 Pancreatic Injuries

Penetrating injuries to the abdomen are the major contributor to pancreatic injuries. Retroperitoneal location of the pancreas protects it from most instances of blunt abdominal trauma. However, in children and young adults (with thin habitus and less abdominal fat), sudden localised force to the upper abdomen causes compression of the pancreas against the spine leading to pancreatic injuries. This usually happens in handle bar injuries to cyclists, direct blow in children or seat belt injuries in a four-wheeler [35]. The body of the pancreas is most commonly injured followed by the head and tail. The clinical and laboratory features of pancreatic injury like abdominal pain, leukocytosis and hyperamylasemia may be subtle and non-specific, limiting their usefulness in early recognition [36]. Thus, imaging plays an essential role in not only detecting parenchymal injury but also helping determine the management plan.

The two most important determinants of outcome following pancreatic injury are the time from injury to definitive diagnosis and the status of the main pancreatic duct (MPD) [37]. For the diagnosis of MPD injuries, CT has sensitivity and specificity of 70–80% [38]. Thus, it needs to be supplemented with MRCP and ERCP in hemodynamically stable patients to improve the outcome of management decision. Various imaging findings seen in pancreatic trauma useful to management are:

CT CT may show a normal pancreas in about 20–40% of patients when it is done within 12 hours of pancreatic trauma [39]. Little change in density and separation of lacerated fragments reduces the sensitivity of detection of pancreatic injuries in early stages. A repeat CT in 24–48 hours with specific pancreatic protocol in cases with high suspicion helps in the detection of specific imaging findings. These include pancreatic contusions (Fig. 17.8), lacerations (including fracture), pancreatic haematoma, focal or diffuse pancreatic oedema, fluid separating the splenic vein and pancreatic parenchyma and vascular injury seen as active extravasation.

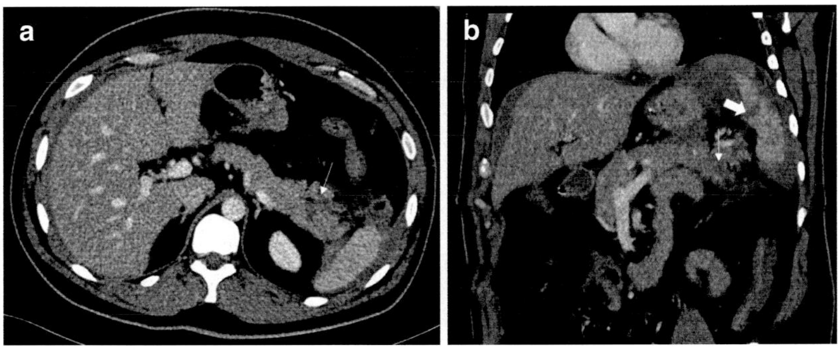

Fig. 17.8 Axial CECT image (**a**) and coronal CECT image (**b**) in an 8-year-old boy after blunt trauma show a contusion in the tail of the pancreas (arrow) with peripancreatic fluid. Lacerations in the spleen (solid arrow) are also seen on the coronal image with perihepatic as well as perisplenic fluid

Specific signs	Non-specific signs
Contusion	Inflammatory changes in peripancreatic region
Laceration	Intraperitoneal/ extraperitoneal fluid
Pancreatic fracture	Thickening of the anterior renal fascia
Haematoma	Fluid in the lesser sac/ mesocolon
Focal or diffuse oedema	Pancreatic ductal dilatation
Fluid between the splenic vein and pancreas	Acute peripancreatic fluid collection
Active extravasation	Fluid in anterior/posterior pararenal spaces

Major contusion is considered when there is hypoenhancement involving greater than 25% of the pancreatic parenchyma. Location and depth of laceration (Figs. 17.9 and 17.10) are important considerations while evaluating the CT in pancreatic injury. Major laceration is usually considered when the injury involves 25–50% of the pancreatic depth. The neck of the pancreas is the most common site of laceration. The spatial relationship of laceration with respect to superior mesenteric vein (SMV) and portal vein axis decides the surgical management. If a major laceration is to the left of SMV, it is usually managed by distal pancreatectomy. A laceration to the right of SMV would require Whipple's procedure. These are then often managed non-operatively except in cases of complete disruption of the head which will require Whipple's surgery.

MRI with MRCP Evaluation of integrity of the pancreatic duct is essential in determining prognosis and management in pancreatic injury. CT has been shown to have suboptimal (43%) sensi-

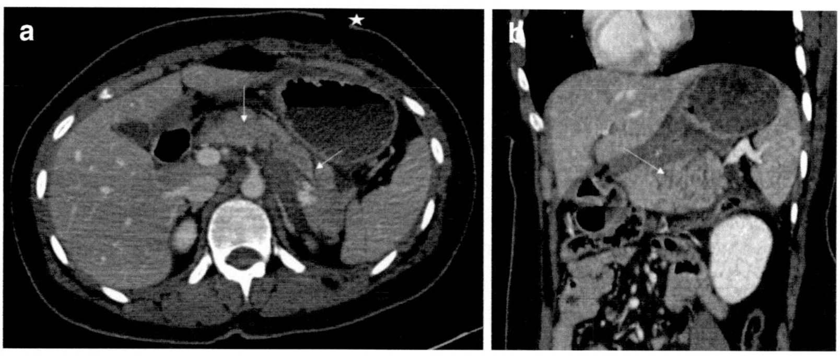

Fig. 17.9 Axial CECT image (**a**) and coronal CECT image (**b**) in a 20-year-old man after penetrating trauma (wound marked with asterisk) show multiple superficial lacerations in the body and the tail of the pancreas (arrows) with perisplenic fluid (haematoma). Haematoma also seen along the track of penetrating injury—along subcutaneous space, anterior abdominal wall and lesser sac

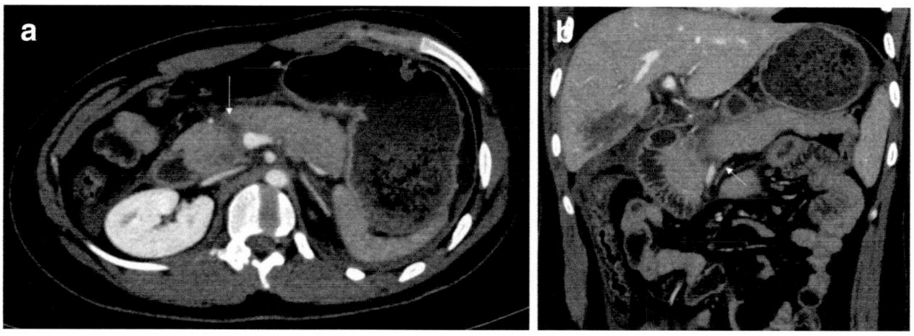

Fig. 17.10 Multiplanar reformatted oblique axial (**a**) and coronal (**b**) images of CECT abdomen in a 30-year-old man with blunt trauma showing a laceration in the neck of the pancreas (arrow) extending across the entire thickness of pancreatic parenchyma. Peripancreatic haematoma also seen with evidence of lacerations in the right lobe of the liver with hemoperitoneum

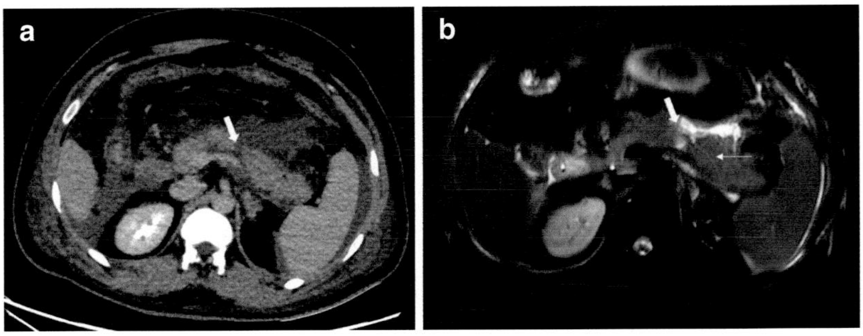

Fig. 17.11 CECT axial (**a**) image in a 38-year-old man with road traffic accident showing laceration (solid arrow) in the body of the pancreas involving more than 50% of the width of pancreatic parenchyma with peripancreatic fluid as well as hemoperitoneum (seen as perihepatic and perisplenic fluid). Axial T2 fat-suppressed image (**b**) clearly depicts the laceration in the body of the pancreas (solid arrow) reaching up to and involving the main pancreatic duct (seen distal to the laceration—arrow) with peripancreatic free fluid

tivity in the detection of pancreatic duct injuries [40]. Hence, MRI with MRCP is usually performed after 48–60 hours of trauma to detect injuries to the pancreatic duct and prevent development of complications. Dynamic secretin-stimulated MRCP is a variation on standard MRCP and can further improve sensitivity and accuracy of detection of pancreatic ductal injuries. It has the advantage over ERCP in demonstration of the pancreatic duct as well as leak even distal to a major laceration or transection which are not seen on ERCP. Also, it is non-invasive, faster and more readily available as compared to ERCP. MRCP has been shown to depict the MPD in the pancreatic body in up to 97% of cases and in the pancreatic tail in up to 83% of cases [41]. Magnetic resonance pancreatograms are acquired by using heavily T2-weighted breath-hold or non-breath hold sequences (Fig. 17.11).

ERCP ERCP is considered as the most accurate investigation in detection of the main pancreatic duct injuries [42]. It involves the advancement of a duodenoscope till the major papilla and then introduction of a cannula into the major papilla. It is followed by injection of contrast under fluoroscopic guidance to visualise the main pancreatic duct. Ductal injury is seen as abrupt termination of MPD or leakage of contrast. ERCP has an advantage over MRCP in enabling image-guided intervention in hemodynamically stable patients in the form of stent insertion in the main pancreatic duct injury. It is helpful in the management of complications like drainage of pseudocyst and diversion of fistula through transpapillary and transmural drainage [42].

Pancreatic injuries are classified according to the AAST-OIS grading of pancreatic injuries [43]. The injuries are classified as follows: *Grade 1*, minor contusion or major laceration without the main pancreatic duct involvement; *Grade 2*, major contusion or major laceration without the main pancreatic duct involvement; *Grade 3*, transection or laceration involving the main pancreatic duct in the body/tail of the pancreas; *Grade 4*, transection or laceration involving the main pancreatic duct/ampulla in the head of the pancreas; *Grade 5*, massive disruption of the pancreatic head.

Like in the case of liver injury, one grade can be advanced (up to Grade 3) for multiple injuries.

17.8 Complications of Pancreatic Trauma

Complications in pancreatic trauma can develop in up to one third of patients. They usually develop when the pancreatic duct is injured and

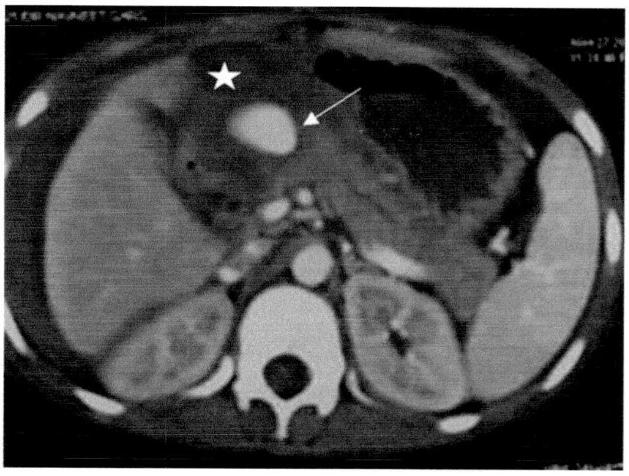

Fig. 17.12 CECT axial image in a young man with road traffic accident showing a large pseudoaneurysm (arrow) in the head of the pancreas with surrounding haematoma (asterisk)

result in prolonged morbidity. Complications include fistula formation (most common), traumatic pancreatitis, pseudocyst formation, abscesses and duct stricture. Leakage of pancreatic enzymes may lead to vessel wall erosion forming pseudoaneurysm (Fig. 17.12) that may complicate with delayed haemorrhage [44]. Prevention and management of complications are imperative to improve prognosis of pancreatic injury, and imaging plays an important role. Follow-up investigations like ultrasound can help in the detection of abscesses and pseudocysts. Fistula and pseudoaneurysms can be detected using cross-sectional investigations like CT and MRI with MRCP. Pseudoaneurysms can be treated with minimally invasive interventional radiological procedures.

17.9 Conclusion

Hepatobiliary and pancreatic trauma is a common emergency that requires prompt diagnosis and management. It is best assessed by contrast-enhanced CT in hemodynamically stable patients. By accurately detecting and characterising these injuries and the associated vascular injuries in addition to evaluating delayed complications, CT has enabled and aided successful non-surgical management of the traumatic injuries. MRI with MRCP is increasingly employed in suspected cases of pancreatic trauma to accurately characterise and grade injuries. The trauma radiologist plays an essential role in selecting the optimal scanning parameters to optimise injury detection and in recognising the range of imaging features typically encountered in upper abdominal trauma, including findings that potentially confound accurate diagnosis. In cases of diagnostic doubt or scenarios where intervention is required, other investigations like hepatobiliary scintigraphy, ERCP, PTBD (in combination with PTC) and DSA should be used judiciously taking into account the clinical condition and tolerability of the trauma patient.

References

1. Dandona R, Kumar GA, Gururaj G, et al. Mortality due to road injuries in the states of India: the Global Burden of Disease Study 1990–2017. Lancet Public Health. 2020;5(2):e86–98. https://doi.org/10.1016/S2468-2667(19)30246-4.
2. Stanescu AL, Gross JA, Bittle M, Mann FA. Imaging of blunt abdominal trauma. Semin Roentgenol. 2006;41(3):196–208. https://doi.org/10.1053/j.ro.2006.05.002.
3. Tinkoff G, Esposito TJ, Reed J, et al. American Association for the Surgery of Trauma Organ Injury Scale I: spleen, liver, and kidney, validation based on the National Trauma Data Bank. J Am Coll Surg. 2008;207(5):646–55. https://doi.org/10.1016/j.jamcollsurg.2008.06.342.
4. Brillantino A, Iacobellis F, Festa P, et al. Non-operative management of blunt liver trauma: safety, efficacy and complications of a standardized treatment protocol. Bull Emerg Trauma. 2019;7(1):49–54. https://doi.org/10.29252/beat-070107.
5. Christmas AB, Wilson AK, Manning B, et al. Selective management of blunt hepatic injuries including nonoperative management is a safe and effective strategy. Surgery. 2005;138(4):606–11. https://doi.org/10.1016/j.surg.2005.07.018.
6. Bala M, Gazalla SA, Faroja M, et al. Complications of high grade liver injuries: management and outcomewith focus on bile leaks. Scand J Trauma Resusc Emerg Med. 2012;20:20. https://doi.org/10.1186/1757-7241-20-20.
7. Extrahepatic bile duct injury in blunt trauma: a systematic review. https://read.qxmd.com/read/31008893/extrahepatic-bile-duct-injury-in-blunt-trauma-a-systematic-review. Accessed 5 Sept 2022.
8. Ball CG, Dixon E, Kirkpatrick AW, Sutherland FR, Laupland KB, Feliciano DV. SAhodrt Reepcoartde of

experience with injuries to the gallbladder. Published online 2010:4.
9. Iacono C, Zicari M, Conci S, et al. Management of pancreatic trauma: a pancreatic surgeon's point of view. Pancreatology. 2016;16(3):302–8. https://doi.org/10.1016/j.pan.2015.12.004.
10. Miller PR, Croce MA, Bee TK, Malhotra AK, Fabian TC. Associated injuries in blunt solid organ trauma: implications for missed injury in nonoperative management. J Trauma. 2002;53(2):238–42; discussion 242–244. https://doi.org/10.1097/00005373-200208000-00008.
11. Körner M, Krötz MM, Degenhart C, Pfeifer KJ, Reiser MF, Linsenmaier U. Current role of emergency US in patients with major trauma. Radiogr Rev Publ Radiol Soc N Am Inc. 2008;28(1):225–42. https://doi.org/10.1148/rg.281075047.
12. Leung V, Sastry A, Woo TD, Jones HR. Implementation of a split-bolus single-pass CT protocol at a UK major trauma centre to reduce excess radiation dose in trauma pan-CT. Clin Radiol. 2015;70(10):1110–5. https://doi.org/10.1016/j.crad.2015.05.014.
13. Linsenmaier U, Wirth S, Reiser M, Körner M. Diagnosis and classification of pancreatic and duodenal injuries in emergency radiology. Radiogr Rev Publ Radiol Soc N Am Inc. 2008;28(6):1591–602. https://doi.org/10.1148/rg.286085524.
14. Wortman JR, Uyeda JW, Fulwadhva UP, Sodickson AD. Dual-energy CT for abdominal and pelvic trauma. Radiogr Rev Publ Radiol Soc N Am Inc. 2018;38(2):586–602. https://doi.org/10.1148/rg.2018170058.
15. Sun EX, Wortman JR, Uyeda JW, Lacson R, Sodickson AD. Virtual monoenergetic dual-energy CT for evaluation of hepatic and splenic lacerations. Emerg Radiol. 2019;26(4):419–25. https://doi.org/10.1007/s10140-019-01687-y.
16. Macari M, Spieler B, Kim D, et al. Dual-source dual-energy MDCT of pancreatic adenocarcinoma: initial observations with data generated at 80 kVp and at simulated weighted-average 120 kVp. AJR Am J Roentgenol. 2010;194(1):W27–32. https://doi.org/10.2214/AJR.09.2737.
17. Lubner M, Menias C, Rucker C, et al. Blood in the belly: CT findings of hemoperitoneum. Radiogr Rev Publ Radiol Soc N Am Inc. 2007;27(1):109–25. https://doi.org/10.1148/rg.271065042.
18. Orwig D, Federle MP. Localized clotted blood as evidence of visceral trauma on CT: the sentinel clot sign. AJR Am J Roentgenol. 1989;153(4):747–9. https://doi.org/10.2214/ajr.153.4.747.
19. Federle MP, Pan KT, Pealer KM. CT criteria for differentiating abdominal hemorrhage: anticoagulation or aortic aneurysm rupture? AJR Am J Roentgenol. 2007;188(5):1324–30. https://doi.org/10.2214/AJR.05.1911.
20. Baghdanian AH, Armetta AS, Baghdanian AA, LeBedis CA, Anderson SW, Soto JA. CT of major vascular injury in blunt abdominopelvic trauma. Radiogr Rev Publ Radiol Soc N Am Inc. 2016;36(3):872–90. https://doi.org/10.1148/rg.2016150160.
21. Hamilton JD, Kumaravel M, Censullo ML, Cohen AM, Kievlan DS, West OC. Multidetector CT evaluation of active extravasation in blunt abdominal and pelvic trauma patients. RadioGraphics. 2008;28(6):1603–16. https://doi.org/10.1148/rg.286085522.
22. Nguyen CT, Nguyen C, Saksobhavivat N, et al. MDCT diagnosis of post-traumatic hepatic arterio-portal fistulas. Emerg Radiol. 2013;20(3):225–32. https://doi.org/10.1007/s10140-012-1092-6.
23. Prasad KR, Kumar A, Gamanagatti S, Chandrashekhara SH. CT in post-traumatic hypoperfusion complex–a pictorial review. Emerg Radiol. 2011;18(2):139–43. https://doi.org/10.1007/s10140-010-0927-2.
24. Kozar RA, Crandall M, Shanmuganathan K, Zarzaur BL, Coburn M, Cribari C, Kaups K, Schuster K, Tominaga GT, AAST Patient Assessment Committee. Organ injury scaling 2018 update: spleen, liver, and kidney. J Trauma Acute Care Surg. 2018;85(6):1119–22. https://doi.org/10.1097/TA.0000000000002058. Erratum in: J Trauma Acute Care Surg. 2019;87(2):512. doi: 10.1097/TA.0000000000002419. PMID: 30462622.
25. Yoon W, Jeong YY, Kim JK, et al. CT in blunt liver trauma. Radiogr Rev Publ Radiol Soc N Am Inc. 2005;25(1):87–104. https://doi.org/10.1148/rg.251045079.
26. Tsai R, Raptis C, Schuerer DJ, Mellnick VM. CT appearance of traumatic inferior vena cava injury. Am J Roentgenol. 2016;207(4):705–11. https://doi.org/10.2214/AJR.15.15870.
27. Gilyard S, Shinn K, Nezami N, et al. Contemporary management of hepatic Trauma: what IRs need to know. Semin Interv Radiol. 2020;37(1):35–43. https://doi.org/10.1055/s-0039-3401838.
28. Erb RE, Mirvis SE, Shanmuganathan K. Gallbladder injury secondary to blunt trauma: CT findings. J Comput Assist Tomogr. 1994;18(5):778–84.
29. LeBedis CA, Bates DDB, Soto JA. Iatrogenic, blunt, and penetrating trauma to the biliary tract. Abdom Radiol NY. 2017;42(1):28–45. https://doi.org/10.1007/s00261-016-0856-y.
30. Chen X, Talner LB, Jurkovich GJ. Gallbladder avulsion due to blunt trauma. AJR Am J Roentgenol. 2001;177(4):822. https://doi.org/10.2214/ajr.177.4.1770822.
31. Melamud K, LeBedis CA, Anderson SW, Soto JA. Biliary imaging: multimodality approach to imaging of biliary injuries and their complications. Radiogr Rev Publ Radiol Soc N Am Inc. 2014;34(3):613–23. https://doi.org/10.1148/rg.343130011.
32. Chiu WC, Wong-You-Cheong JJ, Rodriguez A, Shanmuganathan K, Mirvis SE, Scalea TM. Ultrasonography for interval assessment in the nonoperative management of hepatic trauma. Am Surg. 2005;71(10):841–6.

33. Khalid TR, Casillas VJ, Montalvo BM, Centeno R, Levi JU. Using MR cholangiopancreatography to evaluate iatrogenic bile duct injury. Am J Roentgenol. 2001;177(6):1347–52. https://doi.org/10.2214/ajr.177.6.1771347.
34. Pomerantz BJ. Biliary tract interventions. Tech Vasc Interv Radiol. 2009;12(2):162–70. https://doi.org/10.1053/j.tvir.2009.08.009.
35. Venkatesh SK, Wan JMC. CT of blunt pancreatic trauma: a pictorial essay. Eur J Radiol. 2008;67(2):311–20. https://doi.org/10.1016/j.ejrad.2007.07.003.
36. Potoka DA, Gaines BA, Leppäniemi A, Peitzman AB. Management of blunt pancreatic trauma: what's new? Eur J Trauma Emerg Surg. 2015;41(3):239–50. https://doi.org/10.1007/s00068-015-0510-3.
37. Lee PH, Lee SK, Kim GU, et al. Outcomes of hemodynamically stable patients with pancreatic injury after blunt abdominal trauma. Pancreatology. 2012;12(6):487–92. https://doi.org/10.1016/j.pan.2012.09.006.
38. Odedra D, Mellnick VM, Patlas MN. Imaging of blunt pancreatic trauma: a systematic review. Can Assoc Radiol J J Assoc Can Radiol. 2020;71(3):344–51. https://doi.org/10.1177/0846537119888383.
39. Jeffrey RB, Federle MP, Crass RA. Computed tomography of pancreatic trauma. Radiology. 1983;147(2):491–4. https://doi.org/10.1148/radiology.147.2.6836127.
40. Panda A, Kumar A, Gamanagatti S, et al. Evaluation of diagnostic utility of multidetector computed tomography and magnetic resonance imaging in blunt pancreatic trauma: a prospective study. Acta Radiol Stockh Swed 1987. 2015;56(4):387–96. https://doi.org/10.1177/0284185114529949.
41. Gupta A, Stuhlfaut JW, Fleming KW, Lucey BC, Soto JA. Blunt trauma of the pancreas and biliary tract: a multimodality imaging approach to diagnosis. Radiogr Rev Publ Radiol Soc N Am Inc. 2004;24(5):1381–95. https://doi.org/10.1148/rg.245045002.
42. Debi U, Kaur R, Prasad KK, Sinha SK, Sinha A, Singh K. Pancreatic trauma: a concise review. World J Gastroenterol WJG. 2013;19(47):9003–11. https://doi.org/10.3748/wjg.v19.i47.9003.
43. Moore EE, Cogbill TH, Malangoni MA, Jurkovich GJ, Champion HR, Gennarelli TA, McAninch JW, Pachter HL, Shackford SR, Trafton PG. Organ injury scaling, II: pancreas, duodenum, small bowel, colon, and rectum. J Trauma. 1990;30(11):1427–9. PMID: 2231822.
44. Byrge N, Heilbrun M, Winkler N, et al. An AAST-MITC analysis of pancreatic trauma: staple or sew? Resect or drain? J Trauma Acute Care Surg. 2018;85(3):435–43. https://doi.org/10.1097/TA.0000000000001987.

18 PET/CT in Hepatobiliary Pancreatic Tumours

Sikandar Shaikh

18.1 Hepatic Lesions

18.1.1 HCC

18-Fluoro-2-deoxyglucose (FDG)-positron emission tomography (PET)/computed tomography (CT) is a newer molecular imaging modality which uses glucose as the metabolic contrast agent. The various applications are for the staging, restaging, evaluation of the early disease recurrence, monitoring the response to the treatment, and for the prognosis of the various malignancies. The other important applications are for the diagnosis of the inflammatory diseases. The availability of the routine anatomical modalities like the CT and magnetic resonance imaging (MRI) can help easily diagnose the various tumours of the hepatobiliary pancreatic system and also for the tumour-like lesions. The role of the use of the FDG-PET/CT is fully established now, but despite this, there are many fallacies which limit their precise use in these conditions. The amount of the uptake in these conditions where the primary and secondary malignant lesions involving the hepatic parenchyma show a significant amount of the increased uptake and on the contrary the benign lesions will have a similar amount of the uptake like the background liver parenchyma. Despite this there are many false-negative and false-positive uptake seen in the malignant tumours and also higher amount of the uptake in the benign tumours and various other infective and inflammatory lesions. Again, the amount of the uptake is seen differently in the even similar tumours histologically. The tumour differentiation in some of the tumours is again based on the amount of the uptake which can predict the better prognosis and also the therapeutic response.

Primary hepatobiliary malignancies include various hepatic tumours, cholangiocarcinoma, and gallbladder cancer. Primary hepatic tumours are categorized into malignant or benign [1], which comprises the hepatocellular carcinomas (HCCs), haemangiomas, adenomas, and focal nodular hyperplasia (FNH). Chronic liver disease is the main cause of the increased incidence of the HCC, and hepatitis is one of the common causes [2], followed by alcoholic cirrhosis [3] and other various systemic immune diseases, affecting the entire body such as human immunodeficiency virus [4]. Biliary and gallbladder primary malignant tumours are not that prevalent (<2% of cancer prevalence) but are very difficult to diagnose in the operative stage. Gallbladder cancer has different aetiologies globally, and the common causes are the cholelithiasis and infections like *Salmonella* [5]. The role of PET and PET/CT is very important and well established for the diagnosis, staging, restaging, and

S. Shaikh (✉)
Department of Radiodiagnosis, Shadan Institute of Medical Sciences, Hyderabad, Telangana, India

© The Author(s), under exclusive license to Springer Nature Singapore Pte Ltd. 2025

B. Sureka (ed.), *Hepato-Pancreatico Biliary Imaging*, https://doi.org/10.1007/978-981-95-1699-5_18

follow-up of these malignancies. The availability of various newer hepatic MRI protocols has significantly increased the ability of MRI for the differentiation of various benign and malignant focal hepatic lesions. Diffusion-weighted imaging investigated by Koike et al. [6] is capable of easier differentiation of malignant versus benign lesions by a quantitative parameter of lower apparent diffusion coefficient with increased contrast ratio as compared with adjacent background hepatic parenchyma. With the development of various specific MRI hepatobiliary contrast agents, the lesion detection and characterization have become significantly increased [7]. With the availability of the various MRI techniques, the differentiation and the characterization of the hepatic lesions will become easier in the future. Glucose metabolism in the liver is an important component of the nondietary glucose, for maintaining the glucose homeostasis at the rate of 2.0 mg/kg/min [8]. Various levels of glucose-6-phosphatase (G6Pase) activity and also the glucose transporters (GLUTs) in HCC, and due to this there will be significant change in the amount of the 18F-FDG uptake which is more variable [9–12]. Torizuka et al.'s [9] study revealed that the amount of the FDG uptake in the HCC is based on the HCC differentiation; the higher the grade of HCCs, the higher the FDG uptake (mean [± SD] standardized uptake value [SUV], 6.89 ± 3.39) (Fig. 18.1) as compared with low-grade HCCs (mean SUV, 3.21 ± 0.58) ($p < 0.005$). Because of this the FDG-PET uptake in the scans can detect higher-grade HCCs and less amount of the uptake in the low-grade HCCs, due to the decreased FDG uptake. FDG-PET/CT uptake in the detection of HCC has a significant range of 50–65% [12–16]. Due to this difference, the FDG-PET [14] is not highly sensitive for the diagnosis of the primary HCC.

One of the studies by Khan et al. [13] showed that the sensitivity of FDG-PET for the diagnosis of HCC was 55%, as compared with the contrast-enhanced CT with 90%. Another study by Wudel et al. [15], which has the larger number of FDG-PET evaluation for HCC (n = 91), showed that the sensitivity of FDG-PET for the detection of HCC was 64%. The overall sensitivity of FDG-

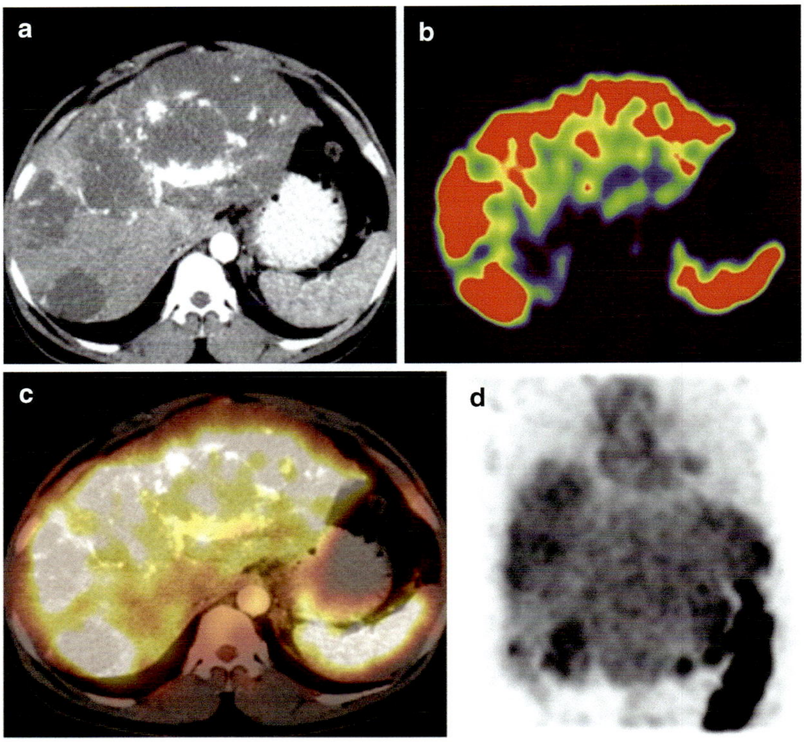

Fig. 18.1 Multiple hypodense lesions seen in both lobes of the liver with peripheral nodular enhancement on CT image **a**, **b**, and **d** showing diffuse increased uptake seen corresponding to the liver lesions which shows high metabolic activity of the lesions. Fused image **c** shows increased uptake corresponding to CT lesions

PET is lower than that of other imaging modalities for HCC, but despite this the FDG uptake will be acting like the biomarker of differentiation. The semiquantitative values of SUVs can only give the opinion of the histopathologic evaluation of the tumour. Shiomi et al. [17] studied and concluded that the SUV ratios (SUV ratio of tumour to non-tumour in the liver) of HCC tumours will be correlating the tumour volume-doubling time ($r = -0.582$; $p = 0.006$). By their technique the cumulative survival rate can be used for the diagnosis for the correct evaluation of the SUV ratio. In this study two groups are formed and divided into two similar group size: group A ($n = 24$) had SUV ratios (here it is defined as the hepatic tumour-to-non-tumour ratio of SUV) of 1.5 or less, and group B ($n = 24$) had the SUV values greater than 1.5. The cumulative survival rate is lower in group B than in group A ($p = 0.026$). One of the studies by the Kong et al. [18] has shown that in patients with HCC of mean SUVs 7 or greater and having the ($p = 0.0003$) on the lower median side in the range of the (4 vs 15 months). The role of FDG-PET/CT is to evaluate tumours better than the conventional CT modality and other modalities, and this has a bigger advantage in evaluating the whole body at one time for the detection of the metastases which can be local or distant [13]. In one of the studies [19], FDG-PET/CT scan for pre-therapy evaluation was done instead of the CT and MRI for the evaluation of extrahepatic metastases. Of the 87 patients, 24 of them had extrahepatic metastases. All these extrahepatic metastases were detected by FDG-PET without performing CT or MRI. Along with the primary evaluation, nodal and skeletal metastases were also detected in four and six patients, respectively. Here the entire tumour, node, and metastasis (TNM) staging which was done based on the conventional modalities such as CT and MRI was changed by the FDG-PET/CT. Ho et al. [20] studies showed that the poorly differentiated HCCs, which are more likely metastatic, are FDG avid; thus, the metastatic foci in the HCCs can be easily detected by the FDG-PET. Wudel et al. [15] showed the sensitivity of the FDG accumulation in the 64% of HCCs which had a significant impact in the work-up of the 26 of 91 patients (28%) with known HCC. All these findings were confirmed with the biopsy ($n = 1$), which detected metastases in 5 cases and 12 cases with the post-therapeutic response to the loco-regional therapy, and thus FDG-PET will be important for staging and management of HCC patients. Thus FDG-PET/CT has shown a significant increased sensitivity for lesion detection, localization, characterization, and also differentiation of these lesions [21]. The role of the triphasic CT is also important in HCC as the 70% of HCCs will be hypodense on plain CT and 20% will be hyperdense on the arterial phase [22]. FDG-PET/CT also has an important role for the detection of the extrahepatic disease in patients with primary HCC. In general, FDG-PET/CT has increased sensitivity for the primary HCC and also for the skeletal metastases evaluation as compared to the multidetector computed tomography (MDCT) and bone scintigraphy. In this study the mean sensitivity and specificity for the diagnosis of bone metastasis were 41.6% and 94.5% for MDCT, 83.3% and 86.1% for FDG-PET/CT, and 52.7% and 83.3% for bone scintigraphy, respectively [23]. Another important role of FDG-PET/CT is for efficacy assessment of chemoembolization therapy in HCC lesions despite the variable and limited uptake in the detection of HCC tumours (Fig. 18.2). Another radiotracer ^{11}C-acetate PET is also used along with the FDG-PET like the dual tracer for the PET/CT scan. Ho et al. showed in one of the studies that the well-differentiated HCCs will have significant accumulation of the ^{11}C-acetate, as compared to the poorly differentiated tumours that will be accumulating the FDG [20]. Delbeke et al. [24] showed that the differential uptake by various lesions by different tracers can identify the lesions better with the more precise diagnosis. Here the accumulation of the tumour by both tracers, and only ^{11}C-acetate, then the possibility of the HCC is more. However, lesions that will show only the FDG accumulation will show more of like the non-HCC malignancy. And the remaining lesions, with no radiotracer uptake by any of these pathologies, show that it is the benign pathology. As there is preferential affinity to

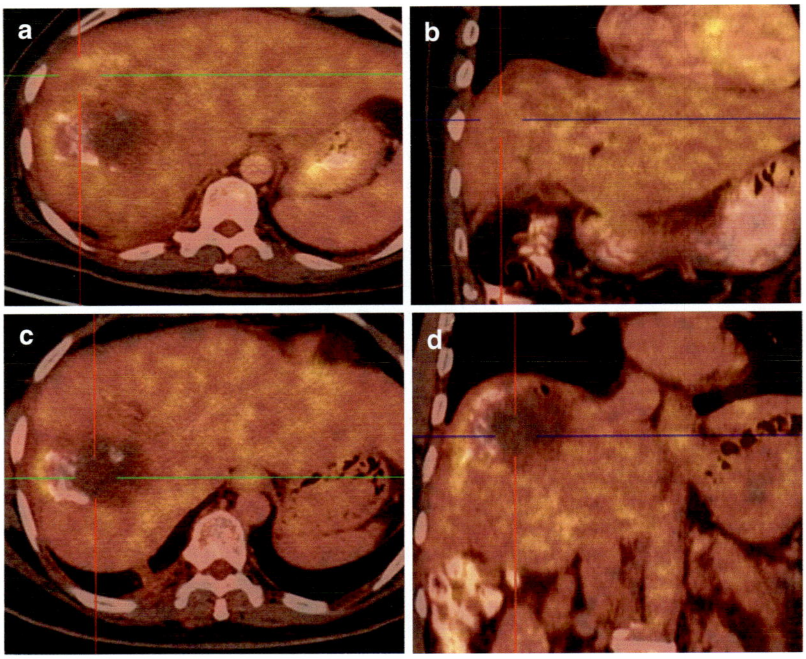

Fig. 18.2 (a–d) Post-TACE fused PET/CT images showing a hypodense lesion with no significant uptake in the liver lesion suggestive of no metabolic activity in the lesion.

different types of HCC lesions, the dual-tracer PET will show the increased sensitivity for the detection of HCC. One of the studies of Ho et al. [20] showed that the 23 HCC lesions were negative for both tracers. The role of the dual-tracer use of the ^{11}C-acetate and FDG-PET/CT [25] showed the significant detection of the primary and metastatic HCC. The sensitivities of FDG, ^{11}C-acetate, and dual-tracer PET/CT were 60.9%, 75.4%, and 82.7%, respectively, in the evaluation of the 110 lesions in 90 patients with known primary HCC. The sensitivities based on the tumour size (1–2, 2–5, and ≥5 cm) were 27.2%, 47.8%, and 92.8%, respectively, for FDG and 31.8%, 78.2%, and 95.2%, respectively, for ^{11}C-acetate [25]. FDG is more sensitive than ^{11}C-acetate in the analysis of extrahepatic metastases (85.7% vs 77%). The ^{11}C-acetate FDG-PET/CT is more sensitive for the detection of primary HCC as compared to the extrahepatic metastases. FDG-PET sensitivity is more sensitive for the poorly differentiated HCC lesions due to their aggressiveness as compared to the metastases [20]. In the staging and to diagnose HCC metastasis, Ho et al. [20] concluded that the role of using the dual-tracer PET/CT shows an increased sensitivity of 98%, a specificity of 86%, a positive predictive value (PPV) of 97%, a negative predictive value (NPV) of 90%, and an accuracy of 96%. FDG-PET is not completely sensitive for HCC detection due to the variable amount of the glucose metabolism, with the sensitivity range of 55–64%, and in this the larger tumours more sensitive than the smaller tumours due to FDG-PET more directly proportional to the grade of the tumour more in the high-grade tumours. The FDG-PET is more sensitive for the evaluation of regional and extrahepatic metastases, and the greater number of metastatic HCCs shows more FDG avidity. The use of the ^{11}C-acetate radiotracer with FDG has shown significantly increased sensitivity for HCC with PET. Benign liver lesions like haemangiomas, FNH, and hepatocellular adenomas (HCA) show increased uptake of FDG as compared to the background liver parenchyma.

18.1.2 The Role of FDG-PET(/CT) in HCC

FDG-PET/CT is more sensitive compared to the conventional imaging modalities for the local tumour recurrence detection and also for the various therapeutic options like radiofrequency ablation. FDG-PET has lower sensitivity for the detection of intrahepatic lesions as HCC tumour differentiation is not precise. The well-differentiated HCC lesions will show the same activity of the normal liver parenchyma, and due to this reason, the tumour detection can be difficult. For intrahepatic tumour recurrence evaluation, the sensitivity is more based on the malignant potential of the lesion [26, 27]. In one of the studies comprising 24 patients, intrahepatic and extrahepatic disease evaluation for follow-up is more precise with FDG-PET in comparison to the CT.

18.1.3 Hepatic Tumours and Tumour-Like Lesions

Malignant tumour, Benign tumour, and Tumour-like lesions are Hepatocellular carcinoma, Hepatocellular adenoma, Intrahepatic cholangiocarcinoma, Hepatic cavernous haemangioma, sclerosed haemangioma, Combined hepatocellular cholangiocarcinoma, Focal nodular hyperplasia, Hepatic angiosarcoma, Angiomyolipoma, Malignant lymphoma, Inflammatory pseudotumour, Neuroendocrine tumour, Pseudolymphoma, Hepatic metastasis, Inflammation, infection, Focal sinusoidal obstruction syndrome, Intratumoural haemorrhage in the acute phase.

The mechanism of the FDG uptake is that FDG is taken up by the cells by GLUTs which is phosphorylated by hexokinase (HK) to FDG-6-phosphate. FDG-6-phosphate is further dephosphorylated by G6Pase and transported outside of cells by GLUT, and this mechanism is important for the maintenance of glucose homeostasis [28]. These GLUTs are seen in various organs and biochemically made up of glycoproteins having 12 isoforms [29]. Hexokinases are of four types having different functions seen in the cell [30]. Mechanism in the normal hepatocyte cells, FDG, or glucose will be taken by GLUT-2 into the cytoplasm, further phosphorylating to HK-IV. This cell-specific enzyme G6Pase is seen in the liver and the kidneys' endoplasmic reticulum [31] as G6Pase Complex; this complex comprises the G6Pase glucose-6-phosphate transporter (G6PT)1, G6PT2, and G6PT3, transporters which will be functioning like transporters of FDG-6-phosphate, FDG, and phosphate, respectively, and can cross the endoplasmic reticulum [32]. The metabolic glycolytic pathway traps the FDG-6-phosphate in the hepatic cells [33]. And the cellular metabolic rate is based on the amount of the uptake of GLUT, HK, and G6Pase [34], having different biological properties [35, 36], like the adenocarcinoma, squamous cell carcinoma, small cell cancer, transitional cell cancer, neuroendocrine tumour (NET), sarcoma, and lymphoma [37]. Different patterns like solid, cystic, and mucinous, tumour differentiation based on the different components like necrosis, degeneration, and haemorrhage can also be quantified.

18.1.4 Factors That Influence FDG-PET/CT Imaging

Characterizing the different hepatic lesions which are based on different technical factors, for example, different artefacts like misregistration, truncation, attenuation correction, and partial volume effect. Misalignment of PET and CT in PET/CT is called misregistration. The FDG metabolic activity of PET images should correspond to CT images, and if this correspondence is not there, then it is known as misregistration [38] leading to many false-negative results. Various causes of the misregistration are breathing artefacts, patient movement, and peristaltic bowel movements which can be seen separately [39]. Truncation artefacts have different sizes in CT (50 cm) and PET (70 cm) based on the field of view, in heavy-built patients and technically different patient positions like the keeping-arm-down position. Due to this the patient's body is seen as beyond the CT field of view and appears truncated. If no attenuation correction is there, then the PET attenuation corrected images will not give correct standardized uptake values. This will lead to streaking artefacts at the margin of the CT image, and the correct data will show higher metabolic activity at the truncation edge leading to the

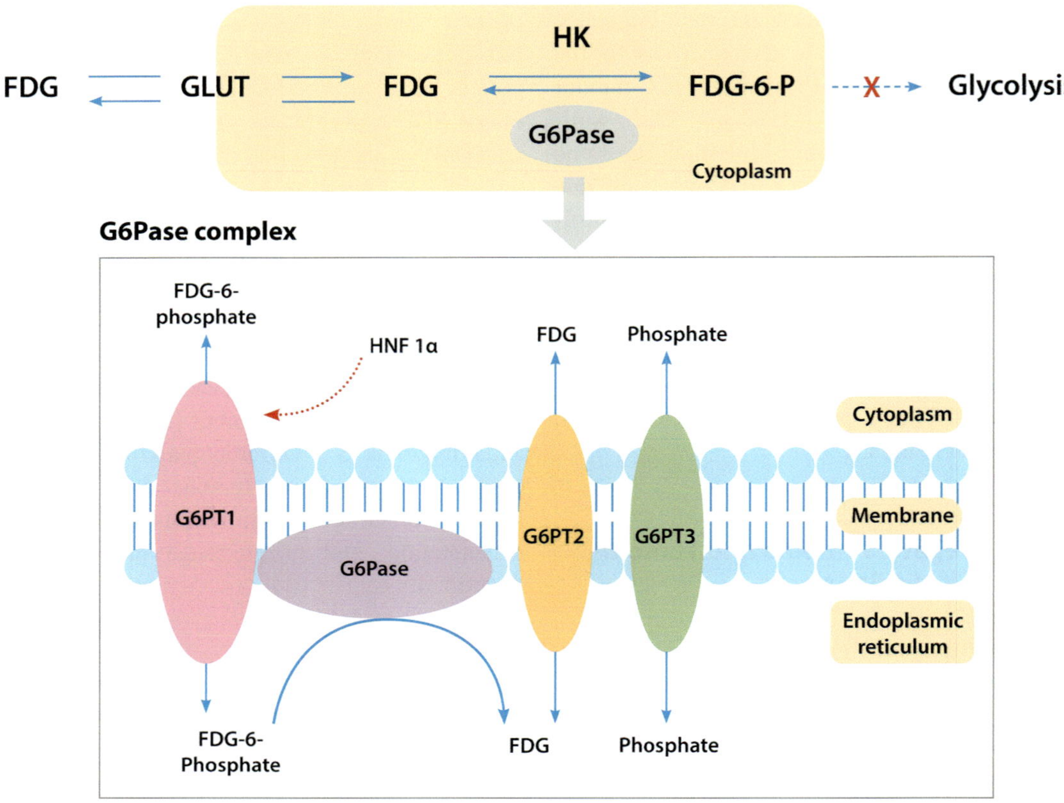

Diagram 18.1 Showing the metabolic activity in the glucose cells

misinterpretation of PET images [39]. This is one of the important reasons hepatic lesions are missed in the CT-based attenuation correction [40]. This attenuation correction is seen in a higher-density areas [41] and also in areas of the low to high photon-attenuating tissue levels where there is no correlation between the PET and CT images [42, 43]. Diaphragmatic areas also show the sharp tissue/air transition which is seen in different positions. This is also seen along the margins of the hepatic parenchyma. The PET signal doesn't have any role in various attenuation correction artefacts [44]. FDG-PET/CT images are based on the qualitative and quantitative parameters depending on the amount of the radiotracer uptake. SUV is a semiquantitative quantification method to quantify the amount of the uptake in various tissues and lesions. Technically the partial volume effect also shows false SUVmax values in the smaller tumours [45]. The size of the lesion will also show the sensitivity of the PET in the hepatic and extrahepatic lesions [46]. This concept shows that FDG-PET is an important modality in HCC patient prognosis [47] (Diagram 18.1).

18.2 Intrahepatic Cholangiocarcinoma

Intrahepatic cholangiocarcinoma (ICC) is the second most common primary liver neoplasm after HCC, which is arising from the epithelium of the bile duct. This ICC is further subclassified into the peripheral type which is arising from small bile ducts and perihilar type which is arising from large bile ducts. These quantifications are based on the location and morphology of the lesion. Approximately 90% of ICCs are having increased FDG uptake in the nodular or mass-forming cholangiocarcinoma seen in the periphery of the lesion [48], and this mass-forming ICC has peripheral rim enhancement seen on CT and/or MRI post-contrast images with ring-like peripheral uptake [49]. The uptake is due to increased expression of GLUT-1 and HK-II [50, 51] . GLUT-1 expression is associated with the FDG uptake, especially in the moderately and poorly differentiated ICC [51]. The perihilar and infiltrating type comprises 10% of all ICCs, resulting in the peripheral and infiltrating type showing the FDG uptake in focal nodular or linear branching pattern [49]. Smaller lesions having higher mucin content predominantly in hilar lesions compared to peripheral lesions [48]. Thus FDG-PET/CT is more accurate in evaluating the nodular type of ICC, compared to the infiltrating type (Fig. 18.3). Due to this the FDG-PET/CT has less sensitivity to evaluate the primary lesion, in comparison to the metastases. And this has a significant impact for the staging on the selection of therapy in 17–30% of patients [52, 53].

Cholangiocellular subtype (also called cholangiocellular carcinoma or bile ductular carcinoma) is being classified as a type of combined hepatocellular cholangiocarcinoma (cHCC-CC) having stem cell features, and it is now classified by the World Health Organization classification criteria (2019) as the small duct type of intrahepatic cholangiocarcinoma [54]. Histologically, the cholangiocellular subtype is described as a well-differentiated adenocarcinoma which has the pattern of the antler-like glands in oedematous, fibrous stroma, and looking like the ductular reaction, this is seen in various acute and chronic liver diseases and also in massive hepatic necrosis. This is the rare entity and the role of the FDG-PET/CT for this subtype are not seen. The biological nature of cholangiocellular subtype has false-negative results of FDG [55], and further evaluation is required for confirmation.

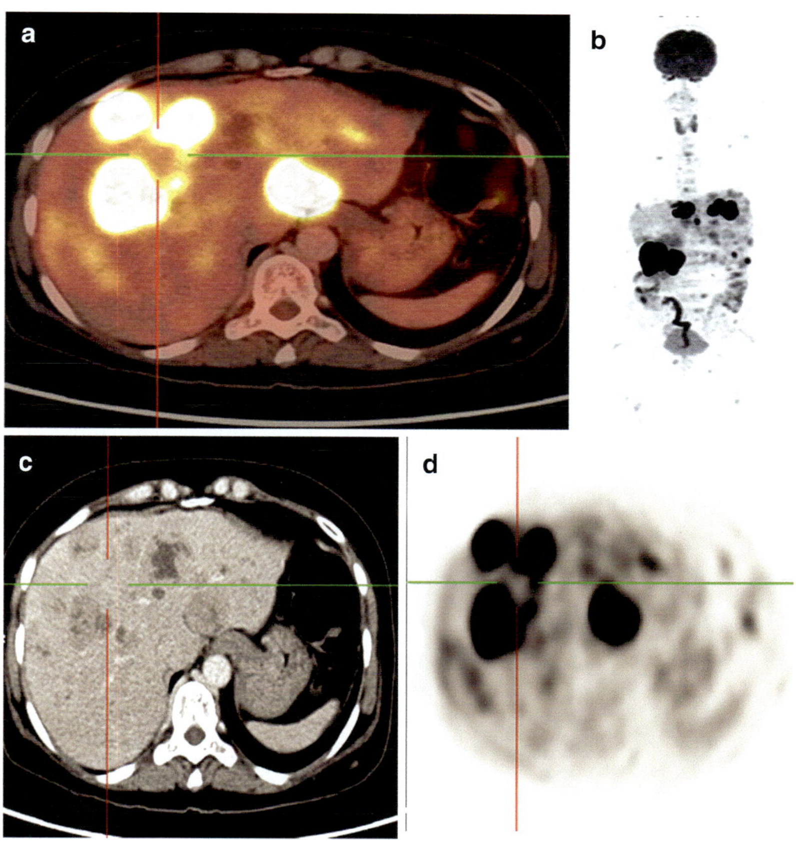

Fig. 18.3 Image **a** fused PET/CT image showing a significant uptake corresponding to hypodense lesions seen in image **c** in both lobes. Image **b** and **d** PET showing corresponding uptake in the lesions

18.3 Combined Hepatocellular Cholangiocarcinoma

cHCC-CC is a primary liver carcinoma comprising both hepatocytic and cholangiocytic differentiation in the same tumour lesion [54]. This is rare and also has a very poor prognosis; the incidence ranges from 1.0 to 4.7% of all primary hepatic tumours. As this is a rare entity, FDG is used for the diagnosis with the pre-treatment tumour-to-normal liver SUV ratio that is an important parameter for the prediction of prognosis [56]. The hepatocytic component will have different degrees of the FDG uptake useful for differentiation and also for the cholangiocytic part showing the higher FDG uptake.

18.4 Hepatic Angiosarcoma

Primary hepatic angiosarcoma is a rare tumour which originates from hepatic endothelial cells and has a very high malignant potential with rapid progression. These lesions are ~1% of all primary hepatic carcinomas and the most common mesenchymal malignancy of the liver. Hepatic angiosarcomas are further classified on the basis of the morphology single mass, mixed massive mass, multiple nodules, and diffuse nodule types, and the combination of all is also the finding seen in many cases. On CT and MRI, these lesions have the indistinct border, with a variable associated with intratumoural haemorrhage. These lesions show the classical centripetal heterogeneous enhancement on CT and MR imaging. High-grade malignant angiosarcoma will show no enhancement due to intratumoural haemorrhage, cystic degeneration, and necrosis [57]. The single lesion and mixed massive mass types of hepatic angiosarcoma show a higher FDG uptake [58, 59] and are still considered as the overexpression of GLUT-1 [57], and the diffuse nodular type shows false accumulation of the FDG activity due to the lower cellular density, intratumoural haemorrhage, and tumoural necrosis [60].

18.5 Malignant Lymphoma

Malignant lymphoma is categorized into Hodgkin's and non-Hodgkin's lymphoma; this will have a wide range of malignant diseases with different histology, variable behavioural patterns, different imaging features, and treatment options. Non-Hodgkin's and Hodgkin's lymphomas are placed as the 13th and 28th most frequent cancers worldwide, respectively, in 2018, with the estimated 509,590 and 79,990 new cases diagnosed and 248,724 and 26,167 deaths respectively. As per the clinical approach, the clinicopathological grading of cases is based on the indolent, aggressive, or highly aggressive system which will be correlating the better management approach with the more precise FDG avidity [61]. The aggressive and highly aggressive non-Hodgkin's lymphomas are the diffuse large B-cell lymphoma; the indolent (low-grade) lymphomas comprise the mucosa-associated lymphoid tissue, chronic lymphocytic leukaemia/small lymphocytic lymphoma, marginal zone lymphoma, and peripheral T-cell lymphoma [62]. The secondary involvement of liver parenchyma is not much uncommon in non-Hodgkin's lymphoma; however, the primary hepatic lymphoma is extremely rare, comprising 0.016% of all non-Hodgkin's lymphoma [63]. The most common subtype of liver parenchyma is the diffuse large B-cell lymphoma [64]. The primary hepatic lymphoma based on the morphological features is classified in the two different types: nodular, which is seen more frequently, and diffuse liver infiltration, which is seen less frequently and also seen as a solitary nodular lesion [64]. The solitary hepatic lesion with very high FDG uptake is more likely suggestive of lymphoma, commonly diffuse large B-cell lymphoma. The diffuse infiltration of primary hepatic lymphoma, which is viewed in CT and MRI, is seen in acute hepatitis [65], and the very high FDG uptake represents lymphoma. In cases of doubts with the FDG PET findings, a percutaneous liver biopsy should be done from the level of the more active area in the lesion. FDG-PET/CT imaging is used for the staging, restaging, assessment of therapeutic response, and early detection of disease recurrence in malignant lymphoma. The degree of FDG uptake corresponds to the aggressiveness of the lesion. Generally, the high FDG uptake is seen in aggressive lymphoma, compared to the indolent lymphoma with less FDG uptake [66]. The important aspect is that the more increased FDG avidity will be more corresponding to the bad prognosis and poor response to treatment [67, 68]. Again, the important aspect to be kept in mind is that the more increased FDG uptake of the low-grade lymphoma will be corresponding to the more higher-grade transformation which is also known as Richter's transformation [69]. GLUT-1 and GLUT-3 are important for the increased uptake in the FDG in the diffuse large B-cell lymphoma and also in the extra nodal natural killer/T-cell lymphoma. The SUVmax values and the GLUT-3 have better prognosis of diffuse large B-cell lymphoma. Hodgkin's lymphoma has higher expression of GLUT-1 and is also related to the amount of the FDG uptake [70–72].

18.6 Primary and Metastatic Neuroendocrine Tumours

Neuroendocrine neoplasms are rare in liver parenchyma and have more heterogeneity as they originate from peptidergic neurons and neuroendocrine cells in the entire body. The common sites for the origin of these tumours are from the gastrointestinal tract, lung, adrenal gland, and thyroid gland. And the most common sites of metastasis are the lymph nodes, liver, spleen, and bone. The primary hepatic neuroendocrine tumours are extremely rare, and the features of the hepatic metastasis have also similar characteristics for the gastroenteropancreatic neuroendocrine tumours. The grade of tumour differentiation is again based on the amount of FDG uptake which shows the amount of aggression in tumour cells, and again GLUT-1 expression is related to the FDG accumulation [73]. The FDG uptake will show the amount of cell differentiation and is lower in the G1 or G2 neoplasms and significantly more in the poorly differentiated neuroendocrine carcinomas. The overall PET/CT for the evaluation of the primary and secondary metastatic neuroendocrine tumours involving the hepatic parenchyma is less with the range of only 36–52% [74, 75] (Fig. 18.4), but despite this the FDG-PET/CT can provide better information [74]. Earlier PET/CT has shown an predictor of the disease-free survival [76], and also the multivariate evaluation has shown that the SUVmax >3 is also an important predictor of disease-free survival [75].

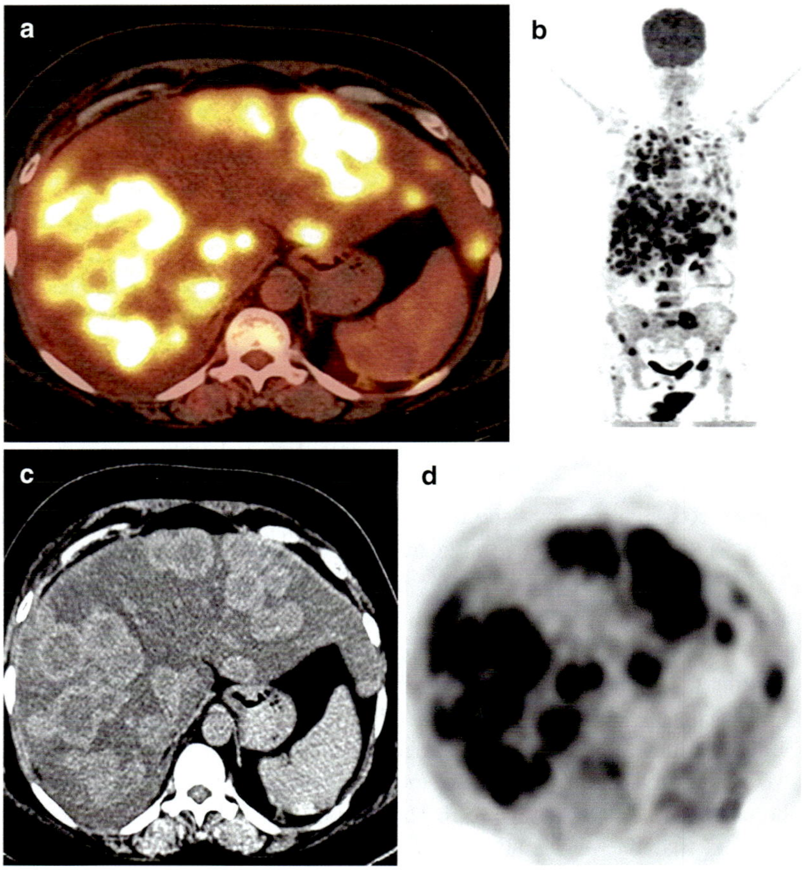

Fig. 18.4 Image **a** fused PET/CT showing a significant uptake in the nodular lesions corresponding to the hypervascular lesions on CT image **b** consistent with high vascularity as well as aggressive lesions. Image **c** and **d** PET showing a corresponding uptake in liver lesions

18.7 Hepatic Metastasis

The metastatic involvement of the liver is more common than the primary liver tumours, and the common sites are the gastrointestinal tract, lung, breast, and pancreas. The precise evaluation, detection, and characterization of hepatic metastases are very important for treatment planning. PET/CT is more superior over CT for the detection of hepatic metastases from the primary cancers [77, 78]. Gadolinium ethoxybenzyl diethylenetriaminepentaacetic acid (Gd-EOB-DTPA)-enhanced MRI is also important for the dynamic contrast-enhanced CT along with the FDGG-PET/CT [79, 80], more focussed for the detection of the smaller lesions. Metastasis has similar features of the primary tumour, with higher uptake of FDG in metastases [79, 80], seen in the overexpression of GLUT-1 in primaries like the lung, pancreas, colorectum, breast, and biliary tract [81]. The amount of FDG uptake is based on the differentiation or histopathologic basis of the tumour [82, 83] (Fig. 18.5). Few of the lesions show the lower amount of the uptake or also the false-negative uptake of FDG. Few of the tumours show the lower glucose metabolism, especially in the well-differentiated lesions like pancreatic adenocarcinomas [84], prostate cancer

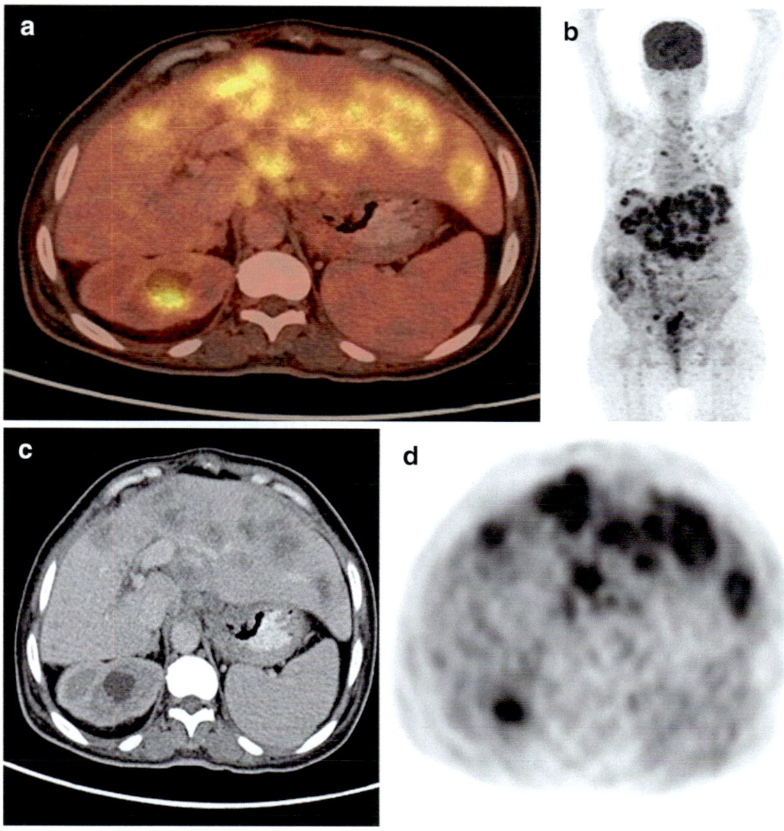

Fig. 18.5 Infiltrative lesion with patchy enhancement seen in image **c** and corresponding uptakes seen in the fused image **a** and PET images **b** and **d** consistent with the intrahepatic cholangiocarcinoma

[85], lung adenocarcinoma [86], bronchioloalveolar carcinoma of the lung [87], and neuroendocrine tumour (G1) [74, 76]. The metabolic activity in these lesions has the relatively lower FDG uptake like the primary tumour, and also the uptake can also be masked due to the background liver uptake. The reason for the lower uptake is the low cellularity due to mucin, cystic component, degeneration, and intratumoural haemorrhage. Cystic tumours, having mucin, degeneration, or cystic change within the tumour, have low volume of the cancer cells, corresponding to the lower FDG uptake in the tissues [87, 88] (Fig. 18.6). Mucinous carcinoma is the most common malignancy to metastases to the liver commonly seen from the gastrointestinal tract comprising approximately 17% of colonic tumours. This is also found in the ovary. These tumours contain clear, gelatinous fluid (mucin) that can be intracellular or extracellular. FDG uptake directly correlates with the number of viable cancer cells, and as mucinous cells, tumours have fewer cancer cells and show decreased FDG avidity; thus PET/CT has a limited role in the mucinous tumours, and the reported sensitivity of the mucinous tumours is 59%.

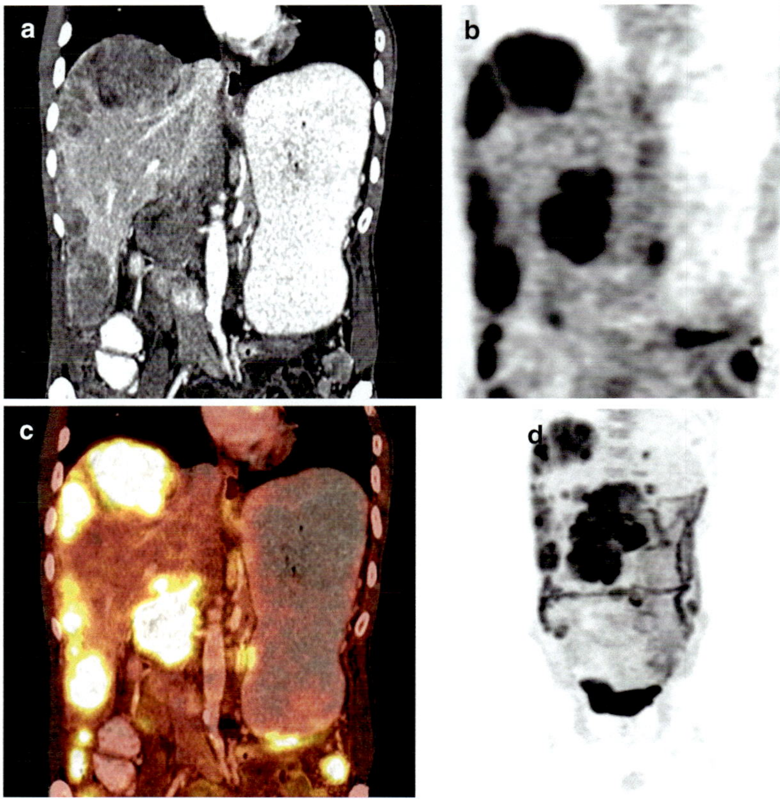

Fig. 18.6 Multiple extrahepatic lesions seen in CT image **c** corresponding to the images **a**, **c**, and **d** which shows a significant metabolic activity suggestive of the extrahepatic metastases with hepatic involvement

18.8 Adenoid Cystic Carcinoma

Adenoid cystic carcinoma (ACC) is a very rare form of adenocarcinoma usually seen in the secretory glands, commonly seen in the major and minor salivary glands of the head and neck, which comprises 5–10% of all salivary gland tumours. They have the potential for the involvement of the nerves and distant metastases by the haematogenous route commonly seen in the lung and bone, which is followed by the brain and liver. The sensitivity of PET/CT for ACC metastases is also rare like the mucinous carcinoma [89]. The intratumoural degeneration or haemorrhage also shows reduced FDG uptake.

Renal cell carcinoma (RCC) is one of the common tumours worldwide. The clear cell RCC (ccRCC) is the most common histologic type. CT is the most commonly used modality for the evaluation of renal tumours and also for the characterization of renal tumours which will be intermediate in ultrasound (US) or CT. FDG-PET/CT is able to diagnose half of the cases [90]. Again, the SUVmax is directly proportional to the grading of the RCC lower in the low-grade and higher in the high-grade lesions. Here the

FDG uptake is based on the expression of GLUT-1 [91, 92], and the significant association is between SUVmax and GLUT-1 expression in ccRCC [92]. The concept here is that lower G6Pase activity due to reduced G6Pase catalytic subunit will show the lower uptake of FDG in RCC. But the expression of G6PTs is significantly variable, and no exact correlation is being found between the tumorous and non-tumorous tissues [93].

18.9 Malignant Melanoma

Malignant melanoma is the important tumour related to the cells containing melanocytes, which are commonly seen in the skin, but can also be seen in other locations like the mouth, intestines, or eye. Due to the higher nodal and distant metastases, it has very poor prognosis and higher recurrence rates. The common metastasis is seen in the lymph nodes (73.6%), then liver (58.3%), brain (54.6%), bone (48.6%), and adrenal glands (46.8%). In the very rare uveal melanoma, the liver is the most common site of the systemic metastasis, thus depicting the varied biological behaviours which is seen between cutaneous and uveal melanoma. PET/CT imaging is the most sensitive and accurate modality for the evaluation of the primary and metastatic lesions of cutaneous melanoma [94], as compared to the uveal melanoma [95, 96]. The GLUT-1 expression is also related to the FDG uptake in the melanoma; despite this 60% of hepatic metastases of uveal melanoma are FDG negative showing that there is no correlation between the expression of GLUT-1 hepatic metastases from cutaneous and uveal melanoma [97]. The lower FDG uptake of glucometabolic disorder may be the reason for these presentations.

18.10 Benign Hepatic Tumours and Tumour-Like Lesions

The majority of benign tumours and non-tumorous lesions show no FDG uptake or minimal uptake in relation to the background liver parenchyma [98]. However the benign tumours and different infective inflammatory lesions show increased uptake as well as false-positive uptake [99–102]. FDG-PET has a role when the routine modalities like CT and MRI have become equivocal for the differentiating benign tumour from malignancies [98, 103].

18.11 Hepatocellular Adenoma

Hepatocellular adenoma (HCA) is a very rare benign liver neoplasm seen in the females off the reproductive age predominantly. It is classified on the basis of the molecular subgroups which are having many risk factors, varied clinical behaviours, different histological presentations, and imaging features also. The hepatocyte nuclear factor-1 α-inactivated HCA, inflammatory HCA, and many HCAs are being linked with the higher risk of malignant transformation and will be associated with the bleeding tendencies showing less but varying amount of metabolic activity [104] (Fig. 18.7). Other imaging protocols like the use of the EOB-enhanced MRI will be able to classify the various subtype and to distinguish the HCA from other hypervascular hepatic tumours.

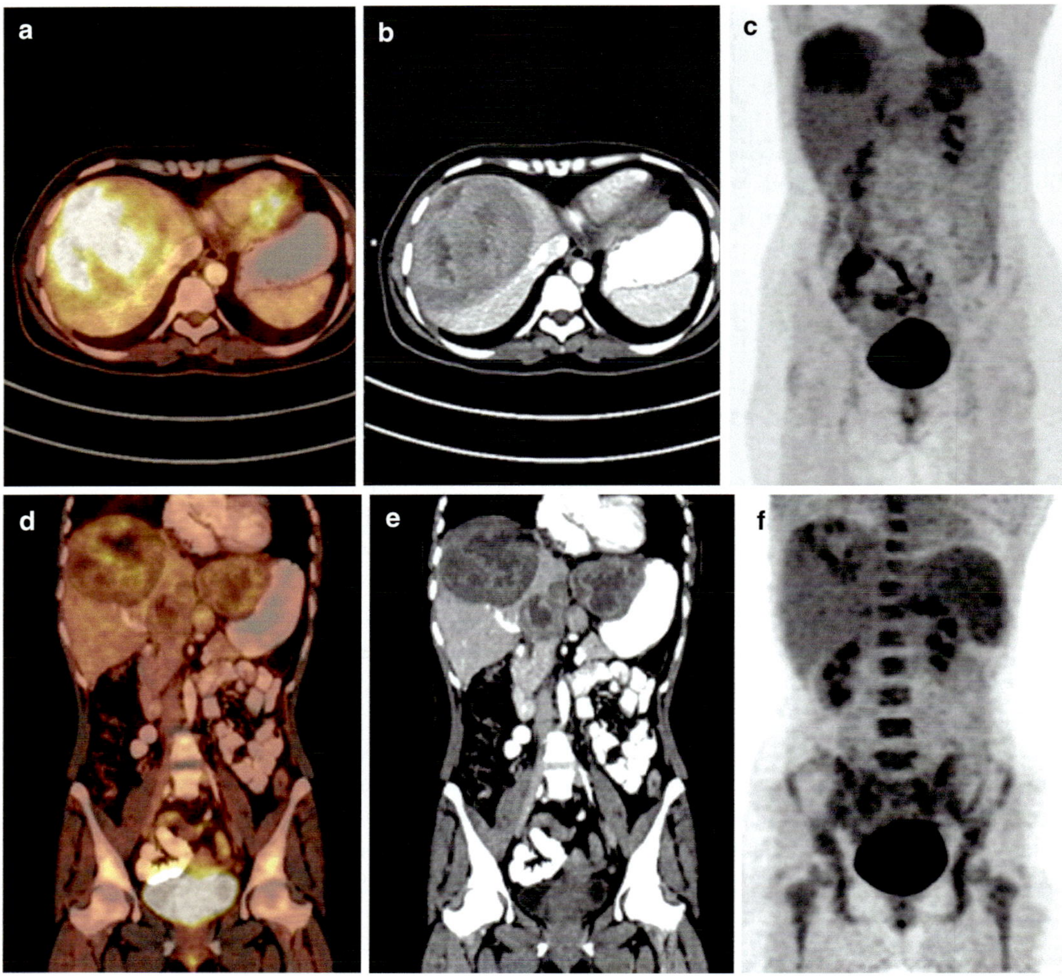

Fig. 18.7 Mild metabolic activity seen in the fused images **a** and **d** corresponding to the CT images **b** and **e** which shows uptake in images **c** and **f** suggestive of the benign lesions—hepatic adenoma

18.12 Hepatic Cavernous Haemangioma and Sclerosed Haemangioma

Cavernous haemangioma is one of the most common benign hepatic tumours with a very high reported incidence as high as 20%. These tumours are composed of different vascular channels which are lined by the single layer of endothelial cells of varying sizes and well supported by a collagenous wall. Most of the haemangiomas, there will be the typical findings [105] on imaging [106]. Haemangiomas FDG uptake will have similar uptake to the background liver [98, 103, 106]. When there are known metastatic lesions and also a larger size of the haemangioma, the lower amount of the uptake on FDG are shown [98, 103]. The different changes which happen in the haemangiomas like the slower blood flow associated with the thrombus, necrosis, fibrosis, calcification, and scar formation. And this when associated with haemangiomas is labelled as the sclerosed haemangioma. These changes which is appending will change the typical findings suppressing the imaging findings on CT and

MRI. And due to this, there are chances of the sclerosed haemangioma to be considered as malignant tumour like the ICC, metastases, and HCC. On FDG-PET imaging, the atypical sclerosed haemangioma has very poor accumulation of FDG, from a malignant tumour [103].

18.13 Focal Nodular Hyperplasia

Focal nodular hyperplasia is the second most common benign hepatic tumour and is due to the hyperplastic response of hepatocytes of the preexisting vascular malformations. On the intravenous contrast-enhanced CT and MRI, the FNH shows homogenous hyperenhancement in the arterial and portal venous phases, which becomes isoenhancement in the delayed or equilibrium phases. The important aspect is that the FNH being benign is treated conservatively needs to be differentiated with the HCC. The majority of FNHs have iso- or hyperintensity which surround the liver parenchyma in the hepatobiliary phase [84, 107]; the hepatobiliary phase imaging differentiates benign from malignant lesions which has the sensitivity of 96.6%, specificity 87.6%, and positive predictive value of 85% [108]. The role of the FDG-PET/CT is not specific for the diagnosis of the FNH and can have the lower FDG uptake with the retention pattern similar to the adjacent normal liver tissue [98, 109]. FNH being the hypervascular lesion will not have the increased glucose metabolism.

18.14 Angiomyolipoma

Angiomyolipoma (AML)/primary hepatic perivascular epithelioid cell tumour is again the benign mesenchymal tumour comprising the blood vessels, smooth muscle cells, and fat. The more the amount of fat in AML, the more it is easily diagnosed on CT and MRI, but the lesser the fat component, the more difficult it will be to diagnose the small lesions. AML also has features similar to the HCC which are hypervascular in the arterial phase and showing washout, mimicking HCC. The early draining vein and the absence of tumour capsule differentiate AML from HCC. The FDG activity in the AML is same as that of the background liver parenchyma [110, 111].

18.15 Inflammatory Pseudotumour

Inflammatory pseudotumour is the rarest condition that can occur anywhere in the body and also seen in the liver. Liver involvement is seen in the proportion of ~0.7% of the focal liver lesions and further characterized by the presence of the inflammatory cells and the area of the fibrosis mimicking the malignant tumour. The cause is not certain and patients present with nonspecific symptoms like the fever, abdominal pain, abdominal discomfort, and leucocytosis. The imaging findings seen in the various routine modalities like ultrasound, CT, and MRI are also nonspecific, which are able to differentiate from the pseudotumour from HCC, ICC, metastasis, and hepatic abscess. Pseudotumour has a higher amount of FDG uptake [112, 113] and becomes difficult to differentiate from the malignancy.

18.16 Pseudolymphoma

Pseudolymphoma is another "reactive lymphoid hyperplasia" or "nodular lymphoid lesion," which is the benign nodular lesion which is characterized histopathologically due to the excessive proliferation of nonneoplastic, polyclonal lymphocytes with active germinal centre [114]. This can be seen in various organs like the skin, orbit, lung, and gastrointestinal tract; however it is very rare in the liver. The occurrence in the liver is more common in the middle-aged females with associated autoimmune disease, malignant tumours, or chronic liver disease. Hepatic pseudolymphoma is difficult to diagnose by ultrasonography, CT, and MRI which are equivocal, and differentiating from the other malignant hepatic tumours is not possible. The median SUVmax is 4.3 (range 3.4–7.2) [115, 116].

18.17 Inflammation and Infection

Inflammatory and infectious liver diseases are many, and the common ones are the hepatic abscess, intrahepatic cholangitis, lymphoproliferative disorders like the immunoglobulin G4 (IgG4)-related systemic disease, sarcoidosis, tuberculosis, and fungal and parasitic infection [117]. FDG-PET/CT is now being used widely for the evaluation of the infection and inflammation for identifying the infective focus source and the extent and severity of disease (Fig. 18.8) and for the therapeutic response assessment [99, 118].

FDG uptake in non-malignant inflammatory conditions gives many false-positive results, especially in the known cases or suspected malignancy [119], and then correlates with the CT and MRI findings. Increased FDG uptake in inflammation and infection causes the increase in GLUT which is seen in the similar fashion like the malignant cells [120] (Fig. 18.9). The inflammatory cells which are activated are seeing the overexpression of GLUT-1 and/or GLUT-3 [121–123]. The GLUT expression for the deoxyglucose is apparently increased due to the cytokines and growth factors, which is not seen in the tumours [124].

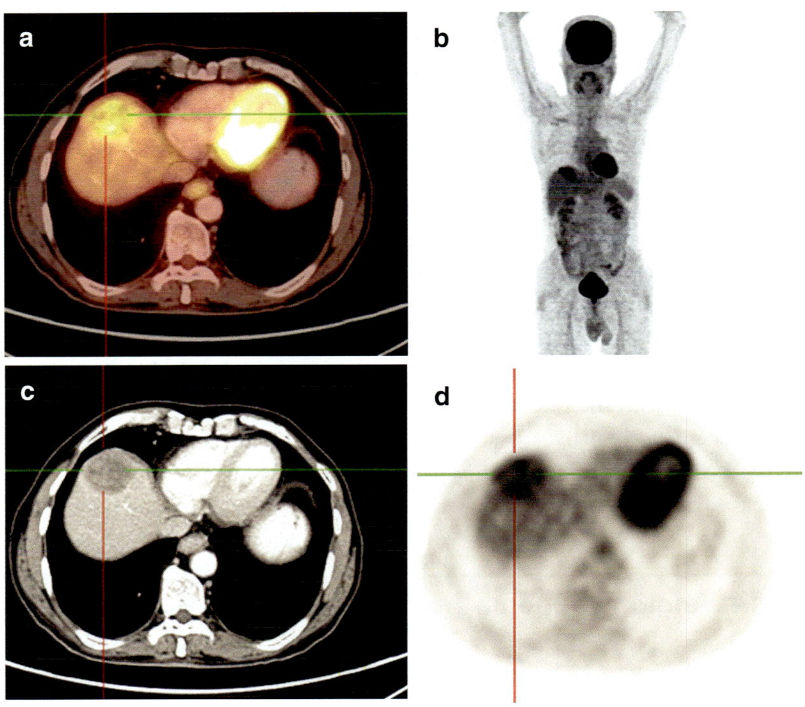

Fig. 18.8 Irregular hypodense lesion seen in CT image **c**, corresponding to the PET image **b** and **d** and fused image **a** suggestive of the chronic organised abscess

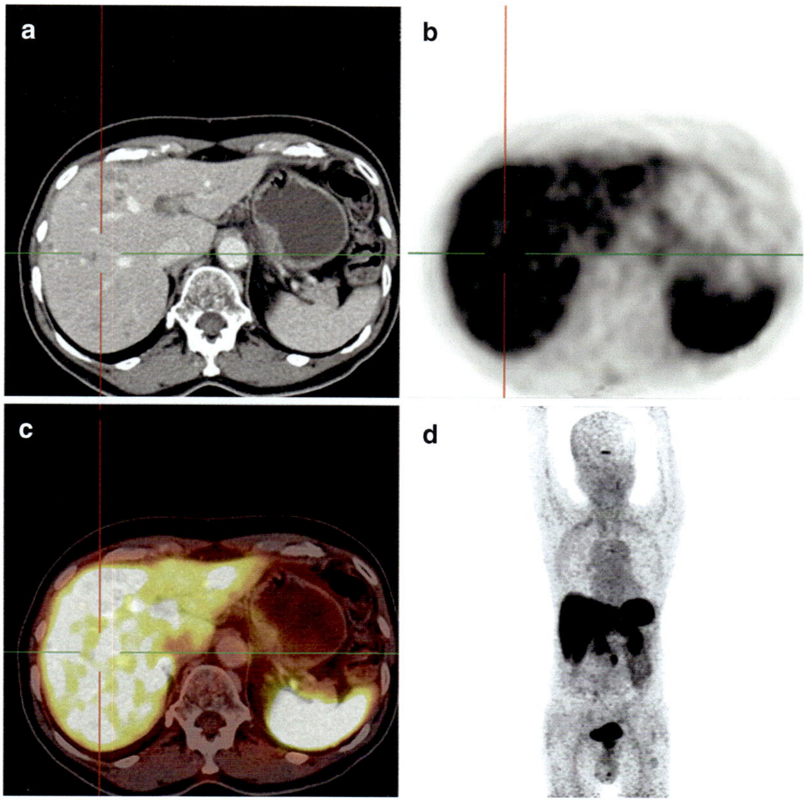

Fig. 18.9 In the setting of the fever of unknown origin, CT image showing multiple hypodensities in image **a** noted with the diffuse uptake in the entire liver parenchyma in the images **b**, **c**, and **d** consistent with hepatitis

18.18 Focal Sinusoidal Obstruction Syndrome

Sinusoidal obstruction syndrome (SOS) is also known as the toxic sinusoidal injury, veno-occlusive disease, or "blue liver syndrome"; this is the common presentation seen as the common vascular pattern of drug-induced liver injury which can be associated with oxaliplatin-based chemotherapy, commonly used for the gastrointestinal malignancy [125]. SOS shows sinusoidal dilatation with congestion, centrilobular vein fibrosis and obstruction, and perisinusoidal fibrosis. These changes are diffusely seen irregularly in the hepatic parenchyma, with the specific imaging features of the diffuse and reticular hypointensity on the hepatobiliary phase of the EOB-enhanced MRI [126]. SOS shows no uptake of FDG due to no glycometabolism. It is also seen as the nodular lesion [127, 128], on FDG-PET/CT imaging that can differentiate it from hepatic metastases along with the combined CT and MR images with contraindication for percutaneous liver biopsy.

18.19 Cholangiocarcinoma

Cholangiocarcinoma has very poor prognosis, and any delay in early diagnosis due to the late presentation will impact on various nonsurgical therapeutic imaging modalities [129]. FDG-PET/CT evaluation doesn't have any specific advantage over the other modalities of the diagnosis of the primary biliary tumours [130, 131]. However for the local and the metastatic work-up, FDG-PET has an important application. The same concept is being used for the FDG accumulation by the increased glucose transporter expression on tumour cells [132]. This type of the presentation is seen in nodular or mass cholangiocarcinomas, which have a significant increased uptake due to the increased expression of glucose transporter-1 [11]. One of the studies by Kluge et al. [133], showing FDG-PET for cholangiocarcinoma in 20 patients with cholangiocarcinoma had sensitivity, specificity, and diagnostic accuracy of 92.3%, 92.9%, and 92.6%, respectively. FDG-PET/CT [132] sensitivity and specificity are more with 94% and 100%, respectively. Thus, the metastatic disease detection with other modalities also has more sensitivity [132]. Another study [130] that showed sensitivity, specificity, PPV, NPV, and accuracy of FDG-PET/CT in primary tumour detection were 84.0%, 79.3%, 92.9%, 60.5%, and 82.9%, respectively. The study by Anderson et al. with 36 patients [134] showed that a significant increased sensitivity for detection with FDG-PET was 85% ($n = 22$) with nodular lesions and 18% ($n = 14$) infiltrating lesions. Infiltrating cholangiocarcinoma with periductal features forms the mass [135], and the uptake is not consistent. FDG-PET can evaluate the nodular cholangiocarcinoma (mass > 1 cm), better and less common for the infiltrating type [132, 134]. The location of the cholangiocarcinoma also has an important role for the detection of these lesions. For the primary hilar or extrahepatic cholangiocarcinoma tumours, the sensitivity is seen as 18–58.8% [132, 134, 136, 137], which is significantly lower than that of peripheral nodular tumours. In one of the studies with 22 patients of the primary sclerosing cholangitis [138], the role of FDG-PET/CT in liver lesions by doing the delayed imaging after 120 minutes can distinguish between hepatic and extrahepatic lesions. The SUVmax which is greater than 3.6 in all the lesions is important. In one of the studies [130], the use of FDG-PET showed a significant amount of uptake in the regional lymph nodal metastases (75.9% vs 60.9%; $p = 0.004$) for the distant metastases (88.3% vs 78.7%; $p = 0.004$) in comparison to CT ($n = 123$). Another study [139] pointed that FDG-PET is more sensitive for lymph nodal metastases in comparison to CT and MRI. In this study the diagnostic accuracies of FDG-PET, CT, and MRI for the detection of lymph node metastasis were 86%, 68%, and 57%; the respective sensitivities were 43%, 43%, and 43%; and the specificities were 100%, 76%, and 64%, respectively. The identification of the occult metastases can be easily done [140–142] for the occult metastases where other imaging modalities are not sensitive [131]. The use of FDG-PET has a significant impact of 17–30% on the management [131, 134, 143] of cholangiocarcinoma patients for the unknown lesions which can be metastatic, and this leads to upstaging [143]. The sensitivity of FDG-PET/CT is based on the morphology of the tumour especially for the diagnosis of the nodular forms which is higher compared to the hilar and infiltrative lesions, and due to this there is a significant impact on patient evaluation and management.

18.20 Multimodality Imaging of the Liver

The overall sensitivity of FDG-PET/CT for the diagnosis of HCC is based on the histological basis as the high-grade lesions are better detected than low-grade lesions. And due to this, the sensitivity of the FDG-PET [144] is not more precise for the primary HCC diagnosis. The HCC's different uptake is due to the different glucose-6-phosphatase in hepatocytes (in addition to differences in GLUT expression). In the malignant cells, glucose-6-phosphatase lower values will result in increased FDG-6-P accumulation. The glucose-6-phosphatase activity in HCCs is based on various degrees of differentiation. The well-differentiated HCCs have higher levels of glucose-6-phosphatase causing dephosphorylation of FDG-6-P resulting in the lower FDG uptake; on the contrary poorly differentiated HCCs have lower glucose6-phosphatase and will be FDG avid [145]. The size criteria of the lesion are also related to the sensitivities of HCC with the detection range of the 27%, 48%, and 93% for tumours which are measuring 1–2, 2–5 cm, and more than 5 cm, respectively [146]. Small lesions are not possible due to lower spatial resolution associated with partial volume effects and also due to respiratory motion. PET is not sensitive for smaller hepatic lesions like HCCs, regenerative nodules, and premalignant dysplastic nodules [147]. And due to all these factors, sensitivity is more in the larger and poorly differentiated tumours. Delayed imaging of the liver parenchyma is very important, where the delayed scans of 2 and 3 hours show more sensitivity. The delay in the normal hepatic parenchyma will have less SUVmax values causing increased SUVmax of normal tissues, resulting in increased tumour-to-normal tissue (T/N) uptake ratio [148, 149].

18.21 The Role of the PET in the Liver Transplantation

HCC is the most common indication for PET/CT in liver transplantation. Surgical resection, high T/N ratio, more than 2, shows the chances of recurrence and poor survival [150] of the patients. Another study presenting the T/N ratio cut-off of 1.15 shows 1-year disease-free survival on multivariate analysis: 94% vs 54% [151]. In one of the single retrospective study of the 43 patients, the pre-transplantation PET was more helpful for the evaluation of the microvascular invasion and also for the recurrences of the tumour. There was the recurrence rate of 50% in PET-positive patients and very less 3.8% in PET-negative patients [152]. The lesions which were beyond the Milan criteria are characterized on the number and the size of lesions, and the negative preoperative PET has very small 3-year recurrence-free survival (80 in comparison with the tumours which meet the Milan criteria. (35%) [152] (Fig. 18.10). Many studies also have shown different criteria for the assessment of FDG-PET for diagnosis and staging of HCC with the extrahepatic metastases [145, 153, 154]. The multidimensional role of FDG-PET/CT in HCC is studied by Wudel et al. [155] who found that 64% of HCCs have FDG and has impacted 26 out of 91 patients (28%) with HCC. Few other roles are biopsy from the large necrotic tumours, detecting distant metastases, monitoring response to treatment with regional therapy, and also for the detection of the recurrence. Thus, FDG-PET/CT images can increase the detection, localization, and dif-

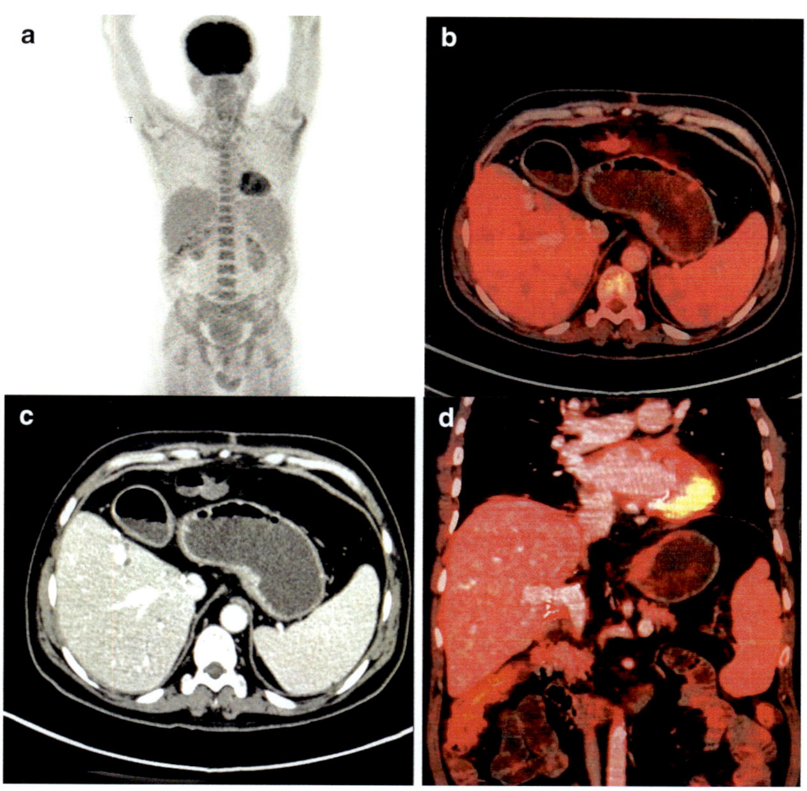

Fig. 18.10 Post-transplant liver showing no uptake in all images with no corresponding CT abnormality suggestive of no post-transplant complications

ferentiation of various physiological versus pathological uptake [156]. CT adds up to 70% of better diagnosis of HCCs which can be seen as hypodense areas on plain CT [156]. Recent study by Wang et al. [157] showed that early dynamic FDG-PET/CT protocol can reflect the physiologic and metabolic information of the tumor.

18.22 Novel Non-FDG-PET Tracers

Due to the lesser sensitivity of FDG for routine diagnosis of HCC, various other biomarkers are being used in HCC and other types of tumour. ^{18}Fluorine-labelled fluorothymidine (FLT) PET commonly detects tumour proliferation, can be used for the detection of HCC in 16 patients, and was reported to show a sensitivity of 69%. FLT also shows reduced survival with high uptakes but can be labelled as insignificant [158]. ^{11}C-acetate PET along with FDG-PET can increase sensitivity for the detection of some HCC tumours, and it complements FDG-PET in a dual-tracer PET scanning approach. Ho et al. [159] showed that well-differentiated HCCs preferentially accumulate ^{11}C-acetate, whereas poorly differentiated tumours tend to preferentially accumulate FDG. Delbeke et al. [160] showed that the use of two radiotracers will narrow the differential diagnosis. In this scenario the accumulation of both tracers or ^{11}C-acetate only then HCC should be favoured in the differential diagnosis [160], and in the cases when the FDG not accumulated then non-HCC malignancy will be favoured. And when this lesion shows a smaller number of attendees that if the lesion is negative for both tracers, then the benign pathology is considered [160]. One of the studies [161] showed that 23 HCC lesions were 100% sensitivity for both radiotracers (^{11}) [146]. The sensitivities of FDG, ^{11}C-acetate, and dual-tracer PET/CT in the detection of 110 lesions in 90 patients with primary HCC were 60.9%, 75.4%, and 82.7%, respectively. ^{11}C-acetate showed the significant increased sensitivity for the detection of primary HCC, but not for the detection of extrahepatic metastases. Ho et al. [162] showed the role of the dual-tracer PET/CT with a sensitivity of 98%, a specificity of 86%, a PPV of 97%, a NPV of 90%, and an accuracy of 96%. PET/CT for restaging after the treatment of HCC [163] showed the significant use of FDG-PET/CT. It showed the overall sensitivity of 89.5%, a specificity of 83.3%, and an accuracy of 88% in detecting HCC recurrence. FDG-PET also showed the increased alpha fetoprotein levels when monitoring the response to therapy, diagnosed extrahepatic metastases, tumour thrombosis in the portal vein, and the extrahepatic metastases in two patients [163].

18.23 Cholangiocarcinoma

Cholangiocarcinoma primary tumour of the bile duct epithelium comprises 2% of all tumours, the second most common primary hepatobiliary cancer after HCC. This type of cancer has a varied presentation with an overlap of many findings. These tumours are classified anatomically based on the location: intrahepatic, perihilar, or extrahepatic. The perihilar lesions at the location of the bifurcation of the hepatic ducts and the intrahepatic cholangiocarcinoma (CCA) lesions arise away from the second-order bile ducts. These lesions are classified by Japanese Liver Cancer Group as exophytic when it is mass-like, infiltrating along the ducts (Klatskin tumours), intraductal (polypoid), or mixed pattern (mass-like and infiltrating). The most common in the perihilar region is the infiltrating type [147]. The 5-year survival is very low 17%, with survival (22–32%) rate of 5 years when the portal or arterial embolization is done which will be followed trisegmentectomy. The preoperative assessment for hepatic and extrahepatic metastases is important [164]. The most common clinical presentation is biliary obstruction causing jaundice in the hilar CCA but not common in the peripheral CCA. Many factors that lead to the diagnosis of CCA are clinical picture, laboratory data, radiological imaging, and histology, also with the differentiating CCA from metastatic adenocarcinoma. Currently, the MRI, including magnetic resonance cholangiopancreatography, CT, endoscopic retrograde cholangiopancreatography, and percutaneous transhepatic cholangiography are various imaging modalities to diagnose CCA. FDG-PET/CT is important in detecting regional and distant metastases in comparison with the conventional imaging [165]. GLUT-1 is not expressed in normal bile ducts but seen in CCA [166, 167]. One of the studies [168] evaluated 20 CCA which showed FDG-PET sensitivity, specificity, and diagnostic accuracy values of 92.3%, 92.9%, and 92.6%, respectively. The primary sclerosing cholangitis [169] on the FDG-PET/CT of the liver showed that delayed scan can differentiate benign strictures from extrahepatic and hilar CCA with the SUVmax of more than 3.6. FDG-PET showed overall values for sensitivity, specificity, PPV, NPV, and accuracy of FDG-PET/CT in primary tumour detection: 84.0%, 79.3%, 92.9%, 60.5%, and 82.9% [170]. FDG-PET/CT in known or suspected recurrent and metastatic cholangiocarcinoma showed sensitivity and specificity to be 94% and 100%, respectively. These results indicate that false-positive cases in this setting are minimal. The sensitivity of FDG-PET/CT in detecting cholangiocarcinoma: hilar and extrahepatic CCA, show lower uptake on FDG PET than peripheral CCA, a finding that may be associated with the smaller size and/or higher mucin content of hilar tumours compared with peripheral ones [172–174]. The peripheral CCA comprises 10% of all CCAs and can show low uptake in the FDG-PET [175, 176]. FDG-PET/CT is more sensitive in detecting primary hilar or extrahepatic CCA tumours in the range of 18–58.8% [171, 177–179], and this is lower in the peripheral nodular tumours.

18.24 Approach to an FDG-Avid Liver Lesion

There are many FDG-avid lesions in the liver, and this needs to be explained in the different planes of trans axial, coronal, and sagittal planes, along with the maximum intensity projections [180]. Misregistration artefacts need to be differentiated with the true intrahepatic lesions. Various other parameters are useful for the evaluation of origin of mass like lt, "claw sign" and the acute angle of the lesion with adjacent liver parenchyma [181]. Contrast-enhanced CT, multiphasic CT, and MRI are particularly useful in the liver, given the poor soft tissue contrast of low-dose unenhanced CT. The distribution of FDG uptake may also be useful in characterizing the nature of the disease [182]. The pattern of the increased metabolic activity can be generalized or segmental in nature, depicting the diffuse process like the inflammation or infections. One of the important studies by G. J. S. Tan et al. shows the FDG-PET/CT evaluation of the liver of the 193 reports of primary liver malignancies such as intrahepatic cholangiocarcinoma or lymphoma demonstrating diffuse FDG uptake [183, 184]. The SUVbw cut-off of greater than 3.5 is important. Evaluation of the infection and inflammation can be done in the generalized pattern with the heterogeneous or focal pattern of involvement by neoplasms.

18.25 Gallbladder Cancer

Gallbladder carcinoma (GBC) is a rare form of cancer with very less prevalence of 2 in 100,000. It is more common in developing countries [185,186]. Various predisposing factors are increased age, female sex, gallstones, obesity, inflammation, smoking, and infection [187]. Histologically adenocarcinoma is the most common histopathologic subtype of gallbladder tumours with a rate of 98%. Clinically GBC is mostly asymptomatic until advanced stages until it produces nonspecific symptoms; they are aggressive in nature showing the rapid progression [188]. Due to the absence of a serosa layer which will be separating the gallbladder from the liver, the local infiltration will cause direct and local hepatic metastases and then by lymphatic dissemination and later by haematogenous spread [189]. They have low rates of survival, and the surgical can be done in vast majority [190]. They are more commonly used for pre-treatment and postoperative staging and also for the nodal and distant metastases [191].

^{18}F-FDG-PET/CT may also play a role as the predictive factor for survival in patients with gallbladder cancer [192, 193] (Fig. 18.11). The role of the SUVmax in PET/CT imaging will be prognostic as SUVmax cut-off of 6.0 was chosen. Patients with SUVmax greater than 6.0 had a median survival of 203 days versus 405 days in patients with SUVmax less than 6.0 (p 5.04). In the multivariate analysis, SUVmax was found to have a hazard ratio of 3.05 with a p-value of 0.04 [194]. In one of the studies, the total lesion glycolysis (TLG), in ^{18}F-FDG-PET/CT, is predictive of overall survival (OS), and metabolic tumor volume (MTV) and SUV are superior for the analysis. Incidental gallbladder carcinoma in the status post-cholecystectomy, and the ^{18}F-FDG-PET/CT will depict the median survival [195]. ^{18}F-FDG-PET/CT is now the important tool for the prognosis and survival in patients with gallbladder cancer [192, 194–196].

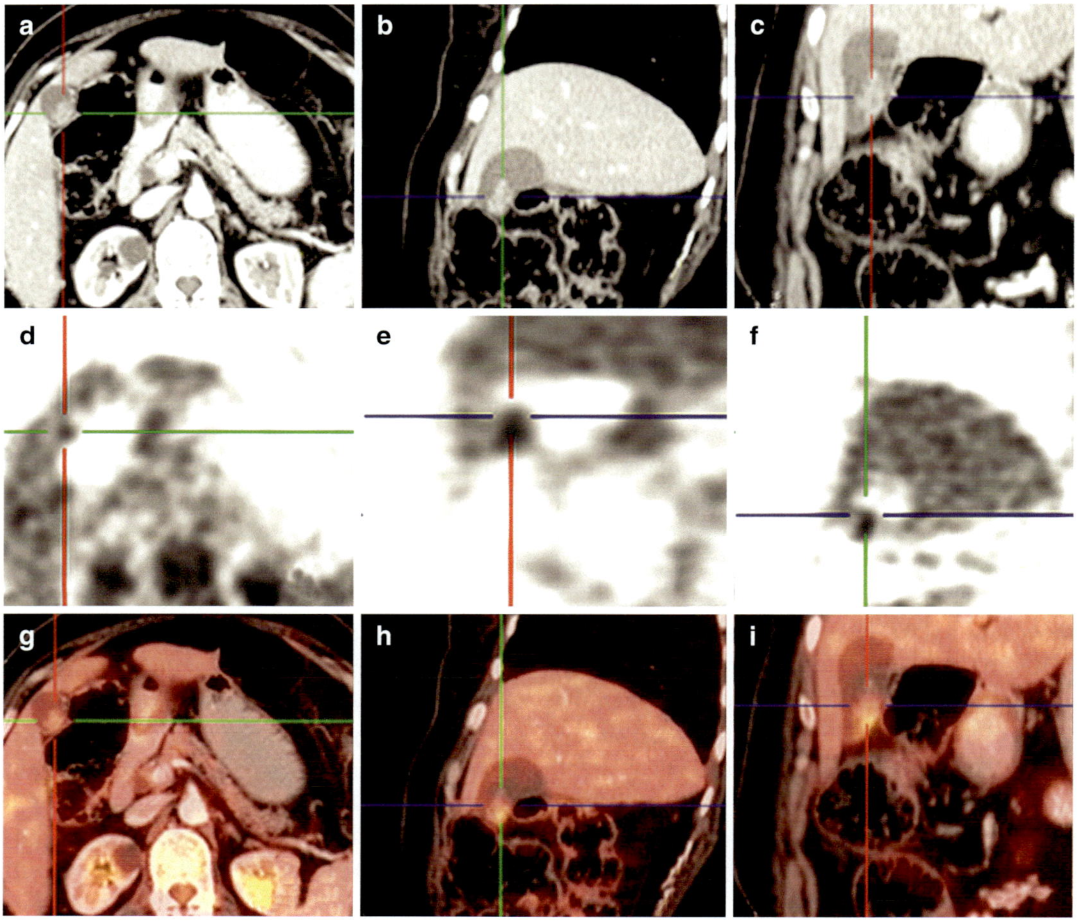

Fig. 18.11 CT images **a**, **b**, and **c** showing a patchily enhancing lesion corresponding to the **d**, **e**, and **f** fused images **g**, **h**, and **i** images for metabolic activity suggestive of the primary lesion

18.26 Pancreas

Positron emission tomography is a functional imaging technique for the evaluation of pancreatic pathologies. PET/CT can easily distinguish normal physiologic uptake from pathologic uptake and can give detailed accurate analysis of the various functional abnormalities with the various false-negative and false-positive findings. PET/CT findings of various pancreatic are important for the evaluation and management of primary pancreatic malignancies and its use in various benign pancreatic disorders; and pancreatic metastases can mimic the primary pancreatic adenocarcinoma, screening for coexisting primary cancers, and limitations and pitfalls of PET/CT imaging modality in the pancreatic lesions.

18.26.1 Primary Pancreatic Malignancies

18.26.1.1 Primary Pancreatic Adenocarcinoma

Pancreatic ductal adenocarcinoma is the commonest type, and the third most frequent malignancy of the gastrointestinal tract, and the fourth leading cause of mortality from cancer. The statistical data shows that only 10–30% of pancreatic cancers are resectable with the 5-year survival rate of 18–20%, and median survival of these patients is 17–21 months [197]. The locally advanced disease has a median survival of 6–10 months. Median survival is 3–6 months. CT, MRI, and endoscopic ultrasound are the main imaging modalities for local involvement of pancreatic cancer.

PET/CT in Preoperative Diagnosis

PET/CT is useful when the pancreatic cancer coexists with chronic pancreatitis and when there is the presence of cystic/complex lesions of the pancreas. Many studies have shown that PET/CT has high rates of sensitivity (85–100%) and specificity (67–99%) for distinguishing benign from malignant pancreatic masses [197] (Fig. 18.12). Stage I disease is confined to the pancreas. Stage II is extended outside the pancreas. Stage III is involved with lymph nodes. Stage IV is characterized by distant metastases. The use of PET is more accurate than CT for metastases (M) staging because it allows better detection of distant metastasis by giving more information with various lesions and for the benign vs malignant or equivocal lesions on CT (Fig. 18.14). Hypervascularity of the thrombus confirms the neoplastic nature with contrast enhancement on CT and MRI and flow signal pattern on Doppler ultrasound. Differential diagnoses of thrombus accumulating a radiotracer on PET are inflammatory and septic venous thrombi frequently accompanied by infectious clinical symptomatology of fever and chills.

18.26.1.2 Benign Pancreatic Disorders

FDG is not a tumour-specific tracer and can show increased uptake in inflammatory cells due to increased glycolytic metabolism. Differentiation between the benign to malignant pathology is needed.

18.26.1.3 Acute Pancreatitis

Acute pancreatitis is an acute inflammatory condition of the pancreas with the invasion of the inflammatory cells (macrophages, neutrophils, T cells) and cytokines released by these cells. Diffuse increased FDG uptake of the pancreas and peripancreatic fat as seen can differentiate benign vs malignant (Fig. 18.13).

18.26.1.4 Autoimmune Pancreatitis

Autoimmune pancreatitis (AIP) is a pancreatic infiltration of the systemic component IgG4-related sclerosing disease. Other organ involvement like salivary glands, lungs, lymph nodes, bile duct system, kidney, retroperitoneum, and prostate are also seen [198]. Significant elevated serum immunoglobulin G (IgG) and IgG4 levels are noted. However, IgG4 is more sensitive than total IgG for diagnosing autoimmune pancreatitis. More IgG4 are seen in this type of pancreatitis and can be misled as cancer especially in the pancreatic head. One of the literatures shows that approximately 3–11% of Whipple procedures are done due to autoimmune pancreatitis misdiagnosed as the pancreatic cancers [199]. So, differ-

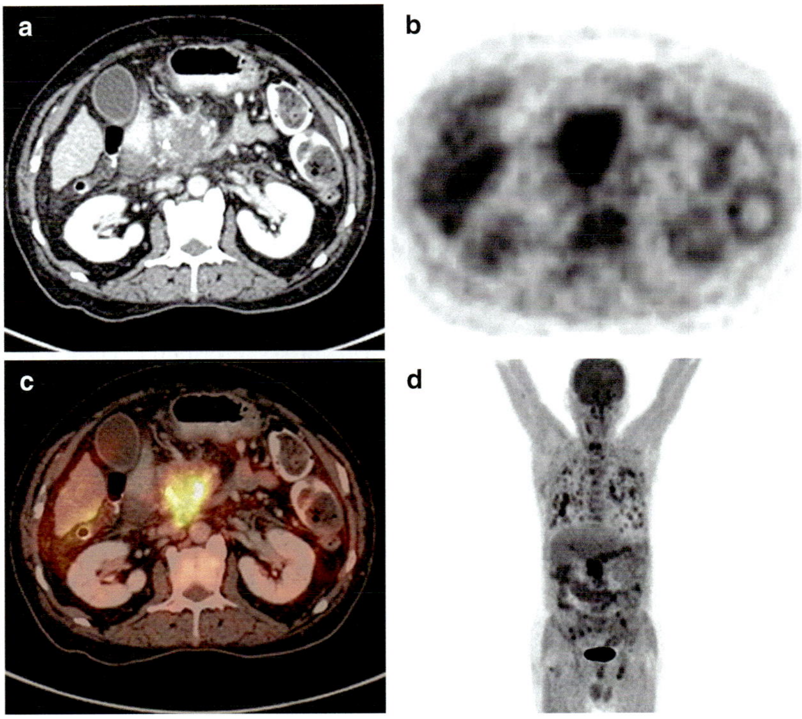

Fig. 18.12 Ill-defined hypodense lesion seen in the pancreatic head and neck in CT image **a** which is corresponding to the metabolically active lesion in images **b**, **c**, and **d** suggestive of the primary pancreatic carcinoma

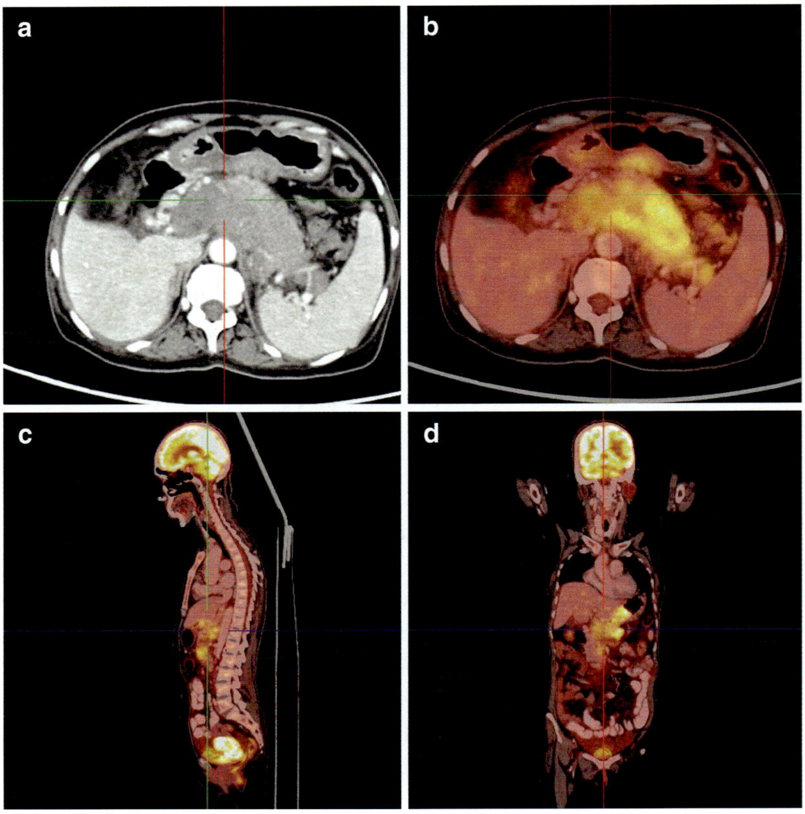

Fig. 18.13 Diffusely bulky hypodense pancreas seen in the CT image **a** corresponding to the images **b**, **c**, and **d** suggestive of acute pancreatitis

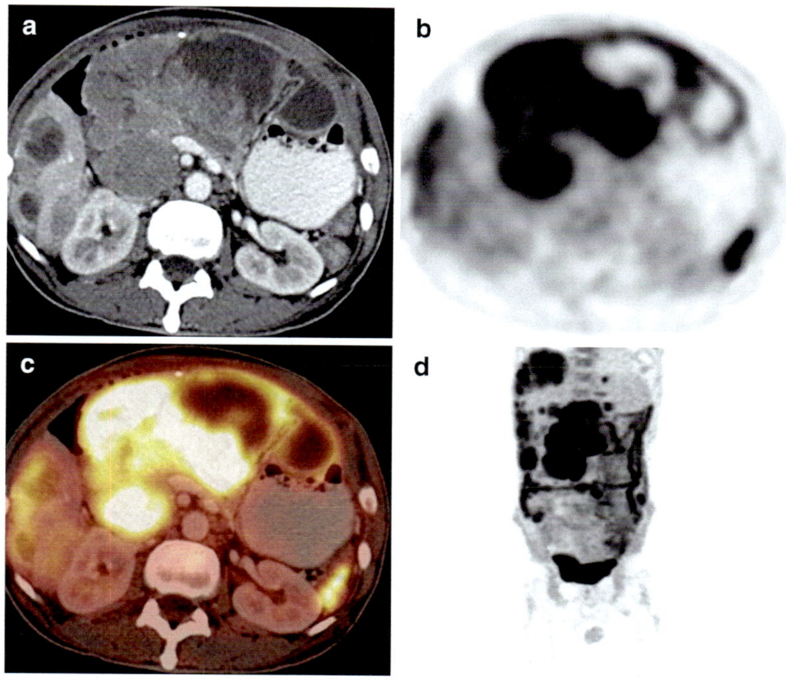

Fig. 18.14 Primary pancreatic lesion showing local infiltration on CT image **a** and corresponding to images **b**, **c**, and **d** showing diffuse increased uptake secondary to the infiltration to adjacent stomach

entiation needs to be done before surgery. On PET/CT imaging, autoimmune pancreatitis diffuse pancreatic uptake with the extrapancreatic involvement like the IgG4-related hypermetabolic lesions. Whole-body PET/CT imaging after the post-steroid therapy can monitor the autoimmune pancreatitis.

18.26.1.5 Pancreatic Metastases

The pancreatic involvement is seen as a single mass (50–73%), diffuse pancreatic enlargement (15–44%), and multiple pancreatic lesions (5–10%) [200]. Pancreatic metastasis will not have pancreatic duct dilation as seen in primary pancreatic cancer. The reason here is that as primary neoplasm arises from ductal epithelium, on the contrary the metastasis involves pancreatic parenchyma. Pancreatic metastasis is seen from head and neck cancer which are usually synchronous/metachronous with the second primary malignancies. Distance metastases and second primary malignancies of the pancreas range from 4% to 25% [201]. Pancreatic metastasis is rare, and PET/CT is the best imaging modality because of its ability to evaluate the whole body [201]. The sensitivity, specificity, and negative predictive value for detecting distance metastases and second primary malignancies were 98%, 93%, and 100%, respectively. The positive predictive value is only 63% [202]. Pancreatic metastasis is most common from lung cancer with the malignancy (18%) involving the pancreas [203]. In lung cancer, small-cell lung cancer is more common than non-small cell lung cancer.

18.26.1.6 Extramedullary Myeloma of the Pancreas

The extramedullary sites of multiple myeloma are predominantly encountered at the head, neck, and upper airways in 80% with rare involvement of the pancreas and presented as multiple lesions. The typical presentation of the pancreatic myeloma is multiple hypoechoic nodules on ultrasound and enhancing lesions on CT and MRI with the biliary obstruction changes. PET/CT will also show the various osseous and extramedullary lesions of multiple myeloma as mentioned in the Durie-Salmon classification of this haematological disorder [204].

18.26.1.7 Lymphoma of the Pancreas

Lymphoma consists of Hodgkin lymphoma (15%) and non-Hodgkin lymphoma (85%), which is less than 10% of all cancers. Non-Hodgkin lymphoma is more aggressive than Hodgkin lymphoma, with a tendency for extranodal involvement. Non-Hodgkin lymphoma is made up of two subtypes: low-grade or aggressive non-Hodgkin lymphoma. Only Hodgkin lymphoma and aggressive non-Hodgkin lymphoma show a high affinity for FDG. One of the studies shows 30% of non-Hodgkin lymphomas which will metastasize to the pancreas [205]. Of the total 70% of pancreatic lymphomas will be responding to the chemotherapy [205].

18.26.1.8 Pancreatic Metastasis from Renal Cell Cancer

Approximately 30% of patients with renal cell cancer have distant metastases at presentation. Three most common metastatic sites are lungs (75%), bone (20%), and liver (18%); pancreatic metastases are rare. Solitary pancreatic metastasis in the known case of the renal cell cancer has 75% and has more better prognosis compared to the primary pancreatic cancer resection [206].

18.26.1.9 Pancreatic Metastasis from Melanoma

Melanoma is the sixth most common cancer in the United States with growing incidence in the last 20 years. The most common metastatic sites are lungs, lymph nodes, gastrointestinal tract, brain, and bone. The pancreatic metastases is less than 5% of patients with distant metastatic sites. Here again PET/CT is used for staging, restaging, and monitoring therapy for stages III and IV and superior to CT as compared to the detection of the distant metastases [207].

18.26.1.10 Coexisting Cancers

Coexisting cancers will be more commonly seen in the high-risk patients due to long duration exposure to carcinogens, mutational genetic predisposition, and immunocompromised/immunodepressed status. As mentioned above, PET/CT, with whole-body assessment, provides a more comprehensive evaluation than other cross-sectional imaging modalities and will diagnose more unanticipated hypermetabolic pathologic processes. PET/CT incidental detection of additional primary malignancies is seen in 5% for general oncologic patients [208]. This can be more in the clinical, imaging, and histopathological follow-up and more thorough with the involved patient groups. The most common PET incidental lesions are colorectal, thyroid, and lung lesions.

18.26.1.11 PET/CT Limitations

PET depends on the target-to-background activity ratio of the tumour; thus it may be limited by several factors. A small lesion size (ampullary carcinoma), a necrotic tumour, or a cancer with low metabolic activity (mucinous adenocarcinoma or neuroendocrine tumour) can cause false-negative results [197]. The hyperglycaemic status causes the decrease in the absorption of FDG due to competitive inhibition. Various benign conditions, such as postoperative changes, inflammation, iatrogenic acute pancreatitis, infection, abscess, and adjacent bowel activity of physiologic origin or induced by diabetic medication, can mimic malignancies. Acute pancreatitis and autoimmune pancreatitis are two benign, inflammatory conditions that can simulate neoplasms as illustrated in the above section, benign pancreatic disorders. PET technical aspects motion artefacts, PET/CT misregistration, and attenuation correction errors related to surgical hardware could cause misinterpretation. Other promising radiotracers, such as ^{18}(F)-fluoro-L-thymidine (a marker for cell proliferation) and ^{68}Ga-labelled somatostatin analogues (peptides with high affinity for neuroendocrine tumours), are currently being evaluated and may have the potential to overcome several above limitations of FDG in detecting different types of pancreatic cancer.

18.26.1.12 Pancreatic Neuroendocrine Tumours

Pancreatic NETs are rare tumours (1% of all pancreatic cancers) arising from endocrine tissues of the pancreas (islet cell tumours). These tumours are aggressive, which is related to different factors, including the grade of malignancy, tumour burden, and presence of metastases, among others [209].

The pancreatic NETs are non-functioning and not associated with hormonal syndrome. SSTRs are overexpressed in the cell surface of pancreatic NETs [210, 211], and the most common subtype is SSTR2 [212]. Due to this aspect, the gamma camera imaging with a radiolabelled form of the somatostatin analogue ^{111}in-DTPA-octreotide is done for the diagnosis of NETs by binding SSTR2 and SSTR4 [213, 214]. The sensitivity of SSTR scintigraphy is reported in the range of 82% to 95%, which is superior when compared with pure anatomic imaging methods, such as CT, MR imaging, and endoscopic US, for identification of islet cell tumours, carcinoids, and their metastases [215–221]. Insulinomas has low SSTR expression in these tumours [222]. Single-photon emission computed tomography (SPECT) with CT provides hybrid anatomic (CT) and functional (SPECT) imaging, enhancing the specificity and increasing the diagnostic confidence for tumour localization [223, 224] (Fig. 18.5). PET using ^{68}Ga-labelled somatostatin analogues is being widely used in recent years with excellent sensitivity and spatial resolution [210, 225–228]. DOTATOC [DOTA-TyI3-octreotide], DOTANOC [DOTA-NaI3-octreotide], DOTATATE [DOTA-Tyr3-octreotide]) are also being used and offer comparable diagnostic accuracy and differing binding affinities for SSTR subtypes [229]. ^{68}Ga-DOTATATE PET/CT is very sensitive when clinical suspicion is there along with the elevated levels of tumour markers, or indeterminate findings for NET in alternative imaging, supporting its use in clinical routine diagnostics [230]. ^{68}Ga-DOTA-labelled somatostatin analogues used for the detection of unsuspected bone lesions have very low incidence of bone lesions in pancreatic NETs [231]. One of the studies by Frilling and colleagues [232] showed the significant impact of ^{68}Ga-DOTATOC PET/CT as compared to the CT and/or MR imaging alone in 31 (59.6%) of the 52 subjects studied with pancreatic NETs. PET/CT ^{68}Ga-DOTATATE PET/CT significantly changed surgical management in one-third of subjects with NETs of the pancreas [233]. A recent study also shows the use of the ^{68}GaDOTATOC PET/MR imaging in subjects with gastroenteropancreatic NETs, with advantages in the characterization of abdominal lesions [234]. Limitations are there for the evaluation of the lung and sclerotic bone lesions and described in one of the studies [235, 236]. Having the higher SUVmax showing the ^{68}Ga-DOTANOC high SUVmax was a risk factor for tumour progression [236].

FDG-PET or PET/CT include imaging-guided biopsy planning, performed with endoscopic US guidance. CT percutaneous route is the common route of biopsy [237, 238]. Benign and malignant lesions can be there in the same patient and tissue sampling to be done [238]. PET/CT images for the intraprocedure CT to guide biopsy in the abdomen are feasible and improves the diagnostic success of CT-guided biopsy [239].

Pancreatitis is a well-known inflammatory process of the pancreas that is easily diagnosed on the basis of clinical, laboratory, and imaging findings. The imaging approach can be misinterpreting it as metastatic or lymphomatous pancreatic involvement. The severity of the disease process is based on the necrosis and can be classified as oedematous or necrotic, with later having bad prognosis [240]. Chronic pancreatitis' common cause is alcohol consumption, and showing the pancreatic duct dilatation and parenchymal atrophy, calcification is a pathognomonic [241].

18.26.1.13 Autoimmune Pancreatitis

Autoimmune pancreatitis is a form of chronic pancreatitis which accounts for 2%–11% of chronic pancreatitis. Type 1 AIP is regarded as part of the immunoglobulin G4 (IgG4)-related disease spectrum [242]. Approximately 30% of patients with pancreatic disease will involve bile ducts, salivary and lachrymal glands, lymph nodes, and retroperitoneal tissue [242–244]. Type I AIP has infiltration of tissues with IgG4-positive plasma cells, fibrosis with subsequent irregular narrowing of the main pancreatic duct, and obliterative phlebitis, as well as increased serum levels of one or more types of immunoglobulins, most commonly IgG4 [242, 245, 246]. Diffuse or focal enlargement of the pancreas and the peripancreatic "halo sign", are seen in the CT and MR imaging [242]. AIP can be diagnosed by the histologic, imaging, and laboratory (i.e., serum IgG4 levels) and post-steroid response to the therapy [246, 247]. Sometimes the AIP mimics like the focal pancreatic neoplasm [242, 247]. The FDG avidity defines the severity of pancreatitis: Diffuse FDG uptake is seen with the low-grade acute or subacute pancreatitis or AIP, with the increased radiotracer usually not seen in chronic pancreatitis [247–250].

18.26.1.14 Limitations of PET in Pancreatic Cancer

Important limitations of PET are the lack of anatomical details for identification of the surgical resectability, vascular infiltration around celiac trunk and superior mesenteric artery, invasion of surrounding organs, metastases to the liver, and differentiating the benign inflammatory processes with the malignancies [251, 252].

18.27 Conclusion

The role of PET in detecting hepatobiliary and pancreatic malignancies is well established but not being commonly used. PET is still not the imaging modality for the early diagnosis of different primary hepatobiliary and pancreatic tumours. Despite a very easy evaluation, the assessment of the primary hepatobiliary and pancreatic lesions is not done. FDG-PET for whole-body staging, restaging, tumour grading, and surveillance in hepatobiliary pancreatic malignancies and occult disease prevents unwarranted surgeries in hepatobiliary and pancreatic cancers. With the availability of many newer radiotracers, the more and more precise evaluation of these tumours will lead to the way of the concept of the personalized medicine.

References

1. Bosch FX, Ribes J, Díaz M, Cléries R. Primary liver cancer: worldwide incidence and trends. Gastroenterology. 2004;127(suppl 1):S5–S16.
2. Oliveri F, Brunetto MR, Actis GC, Bonino F. Pathobiology of chronic hepatitis virus infection and hepatocellular carcinoma (HCC). Ital J Gastroenterol. 1991;23:498–502.
3. Fabris C, Toniutto P, Falleti E, et al. MTHFR C677T polymorphism and risk of HCC in patients with liver cirrhosis: role of male gender and alcohol consumption. Alcohol Clin Exp Res. 2009;33:102–7.
4. Murillas J, Del Río M, Riera M, et al. Increased incidence of hepatocellular carcinoma (HCC) in HIV-1 infected patients. Eur J Intern Med. 2005;16:113–5.
5. Randi G, Franceschi S, La Vecchia C. Gallbladder cancer worldwide: geographical distribution and risk factors. Int J Cancer. 2006;118:1591–602.
6. Koike N, Cho A, Nasu K, et al. Role of diffusion-weighted magnetic resonance imaging in the differential diagnosis of focal hepatic lesions. World J Gastroenterol. 2009;15:5805–12.
7. Seale MK, Catalano OA, Saini S, Hahn PF, Sahani DV. Hepatobiliary-specific MR contrast agents: role in imaging the liver and biliary tree. Radiographics. 2009;29:1725–48.
8. Raddatz D, Ramadori G. Carbohydrate metabolism and the liver: actual aspects from physiology and disease. Z Gastroenterol. 2007;45:51–62.
9. Torizuka T, Tamaki N, Inokuma T, et al. In vivo assessment of glucose metabolism in hepatocellular carcinoma with FDG-PET. J Nucl Med. 1995;36:1811–7.
10. Salem N, MacLennan GT, Kuang Y, et al. Quantitative evaluation of 2-deoxy-2[F-18]fluoro-Dglucose-positron emission tomography imaging on the woodchuck model of hepatocellular carcinoma with histological correlation. Mol Imaging Biol. 2007;9:135–43.
11. Lee JD, Yang WI, Park YN, et al. Different glucose uptake and glycolytic mechanisms between hepatocellular carcinoma and intrahepatic massforming cholangiocarcinoma with increased (18) F-FDG uptake. J Nucl Med. 2005;46:1753–9.
12. Roh MS, Jeong JS, Kim YH, Kim MC, Hong SH. Diagnostic utility of GLUT1 in the differential diagnosis of liver carcinomas. Hepato-Gastroenterology. 2004;51:1315–8.
13. Khan MA, Combs CS, Brunt EM, et al. Positron emission tomography scanning in the evaluation of hepatocellular carcinoma. J Hepatol. 2000;32:792–7.
14. Ho CL, Yu SC, Yeung DW. 11C-acetate PET imaging in hepatocellular carcinoma and other liver masses. J Nucl Med. 2003;44:213–21.
15. Wudel LJ Jr, Delbeke D, Morris D, et al. The role of [18F]fluorodeoxyglucose positron emission tomography imaging in the evaluation of hepatocellular carcinoma. Am Surg 2003; 69:117–124, discussion 124–126.
16. Rose AT, Rose DM, Pinson CW, et al. Hepatocellular carcinoma outcomes based on indicated treatment strategy. Am Surg. 1998;64:1128–34. discussion 1134–5
17. Shiomi S, Nishiguchi S, Ishizu H, et al. Usefulness of positron emission tomography with fluorine-18-fluorodeoxyglucose for predicting outcome in patients with hepatocellular carcinoma. Am J Gastroenterol. 2001;96:1877–80.
18. Kong YH, Han CJ, Lee SD, et al. Positron emission tomography with fluorine-18-fluorodeoxyglucose is useful for predicting the prognosis of patients with

hepatocellular carcinoma (in Korean). Korean J Hepatol. 2004;10:279–87.
19. Yoon KT, Kim JK, Kim do Y, et al. Role of 18Ffluorodeoxyglucose positron emission tomography in detecting extrahepatic metastasis in pretreatment staging of hepatocellular carcinoma. Oncology. 2007;72(suppl 1):104–10.
20. Ho CL, Chen S, Yeung DW, Cheng TK. Dualtracer PET/CT imaging in evaluation of metastatic hepatocellular carcinoma. J Nucl Med. 2007;48:902–9.
21. Czernin J, Schelbert HR. PET/CT in cancer patient management: introduction. J Nucl Med. 2007;48(suppl 1):2S–3S.
22. Iannaccone R, Piacentini F, Murakami T, et al. Hepatocellular carcinoma in patients with nonalcoholic fatty liver disease: helical CT and MR imaging findings with clinical-pathologic comparison. Radiology. 2007;243:422–30.
23. Kawaoka T, Aikata H, Takaki S, et al. FDG positron emission tomography/computed tomography for the detection of extrahepatic metastases from hepatocellular carcinoma. Hepatol Res. 2009;39:134–42.
24. Delbeke D, Pinson CW. 11C-acetate: a new tracer for the evaluation of hepatocellular carcinoma. J Nucl Med. 2003;44:222–3.
25. Park JW, Kim JH, Kim SK, et al. A prospective evaluation of 18F-FDG and 11C-acetate PET/CT for detection of primary and metastatic hepatocellular carcinoma. J Nucl Med. 2008;49:1912–21.
26. Wang XY, Chen D, Zhang XS, et al. Value of 18F-FDG-PET/CT in the detection of recurrent hepatocellular carcinoma after hepatectomy or radiofrequency ablation: a comparative study with contrast-enhanced ultrasound. J Dig Dis. 2013;14(8):433–8.
27. Paudyal B, Oriuchi N, Paudyal P, et al. Early diagnosis of recurrent hepatocellular carcinoma with 18F-FDG PET after radiofrequency ablation therapy. Oncol Rep. 2007;18(6):1469–73.
28. Raddatz D, Ramadori G. Carbohydrate metabolism and the liver: actual aspects from physiology and disease. Z Gastroenterol. 2007;45(1):51–62.
29. Mueckler M, Thorens B. The SLC2 (GLUT) family of membrane transporters. Mol Asp Med. 2013;34(2–3):121–38.
30. Wilson JE. Hexokinases. Rev Physiol Biochem Pharmacol. 1995;126:65–198.
31. van Schaftingen E, Gerin I. The glucose-6-phosphatase system. Biochem J. 2002;362(Pt 3):513–32.
32. Burchell A. Molecular pathology of glucose-6-phosphatase. FASEB J. 1990;4(12):2978–88.
33. Pauwels EK, Ribeiro MJ, Stoot JH, McCready VR, Bourguignon M, Maziere B. FDG accumulation and tumor biology. Nucl Med Biol. 1998;25(4):317–22.
34. Jadvar H, Alavi A, Gambhir SS. 18F-FDG uptake in lung, breast, and colon cancers: molecular biology correlates and disease characterization. J Nucl Med. 2009;50(11):1820–7.
35. Kim BT, Kim Y, Lee KS, Yoon SB, Cheon EM, Kwon OJ, et al. Localized form of bronchioloalveolar carcinoma: FDG PET fndings. AJR Am J Roentgenol. 1998;170(4):935–9.
36. Jadvar H, Segall GM. False-negative fuorine-18-FDG PET in metastatic carcinoid. J Nucl Med. 1997;38(9):1382–3.
37. Schuurbiers OC, Meijer TW, Kaanders JH, Looijen-Salamon MG, de Geus-Oei LF, van der Drift MA, et al. Glucose metabolism in NSCLC is histology-specifc and diverges the prognostic potential of 18FDG-PET for adenocarcinoma and squamous cell carcinoma. J Thorac Oncol. 2014;9(10):1485–93.
38. Blake MA, Singh A, Setty BN, Slattery J, Kalra M, Maher MM, et al. Pearls and pitfalls in interpretation of abdominal and pelvic PET-CT. Radiographics. 2006;26(5):1335–533.
39. Sureshbabu W, Mawlawi O. PET/CT imaging artifacts. J Nucl Med Technol. 2005;33(3):156–61.
40. Dizendorf E, Hany TF, Buck A, Von Schulthess GK, Burger C. Cause and magnitude of the error induced by oral CT contrast agent in CT-based attenuation correction of PET emission studies. J Nucl Med. 2003;44(5):732–8.
41. Goerres GW, Ziegler SI, Burger C, Berthold T, Von Schulthess GK, Buck A. Artifacts at PET and PET/CT caused by metallic hip prosthetic material. Radiology. 2003;226(2):577–84.
42. Goerres GW, Burger C, Kamel E, Seifert B, Kaim AH, Buck A, et al. Respiration-induced attenuation artifact at PET/CT: technical considerations. Radiology. 2003;226(3):906–910. 716 Japanese Journal of Radiology (2020) 38:697–718 1 3
43. Nakamoto Y, Tatsumi M, Cohade C, Osman M, Marshall LT, Wahl RL. Accuracy of image fusion of normal upper abdominal organs visualized with PET/CT. Eur J Nucl Med Mol Imaging. 2003;30(4):597–602.
44. Vogel WV, van Dalen JA, Wiering B, Huisman H, Corstens FH, Ruers TJ, et al. Evaluation of image registration in PET/CT of the liver and recommendations for optimized imaging. J Nucl Med. 2007;48(6):910–9.
45. Soret M, Bacharach SL, Buvat I. Partial-volume effect in PET tumor imaging. J Nucl Med. 2007;48(6):932–45.
46. Kawaoka T, Aikata H, Takaki S, Uka K, Azakami T, Saneto H, et al. FDG positron emission tomography/computed tomography for the detection of extrahepatic metastases from hepatocellular carcinoma. Hepatol Res. 2009;39(2):134–42.
47. Sun DW, An L, Wei F, Mu L, Shi XJ, Wang CL, et al. Prognostic significance of parameters from pretreatment (18)F-FDG PET in hepatocellular carcinoma: a meta-analysis. Abdom Radiol (NY). 2016;41(1):33–41.
48. Anderson CD, Rice MH, Pinson CW, Chapman WC, Chari RS, Delbeke D. Fluorodeoxyglucose PET imaging in the evaluation of gallbladder carci-

noma and cholangiocarcinoma. J Gastrointest Surg. 2004;8(1):90–7.
49. Kim YJ, Yun M, Lee WJ, Kim KS, Lee JD. Usefulness of 18FFDG PET in intrahepatic cholangiocarcinoma. Eur J Nucl Med Mol Imaging. 2003;30(11):1467–72.
50. Lee JD, Yang WI, Park YN, Kim KS, Choi JS, Yun M, et al. Different glucose uptake and glycolytic mechanisms between hepatocellular carcinoma and intrahepatic mass-forming cholangiocarcinoma with increased (18) F-FDG uptake. J Nucl Med. 2005;46(10):1753–9.
51. Suzuki H, Komuta M, Bolog A, Yokobori T, Wada S, Araki K, et al. Relationship between 18-F-fuoro-deoxy-D-glucose uptake and expression of glucose transporter 1 and pyruv-ate kinase M2 in intrahepatic cholangiocarcinoma. Dig Liver Dis. 2015;47(7):590–6.
52. Jadvar H, Henderson RW, Conti PS. [F-18] fuorodeoxyglucose positron emission tomography and positron emission tomography: computed tomography in recurrent and metastatic cholangiocarcinoma. J Comput Assist Tomogr. 2007;31(2):223–8.
53. Corvera CU, Blumgart LH, Akhurst T, DeMatteo RP, D'Angelica M, Fong Y, et al. 18F-fuorodeoxyglucose positron emission tomography infuences management decisions in patients with biliary cancer. J Am Coll Surg. 2008;206(1):57–655.
54. Paradis V, Fukayama M, Park YN, Schirmacher P. Tumors of the liver and intrahepatic bile ducts. In: WHO classifcation of tumours editorial board. WHO classification of tumours of the digestive system. 5th ed. Lyon: IARC; 2019. p. 215–64.
55. Mori N, Ichikawa T, Hashimoto J, Yamashita T, Yamada M, Hirabayashi K, et al. Cholangiolocellular carcinoma of the liver exhibiting high F-18 FDG uptake. Tokai J Exp Clin Med. 2016;41(2):60–4.
56. Lim CH, Moon SH, Cho YS, Choi JY, Lee KH, Hyun SH. Prognostic value of 18F-fuorodeoxyglucose positron emission tomography/computed tomography in patients with combined hepatocellular-cholangiocarcinoma. Eur J Nucl Med Mol Imaging. 2019;46(8):1705–12.
57. Yi LL, Zhang JX, Zhou SG, Wang J, Huang YQ, Li J, et al. CT and MRI studies of hepatic angiosarcoma. Clin Radiol 2019;74(5):406.e1–406.e8.
58. Kamatani T, Iguchi H, Okada T, Yamazaki H, Tsunoda H, Watanabe M, et al. Co-registered positron emission tomography/computed tomography and gadolinium-ethoxybenzyldiethylenetriaminepen taacetic acid magnetic resonance imaging Japanese Journal of Radiology (2020) 38:697–718 717 1 3 features of multiple angiosarcoma of the liver. Hepatol Res. 2014;44(10):E297–303.
59. Maeda T, Tateishi U, Hasegawa T, Ojima H, Arai Y, Sugimura K. Primary hepatic angiosarcoma on coregistered FDG PET and CT images. AJR Am J Roentgenol. 2007;188(6):1615–7.
60. Mark L, Delmore F, Creech JL Jr, Ogden LL II, Fadell EH, Songster CL, et al. Clinical and morphologic features of hepatic angiosarcoma in vinyl chloride workers. Cancer. 1976;37(1):149–63.
61. Cronin CG, Swords R, Truong MT, Viswanathan C, Rohren E, Giles FJ, et al. Clinical utility of PET/CT in lymphoma. AJR Am J Roentgenol. 2010;194(1):W91–W103.
62. Weiler-Sagie M, Bushelev O, Epelbaum R, Dann EJ, Haim N, Avivi I, et al. (18)F-FDG avidity in lymphoma readdressed: a study of 766 patients. J Nucl Med. 2010;51(1):25–30.
63. Avlonitis VS, Linos D. Primary hepatic lymphoma: a review. Eur J Surg. 1999;165(8):725–9.
64. Ohsawa M, Aozasa K, Horiuchi K, Kataoka M, Hida J, Shimada H, et al. Malignant lymphoma of the liver. Report of five cases and review of the literature. Dig Dis Sci. 1992;37(7):1105–9.
65. Lee JA, Jeong WK, Min JH, Kim J. Primary hepatic lymphoma mimicking acute hepatitis. Clin Mol Hepatol. 2013;19(3):320–3.
66. Juweid ME, Cheson BD. Role of positron emission tomography in lymphoma. J Clin Oncol. 2005;23(21):4577–80.
67. Noy A, Schöder H, Gönen M, Weissler M, Ertelt K, Cohler C, et al. The majority of transformed lymphomas have high SUVs on positron emission tomography (PET) scanning similar to diffuse large B-cell lymphoma (DLBCL). Ann Oncol. 2009;20(3):508–12.
68. Rodriguez M, Rehn S, Ahlström H, Sundström C, Glimelius B. Predicting malignancy grade with PET in non-Hodgkin's lymphoma. J Nucl Med. 1995;36(10):1790–6.
69. Tsimberidou AM, Wierda WG, Plunkett W, Kurzrock R, O'Brien S, Wen S, et al. Phase I-II study of oxaliplatin, fudarabine, cytarabine, and rituximab combination therapy in patients with Richter's syndrome or fudarabine-refractory chronic lymphocytic leukemia. J Clin Oncol. 2008;26(2):196–203.
70. Liu YM, Zhai XM, Wu YW. Biological correlation between glucose transporters, Ki-67 and 2-deoxy-2-[18F]-fuoro-d-glucose uptake in diffuse large B-cell lymphoma and natural killer/T-cell lymphoma. Genet Mol Res. 2016;15(2)
71. Hirose Y, Suefuji H, Kaida H, Hayakawa M, Hattori S, Kurata S, et al. Relationship between 2-deoxy-2-[(18)F]-fuoro-d-glucose uptake and clinicopathological factors in patients with diffuse large B-cell lymphoma. Leuk Lymphoma. 2014;55(3):520–5.
72. Shim HK, Lee WW, Park SY, Kim H, Kim SE. Relationship between FDG uptake and expressions of glucose transporter type 1, type 3, and hexokinase-II in Reed-Sternberg cells of Hodgkin lymphoma. Oncol Res. 2009;17(7):331–7.
73. Benzerdjeb N, Berna P, Sevestre H. GLUT1: a novel tool reflecting proliferative activity of lung neuroendocrine tumors? Pathol Int. 2017;67(1):32–6.
74. Binderup T, Knigge U, Loft A, Mortensen J, Pfeifer A, Federspiel B, et al. Functional imaging of neuroendocrine tumors: a head-to-head comparison of somatostatin receptor scintigraphy, 123I-MIBG

scintigraphy, and 18F-FDG PET. J Nucl Med. 2010;51(5):704–12.
75. Garin E, Le Jeune F, Devillers A, Cuggia M, de Lajarte-Thirouard AS, Bouriel C, et al. Predictive value of 18F-FDG PET and somatostatin receptor scintigraphy in patients with metastatic endocrine tumors. J Nucl Med. 2009;50(6):858–64.
76. Binderup T, Knigge U, Loft A, Federspiel B, Kjaer A. 18F-fuorodeoxyglucose positron emission tomography predicts survival of patients with neuroendocrine tumors. Clin Cancer Res. 2010;16(3):978–85.
77. D'souza MM, Sharma R, Mondal A, Jaimini A, Tripathi M, Saw SK, et al. Prospective evaluation of CECT and 18F-FDG-PET/ CT in detection of hepatic metastases. Nucl Med Commun. 2009;30(2):117–25.
78. Arulampalam TH, Francis DL, Visvikis D, Taylor I, Ell PJ. FDGPET for the pre-operative evaluation of colorectal liver metastases. Eur J Surg Oncol. 2004;30(3):286–91.
79. Sivesgaard K, Larsen LP, Sørensen M, Kramer S, Schlander S, Amanavicius N, et al. Diagnostic accuracy of CE-CT, MRI and FDG PET/CT for detecting colorectal cancer liver metastases in patients considered eligible for hepatic resection and/ or local ablation. Eur Radiol. 2018;28(11):4735–47.
80. Lincke T, Zech CJ. Liver metastases: detection and staging. Eur J Radiol. 2017;97:76–82.
81. Zimmerman RL, Fogt F, Burke M, Murakata LA. Assessment of Glut-1 expression in cholangiocarcinoma, benign biliary lesions and hepatocellular carcinoma. Oncol Rep Oncol Rep. 2002;9(4):689–92.
82. Pinilla I, Rodríguez-Vigil B, Gómez-León N. Integrated FDG PET/CT: utility and applications in clinical oncology. Clin Med Oncol. 2008;2:181–98.
83. Poeppel TD, Krause BJ, Heusner TA, Boy C, Bockisch A, Antoch G. PET/CT for the staging and follow-up of patients with malignancies. Eur J Radiol. 2009;70(3):382–92.
84. Wang Z, Chen JQ, Liu JL, Qin XG, Huang Y. FDG-PET in diagnosis, staging and prognosis of pancreatic carcinoma: a meta-analysis. World J Gastroenterol. 2013;19(29):4808–17.
85. Liu Y. Role of positron emission tomography with fuorodeoxyglucose in prostate cancer. Oncol Lett. 2014;7(6):2013–8.
86. Iwano S, Ito S, Tsuchiya K, Kato K, Naganawa S. What causes false-negative PET findings for solid-type lung cancer? Lung Cancer. 2013;79(2):132–6.
87. Higashi K, Clavo AC, Wahl RL. Does FDG uptake measure proliferative activity of human cancer cells? In vitro comparison with DNA flow cytometry and tritiated thymidine uptake. J Nucl Med. 1993;34(3):414–9.
88. Berger KL, Nicholson SA, Dehdashti F, Siegel BA. FDG PET evaluation of mucinous neoplasms: correlation of FDG uptake with histopathologic features. AJR Am J Roentgenol. 2000;174(4):1005–8.
89. Picchia S, Riddell A, Terlizzo M, Bali MA. Liver metastasis from adenoid cystic carcinoma: imaging and histologic features. Curr Probl Cancer. 2019;43(4):331–5.
90. Takahashi M, Kume H, Koyama K, Nakagawa T, Fujimura T, Morikawa T, et al. Preoperative evaluation of renal cell carcinoma by using 18F-FDG PET/ CT. Clin Nucl Med. 2015;40(12):936–40.
91. Ozerlat I. Kidney cancer: targeted therapy of glucose uptake via GLUT1 kills RCC cells. Nat Rev Urol. 2011;8(9):471.
92. Chan DA, Sutphin PD, Nguyen P, Turcotte S, Lai EW, Banh A, et al. Targeting GLUT1 and the Warburg effect in renal cell carcinoma by chemical synthetic lethality. Sci Transl Med. 2011;3(94):94ra70.
93. Schmoll D, Balabanov S, Schwarck D, Burchell A, Kleist B, Zimmermann U, et al. Differential expression of the subunits of the glucose-6-phosphatase system in the clear cell type of human renal cell carcinoma—no evidence for an overexpression of protein kinase B. Cancer Lett. 2001;167(1):85–90.
94. Macfarlane DJ, Sondak V, Johnson T, Wahl RL. Prospective evaluation of 2-fuorine-[18F]-fuoro-2-deoxy-d-glucose positron emission tomography in staging of regional lymph nodes in patients with cutaneous malignant melanoma. J Clin Oncol. 1998;16(5):1770–6.
95. Lucignani G, Paganelli G, Modorati G, Pieralli S, Rizzo G, Magnani P, et al. MRI, antibody-guided scintigraphy, and glucose metabolism in uveal melanoma. J Comput Assist Tomogr. 1992;16(1):77–83.
96. Spraul CW, Lang GE, Lang GK. Value of positron emission tomography in the diagnosis of malignant ocular tumors. Ophthalmologica. 2001;215(3):163–8.
97. Strobel K, Bode B, Dummer R, Veit-Haibach P, Fischer DR, Imhof L, et al. Limited value of 18F-FDG PET/CT and S-100B tumour marker in the detection of liver metastases from uveal melanoma compared to liver metastases from cutaneous melanoma. Eur J Nucl Med Mol Imaging. 2009;36(11):1774–822.
98. Sacks A, Peller PJ, Surasi DS, Chatburn L, Mercier G, Subramaniam RM. Value of PET/CT in the management of primary hepatobiliary tumors, part 2. AJR Am J Roentgenol. 2011;197(2):W260–W265265.
99. Love C, Tomas MB, Tronco GG, Palestro CJ. FDG PET of infection and inflammation. Radiographics. 2005;25(5):1357–68.
100. Magini G, Farsad M, Frigerio M, Serra C, Colecchia A, Jovine E, et al. C-11 acetate does not enhance usefulness of F-18 Japanese Journal of Radiology 1 3 FDG PET/CT in differentiating between focal nodular hyperplasia and hepatic adenoma. Clin Nucl Med Clin Nucl Med. 2009;34(10):659–65.
101. Ozaki K, Harada K, Terayama N, Matsui O, Saitoh S, Tomimaru Y, et al. Hepatocyte nuclear factor 1α-inactivated hepatocellular adenomas exhibit high (18)F-fudeoxyglucose uptake associated with

glucose-6-phosphate transporter inactivation. Br J Radiol. 2016;89(1063):20160265.
102. Lee SY, Kingham TP, LaGratta MD, Jessurun J, Cherqui D, Jarnagin WR, et al. PET-avid hepatocellular adenomas: incidental findings associated with HNF1-α mutated lesions. HPB (Oxford). 2016;18(1):41–8.
103. Delbeke D, Martin WH, Sandler MP, Chapman WC, Wright JK Jr, Pinson CW. Evaluation of benign vs malignant hepatic lesions with positron emission tomography. Arch Surg. 1998;133:510–5. discussion 515–6
104. Nault JC, Paradis V, Cherqui D, Vilgrain V, Zucman-Rossi J. Molecular classifcation of hepatocellular adenoma in clinical practice. J Hepatol. 2017;67(5):1074–83.
105. Vilgrain V, Boulos L, Vullierme MP, Denys A, Terris B, Menu Y. Imaging of atypical hemangiomas of the liver with pathologic correlation. Radiographics. 2000;20(2):379–97.
106. Shimada K, Nakamoto Y, Isoda H, Saito H, Arizono S, Shibata T, et al. FDG PET for giant cavernous hemangioma: important clue to differentiate from a malignant vascular tumor in the liver. Clin Nucl Med. 2010;35(12):924–6.
107. Mohajer K, Frydrychowicz A, Robbins JB, Loefer AG, Reed TD, Reeder SB. Characterization of hepatic adenoma and focal nodular hyperplasia with gadoxetic acid. J Magn Reson Imaging. 2012;36(3):686–96.
108. Grazioli L, Bondioni MP, Haradome H, Motosugi U, Tinti R, Frittoli B, et al. Hepatocellular adenoma and focal nodular hyperplasia: value of gadoxetic acid-enhanced MR imaging in differential diagnosis. Radiology. 2012;262(2):520–9.
109. Morana G, Grazioli L, Kirchin MA, Bondioni MP, Faccioli N, Guarise A, et al. Solid hypervascular liver lesions: accurate identification of true benign lesions on enhanced dynamic and hepatobiliary phase magnetic resonance imaging after gadobenate dimeglumine administration. Investig Radiol. 2011;46(4):225–39.
110. Wang X, Wang J, Cheng X, Li F, Huo L. Hepatic Angiomyolipoma having FDG uptake at the similar level of the Normal liver parenchyma. Clin Nucl Med. 2019;44(7):599–601.
111. Lee SJ, Kim SY, Kim KW, Shin YM, Kim HJ, Lee JS, et al. Hepatic angiomyolipoma with minimal fat, mimicking hepatocellular carcinoma. Clin Mol Hepatol. 2012;18(3):330–5.
112. Matsuo Y, Sato M, Shibata T, Morimoto M, Tsuboi K, Shamoto T, et al. Inflammatory pseudotumor of the liver diagnosed as metastatic liver tumor in a patient with a gastrointestinal stromal tumor of the rectum: report of a case. World J Surg Oncol. 2014;12:140.
113. Chong A, Jeong SY, Min JJ. Inflammatory pseudotumours resembling multiple hepatic metastases and their complete regression, as revealed by 18F-FDG PET/CT. Eur J Nucl Med Mol Imaging. 2009;36(7):1199–200.
114. Sharif S, Murphy M, Loda M, Pinkus GS, Khettry U. Nodular lymphoid lesion of the liver: an immune-mediated disorder mimicking low-grade malignant lymphoma. Am J Surg. 1999;23:302–8.
115. Lin E. Reactive lymphoid hyperplasia of the liver identified by FDG PET. Clin Nucl Med. 2008;33:419–20.
116. Lv A, Liu W, Qian HG, Leng JH, Hao CY. Reactive lymphoid hyperplasia of the liver mimicking hepatocellular carcinoma: incidental finding of two cases. Int J Clin Exp Pathol. 2015;8:5863–9.
117. Tan GJ, Berlangieri SU, Lee ST, Scott AM. FDG-PET/CT in the liver: lesions mimicking malignancies. Abdom Imaging. 2014;39(1):187–95.
118. Vaidyanathan S, Patel CN, Scarsbrook AF, Chowdhury FU. FDGPET/CT in infection and inflammation—current and emerging clinical applications. Clin Radiol. 2015;70(7):787–800.
119. Zhuang H, Alavi A. 18-fuorodeoxyglucose positron emission tomographic imaging in the detection and monitoring of infection and inflammation. Semin Nucl Med. 2002;32:47–59.
120. Paik JY, Lee KH, Choe YS, Choi Y, Kim BT. Augmented 18FFDG uptake in activated monocytes occurs during the priming process and involves tyrosine kinases and protein kinase C. J Nucl Med. 2004;45:124–8.
121. Meller J, Sahlmann CO, Scheel AK. 18F-FDG PET and PET/ CT in fever of unknown origin. J Nucl Med. 2007;48(1):35–45.
122. Mochizuki T, Tsukamoto E, Kuge Y, Kanegae K, Zhao S, Hikosaka K, et al. FDG uptake and glucose transporter subtype expressions in experimental tumor and inflammation models. J Nucl Med. 2001;42(10):1551–5.
123. Zhao S, Kuge Y, Tsukamoto E, Mochizuki T, Kato T, Hikosaka K, et al. Fluorodeoxyglucose uptake and glucose transporter expression in experimental inflammatory lesions and malignant tumours: effects of insulin and glucose loading. Nucl Med Commun. 2002;23(6):545–50.
124. Kubota R, Yamada S, Kubota K, Ishiwata K, Tamahashi N, Ido T. Intratumoral distribution of fluorine-18-fuorodeoxyglucose in vivo: high accumulation in macrophages and granulation tissues studied by microautoradiography. J Nucl Med. 1992;33:1972–80.
125. DeLeve LD, Shulman HM, McDonald GB. Toxic injury to hepatic sinusoids: sinusoidal obstruction syndrome (venoocclusive disease). Semin Liver Dis. 2002;22:27–422.
126. Shin NY, Kim MJ, Lim JS, Park MS, Chung YE, Choi JY, et al. Accuracy of gadoxetic acid-enhanced magnetic resonance imaging for the diagnosis of sinusoidal obstruction syndrome in patients with chemotherapy-treated colorectal liver metastases. Eur Radiol. 2012;22(4):864–71.
127. Kawai T, Yamazaki S, Iwama A, Higaki T, Sugitani M, Takayama T. Focal sinusoidal obstruction syndrome caused by Oxaliplatin-induced chemotherapy: a case report. Hepat Mon. 2016;16(9):e37572.

128. Choi JH, Won YW, Kim HS, Oh YH, Lim S, Kim HJ. Oxaliplatin-induced sinusoidal obstruction syndrome mimicking metastatic colon cancer in the liver. Oncol Lett. 2016;11(4):2861–4.
129. Plengsuriyakarn T, Matsuda N, Karbwang J, Viyanant V, Hirayama K, Na-Bangchang K. Anticancer activity of Atractylodeslancea (Thunb.) DC in a hamster model and application of PET-CT for early detection and monitoring progression of Cholangiocarcinoma. Asian Pac J Cancer Prev. 2015;16(15):6279–84. [Crossref]
130. Wells ML, Venkatesh SK, Chandan VS, Fidler JL, Fletcher JG, Johnson GB, Hough DM, Roberts LR. Biphenotypic hepatic tumors: imaging findings and review of literature. Abdom Imaging. 2015;40(7):2293–305. [Crossref]
131. Kaye TL, Ashley Guthrie J. Imaging the liver and biliary tract. Medicine. 2015;43(10):562–7. [Crossref]
132. Ercolani G, Dazzi A, Giovinazzo F, Ruzzenente A, Bassi C, Guglielmi A, Scarpa A, D'Errico A, Pinna AD. Intrahepatic, peri-hilar and distal cholangiocarcinoma: three different locations of the same tumor or three different tumors? Eur J Surg Oncol. 2015;41(9):1162–9. [Crossref]
133. Parikh U, Marcus C, Sarangi R, Taghipour M, Subramaniam RM. FDG PET/CT in pancreatic and hepatobiliary carcinomas. PET Clinics. 2015;10(3):327–43. [Crossref]
134. Gavra M, Syed R, Fraioli F, Afaq A, Bomanji J. PET/MRI in the upper abdomen. Semin Nucl Med. 2015;45(4):282–92. [Crossref]
135. Song J-Y, Lee YN, Kim YS, Kim SG, Jin SJ, Park JM, Choi GS, Chung JC, Lee MH, Cho YH, Choi MH, Kim DC, Choi HJ, Moon JH, Lee SH, Jeong SW, Jang JY, Kim HS, Kim BS. Predictability of preoperative 18F-FDG PET for histopathological differentiation and early recurrence of primary malignant intrahepatic tumors. Nucl Med Commun. 2015;36(4):319–27. [Crossref]
136. Plengsuriyakarn T, Karbwang J, Na-Bangchang K. Anticancer activity using positron emission tomography-computed tomography and pharmacokinetics of β -eudesmol in human cholangiocarcinoma xenografted nude mouse model. Clin Exp Pharmacol Physiol. 2015;42(3):293–304. [Crossref]
137. Lee SY, Peter Kingham T, LaGratta MD, Jessurun J, Cherqui D, Jarnagin WR, Kluger MD. PET-avid hepatocellular adenomas: incidental findings associated with HNF1-α mutated lesions. HPB. 2015;18(1):41–8. [Crossref]
138. Bellissimo F. Diagnostic and therapeutic management of hepatocellular carcinoma. World J Gastroenterol. 2015;21(42):12003. [Crossref]
139. Santiago JFY. Rare or unusual primary malignancies. Springer. p. 49–73. [Crossref]
140. Chirindel A, Alluri KC, Tahari AK, Chaudhry M, Wahl RL, Lodge MA, Subramaniam RM. Liver standardized uptake value corrected for lean body mass at FDG PET/CT. Clin Nucl Med. 2015;40(1):e17–22. [Crossref] Downloaded from www.ajronline.org by 117.195.237.192 on 10/22/21 from IP address 117.195.237.192. Copyright ARRS. For personal use only; all rights reserved
141. Nakashima T, Takayama Y, Nishie A, Asayama Y, Baba S, Yamashita Y, Shirabe K, Kubo Y, Hida T, Honda H. Hepatocellular adenoma showing high uptake of 18Ffluorodeoxyglucose (FDG) via an increased expression of glucose transporter 2 (GLUT-2). Clin Imaging. 2014;38(6):888–91. [Crossref]
142. Ahn SY, Lee JM, Joo I, Lee ES, Lee SJ, Cheon GJ, Han JK, Choi BI. Prediction of microvascular invasion of hepatocellular carcinoma using gadoxetic acid-enhanced MR and 18F-FDG PET/CT. Abdom Imaging. 2014;40(4):843–51. [Crossref]
143. Paidpally V, Chirindel A, Chung CH, Richmon J, Koch W, Quon H, Subramaniam RM. FDG volumetric parameters and survival outcomes after definitive Chemoradiotherapy in patients with recurrent head and neck squamous cell carcinoma. Am J Roentgenol. 2014;203(2):W139–45. [Abstract] [Full Text] [PDF] [PDF Plus]

Multimodality Imaging of Liver 144 to 179

144. Cho E, Jun CH, Kim BS, Son DJ, Choi WS, Choi SK. 18F-FDG PET CT as a prognostic factor in hepatocellular carcinoma. Turk J Gastroenterol. 2015;26:344–50.
145. Asman Y, Evenson AR, Even-Sapir E, Shibolet O. [18F]fludeoxyglucose positron emission tomography and computed tomography as a prognostic tool before liver transplantation, resection, and loco-ablative therapies for hepatocellular carcinoma. Liver Transpl. 2015;21:572–80.
146. Boellaard R, Delgado-Bolton R, Oyen WJ, Giammarile F, Tatsch K, Eschner W, et al. FDG PET/CT: EANM procedure guidelines for tumour imaging: version 2.0. Eur J Nucl Med Mol Imaging. 2015;42(2):328–54.
147. Na SJ, Oh JK, Hyun SH, Lee JW, Hong IK, Song BI, et al. 18F-FDG PET/CT can predict survival of advanced hepatocellular carcinoma patients: a multicenter retrospective cohort study. J Nucl Med. 2017;58(5):730–6.
148. Roberts LR, Sirlin CB, Zaiem F, Almasri J, Prokop LJ, Heimbach JK, et al. Imaging for the diagnosis of hepatocellular carcinoma: a systematic review and meta-analysis. Hepatology. 2018;67(1):401–21.
149. Hennedige T, Venkatesh SK. Imaging of hepatocellular carcinoma: diagnosis, staging and treatment monitoring. Cancer Imaging. 2013;12:530–47.
150. Lin CY, Liao CW, Chu LY, Yen KY, Jeng LB, Hsu CN, et al. Predictive value of 18F-FDG PET/CT for vascular invasion in patients with hepatocellular carcinoma before liver transplantation. Clin Nucl Med. 2017;42:e183–7.
151. Boussouar S, Itti E, Lin SJ, Decaens T, Evangelista E, Chiaradia M, et al. Functional imaging of hepa-

tocellular carcinoma using diffusion-weighted MRI and (18)F-FDG PET/CT in patients on waiting-list for liver transplantation. Cancer Imaging. 2016;16:4.
152. Hong G, Suh KS, Suh SW, Yoo T, Kim H, Park MS, Choi Y, Paeng JC, Yi NJ, Lee KW. Alpha-fetoprotein and (18)F-FDG positron emission tomography predict tumor recurrence better than Milan criteria in living donor liver transplantation. J Hepatol. 2016;64:852–9.
153. Lee SD, Lee B, Kim SH, Joo J, Kim SK, Kim YK, Park SJ. Proposal of new expanded selection criteria using total tumor size and (18) F-fluorodeoxyglucose – positron emission tomography/computed tomography for living donor liver transplantation in patients with hepatocellular carcinoma: the National Cancer Center Korea criteria. World J Transplant. 2016;6:411–22.
154. Bailly M, Venel Y, Orain I, Salamé E, Ribeiro MJ. 18F-FDG PET in liver transplantation setting of hepatocellular carcinoma: predicting histology? Clin Nucl Med. 2016;41:e126–9.
155. Lin CY, Liao CW, Chu LY, Yen KY, Jeng LB, Hsu CN, Lin CL, Kao CH. Predictive value of 18F-FDG PET/CT for vascular invasion in patients with hepatocellular carcinoma before liver transplantation. Clin Nucl Med. 2017;42:e183–7.
156. Marrero JA, Ahn J, Rajender Reddy K. ACG clinical guideline: the diagnosis and management of focal liver lesions. Am J Gastroenterol. 2014;109:1328–47. https://doi.org/10.1038/ajg.2014.213.
157. Wang Y, Yang Y, Li J, Cheng D, Xu H, Huang J. Dynamic FDG PET/CT imaging: quantitative assessment, advantages and application in the diagnosis of malignant solid tumors. Front Oncol. 2025;15:1539911. https://doi.org/10.3389/fonc.2025.1539911.
158. Omata M, Cheng AL, Kokudo N, Kudo M, Lee JM, Jia J, et al. Asia-Pacific clinical practice guidelines on the management of hepatocellular carcinoma: a 2017 update. Hepatol Int. 2017;11:317–70.
159. Ho CL, Yu SC, Yeung DW. 11C-acetate PET imaging in hepatocellular carcinoma and other liver masses. J Nucl Med. 2003 ;44:213–21. https://pubmed.ncbi.nlm.nih.gov/12571212/.
160. Hwang KH, Choi DJ, Lee SY, et al. Evaluation of patients with hepatocellular carcinomas using [(11) C]acetate and [(18)F]FDG PET/CT: a preliminary study. Appl Radiat Isot. 2009;67:1195–8. https://doi.org/10.1016/j.apradiso.2009.02.011.
161. Cheung TT, Ho CL, Lo CM, et al. 11C-acetate and 18F-FDG PET/CT for clinical staging and selection of patients with hepatocellular carcinoma for liver transplantation on the basis of Milan criteria: surgeon's perspective. J Nucl Med. 2013;54:192–200. https://doi.org/10.2967/jnumed.112.107516.
162. Liu D, Khong PL, Gao Y, et al. Radiation dosimetry of whole-body dual-tracer 18F-FDG and 11C-acetate PET/CT for hepatocellular carcinoma. J Nucl Med. 2016;57:907–12. https://doi.org/10.2967/jnumed.115.165944.
163. Ho CL, Chen S, Yeung DW, et al. Dual-tracer PET/CT imaging in evaluation of metastatic hepatocellular carcinoma. J Nucl Med. 2007;48:902–9. https://doi.org/10.2967/jnumed.106.036673.
164. Ho CL, Yu SC, Yeung DW. 11C-acetate PET imaging in hepatocellular carcinoma and other liver masses. J Nucl Med. 2003;44:213–21.
165. Ong LC, Jin Y, Song IC, Yu S, Zhang K, Chow PK. 2-[18F]-2-deoxy-D-glucose (FDG) uptake in human tumor cells is related to the expression of GLUT-1 and hexokinase II. Acta Radiol. 2008;49:1145–53.
166. Zhao S, Kuge Y, Mochizuki T, Takahashi T, Nakada K, Sato M, Takei T, Tamaki N. Biologic correlates of intratumoral heterogeneity in 18F-FDG distribution with regional expression of glucose transporters and hexokinase-II in experimental tumor. J Nucl Med. 2005;46:675–82.
167. Zimmerman RL, Burke M, Young NA, Solomides CC, Bibbo M. Diagnostic utility of Glut-1 and CA 15-3 in discriminating adenocarcinoma from hepatocellular carcinoma in liver tumors biopsied by fine-needle aspiration. Cancer. 2002;96:53–7.
168. Lee JD, Yang WI, Park YN, Kim KS, Choi JS, Yun M, Ko D, Kim TS, Cho AE, Kim HM, Han KH, Im SS, Ahn YH, Choi CW, Park JH. Different glucose uptake and glycolytic mechanisms between hepatocellular carcinoma and intrahepatic mass-forming cholangiocarcinoma with increased (18)F-FDG uptake. J Nucl Med. 2005;46:1753–9.
169. Siqueira E, Schoen RE, Silverman W, et al. Detecting cholangiocarcinoma in patients with primary sclerosing cholangitis. Gastrointest Endosc. 2002;56:40–7.
170. Albazaz R, Patel CN, Chowdhury FU, Scarsbrook AF. Clinical impact of FDG PET-CT on management decisions for patients with primary biliary tumours. Insights Imaging. 2013;4:691–700. https://doi.org/10.1007/s13244-013-0268-2.
171. Annunziata S, Caldarella C, Pizzuto DA, Galiandro F, Sadeghi R, Giovanella L, et al. Diagnostic accuracy of fluorine-18-fluorodeoxyglucose positron emission tomography in the evaluation of the primary tumor in patients with cholangiocarcinoma: a meta-analysis. Biomed Res Int. 2014;2014:247693. https://doi.org/10.1155/2014/247693.
172. Fujita N, Asayama Y, Nishie A, Ishigami K, Ushijima Y, Takayama Y, et al. Mass-forming intrahepatic cholangiocarcinoma: enhancement patterns in the arterial phase of dynamic hepatic CT – correlation with clinicopathological findings. Eur Rad. 2016;27:498.
173. Park TG, Yu YD, Park BJ, Cheon GJ, Oh SY, Kim DS, et al. Implication of lymph node metastasis detected on 18F-FDG PET/CT for surgical planning in patients with peripheral intrahepatic cholangiocarcinoma. Clin Nucl Med. 2014;39:1–7. https://doi.org/10.1097/RLU.0b013e3182867b99.
174. Olthof SC, Othman A, Clasen S, Schraml C, Nikolaou K, Bongers M. Imaging of cholangiocarcinoma. Visc Med. 2016;32:402–10.

175. Moon CM, Bang S, Chung JB. The role of (18) F-fluorodeoxyglucose positron emission tomography in the diagnosis, staging, and follow-up of cholangiocarcinoma. Surg Oncol. 2011;20:e10–7.
176. Fritscher-Ravens A, Bohuslavizki KH, Broering DC, Jenicke L, Schafer H, Buchert R, et al. FDG PET in the diagnosis of hilar cholangiocarcinoma. Nucl Med Commun. 2001;22:1277–85.
177. Cho KM, Oh DY, Kim TY, Lee KH, Han SW, Im SA, et al. Metabolic characteristics of advanced biliary tract cancer using F-18-Fluorodeoxyglucose positron emission tomography and their clinical implications. Oncologist. 2015;20:926–33. https://doi.org/10.1634/theoncologist.2014-0356.
178. Jo I, Won KS, Kim SH, Song B-I, Kang YN, Kim JY. Catheter tract implantation metastasis diagnosed by F-18 FDG PET/CT after percutaneous Transhepatic biliary drainage for hilar Cholangiocarcinoma. Nucl Med Mol Imaging. 2014;48:326–7.
179. Reinhardt MJ, Strunk H, Gerhardt T, Roedel R, Jaeger U, Bucerius J, et al. Detection of Klatskin's tumor in extrahepatic bile duct strictures using delayed 18F-FDG PET/CT: preliminary results for 22 patient studies. J Nucl Med. 2005;46:1158–63.
180. Boellaard R, O'Doherty MJ, Weber WA, et al. FDG PET and PET/CT: EANM procedure guidelines for tumour PET imaging: version 1.0. Eur J Nucl Med Mol Imaging. 2010;37:181–200.
181. Routhier JR, Woodfield CA, Mayo-Smith WW. AJR teaching file: fat-containing retroperitoneal mass presenting with acute flank pain. AJR Am J Roentgenol. 2009;192:S122–4.
182. Vogel WV, Oyen WJ, Barentsz JO, Kaanders JH, Corstens FH. PET/CT: panacea, redundancy, or something in between? J Nucl Med. 2004;45(Suppl 1):15S–24S.
183. Kim YJ, Yun M, Lee WJ, Kim KS, Lee JD. Usefulness of 18F-FDG PET in intrahepatic cholangiocarcinoma. Eur J Nucl Med Mol Imaging. 2003;30:1467–72.
184. Lam WW, Osmany S. Biliary non-Hodgkin lymphoma detected by F-18 FDG PET/CT. Clin Nucl Med. 2009;34:791–2.
185. Delbeke D, et al. Procedure guideline for tumor imaging with 18F-FDG PET/CT 1.0. J Nucl Med. 2006;47(5):885–95.
186. Koh T, Taniguchi H, Yamaguchi A, Kunishima S, Yamagishi H. Differential diagnosis of gallbladder cancer using positron emission tomography with fluorine-18-labeled fluoro-deoxyglucose (FDG-PET). J Surg Oncol. 2003;84:74–81. https://doi.org/10.1002/jso.10295.
187. Kim J, Ryu JK, Kim C, Paeng JC, Kim YT. Is there any role of positron emission tomography computed tomography for predicting resectability of gallbladder cancer? J Korean Med Sci. 2014;29:680–4. https://doi.org/10.3346/jkms.2014.29.5.680.
188. Ramos-Font C, Gómez-Rio M, Rodríguez-Fernández A, Jiménez-Heffernan A, Sánchez Sánchez R, Llamas-Elvira JM. Ability of FDG-PET/CT in the detection of gallbladder cancer. J Surg Oncol. 2014;109(03):218–24.
189. European Association of Nuclear Medicine (EANM), Boellaard R, Delgado-Bolton R, Oyen WJG. FDG PET/CT: EANM procedure guidelines for tumour imaging: version 2.0. Eur J Nucl Med Mol Imaging. 2015;42(02):328–54.
190. Ma KW, Cheung TT, She WH. Diagnostic and prognostic role of 18-FDG PET/CT in the management of resectable biliary tract cancer. World J Surg. 2018;42(03):823–34.
191. Kim J, Ryu JK, Kim C, Paeng JC, Kim Y-T. Is there any role of positron emission tomography computed tomography for predicting resectability of gallbladder cancer? J Korean Med Sci. 2014;29(05):680–4.
192. Yoo J, Choi JY, Lee KT, et al. Prognostic significance of volume-based metabolic parameters by (18)FFDG PET/CT in gallbladder carcinoma. Nucl Med Mol Imaging. 2012;46(3):201–6.
193. Donohue JH. Present status of the diagnosis and treatment of gallbladder carcinoma. J Hepatobiliary Pancreat Surg. 2001;8(6):530–4.
194. Hwang JP, Lim I, Na II, et al. Prognostic value of suvmax measured by fluorine-18 fluorodeoxyglucose positron emission tomography with computed tomography in patients with gallbladder cancer. Nucl Med Mol Imaging. 2014;48(2):114–20.
195. Butte and colleagues. T he role of PET-CT in patients with incidental gallbladder cancer. HPB (Oxford). 2009;11(7):585–91.
196. Redondo F, Butte J, Lavados H, et al. 18F-FDG PET/CT performance and prognostic value in patients with incidental gallbladder carcinoma. J Nucl Med. 2012;53(515):515.
197. Delbeke D, Martin WH. PET and PET/CT for pancreatic malignancies. Surg Oncol Clin N Am. 2010;19:235–54. [PMID 20159513]
198. Kamisawa T, Okamoto A. IgG4-related sclerosing disease. World J Gastroenterol. 2008;14:3948–55. [PMID 18609677]
199. Abraham SC, Wilentz RE, Yeo CJ, Sohn TA, Cameron JL, Boitnott JK, et al. Pancreaticoduodenectomy (Whipple resections) in patients without malignancy: are they all 'chronic pancreatitis'? Am J Surg Pathol. 2003;27:110–20. [PMID 12502933]
200. Tsitouridis I, Diamantopoulou A, Michaelides M, Arvanity M, Papaioannou S. Pancreatic metastases: CT and MRI findings. Diagn Interv Radiol. 2010;16:45–51. [PMID 20027546]
201. Jerjes W, Upile T, Petrie A, Riskalla A, Hamdoon Z, Vourvachis M, et al. Clinicopathological parameters, recurrence, locoregional and distant metastasis in 115 T1-T2 oral squamous cell carcinoma patients. Head Neck Oncol. 2010;2:9. [PMID 20406474]
202. Kim SY, Roh JL, Yeo NK, Kim JS, Lee JH, Choi SH, Nam SY. Combined 18F-fluorodeoxyglucose-positron emission tomography and computed tomography as a primary screening method for detecting second primary cancers and distant metastases in

patients with head and neck cancer. Ann Oncol. 2007;18:1698–703. [PMID 17716985]
203. Adsay NV, Andea A, Basturk O, Kilinc N, Nassar H, Cheng JD. Secondary tumors of the pancreas: an analysis of a surgical and autopsy database and review of the literature. Virchows Arch. 2004;444:527–35. [PMID 15057558]
204. Durie BG. The role of anatomic and functional staging in myeloma: description of Durie/Salmon plus staging system. Eur J Cancer. 2006;42:1539–43. [PMID 16777405]
205. Webb TH, Lillemoe KD, Pitt HA, Jones RJ, Cameron JL. Pancreatic lymphoma. Is surgery mandatory for diagnosis or treatment? Ann Surg. 1989;209:25–30. [PMID 2910212]
206. Sohn TA, Yeo CJ, Cameron JL, Nakeeb A, Lillemoe KD. Renal cell carcinoma metastatic to the pancreas: results of surgical management. J GastrointestSurg. 2000;5:346–51. [PMID 11985973]
207. Reinhardt MJ, Joe AY, Jaeger U, Huber A, Matthies A, Bucerius J, et al. Diagnostic performance of whole body dual modality 18FFDG PET/CT imaging for N- and M-staging of malignant melanoma: experience with 250 consecutive patients. J Clin Oncol. 2006;24:1178–87. [PMID 16505438]
208. Choi JY, Lee KS, Kwon OJ, Shim YM, Baek CH, Park K, et al. Improved detection of second primary cancer using integrated (18F) fluorodeoxyglucose positron emission tomography and computed tomography for initial tumor staging. J Clin Oncol. 2005;23:7654–9. [PMID 16234527]
209. Yao JC, Hassan M, Phan A, et al. One hundred years after "carcinoid": epidemiology of and prognostic factors for neuroendocrine tumors in 35,825 cases in the United States. J Clin Oncol. 2008;26(18):3063–72.
210. Buchmann I, Henze M, Engelbrecht S, et al. Comparison of 68Ga-DOTATOC PET and 111InDTPAOC (Octreoscan) SPECT in patients with neuroendocrine tumours. Eur J Nucl Med Mol Imaging. 2007;34(10):1617–26.
211. Treglia G, Castaldi P, Rindi G, et al. Diagnostic performance of Gallium-68 somatostatin receptor PET and PET/CT in patients with thoracic and gastroenteropancreatic neuroendocrine tumours: a meta-analysis. Endocrine. 2012;42(1):80–7.
212. Hoyer D, Bell GI, Berelowitz M, et al. Classification and nomenclature of somatostatin receptors. Trends Pharmacol Sci. 1995;16(3):86–8.
213. Krenning EP, Kwekkeboom DJ, Bakker WH, et al. Somatostatin receptor scintigraphy with [111InDTPA-D-Phe1]- and [123I-Tyr3]-octreotide: the Rotterdam experience with more than 1000 patients. Eur J Nucl Med. 1993;20(8):716–31.
214. Kwekkeboom DJ, Krenning EP. Somatostatin receptor imaging. Semin Nucl Med. 2002;32(2):84–91.
215. Alexander HR, Fraker DL, Norton JA, et al. Prospective study of somatostatin receptor scintigraphy and its effect on operative outcome in patients with Zollinger-Ellison syndrome. Ann Surg. 1998;228(2):228–38.
216. Cadiot G, Lebtahi R, Sarda L, et al. Preoperative detection of duodenal gastrinomas and peripancreatic lymph nodes by somatostatin receptor scintigraphy. Groupe D'etude Du syndrome De Zollinger-Ellison. Gastroenterology. 1996;111(4):845–54.
217. de Kerviler E, Cadiot G, Lebtahi R, et al. Somatostatin receptor scintigraphy in forty-eight patients with the Zollinger-Ellison syndrome. GRESZE: Groupe d'Etude du syndrome de Zollinger-Ellison. Eur J Nucl Med. 1994;21(11):1191–7.
218. Gibril F, Reynolds JC, Doppman JL, et al. Somatostatin receptor scintigraphy: its sensitivity compared with that of other imaging methods in detecting primary and metastatic gastrinomas. A prospective study. Ann Intern Med. 1996;125(1):26–34.
219. Jensen RT, Gibril F, Termanini B. Definition of the role of somatostatin receptor scintigraphy in gastrointestinal neuroendocrine tumor localization. Yale J Biol Med. 1997;70(5–6):481–500.
220. Termanini B, Gibril F, Reynolds JC, et al. Value of somatostatin receptor scintigraphy: a prospective study in gastrinoma of its effect on clinical management. Gastroenterology. 1997;112(2):335–47. 14 Pinho & Subramaniam
221. Joseph S, Wang YZ, Boudreaux JP, et al. Neuroendocrine tumors: current recommendations for diagnosis and surgical management. Endocrinol Metab Clin N Am. 2011;40(1):205–31. x
222. McKenna LR, Edil BH. Update on pancreatic neuroendocrine tumors. Gland Surg. 2014;3(4):258–75.
223. Krausz Y, Keidar Z, Kogan I, et al. SPECT/CT hybrid imaging with 111In-pentetreotide in assessment of neuroendocrine tumours. Clin Endocrinol. 2003;59(5):565–73.
224. Even-Sapir E, Keidar Z, Sachs J, et al. The new technology of combined transmission and emission tomography in evaluation of endocrine neoplasms. J Nucl Med. 2001;42(7):998–1004.
225. Lee I, Paeng JC, Lee SJ, et al. Comparison of diagnostic sensitivity and quantitative indices between (68) Ga-DOTATOC PET/CT and (111)in-Pentetreotide SPECT/CT in neuroendocrine tumors: a preliminary report. Nucl Med Mol Imaging. 2015;49(4):284–90.
226. Schreiter NF, Bartels AM, Froeling V, et al. Searching for primaries in patients with neuroendocrine tumors (NET) of unknown primary and clinically suspected NET: evaluation of Ga-68 DOTATOC PET/CT and in-111 DTPA octreotide SPECT/CT. Radiol Oncol. 2014;48(4):339–47.
227. Schmid-Tannwald C, Schmid-Tannwald CM, Morelli JN, et al. Comparison of abdominal MRI with diffusion-weighted imaging to 68Ga-DOTATATE PET/CT in detection of neuroendocrine tumors of the pancreas. Eur J Nucl Med Mol Imaging. 2013;40(6):897–907.
228. Sharma P, Arora S, Dhull VS, et al. Evaluation of (68)Ga-DOTANOC PET/CT imaging in a large

exclusive population of pancreatic neuroendocrine tumors. Abdom Imaging. 2015;40(2):299–309.
229. Brooks JC, Shavelle RM, Vavra-Musser KN. Life expectancy in pancreatic neuroendocrine cancer. Clin Res Hepatol Gastroenterol. 2019;43(1):88–97. https://doi.org/10.1016/j.clinre.2018.08.005.
230. Vinjamuri S, Gilbert TM, Banks M, McKane G, Maltby P, Poston G, et al. Peptide receptor radionuclide therapy with (90)Y-DOTATATE/(90)Y-DOTATOC in patients with progressive metastatic neuroendocrine tumours: assessment of response, survival and toxicity. Br J Cancer. 2013;108(7):1440–8. https://doi.org/10.1038/bjc.2013.103.
231. McKenna LR, Edil BH. Update on pancreatic neuroendocrine tumors. Gland Surg. 2014;3(4):258–75. https://doi.org/10.3978/j.issn.2227-684X.2014.06.03.
232. Halfdanarson TR, Rabe KG, Rubin J, Petersen GM. Pancreatic neuroendocrine tumors (Pnets): incidence, prognosis and recent trend toward improved survival. Ann Oncol. 2008;19(10):1727–33.
233. Srirajaskanthan R, Kayani I, Quigley AM, Soh J, Caplin ME, Bomanji J. The role of 68Ga-DOTATATE PET in patients with neuroendocrine tumors and negative or equivocal findings on 111In-DTPA-octreotide scintigraphy. J Nucl Med. 2010;51(6):875–82.
234. Panagiotidis E, Alshammari A, Michopoulou S, Skoura E, Naik K, Maragkoudakis E, et al. Comparison of the impact of 68Ga-DOTATATE and 18F-FDG PET/CT on clinical management in patients with neuroendocrine tumors. J Nucl Med. 2017;58(1):91–6.
235. Sharma P, Arora S, Dhull VS, Naswa N, Kumar R, Ammini AC, et al. Evaluation of (68)Ga-DOTANOC PET/CT imaging in a large exclusive population of pancreatic neuroendocrine tumors. Abdom Imaging. 2015;40(2):299–309.
236. Schmid-Tannwald C, Schmid-Tannwald CM, Morelli JN, Neumann R, Haug AR, Jansen N, et al. Comparison of abdominal MRI with diffusion-weighted imaging to 68Ga-DOTATATE PET/CT in detection of neuroendocrine tumors of the pancreas. Eur J Nucl Med Mol Imaging. 2013;40(6):897–907.
237. Falconi M, Eriksson B, Kaltsas G, Bartsch DK, Capdevila J, Caplin M, et al. Enets consensus guidelines update for the management of patients with functional pancreatic neuroendocrine tumors and non-functional pancreatic neuroendocrine tumors. Neuroendocrinology. 2016;103(2):153–71.
238. Tyng CJ, Almeida MF, Barbosa PN, et al. Computed tomography-guided percutaneous core needle biopsy in pancreatic tumour diagnosis. World J Gastroenterol. 2015;21:3579–86.
239. Gupta S, Madoff DC. Image-guided percutaneous needle biopsy in cancer diagnosis and staging. Tech Vasc Interv Radiol. 2007;10:88–101.
240. Dong A, Dong H, Zhang L, Zuo C. Hypermetabolic lesions of the pancreas on FDG PET/CT. Clin Nucl Med. 2013;38:e354–66. https://doi.org/10.1097/RLU.0b013e3182708503.
241. Balink H, Tan SS, Veeger NJ, Holleman F, van Eck-Smit BL, Bennink RJ, et al. (1)(8)F-FDG PET/CT in inflammation of unknown origin: a cost-effectiveness pilot-study. Eur J Nucl Med Mol Imaging. 2015;42:1408–13. https://doi.org/10.1007/s00259-015-3010-0.
242. Vlachou PA, Khalili K, Jang HJ, Fischer S, Hirschfield GM, Kim TK. IgG4-related sclerosing disease: autoimmune pancreatitis and extrapancreatic manifestations. Radiographics. 2011;31(5):1379–402.
243. Kamisawa T, Takum K, Anjiki H, et al. FDG-PET/CT findings of autoimmune pancreatitis. Hepato-Gastroenterology. 2010;57(99–100):447–50.
244. Zen Y, Nakanuma Y. IgG4-related disease: a cross-sectional study of 114 cases. Am J Surg Pathol. 2010;34(12):1812–9.
245. Finkelberg DL, Sahani D, Deshpande V, Brugge WR. Autoimmune pancreatitis. N Engl J Med. 2006;355(25):2670–6.
246. Chari ST, Smyrk TC, Levy MJ, et al. Diagnosis of autoimmune pancreatitis: the Mayo Clinic experience. Clin Gastroenterol Hepatol. 2006;4(8):1010–6. quiz 934
247. Lee TY, Kim MH, Park H, et al. Utility of 18FFDG PET/CT for differentiation of autoimmune pancreatitis with atypical pancreatic imaging findings from pancreatic cancer. AJR Am J Roentgenol. 2009;193(2):343–8.
248. Cheng MF, Guo YL, Yen RF, Chen YC, Ko CL, Tien YW, et al. Clinical utility of FDG PET/CT in patients with autoimmune pancreatitis: a case-control study. Sci Rep. 2018;8:3651–8. https://doi.org/10.1038/s41598-018-21996-5.
249. Kamisawa T, Okamoto A. Autoimmune pancreatitis: proposal of IgG4-related sclerosing disease. J Gastroenterol. 2006;41:613–25. https://doi.org/10.1007/s00535-006-1862-6.
250. Cheng G, Torigian DA, Zhuang H, Alavi A. When should we recommend use of dual time-point and delayed time-point imaging techniques in FDG PET? Eur J Nucl Med Mol Imaging. 2013;40:779–87. https://doi.org/10.1007/s00259-013-2343-9.
251. Strobel K, Heinrich S, Bhure U, et al. Contrast-enhanced 18F-FDG PET/CT: 1-stop-shop imaging for assessing the resectability of pancreatic cancer. J Nucl Med. 2008;49(9):1408–13.
252. Zhang J, Zuo CJ, Jia NY, Wang JH, Hu SP, Yu ZF, et al. Cross-modality PET/CT and contrast-enhanced CT imaging for pancreatic cancer. World J Gastroenterol. 2015;21:2988–96. https://doi.org/10.3748/wjg.v21.i10.2988.

Surgical Techniques in Hepato-biliary Pathologies

19

Ankit Jain, Jeewan Ram Vishnoi, and Sanjeev Misra

19.1 Anatomy of the Liver from the Surgical Perspective

The foundation of modern liver surgery was laid by the pioneering independent anatomical works of Couinaud [1] and Healey [2, 3]. By using the corrosion casting method, both subdivided the liver into components, separated by watershed regions. While Couinaud used portal vein ramifications for subdividing, Healey used hepatic artery and bile ducts to define the liver anatomy. The branching pattern of the portal vein, hepatic artery, and bile duct is identical on the right side, resulting in identical categorization of second-order and third-order divisions. However, on the left side, the left portal vein divides into an umbilical branch (to segments 3 and 4) and a branch to segment 2, whereas the left hepatic artery and bile duct divide into medial (segment 4) and lateral branches (segments 2 and 3).

In order to avoid confusion over the different terms, the International Hepato-Pancreato Biliary Association (IHPBA) came up with "The Brisbane 2000 terminology of Liver Anatomy and Resections" [4]. They adopted the division of the liver based on hepatic artery and bile duct ramifications. The liver has been divided and subdivided into three levels or divisions (Fig. 19.1). The first-order division bisects the liver into the right and left *liver* (or *hemi-livers*). The second-order arterial and bile duct pedicles divide the right liver into right anterior and right posterior *sections*, whereas the left liver is subdivided into left medial and left lateral *sections*. The third-order divisions have been termed as *segments (Sg)*. As second-order division of the left liver based on the portal vein is also anatomically correct, therefore, alternative sub-classification of the left liver has been added as an addendum.

The hepatoduodenal ligament consists of a hepatic artery proper, portal vein, and the bile duct encased by a layer of the fibrous connective tissue known as the Walaeus or Glisson sheath. Together these form the "Glissonean pedicle (GP)." At the hepatic hilum, the main pedicle divides into three secondary GP, which can be approached extrahepatically. Based on this, Takasaki divided the liver into three "segments," namely, the right, middle, and left segments with an additional caudate area (Fig. 19.2). The boundaries between these segments are traversed by the right and the middle hepatic veins. The

A. Jain
Department of Surgical Oncology, AIIMS Bhopal, Bhopal, India

J. R. Vishnoi (✉)
Department of Surgical Oncology, AIIMS Jodhpur, Jodhpur, India

S. Misra
Department of Surgical Oncology, AIIMS Jodhpur, Jodhpur, India

Atal Bihari Vajpayee Medical University, Lucknow, India

© The Author(s), under exclusive license to Springer Nature Singapore Pte Ltd. 2025

B. Sureka (ed.), *Hepato-Pancreatico Biliary Imaging*, https://doi.org/10.1007/978-981-95-1699-5_19

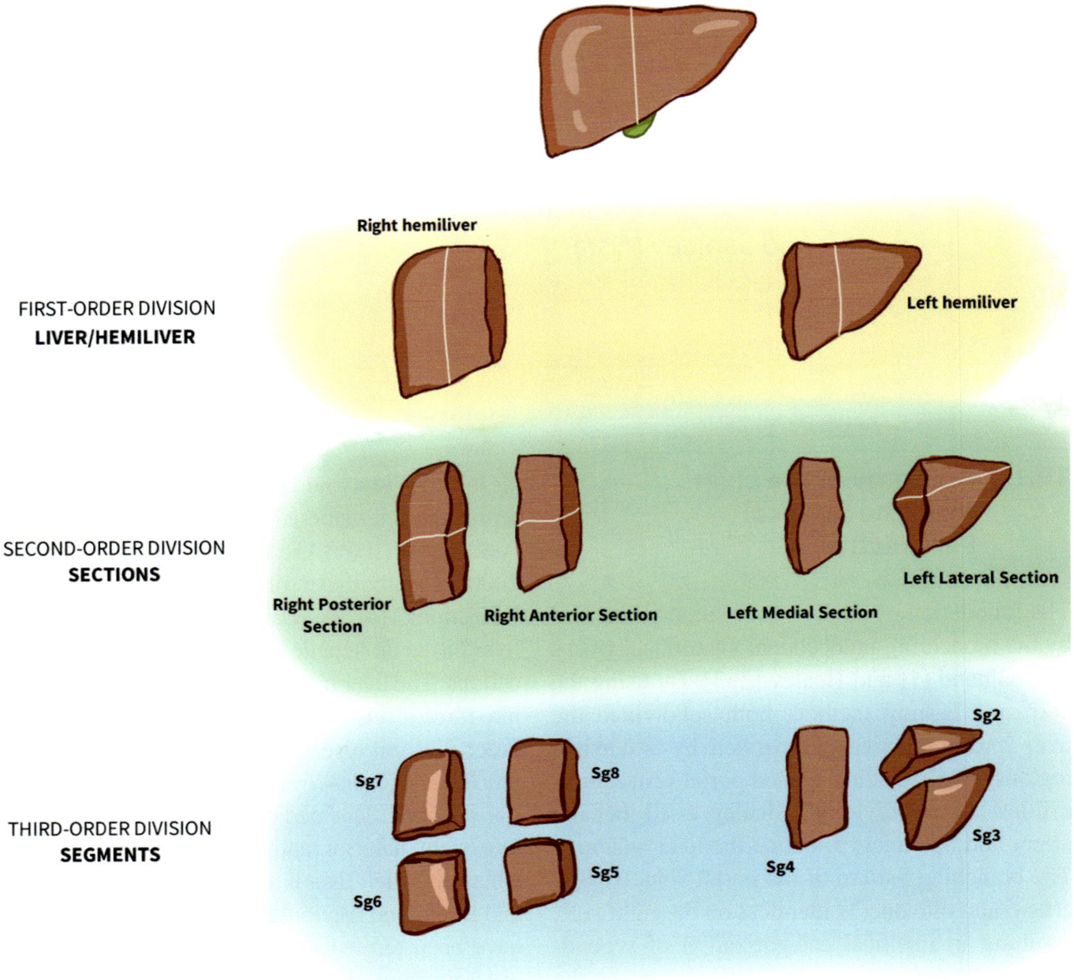

Fig. 19.1 Brisbane 2000 anatomical definitions

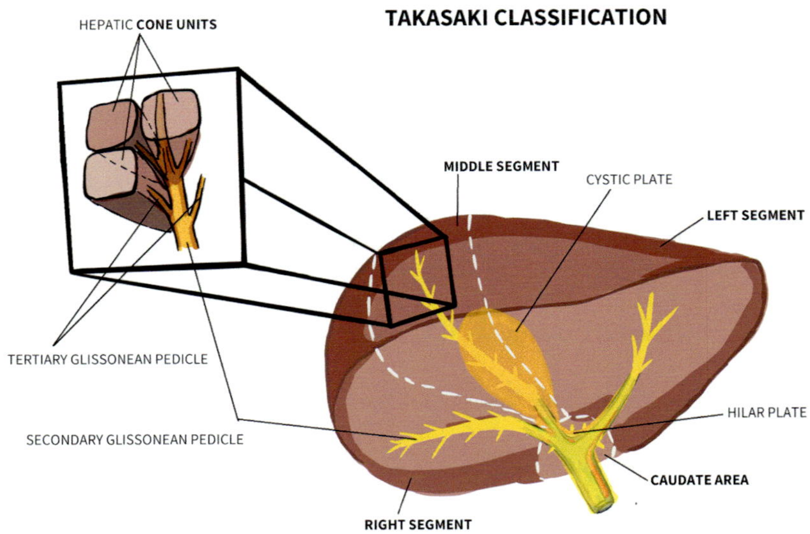

Fig. 19.2 Takasaki classification of hepatic anatomy

right and middle segments correspond to the right posterior and right anterior sections of the Brisbane 2000 terminology, whereas the left hemi-liver is defined as the left segment. Each secondary GP gives out multiple tertiary pedicles. Interestingly, the volume supplied by these tertiary pedicles does not correspond to Couinaud's definition of segments. Instead, they represent smaller subsegmental units, referred to as the "cone units of liver" [5, 6].

19.2 Types of Liver Resection

Liver resection can be broadly classified into anatomic and non-anatomic liver resections (NALR). Anatomic liver resection (ALR) involves resection of the hepatic territory defined by a clear inflow pedicle. Depending upon the level of pedicle occlusion, ALR can range from extended hemi-hepatectomy to subsegmental resections of the hepatic cone unit [7]. In contrast, liver parenchyma is resected without identifying the inflow pedicle in NALR, usually with a predefined surgical resection margin. The NALR is "lesion-centric" with the goal of preserving the hepatic parenchyma to prevent postoperative liver insufficiency.

Anatomic liver resections have been classified within the Brisbane 2000 terminology (Fig. 19.3). Resection of the lobe or hemi-liver has been termed as "hepatectomy" or "hemi-hepatectomy." The terms "sectionectomy" and "segmentectomy" have been used to describe resection of section and segment, respectively [4].

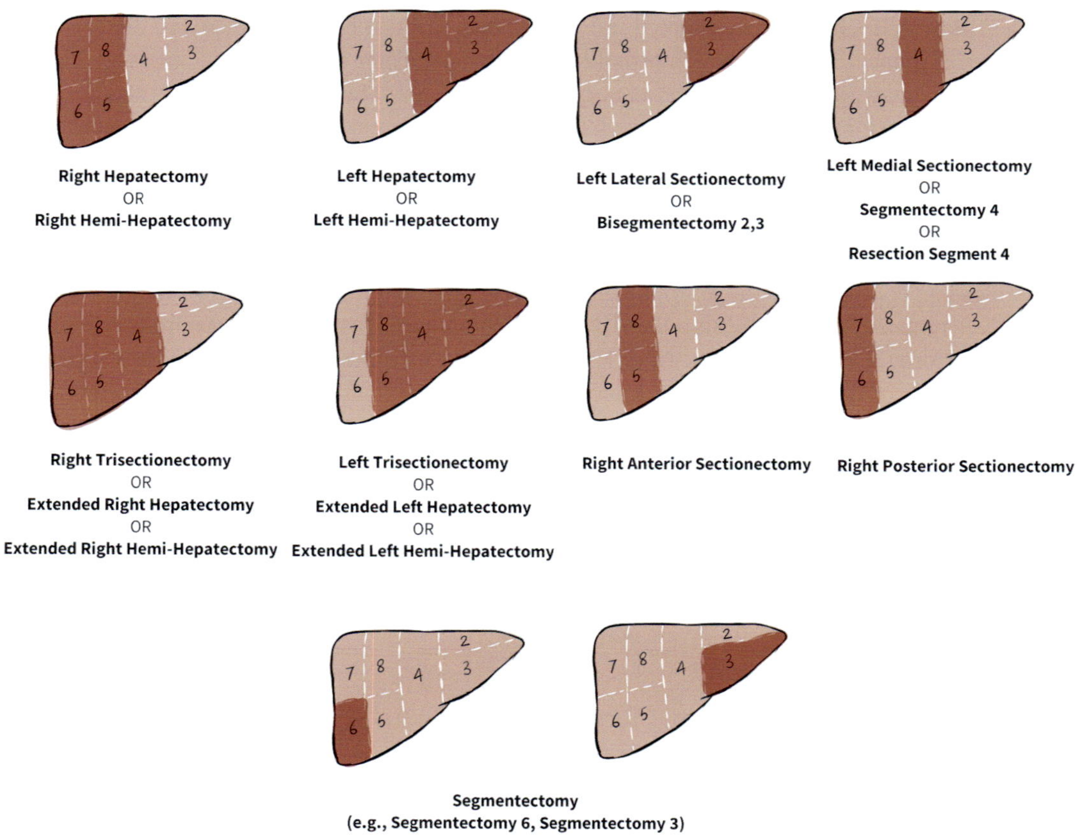

Fig. 19.3 Brisbane 2000 classification of hepatic resection

19.3 Preoperative Considerations

Evaluation begins with the assessment of the liver function. Child-Pugh-Turcotte (CTP) score is one of the simplest and the most used systems for classifying the severity of hepatic dysfunction. CTP score utilizes five parameters, namely, encephalopathy, bilirubin, ascites, albumin, and prothrombin time. The scores range from 5 to 15 and are grouped into three categories: A, B, and C. While liver resections can be performed in CTP-A group, they are not tolerated well in CTP-B and CTP-C groups.

Cross-sectional imaging plays a critical role in the planning of liver surgery. The main goal of imaging in this context includes accurate delineation and localization of the hepatic lesions, identification of any anatomic variation, planning of surgical resection, and estimation of the future liver remnant (FLR). In patients with a normal liver, a FLR of ≥20% has been considered safe as per current evidence. However, this threshold is higher in patients with a diseased liver, e.g., cirrhosis, and those exposed to systemic therapy for cancer prior to hepatic resection [8].

In patients requiring significant liver resections, preoperative portal vein embolization (PVE) results in atrophy of the part of the liver to be resected and compensatory hypertrophy of the future liver remnant, thus decreasing the risk of post-hepatectomy liver insufficiency. After PVE, if FLR is ≤20% or the degree of hypertrophy is ≤5%, then the patient is not a candidate for hepatic resection [9].

19.4 Approach to Hepatic Inflow

Hilar approach, also known variously as the *intrafascial approach* or the *control method*, was first introduced by Honjo and Lortat-Jacob in the early 1950s. It involves dissection of the hepatoduodenal ligament and the hepatic hilum, identification and skeletonization of the elements of the portal triad, and subsequent ligation of these elements individually at a level depending on the part of the liver to be resected. However, Bismuth and Couinaud noted that this technique can be associated with an increased risk of the remaining liver's vascular and bile duct injury due to inaccurate identification of the anatomic variations [10].

In the Glissonean approach (also known as Takasaki's procedure), the GP is ligated without opening and dissecting the Walaeus sheath (Fig. 19.4). As pointed out previously, the secondary GP can be approached and dissected out extrahepatically without opening the hepatic parenchyma. This allows the performance of left hemi-hepatectomy, right anterior sectionectomy, and right posterior sectionectomy. This approach is the simple *extrafascial approach*. However, exposure of tertiary GP which lies deep within the hepatic parenchyma requires dissection of the liver parenchyma at the border in between the sections as the first step. The commonly described *extrafascial transfissural approach* involves opening the main portal fissure or the umbilical fissure, with exposure of the hilar plate or umbilical plate, respectively. This allows subsequent

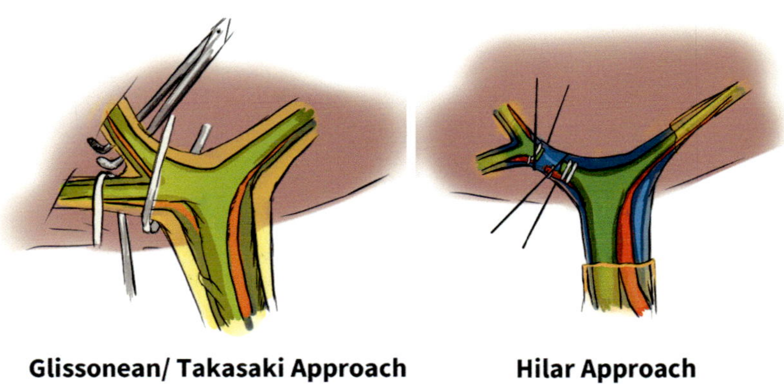

Fig. 19.4 Approach to hepatic inflow

identification of tertiary GP and performance of segmental resections (esp. for Sg4, Sg 5, and Sg8) [10].

19.5 Mode of Liver Parenchyma Transection

The underlying basis of liver transaction revolves around the division of liver parenchyma, ligation or suturing of small vessels on the hepatic cut surface, electrocauterizing even smaller vessels, achieving hemostasis, identification of any bile leak, and ligation of any exposed small biliary radicles. Liver transaction has been traditionally performed by fracturing the liver parenchyma between the fingers. A little improvement over this in terms of accuracy is by using arterial clamps to crush the liver and divide the exposed vessels and bile ducts. This "crush-clamp" technique has served as a reference method against which all other methods have been compared.

Newer techniques include dissection of the liver using ultrasound (Cavitron Ultrasonic Surgical Aspirator, CUSA), water-jet, vessel sealing devices (bipolar/ultrasonic-based), saline-linked radiofrequency sealers, radiofrequency probes, and vascular staplers. These techniques offer different advantages over the conventional technique and can be used either singly or in combination with each other [11].

19.6 Vascular Control

The liver receives nearly 25% of the cardiac output, which amounts to approximately 800–1200 mL/min. Nearly 75% of this blood is supplied by the portal vein and the remaining by the hepatic artery. Blood from the liver then drains into the inferior vena cava (IVC) through the hepatic veins. One of the most significant challenges encountered during hepatic surgery is intraoperative bleeding. Bleeding can occur during dissection, hepatic parenchyma transection, or revascularization.

In order to decrease the amount of blood loss during hepatic surgery, three approaches can be considered:

1. Occlusion of hepatic inflow (selective or non-selective)
2. Combined occlusion of hepatic inflow and outflow
3. Lowering down of Central Venous Pressure

Pringle maneuver, first described in 1908, involves temporary compression of the hepatoduodenal ligament with vascular clamps or soft tourniquets, thus resulting in total hepatic inflow occlusion. As the liver derives its oxygen supply equally from the portal vein and hepatic artery, ligation of inflow portends exposure of the liver to ischemic injury. Furthermore, on release of occlusion, reperfusion of the liver results in sterile inflammatory response and hepatocellular injury, resulting in a condition known as hepatic ischemia/reperfusion injury (HIRI). The non-diseased liver has been shown to tolerate up to 65 minutes of ischemia. Diseased livers resulting from cirrhosis or chemotherapy-induced hepatic changes are more prone to development of HIRI. The amount of adenosine triphosphate depletion and oxidative stress is directly proportional to the duration of ischemia [12].

However, significant blood loss from backflow from hepatic veins can still occur despite the inflow ligation. Also, if a tumor is infiltrating the retrohepatic IVC, then resection of the IVC can be considered. In such cases, inflow occlusion by Pringle maneuver, clamping of infrahepatic IVC above renal and adrenal veins, and suprahepatic IVC above the hepatic veins can be considered. This is known as total vascular exclusion (TVE). In addition to decreasing blood loss, TVE allows the use of in situ hypothermic perfusion of the liver, which decreases the metabolic demand of the liver and thus decreasing ischemic injury [12].

19.7 Technique of Hepatic Resections

The patient is kept in a supine position. Hepatic resections can be performed either by open technique or by the use of modern minimal invasive approaches depending upon the surgeon's preference and expertise. In the open technique, generous exposure of the right upper quadrant is required and can be achieved by various abdominal incisions, e.g., thoracoabdominal, Makuuchi incision and its modifications, T-shaped incisions, right subcostal with vertical midline incision, etc. Self-retaining retractors provide excellent exposure and are generally recommended. After ruling out any extrahepatic disease by visual inspection of the abdominal cavity, the liver is mobilized by taking down its peritoneal attachments. Division of the round and the falciform ligaments up to the anterior surface of hepatic veins and suprahepatic IVC offers excellent exposure of the superior aspect of the liver. For right-sided hepatic resections, further mobilization of the right lobe of the liver can be achieved by dividing the right coronary and triangular ligament. Similarly, division of the gastrohepatic ligament after ascertaining the absence of any accessory or replaced left hepatic artery allows exposure of the caudate lobe and the ability to loop the hepatoduodenal ligament for the Pringle maneuver.

For right hepatectomy, exposure and control of the right hepatic vein are obtained by mobilizing the right liver anteriorly and rotated to the left, carefully dissecting, and ligating the short hepatic veins draining directly into the IVC and dividing the retrocaval or Makuuchi ligament. Cholecystectomy is performed with the gallbladder either removed or left attached with the cystic duct for retraction purposes. The next step is to approach the hepatic inflow by either the hilar or the Takasaki's technique. For right or left hepatectomy, the first-order Glissonean pedicle on the ipsilateral side is ligated. This results in the creation of a line of demarcation over the liver surface between the ischemic and non-ischemic lobe of the liver. Pringle maneuver can be carried out prior to proceeding to hepatic parenchyma transaction to decrease the amount of blood loss. Hepatic parenchyma transection is then carried out and the specimen is removed.

For sectionectomy, the inflow is ligated at second-order division. Segmentectomies are achieved by temporary occlusion of second-order divisions to create a line of vascular demarcations, parenchymal transections, and unroofing of third-order pedicles allowing them to be separately ligated. Subsegmental resections utilize Takasaki's cone unit concept. Intraoperative ultrasound is used to localize the tertiary branches from the second-order divisions. Then the target branch is compressed between the ultrasound probe and the surgeon's fingers, causing ischemic demarcation of the target area. The target area is then marked, and hepatic transection is carried out with subsequent ligation of the tertiary draining branch.

19.8 Perihilar Cholangiocarcinoma

Perihilar cholangiocarcinoma (pCCA) is an aggressive neoplasm characterized by perineural invasion and periductal lymphatic spread, with the ability to spread longitudinally along bile ducts to involve the intrahepatic sectoral and segmental bile ducts. Radial growth of the disease leads to infiltration into surrounding structures, namely, hepatic artery, portal vein, adjacent hepatic parenchyma, and inferior vena cava. Ipsilateral portal venous infiltration can lead to lobar atrophy.

As the surgery for pCCA is technically challenging and associated with significant morbidity, careful selection of patients is necessary. Important factors precluding a patient from surgical resection include medically unfit for surgery, presence of non-satellite hepatic or distant metastases, involvement of non-regional lymph nodes, bilateral segmental ductal involvement, ipsilateral segmental ductal involvement with contralateral involvement of vascular inflow or unilateral atrophy with contralateral segmental ductal involvement and/or hepatic inflow involvement, and inadequate future liver remnant [9, 13].

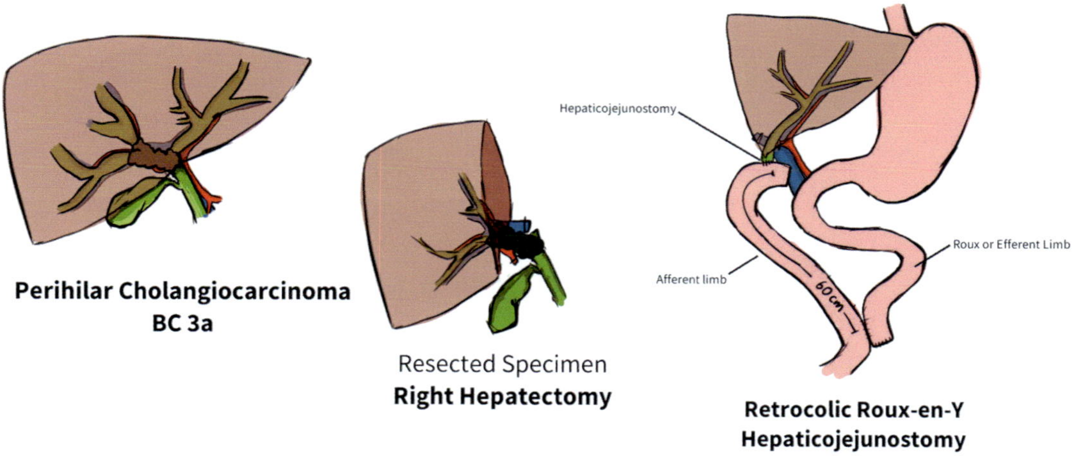

Fig. 19.5 Right hepatectomy performed for Bismuth-Corlette type 3a cholangiocarcinoma and reconstruction with retrocolic Roux-en-Y hepaticojejunostomy

Helical high-resolution triple-phase contrast computed tomography with a section thickness of 2.5 mm and reconstruction at 1.25 mm has relatively high accuracy in predicting resectability. Magnetic resonance imaging with magnetic resonance cholangiopancreatography better delineates the intrahepatic extension of pCCA but is very poor in the prediction of vascular invasion. Positron emission tomography/computed tomography is of limited value in the evaluation of primary tumors as pCCA is generally not fludeoxyglucose-avid. However, despite adequate preoperative imaging, 20–50% of patients are found to have unresectable disease upon exploration [9].

The main goal of surgery in pCCA is to achieve a margin-negative resection (R0) as it is the most important criterion for long-term survival. Due to the proximity of hilar structures, IVC, and the aim of preserving functionally adequate remnant liver, margins are often microscopically positive (R1), especially at the bile duct margins. The extent of resection depends upon the degree of involvement of biliary disease and future liver remnant. Generally, ipsilateral hemi-hepatectomy is performed. Extended resections including trisectionectomy are usually considered in events where negative margins are unlikely to be achieved by hemi-hepatectomy. As per current evidence, the caudate lobe is concurrently involved in pCCA; hence it is prudent to include the caudate lobe in hepatectomies for pCCA [14]. Biliary reconstruction is generally carried out in a retrocolic Roux-en-Y hepaticojejunostomy with preferable ≈60 cm length of the afferent limb (Fig. 19.5).

19.9 Carcinoma Gallbladder

Radical cholecystectomy has been the mainstay in the treatment of ≥pT1b gallbladder carcinoma and has demonstrated significant improvements in survival outcomes in comparison to simple cholecystectomy. A diagnostic laparoscopy is performed to look for any peritoneal deposits and to ascertain resectability. Once resectability is confirmed, the abdomen is entered typically by the right subcostal incision which can be extended across the midline. A generous Kocher's maneuver is performed, and the infrarenal aortocaval lymph node is excised and sent for frozen section. If the frozen section is negative for malignancy, then retroduodenal lymph nodes are dissected out. The gastrohepatic ligament is divided, and the lymph nodes around celiac axis and the common hepatic artery are removed. Lymph nodes within the hepatoduodenal ligament are removed, thus skeletonizing the bile duct, hepatic artery proper, and the portal vein. The cystic duct is ligated close

Fig. 19.6 Radical cholecystectomy

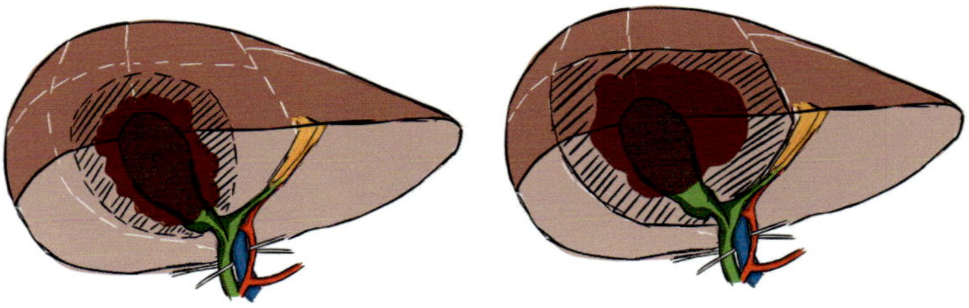

Non-Anatomic Radical Cholecystectomy **Radical Cholecystectomy with Anatomic Segment 4b and 5 Resection**

to the CBD, and the cystic duct margin is sent for frozen section. If cystic duct margin is positive, then CBD resection is concurrently performed, and biliary-enteric reconstruction is performed with Roux-en-Y hepaticojejunostomy. For non-anatomic resection, a wedge resection of the gallbladder fossa with a 2-cm margin of the normal liver is resected en bloc with the gallbladder (Fig. 19.6). However, in anatomic resection, which is usually indicated for T2–T3 tumors, segments 4b and 5 are removed en bloc. If hepatic hilar confluence is involved, then a right hepatectomy or right trisectionectomy can be considered [15].

References

1. Le Foie CC. Études anatomiques et chirurgicales. Paris: Masson & Cie; 1957.
2. Healey JE, Schroy PC. Anatomy of the biliary ducts within the human liver; analysis of the prevailing pattern of branchings and the major variations of the biliary ducts. AMA Arch Surg [Internet]. 1953 [cited 2023 Aug 19];66(5):599–616. Available from: https://pubmed.ncbi.nlm.nih.gov/13039731/.
3. Healey JEJ. Clinical anatomic aspects of radical hepatic surgery. J Int Coll Surg. 1954;22(5 Sect. 1):542–50.
4. Strasberg SM, Belghiti J, Clavien PA, Gadzijev E, Garden JO, Lau WY, et al. The Brisbane 2000 terminology of liver anatomy and resections. HPB. 2000;2(3):333–9.
5. Takasaki K. Glissonean pedicle transection method for hepatic resection: a new concept of liver segmentation. J Hepato-Biliary-Pancreat Surg. 1998;5(3):286–91.
6. Takasaki K, Yamamoto M. Surgical anatomy of the liver in the Glissonean pedicle approach: what we need to know. In: Venous embolization of the liver. London: Springer London; 2011. p. 23–7.
7. Makuuchi M, Hasegawa H, Yamazaki S. Ultrasonically guided subsegmentectomy. Surg Gynecol Obstet. 1985;161(4):346–50.
8. Guglielmi A, Ruzzenente A, Conci S, Valdegamberi A, Iacono C. How much remnant is enough in liver resection? Dig Surg [Internet]. 2012 [cited 2023 Aug 27];29(1):6–17. Available from: https://pubmed.ncbi.nlm.nih.gov/22441614/.
9. Mansour JC, Aloia TA, Crane CH, Heimbach JK, Nagino M, Vauthey JN. Hilar Cholangiocarcinoma: expert consensus statement. HPB (Oxford) [Internet]. 2015 [cited 2023 Aug 26];17(8):691. Available from: https://pubmed.ncbi.nlm.nih.gov/26172136/.
10. Yamamoto M, Ariizumi S. Glissonean pedicle approach in liver surgery. Ann Gastroenterol Surg [Internet]. 2018 [cited 2023 Aug 14];2(2):124. Available from: https://pubmed.ncbi.nlm.nih.gov/29863152/.
11. Aragon RJ, Solomon NL. Techniques of hepatic resection. J Gastrointest Oncol [Internet]. 2012 [cited 2023 Aug 24];3(1):28–40. Available from: https://jgo.amegroups.org/article/view/297/html.
12. Van Gulik TM, De Graaf W, Dinant S, Busch ORC, Gouma DJ. Vascular occlusion techniques during liver resection. Dig Surg [Internet]. 2007 [cited 2023 Aug 25];24(4):274–81. Available from: https://doi.org/10.1159/000103658.
13. Schulick RD. Criteria of unresectability and the decision-making process. HPB (Oxford) [Internet]. 2008 [cited 2023 Aug 26];10(2):122. Available from: https://pubmed.ncbi.nlm.nih.gov/18773070/.
14. Malago M, Frilling A, Li J, Lang H, Broelsch C. Cholangiocellular carcinoma – the role of caudate lobe resection and mesohepatectomy. HPB. 2008;10(3):179–82.
15. Miyazaki M, Shimizu H, Ohtsuka M, Yoshidome H, Kato A, Yoshitomi H, et al. Hepatic S4a + S5 and bile duct resection for gallbladder carcinoma. J Hepatobiliary Pancreat Sci [Internet]. 2012 [cited 2023 Aug 27];19(3):225–9. Available from: https://pubmed.ncbi.nlm.nih.gov/22374509/.

Hardware in Hepato-pancreatico-biliary Interventions

20

Pawan Kumar Garg, Samarth Gowda, and Pushpinder Singh Khera

20.1 Introduction

Interventional radiology (IR) is an essential medical specialty that deals with the management of various hepato-pancreatico-biliary (HPB) pathologies in a minimally invasive way. The spectrum of interventions can be broadly categorized into non-vascular and vascular interventions (Table 20.1).

The non-vascular interventions include percutaneous biopsy and aspiration of various lesions for histopathological and microbiological analysis; liver abscess drainage [1]; percutaneous drainage of peripancreatic and postoperative collections; percutaneous aspiration, instillation, and re-aspiration (PAIR) procedure for hydatid cyst; percutaneous transhepatic cholangiography (PTC) and percutaneous transhepatic biliary drainage (PTBD) [2, 3]; percutaneous cholecystostomy; ablation of the liver, biliary, and pancreatic primary or metastatic tumors; etc.

The vascular interventions include transarterial chemoembolization (TACE) for hepatocellular carcinoma; pre-operative portal vein embolization (PVE) for extended right hepatectomy patients with small future liver remnant volume; hepatic venous pressure gradient (HVPG) for indirect measurement of portal hypertension; transjugular liver biopsy (TJLB); hepatic venoplasty and stenting; transjugular intrahepatic portosystemic shunt (TIPS) for portal hypertension and direct intrahepatic portosystemic shunt (DIPS) for Budd-Chiari syndrome; balloon-occluded retrograde transvenous obliteration (BRTO) for isolated gastric variceal bleed

Table 20.1 Various interventional radiology procedures

Non-vascular procedures	Vascular procedures
Percutaneous biopsy and fine needle aspiration	Transarterial chemoembolization (TACE) for hepatocellular carcinoma
Liver abscess drainage	Pre-operative portal vein embolization (PVE)
Percutaneous drainage of collections	Hepatic venous pressure gradient (HVPG)
Percutaneous aspiration, instillation, and re-aspiration (PAIR)	Transjugular liver biopsy (TJLB)
Percutaneous cholecystostomy	Hepatic vein and inferior vena cava (IVC) venoplasty and stenting
Percutaneous transhepatic cholangiography (PTC)	Embolization of pseudoaneurysm
Percutaneous transhepatic biliary drainage (PTBD) and biliary stenting	Transjugular intrahepatic portosystemic shunt (TIPS) and direct intrahepatic portosystemic shunt (DIPS)
Ablation of tumors	Balloon-occluded retrograde transvenous obliteration (BRTO)

P. K. Garg (✉) · S. Gowda · P. S. Khera
Department of Diagnostic and Interventional Radiology, AIIMS Jodhpur, Jodhpur, India

© The Author(s), under exclusive license to Springer Nature Singapore Pte Ltd. 2025
B. Sureka (ed.), *Hepato-Pancreatico Biliary Imaging*, https://doi.org/10.1007/978-981-95-1699-5_20

[4], inferior vena cava (IVC) venoplasty and stenting; embolization of pseudoaneurysms/foci of arterial active extravasation secondary to trauma, post-surgery, or pancreatitis; etc.

20.2 Hardware for Interventional Radiology Procedures

20.2.1 Puncture Needle (Fig. 20.1a)

Puncture needles are used to access the blood vessel, biliary radicle, or abscess cavity. The needles are then exchanged with the guidewire for the final placement of either vascular access sheath or pigtail catheter using the Seldinger technique.

The puncture needles are available in different sizes and lengths. The size of the needle is measured in G (gauge), which is an internationally used scale. The bigger the number of gauge, the smaller the diameter of the needle.

The needle's length depends upon the target vessel's depth or structure. Commonly used in IR are Chiba needles, which have a beveled tip angle of 30°, as described originally. It is available in 18–25 G sizes.

The 21 G needle is used to puncture small-sized vessels, in pediatric patients and small caliber biliary radicles. The 21 G needle allows the passage of a 0.018-inch-sized guidewire, while the 18 G needle is used in bigger vessels in adult or large abscess cavities, allowing the passage of a 0.035-inch guidewire. Needles with echogenic tips are also available, which have better visualization on ultrasound.

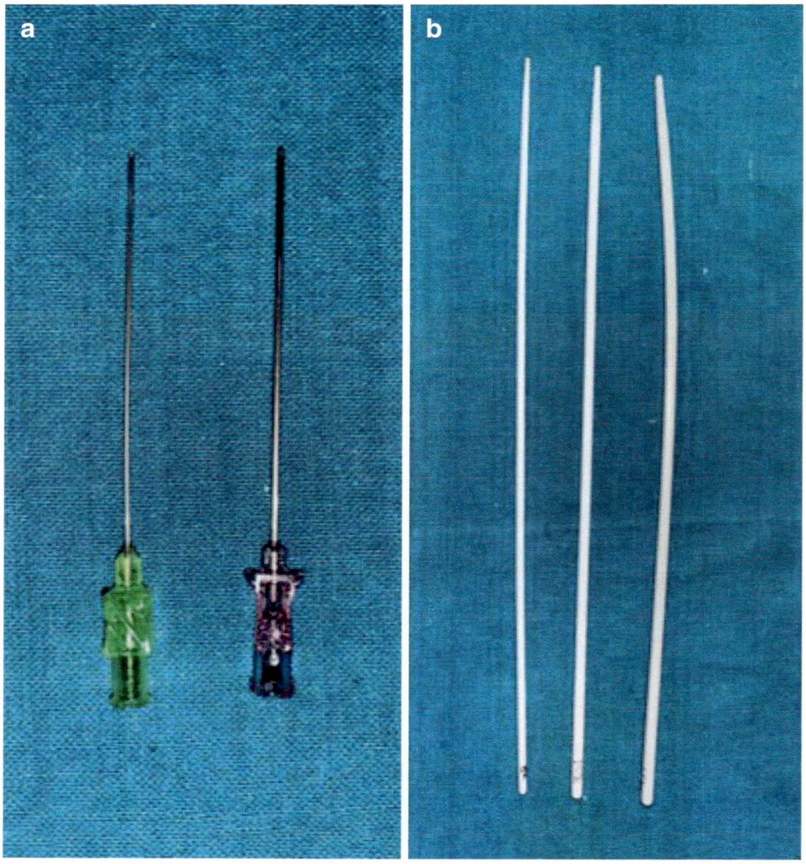

Fig. 20.1 (**a**) Puncture needle of size 21 G (green) and 18 G (pink). (**b**) Fascial dilators of size 8, 10, and 12 Fr

20.2.2 Fascial Dilators (Fig. 20.1b)

Fascial dilators are tapered tip hollow catheters made up of soft polyethylene material. These dilators are used to dilate the percutaneous tract before placement of a large-size vascular sheath, device, or pigtails over the guidewire using Seldinger techniques. These are available in various sizes ranging from 6 to 24 French.

20.2.3 Vascular Access Sheath (Fig. 20.2)

The vascular sheath is an access sheath with a hemostatic one-way valve that allows the introduction of catheters and wires but prevents blood from exiting. Also, it has a sidearm that allows saline flush and infusion to prevent clotting within the lumen of the sheath. The sheath is available in various sizes and lengths. The diameter is expressed in French (Fr). Three French is equal to 1 millimeter (mm). The commonly used sheath sizes are 5 and 6 Fr for diagnostic vascular purposes.

The vascular sheaths are available in various lengths, like 7, 11, 16, and 50–100 centimeters (cm). The required length varies depending on various procedures.

The vascular access sheath can be used in non-vascular procedures like PTBD to maintain the access site and during biliary stenting.

20.2.4 Guidewire (Fig. 20.3a)

Guidewires are wires that serve as a guide for the negotiation of catheters within the vessels and abscess cavities and provide support for the entry of large bore catheters, sheaths, etc. The guidewires are available in different sizes and made up of different materials.

The guidewires are divided based on size, length, tip shape, and material property. The guidewires are available in various sizes, like 0.035, 0.038, 0.014, and 0.018 inches in diameter and 80, 150, 260, and 300 cm in length. The 5 Fr catheters allow 0.038-inch guidewires, while 4 Fr diagnostic catheters allow 0.035-inch guidewires. The 0.014- and 0.018-inch wire is compatible with microcatheters.

The guidewire is available in straight tip or J-tip shape. The J-tip wire is commonly used and is less traumatic. The straight-tip wire is used to cross tight strictures or stenosis and is more traumatic.

The polytetrafluoroethylene (PTFE)-coated wires are hydrophilic and slide easily when in

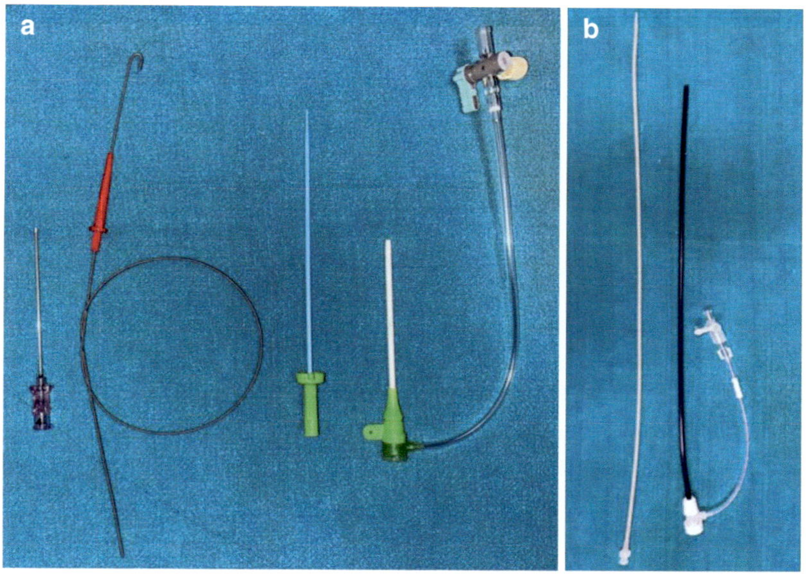

Fig. 20.2 (**a**) Vascular access sheath set containing a puncture needle, guidewire, inner dilator, sheath with a hemostatic valve, and side arm. (**b**) Long vascular access sheath with a dilator

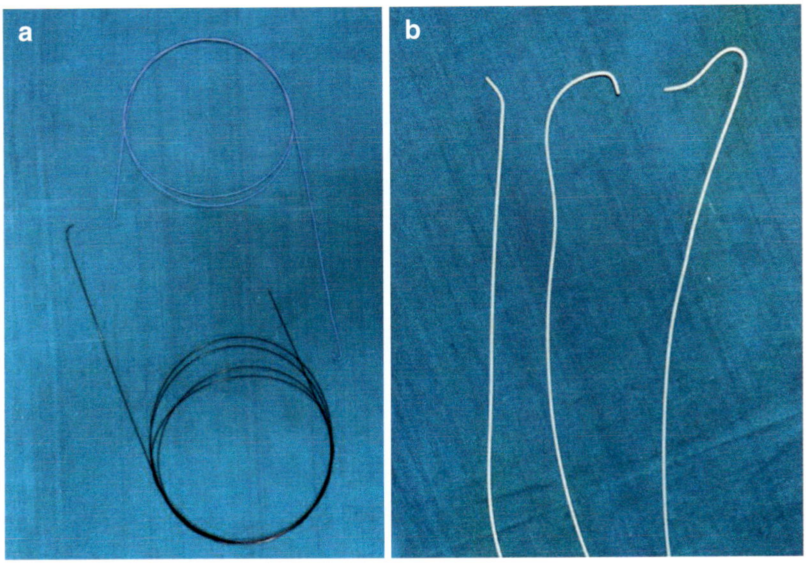

Fig. 20.3 (**a**) J-tip guidewire, hydrophilic (black) and stiffer, Amplatz (blue). (**b**) Diagnostic catheters: vertebral shape with a single curve, Cobra 1 with the double curve in the same direction, and Simmon 1 catheter with the reverse curve

contact with saline and blood. These hydrophilic wires are helpful to negotiate the difficult curves of vessels. The other type of wire is Amplatz, which is stiffer and helps negotiate bulky devices like balloons and stents.

20.2.5 Diagnostic Catheters (Fig. 20.3b)

The catheters are hollow tubes with different shapes at the tip. The wire catheter combinations are used to negotiate difficult anatomy. The common diagnostic catheters are available in 4–6 Fr sizes.

The shapes of catheters are classified as single curve, double curve in same direction, and double curve in opposite directions. Commonly used catheters are Cobra (C), Simmons (Sim), Multipurpose (MPA), Head Hunter (H), Vertebral, Renal Double Curve (RDC), and Picard. Catheter shapes can be advantageous while cannulating the ostium of vessels, which are often oriented in different directions.

20.2.6 Micropuncture Access Set (Fig. 20.4)

Micropuncture access set is used to gain access to small arteries and veins, especially in pediatric patients. This is also useful in radial access and pedal access. It consists of an echogenic tip micropuncture needle of 21 G, a soft J-tip 0.018-inch wire, and a coaxial catheter pair of 10 cm in length, available in 4 and 5 Fr sizes. The micropuncture needle is used to access the vessel, followed by wire and coaxial catheter insertion using the Seldinger technique. The inner catheter is removed, and a 0.035-inch wire is placed through the outer catheter.

Neff percutaneous access set is similar to the micropuncture access set and is used mainly for non-vascular procedures like percutaneous transhepatic biliary access and percutaneous nephrostomy. It has a 15-cm-long 22 G needle, a long-length 0.018-inch wire with a triaxial sheath of 7 Fr size, having an introducer catheter, and a metallic stiffener cannula.

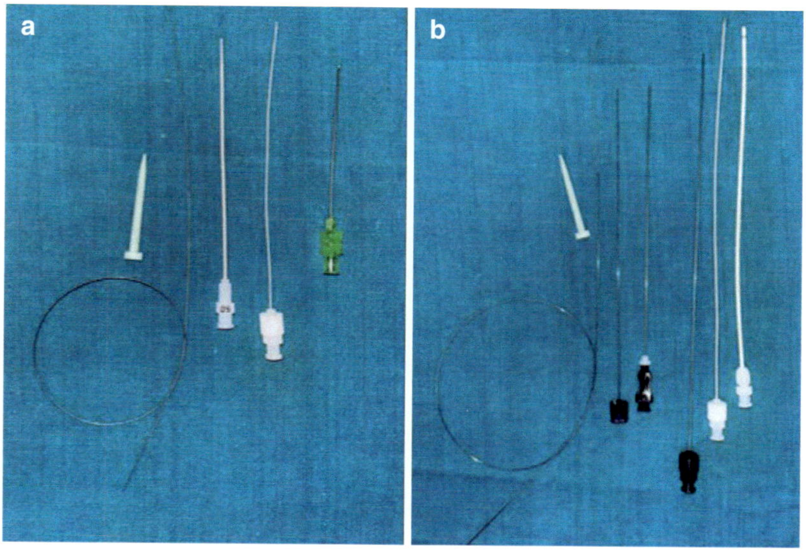

Fig. 20.4 (**a**) Micropuncture access set, containing a soft J-tip microwire, coaxial catheter pair of 5 Fr, and micropuncture needle. (**b**) Neff percutaneous access set containing a long-length J-tip microwire 22 G, a 15-cm-long Chiba needle with a trocar, and a triaxial sheath of 7 Fr size, having an introducer catheter, and a metallic stiffener cannula.

20.2.7 Drainage Catheter (Fig. 20.5)

Percutaneous drainage of liver abscesses and infected collections is beneficial for quickly draining out the infected fluid, which further helps in faster patient recovery and avoids the need for open surgical procedures.

The drainage catheters are available in various shapes. The common types of catheters are pigtail shape, Malecot type having flower-shaped catheters, and internal-external biliary catheters for biliary drainage.

The pigtail catheter has the shape of a pigtail, which, once inserted and formed, holds the catheter in place. The pigtail catheter has multiple holes at and near the tip to drain the fluid. The pigtail catheter is available for single-time placement using a metallic trocar or after serial tract dilatation using the Seldinger technique.

The Malecot catheter has a flower shape at the tip with end holes for fluid drainage. The catheter is straightened using an inner straightener for placement.

The catheters are available from 5 to 28 Fr size. The catheter's size depends upon the content's thickness and consistency.

The internal-external biliary drainage catheter is a long-length catheter designed to drain bile externally into a drainage bag and internally into the duodenum after placement. This is available from 5 to 12 Fr size.

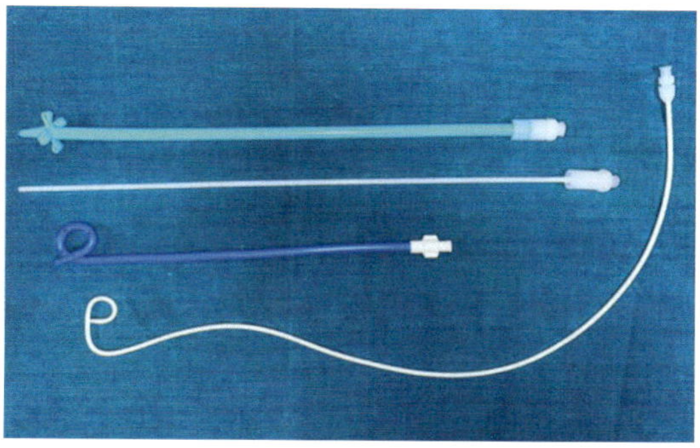

Fig. 20.5 Drainage catheters of different shapes with multiple holes: Malecot catheter (green) with a dilator, pigtail catheter (blue), and internal-external biliary drainage catheter of long length (white)

20.2.8 Biopsy Needle (Fig. 20.6)

The biopsy needle obtains a small piece of a representative tissue from any tumor or parenchyma for pathological or microbiological evaluation. Commonly performed percutaneous biopsy procedures are for liver, gallbladder, or pancreatic tumors. Liver biopsy is also indicated in diffuse liver disease for etiological workup. The biopsy

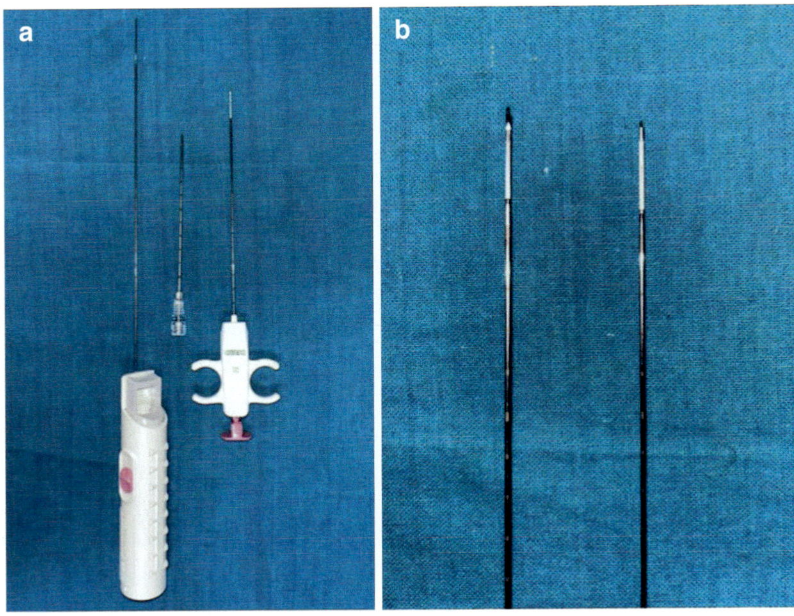

Fig. 20.6 (**a**) Percutaneous biopsy needle: automatic (larger) and semiautomatic (smaller) type with a coaxial needle. (**b**) The cutting throw of both needles is of similar type

needle is available in sizes 14–20 G; 18 and 20 G are commonly used.

Based on the tissue-cutting mechanism, the biopsy needle can be divided into fully automatic and semiautomatic. The biopsy needle consists of an inner needle with a tissue throw and an outer cutting needle.

In the automatic biopsy needle, the tip penetrates a length of 22 mm and hence must be placed at the edge of the lesion. Upon firing the needle, the inner needle first slides out, followed immediately by the outer cutting needle, to cut the tissue within the throw. The throw size is 20 mm, and the biopsy needle is available in different lengths, like 10, 16, and 20 cm.

In a semiautomatic biopsy needle, the inner needle is placed within the lesion, and on firing, only the outer cutting needle will slide. The advantage of this is that it allows for the biopsy of small lesions and lesions with nearby vascular structures. In a semiautomatic biopsy needle, 10-mm and 20-mm-size throw are available. This is also available in different lengths like 10, 16, and 20 cm.

The coaxial biopsy technique is used in which an outer coaxial needle is placed into the lesion or liver, through which the biopsy needle is positioned to take multiple cores with a single puncture of the liver capsule or lesion. This technique prevents complications due to multiple capsular punctures. In post-biopsy bleeding, the same coaxial needle can be used to inject gelfoam or any other embolizing agent.

20.2.9 Balloon Catheter and Inflation Device (Fig. 20.7a)

The balloon catheter is a catheter with an inflatable balloon near the tip. This is used to open up stenotic areas within vessels or biliary strictures. Balloon catheters are divided based on compatible delivery guidewires like 0.035 or 0.018 inches.

The balloon catheters are available in different sizes and lengths based on the vessel diameter and size of stenosis. Commonly used are 4–10 mm balloons; however, large-size balloons are also available for procedures such as IVC venoplasty.

The inflation device uses a diluted contrast mixture to inflate the balloon with precise pres-

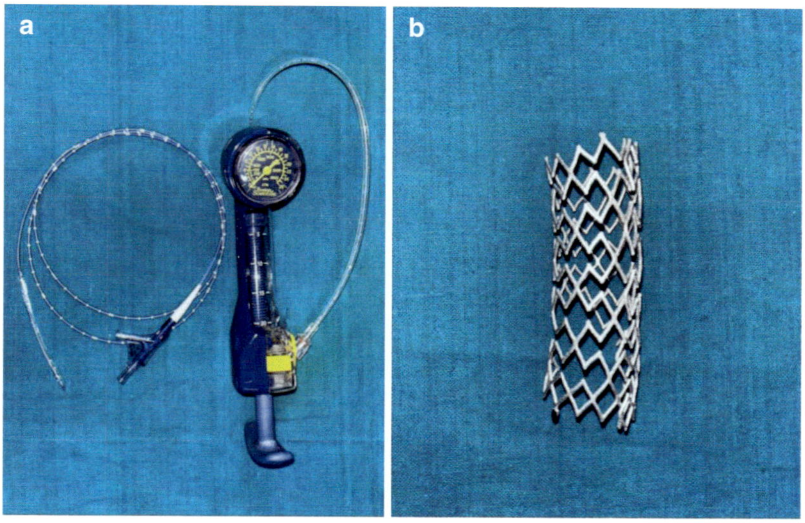

Fig. 20.7 (**a**) Balloon catheter with two hubs, one for wire passage and the other for balloon inflation. Inflation device with pressure measurement display. (**b**) The metallic stent of open-cell-type design

sure to prevent under- and overinflation. Each balloon inflates to its intended size at a pre-fixed pressure called nominal burst pressure and ruptures at a pre-fixed pressure called the rated burst pressure; both are provided within the balloon package by the vendor.

20.2.10 Metallic Stent (Fig. 20.7b)

The stent is a metallic scaffolding intended to keep the vessel or bile duct open. The stent is used in hepatic vein, IVC stenting, DIPS/TIPS, or biliary stenting. Stents are commonly made up of nitinol (nickel-titanium alloy) or cobalt chromium.

The stent is divided into open cell versus closed cell, self-expanding versus balloon-expandable stent, and uncovered versus covered stent.

All the stent cells are interconnected in closed-cell stents, resulting in smaller cell sizes, whereas in open-cell stents, the cell size is larger. The closed-cell stent has more radial force.

The self-expanding stent expands on simple unsheathing, while the balloon-mounted stent requires a balloon to expand. The balloon-mounted stent has the highest radial force and is used for precise deployment in ostial legions.

The covered stent has a metallic stent covered with an impermeable layer of either expanded polytetrafluoroethylene (ePTFE) or Dacron material.

20.2.11 Embolizing Agents (Fig. 20.8)

Embolizing agents can be divided into temporary and permanent agents. Temporary embolizing agents include gelfoam and autologous blood clots. Permanent embolizing agents are divided into particulate, metallic, and liquid agents.

Particulate embolization material includes polyvinyl alcohol (PVA) particles, embosphere, and microspheres. The metallic embolizing agents include coils and vascular plugs. The liquid embolizing agents include N-butyl cyanoacrylate (NBCA) or glue and onyx.

Metallic embolizing agents like coils and vascular plugs are commonly used to occlude vessels proximally. Based on the delivery mechanism, the coils are either pushable or detachable.

The pushable coils are made of platinum wire with synthetic fibers in a spring shape, preloaded in a cartridge, and pushed using wires. These are made up of 0.035-inch or 0.018-inch wire and are delivered through compatible catheters. The

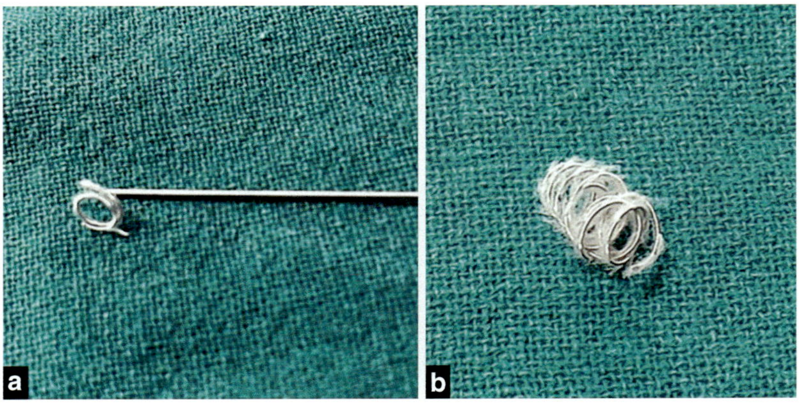

Fig. 20.8 (**a**) and (**b**) 0.018-inch size pushable coil with thrombogenic fibers

detachable coils are meant for precise deployment and are detached mechanically or electronically.

The vascular plug is a metallic cylinder that is compressed in a sheath, which will expand after deployment and take its shape and size. These are made of nitinol wire mesh. These are available in cylinder or disk-like shapes.

20.2.12 Liquid Embolizing Agents

Liquid embolic agents include NBCA glue and onyx. NBCA is commonly used for peripheral and HPB interventions [5]. It is mixed with lipiodol to achieve the different concentrations of glue. Glue lipiodol mixture will polymerize when it comes in contact with saline or blood. More concentrated glue will polymerize early compared with less concentrated glue. The 5% dextrose solution is used to flush the catheter before the glue injection to prevent polymerization within the catheter itself.

Onyx is an ethylene vinyl alcohol copolymer dissolved in dimethyl sulfoxide (DMSO) [6]. It precipitates when it comes in contact with an aqueous solution like blood, saline, etc. Special DMSO-compatible catheters are required to inject the onyx into the target location.

Lipiodol is an ethiodized poppy seed oil containing 4.8 gm of iodine per 10 ml. It is used with glue for embolization and chemotherapeutic drugs like doxorubicin or epirubicin to make water in oil emulsion during TACE for hepatocellular carcinoma.

20.2.13 Particulate Embolizing Agents (Fig. 20.9a,b)

The particulate embolizing agents are used to embolize the distal bed of parenchyma or tumor. These are used in case of tumor embolization or portal vein embolization. PVA are available in different sizes and are a mixture of a range of particles. Embospheres are more spherical and regular in shape and have a uniform range of particle sizes.

20.2.14 Transjugular Liver Biopsy Set (Fig. 20.10a)

Transjugular liver biopsy is indicated when percutaneous liver biopsy is not possible, like in the cases of gross ascites and deranged coagulation

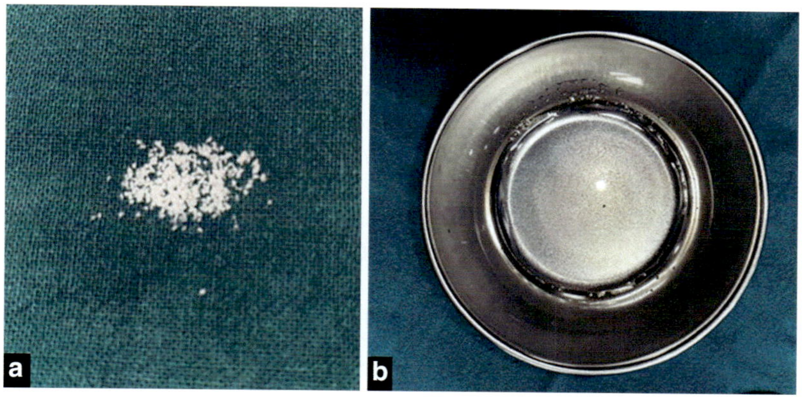

Fig. 20.9 (**a**) PVA particles of 300–500 micrometer size. (**b**) Relatively uniform sized Embosphere of 300 micrometer, mixed with contrast in a bowl

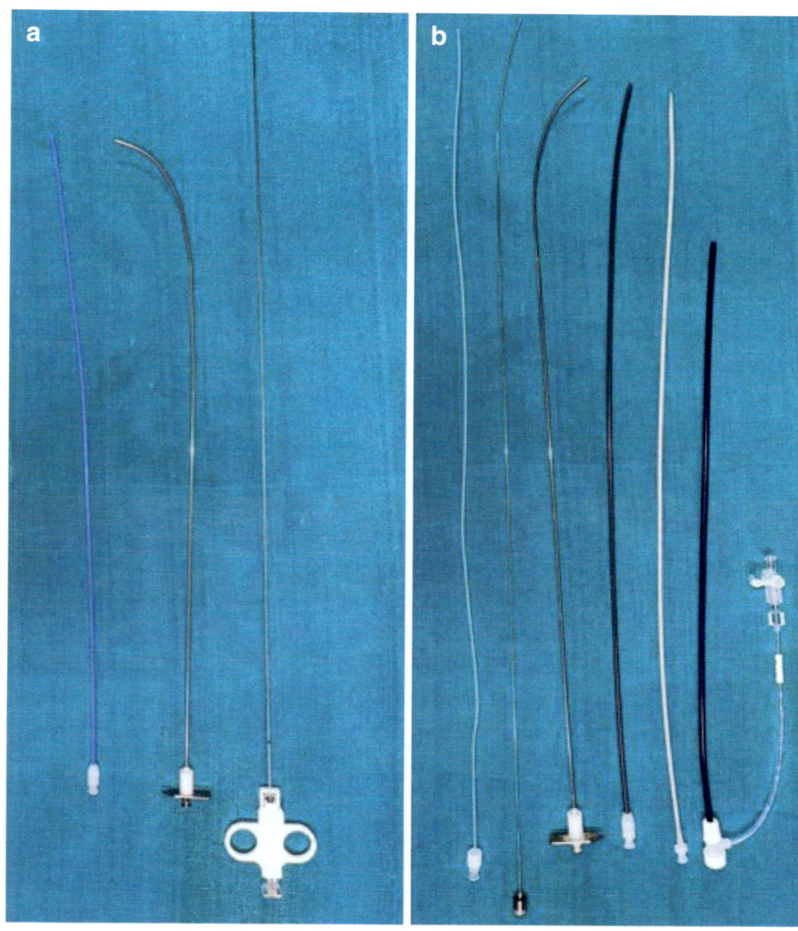

Fig. 20.10 (**a**) TJLB set containing 7-Fr-long vascular sheath with 14 G stiffening metallic cannula and long biopsy needle of 18 and 19 G sizes and 20 mm throw length. (**b**) Rösch-Uchida Transjugular Liver Access Set (RUPS) set containing trocar stylet covered with a 5 Fr catheter, stiffening cannula with a 10 Fr catheter, and 10-Fr-long vascular sheaths with a dilator.

profile of the patient. Here, the biopsy is taken through the hepatic vein into the liver parenchyma.

The commonly used TJLB set is Liver Access and Biopsy Sets (LABS) by Cook Medical [7]. This LABS set consists of a 7-Fr-long vascular sheath with a hemostatic valve and sidearm for the flush.

The 14 G stiffening metallic cannula provides stability and wedges the tip into the parenchyma. The biopsy needle is similar to a percutaneous biopsy needle with a long shaft and is available in 18 and 19 G sizes and 20 mm throw length.

20.2.15 Transjugular Intrahepatic Portosystemic Shunt Set (Fig. 20.10b)

In TIPS, a shunt is created between the portal vein and hepatic vein to reduce the portal pressure in cases of portal hypertension. The common indications include refractory ascites, refractory hydrothorax, and recurrent or failed esophageal variceal bleeding. Sometimes, in cases of Budd-Chiari syndrome, a shunt is created between the portal vein and IVC, which is directly called a DIPS.

Two commonly used hardware are the Ring Transjugular Intrahepatic Access Set (RING) and the RUPS developed by Cook Medical.

The Ring set was launched in 1992 by Dr. Ernie Ring, who used the Colapinto needle invented by Dr. Ronald F. Colapinto [8]. The set contains the 9/10 French and 38.5-cm-long vascular sheath with a dilator. Inside the sheath goes a 16 G and 50.5-cm-long Ross Modified Colapinto Needle covered with a 9/10 French catheter. A Colapinto needle punctures the portal vein, and sequentially introduced sheath is placed into the portal vein [9].

The RUPS set was launched in 1992 by Dr. Josef Rösch and Barry Uchida, a former X-ray technician [10]. The set contains the outer most 10 French and 40-cm-long vascular sheath with a dilator. Inside the sheath goes a stiffening cannula of 14 G and 51.5 cm length covered with a 10 Fr catheter. Through the stiffening cannula goes a 0.038-inch size and 62.5-cm length trocar stylet covered with a 5 Fr catheter. This set uses a trocar stylet to puncture the portal vein, and sequentially stiffening cannula and introducer sheath are placed into the portal vein.

20.3 Conclusion

The HPB interventions are continuously increasing and help in the minimally invasive management of various pathologies. The knowledge of various hardware used for HPB intervention is essential to perform these interventions safely.

References

1. Kumar S, Midha NK, Ahari K, Kumar D, Gopalakrishnan M, Kumar B, Bohra GK, Garg P, Sureka B, Garg MK. Role of pigtail catheter drainage versus percutaneous needle aspiration in the management of liver abscess: a retrospective analysis. Cureus. 2021;13(12).
2. Yadav A, Condati NK, Mukund A. Percutaneous transhepatic biliary interventions. Journal of Clinical Interventional Radiology ISVIR. 2018;2(01):27–37.
3. Ahmed O, Mathevosian S, Arslan B. Biliary interventions: tools and techniques of the trade, access, cholangiography, biopsy, cholangioscopy, cholangioplasty, stenting, stone extraction, and brachytherapy. In Seminars in interventional radiology 2016;33(04):pp. 283–90. Thieme Medical Publishers.
4. Khera PS, Garg PK, Tiwari S, Bhargava N, Yadav T, Sureka B, Ghosh T, Babu S, Dadhich S, Singh S. Retrograde Transvenous Obliteration of Gastric Varices using Sodium Tetradecyl Sulphate: Technical Considerations and Results from a Single Institution Retrospective Study. Journal of Clinical Interventional Radiology ISVIR. 2021;6(01):10–7.
5. Hill H, Chick JF, Hage A, Srinivasa RN. N-butyl cyanoacrylate embolotherapy: techniques, complications, and management. Diagnostic and Interventional Radiology. 2018;24(2):98
6. https://europe.medtronic.com/xd-en/healthcare-professionals/products/cardiovascular/peripheral-embolization/onyx-liquid-embolic-system.html.
7. https://www.cookmedical.com/products/de7165fe-69af-46bb-9635-b1f79bdb8d0c/.
8. https://www.cookmedical.com/interventional-radiology/transforming-ideas-into-devices-the-ingenuity-of-cook-and-medical-practitioner-innovations/.
9. https://www.cookmedical.com/products/ir_rtps_webds/.
10. https://www.cookmedical.com/products/ir_rups_webds/#.

Interventional Radiology in the Biliary Tree, Liver, and Pancreas

21

Matilde Bariani, Francesca Mambrin, and Alberto Contro

21.1 Biliary Interventions

21.1.1 Indications

Indications for percutaneous biliary interventions are:

- Diagnosis and treatment of a stricture (benign or malignant) and its most common complications, high bilirubin and pruritus.
- Removal of biliary stones.
- Treatment of biliary leaks.

21.1.1.1 Biliary Tree Obstructions

Biliary Strictures

Biliary strictures can be differentiated in low (below the cystic duct insertion) and high (above the cystic duct insertion).

Low strictures are usually managed endoscopically, and percutaneous treatment is the second choice if endoscopy is impossible or fails. The most common causes of failed endoscopy are congenital anatomic anomalies, such as the presence of duodenal diverticulum, or post-surgery (e.g., after Roux-loop bilio-enteric bypass).

High strictures are managed through percutaneous interventions [1].

Strictures can have a benign or malignant cause. If it is impossible to identify it with pre-procedural imaging, an intraprocedural biopsy is suggested. Two techniques can be used, brushing or forceps biopsy. Forceps biopsy is preferred to brushing thanks to its higher sensitivity (78 vs 61%) and negative predictive value (30 vs 19%) [2].

Malignant Biliary Strictures

Strictures can be due to primitive biliary neoplasms (cholangiocarcinoma), primitive hepatic neoplasms, or metastatic tumors.

Cholangiocarcinoma is a rare neoplasm (less than 2% of all malignancies), but it is the most common tumor of the biliary system. It can be classified according to its origin as intrahepatic (originating beyond the second-order biliary ducts), perihilar (Klatskin tumor), or distal to the junction of the cystic duct.

The Bismuth-Corlette classification describes perihilar cholangiocarcinoma biliary tree involvement:

- I: hepatic duct below the confluence.
- II: right and left hepatic duct confluence.
- IIIa: extent to the right hepatic duct.
- IIIb: extent to the left hepatic duct.
- IV: extent in right and left hepatic ducts or multifocal disease [3].

M. Bariani · F. Mambrin · A. Contro (✉)
Institute of Radiology, Azienda Ospedaliera Universitaria Integrata di Verona, Verona, Italy

© The Author(s), under exclusive license to Springer Nature Singapore Pte Ltd. 2025

B. Sureka (ed.), *Hepato-Pancreatico Biliary Imaging*, https://doi.org/10.1007/978-981-95-1699-5_21

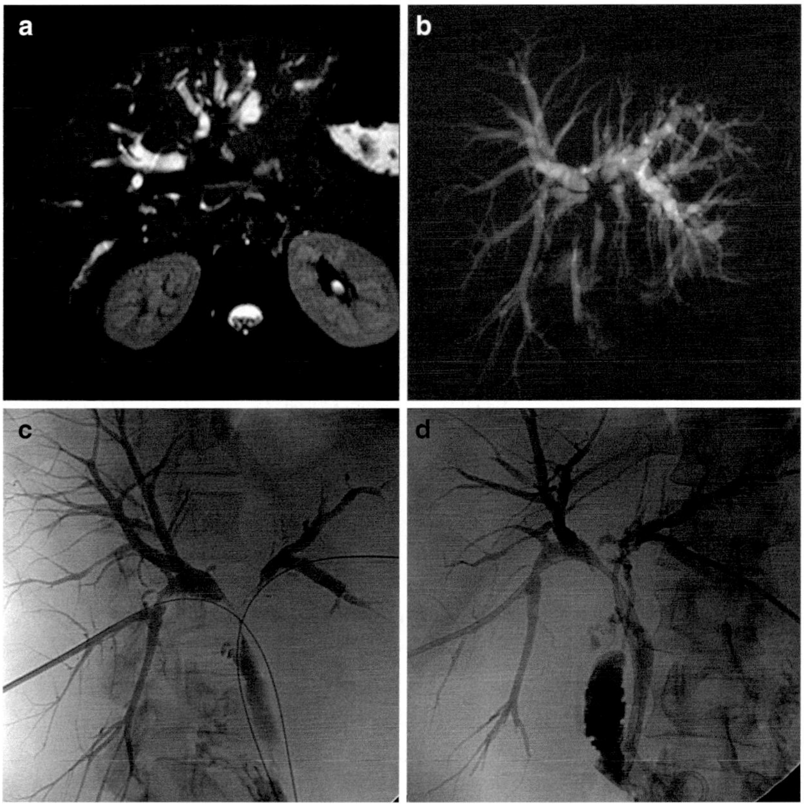

Fig. 21.1 A 42-year-old woman with type IV Klatskin cholangiocarcinoma. (**a**, **b**) T2-weighted fat-saturated MRI (**a**) and MRCP (**b**) show massive dilation of intrahepatic biliary ducts due to infiltration of the biliary confluence and first-grade biliary ducts. No clear mass is discernible. (**c**) Cholangiography confirms the stenosis, and (**d**) two drainages are positioned to drain both hepatic lobes, palliating jaundice and preventing cholangitis

Biliary drainage with stents or external-internal drainages can be used for palliation of jaundice in non-operable neoplasms and to treat cholangitic patients (Fig. 21.1).

The procedure is controversial as bridge treatment in non-septic patients candidate to surgery: some authors think it increases the risk of tumor seeding, cholangitis, and peri-operative infection. A large multicenter European study by Farges et al. showed a clear benefit in lowering bilirubin levels below 2.92 mg/dl before resection [4, 5].

Benign Biliary Strictures

Benign biliary strictures can be focal or diffuse.

Focal strictures (Fig. 21.2) are due to iatrogenic damage (they are common after the creation of a biliary-enteric anastomosis), trauma, radiation therapy, pancreatitis, and biliary stones.

Diffuse strictures are caused by cholangitis, ischemia, and sclerosing cholangitis.

Percutaneous treatment allows to go below the stenotic biliary tract and to perform balloon dilation of the stricture (bilioplasty) in multiple sessions. An external-internal drainage is usually left across the stenosis between the sessions.

Contraindications to the treatment are long segments and multiple strictures and patients with a newly surgically performed bilio-enteric anastomosis because often the stenosis is due to edema which resolves spontaneously after 1–2 weeks.

A cholangiogram is performed to assess the treatment outcome. If the stricture has resolved, an external drainage should be left for 1–2 weeks after percutaneous transhepatic biliary drainage (PTBD) removal, to allow easy reintervention in case of recurrence of the pathology [6, 7].

Biliary Stones

Endoscopic retrograde cholangiopancreatography (ERCP) is the preferred method used to treat

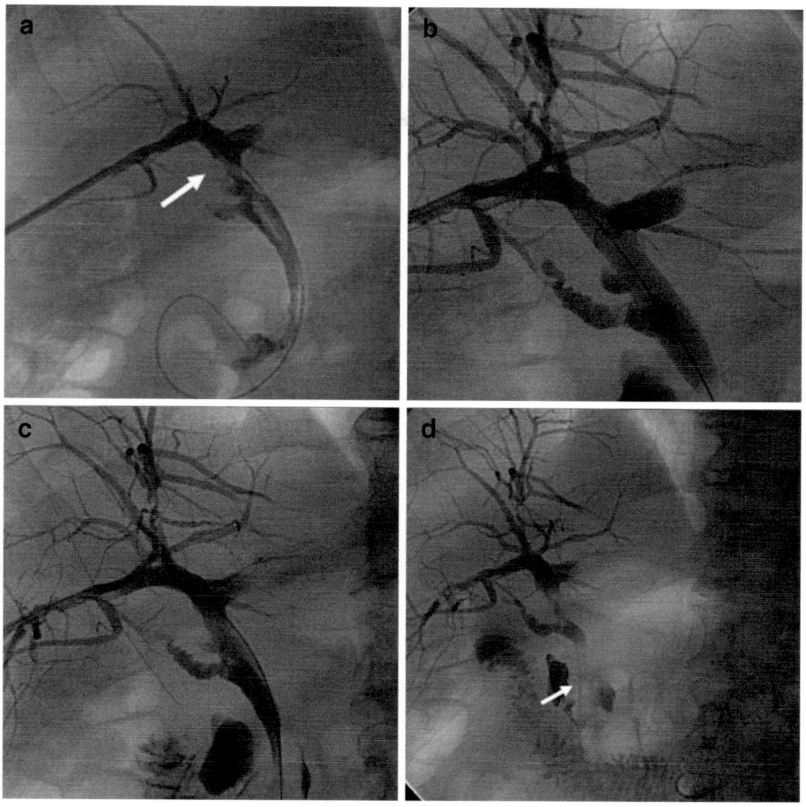

Fig. 21.2 A 74-year-old man treated with cholecystectomy complicated by left hepatic lobe necrosis and hepatic duct stenosis. (**a**) Cholangiography shows stenosis of the common hepatic duct (arrow). (**b**) Stenosis dilation is performed with an angioplasty balloon. (**c**) Cholangiography after dilation shows the resolution of the stenosis (**d**), and only a small catheter (arrow) is left in site for some days to control the complete resolution of symptoms before declaring the patient is healed

extrahepatic stones. Percutaneous intervention is indicated in case of failed endoscopy or intrahepatic stones.

Stones can be divided into brown stones and cholesterol calcified stones.

Pigmented (brown) stones form in case of biliary stasis and are softer than calcified ones. They can be removed by being pushed in the duodenum through balloon maceration and sweep of the duct (Fig. 21.3) or with a stone retrieval device (basket).

Calcified cholesterol stones are harder and can't be easily macerated. Stones measuring <5 mm can be swept into the duodenum, and larger ones require papillotomy (if they measure 5–10 mm) or lithotripsy [8].

Cholangitis

Acute cholangitis is a life-threatening medical emergency caused by retrograde infection of the biliary tree in the setting of complete or partial biliary obstruction.

Tokyo guidelines (2013 and 2018) define diagnostic criteria for cholangitis:

- Systemic inflammation: fever higher than 38 °C and laboratory evidence of inflammation.
- Cholestasis: jaundice (bilirubin >2 mg/dl) and abnormal liver function tests.
- Imaging: biliary dilation and evidence of obstruction.

Diagnosis is suspected if one criterion of systemic inflammation and one of imaging or cholestasis are present.

A definite diagnosis can be made if one criterion of systemic inflammation, one of cholestasis, and one of imaging are met [9].

Tokyo guidelines also divide cholangitis into three grades based on the initial response to medical treatment and organ dysfunction. Each grade has its indications to perform percutaneous biliary drainage:

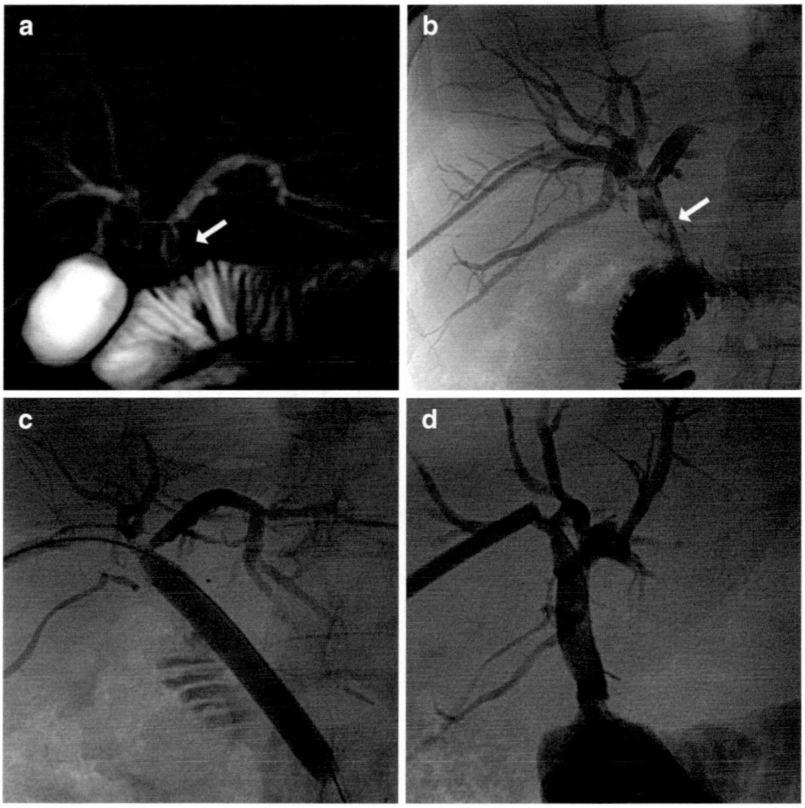

Fig. 21.3 A 62-year-old woman with stones in the hepatic duct after confection of bilio-enteric anastomosis. (**a**, **b**) MRCP (**a**) and cholangiography (**b**) demonstrate filling defects in the hepatic duct (arrows). (**c**) Balloon sweeping and bilioplasty are performed, and stones are removed with (**d**) normalization of the biliary tree

- Grade I (mild cholangitis): patients do not have organ dysfunction or symptoms described below. They should receive medical treatment. Biliary drainage should be performed if after 24 hours there's no response to medical treatment.
- Grade II (moderate): patients present with any two: white blood count >12,000/mm or <4000/mm, high fever (≥39 °C), age ≥75 years old, bilirubin ≥5 mg/dl, and hypo-albuminemia. Biliary drainage should be performed immediately, with the beginning of medical treatment.
- Grade III (severe): patients suffer from organ failure and should receive emergent biliary drainage, immediate medical treatment, and general supportive care [9, 10].

21.1.1.2 Biliary Duct Injuries

Biliary duct injuries represent a complication of hepatobiliary surgery or abdominal trauma. The most common sites of injury are the remnant of the cystic duct and ducts of Luschka after cholecystectomy.

Small leaks may resolve with conservative management, while larger leaks must be treated with drainage of the biloma and biliary reconstruction.

The International Study Group of Liver Surgery classifies leakages in three grades according to the impact they have on the clinical management of the patient:

- Grade A requires no or little changes in the management.
- Grade B requires changes in the management without necessity or relaparotomy or grade A leakages that last longer than a week.
- Grade C requires relaparotomy.

Percutaneous treatment is suggested in type B leakages [11].

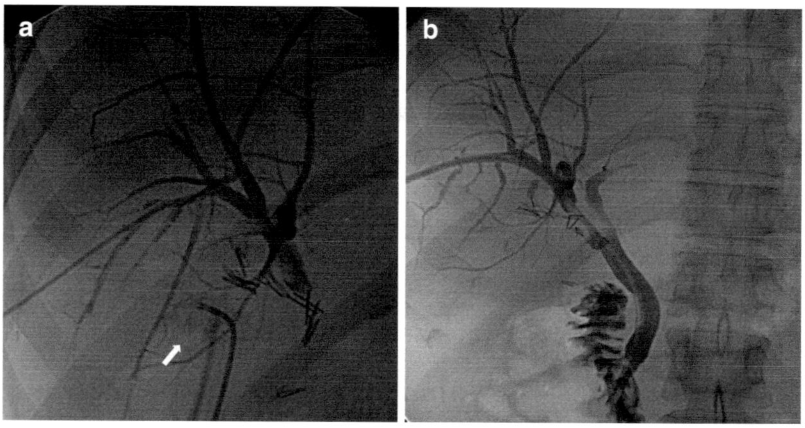

Fig. 21.4 A 47-year-old woman with biliary stenosis and fistula after cholecystectomy. (**a**) Cholangiography shows right hepatic duct stenosis and a small fistula that creates a collection in the cholecystic fossa (arrow, drained by the drainage shown in the picture). (**b**) PTBD is positioned to recreate normal biliary anatomy

Based on their anatomical characteristics, three different biliary leakage categories can be defined as useful to plan intervention:

- Direct communication: bile ducts upstream directly communicate with bile ducts downstream the leak. PTBD is the choice treatment for this type of leakage (Fig. 21.4).
- Indirect communication: bile ducts upstream and downstream the leak communicate through a bile collection. These leaks can be treated with a combined endoscopic and percutaneous rendezvous: bile leak is reached with a percutaneous catheter and an endoscopic approach through the intestine. The percutaneous catheter is then caught up from the endoscopic route and brought into the bowel loop.
- No communication: upstream and downstream bile ducts are completely excluded from each other. These leakages are generally considered grade 3, requiring surgical relaparotomy, but in some specialized centers, a percutaneous approach to reconstruct the biliary tree has been made with success [12].

Preprocedural

Before any biliary intervention, the clinical history of the patient must be investigated, and the biliary tree should be studied through imaging.

Ultrasonography (US) is the first-line imaging, which identifies biliary dilation and may determine the level of the obstruction causing it. Second-line techniques (computed tomography (CT) and magnetic resonance imaging (MRI) with magnetic resonance cholangiopancreatography (MRCP)) allow to identify the cause of the dilation.

Any biliary intervention is at best a clean-contaminated procedure: prophylactic antibiotics are indicated in all patients before intervention and should be continued for at least 48 hours after the procedure.

Coagulation parameters must be checked before intervention and, if necessary, corrected.

Contraindications are uncorrected coagulopathy and multisegmental obstructions. Ascites is a relative contraindication, easily corrected performing paracentesis.

An atrophic hepatic lobe (both biliary tree and portal vein are infiltrated) should not be drained unless cholangitis occurs.

21.1.2 Techniques

21.1.2.1 Percutaneous Transhepatic Cholangiography

Percutaneous transhepatic cholangiography is a diagnostic technique used to evaluate the biliary tree. Currently, it has been replaced by ERCP and MRCP, and it is rarely performed. The biliary tree is usually accessed through the right hepatic lobe.

Materials

In biliary interventions, the Chiba needle is generally used as an access needle. It is 15 cm long and has a 22 gauge diameter with a central sharp stylet that can be removed to inject contrast or insert a guidewire.

Procedure

The patient is positioned supine on the fluoroscopic table. After sterilization of the right flank and administration of sedoanalgesia, percutaneous access is performed with a Chiba needle on the midaxillary line. The needle is inserted under fluoroscopic guidance toward the 12th vertebral body. The stylet of the needle is removed, and a contrast-filled syringe is attached to the hub. The needle is slowly withdrawn while injecting contrast media to search for a bile duct. Contrast media in a bile duct flows slowly, like melted wax, allowing the differentiation from portal branches, hepatic vein, and arterial branches (it flows away rapidly). If a bile duct is not entered on the first attempt, other attempts can be made moving the needle in a fan shape. When a bile duct is entered, contrast media is injected to delineate the biliary tree. Radiograph projections are obtained in anteroposterior and both oblique views.

21.1.2.2 Percutaneous Transhepatic Biliary Drainage

Percutaneous transhepatic biliary drainage is an image-based technique used to drain a biliary tract through percutaneous access.

Materials

- Guidewires.
- Catheters.
- Dilators: short catheters of stiff plastic used to spread soft tissues for better access to other devices.
- Biliary drainages: they can be external or external-internal. External ones drain bile in an external bag. They are used only if impassable stenosis or severe cholangitis occurs (the less the biliary tree is manipulated, the least sepsis is likely to occur). They can cause important fluid loss and electrolyte imbalance. External-internal has proximal and terminal side holes that should be positioned above and below the biliary obstruction. The distal extremity is positioned in the duodenum, allowing both external and duodenal bile drainage. They are preferred since they maintain physiological bile drainage in the duodenum and are less easily dislocated than external catheters.

Drainages must be flushed daily to prevent occlusion and need to be replaced every few months.

Procedure

- *Right-Sided Biliary Drainage*

The patient is prepared as described to perform a cholangiography. The technique is the same until the biliary tree is opacified by contrast; if a favorable biliary duct is entered (preferred one is the duct draining S6), a soft guidewire is inserted through the needle and moved toward the hilum. A catheter is then placed on the guidewire, and they are manipulated to cross the stenosis and reach the intestine. The guidewire is exchanged with a stiffer one, and the catheter removed. The percutaneous tract is dilated with a dilator, and an external-internal (or only external) biliary drainage is positioned.

- *Left-Sided Biliary Drainage*

This procedure can be more challenging due to the anatomy of the left lobe, its proximity to the heart, and its relationship with the sternum. US guide is used to detect and guide the needle into a biliary duct through the inverted "V" formed by the sternum and medial edges of the ribs. The preferred biliary duct is the one draining S3.

Drainages must be fixed to the patient's skin to prevent their displacement.

21.1.2.3 Internal Biliary Stenting

Internal biliary stents are used to manage malignant biliary tree stenosis if no other treatment is possible. Rarely they can be used to treat benign stenosis if other previously performed treatments failed.

Materials

Self-expanding metallic stents are the most utilized.

Bare metallic stents with narrow spaces between the wire mesh are used in oncologic patients with short life expectancy (6–8 months) to palliate a malignant biliary obstruction. They cannot be removed.

Covered metallic stents are preferred for the treatment of benign strictures because they can be removed or exchanged. They are generally used in the lower common biliary duct not to cover biliary branches. Obstruction of the cystic duct is avoided thanks to the presence of small holes in the proximal extremity of the stent.

Biodegradable stents made of polydioxanone are sometimes used as a last resource in benign strictures which do not resolve with balloon dilation. They degrade in 3–6 months (Fig. 21.5) [13].

Procedure

Stents are loaded on the end of a delivery catheter, compressed by a sheath. The stent deploys from distal to proximal once delivered by the operator by withdrawing the sheath. It is important to overstent a malignant stricture by positioning the end of the stent 2–3 mm above the proximal tumor edge, to prevent rapid tumor growth inside its lumen.

If both liver lobes need to be drained, stents can be placed at the hilum with a T or Y configuration. A small safety catheter should be left inside the stent for the first week; it can be removed after stent patency is proved with a cholangiogram.

Complications

Potential major complications of PTBD are pneumothorax, bleeding, biliary sepsis, cholecystitis, and pancreatitis. Bile peritoneum occurs if the bile leaks into the abdomen.

Venous bleeding can be easily treated by repositioning the catheter moving its side holes away from the vein branch.

Arterial bleedings should be suspected if there is pulsatile bleeding, if blood leaks around the catheter, and if hematocrit lowers. Arteriography should be performed, and the bleeding/pseudoaneurysm site must be embolized.

Stents can also migrate or occlude, with consequent development of cholangitis [1, 14].

21.1.2.4 Percutaneous Cholecystostomy

Indications

Percutaneous cholecystostomy is a means to provide treatment in patients with calculous and acalculous cholecystitis noncandidate to surgery because of their clinical conditions or comorbidi-

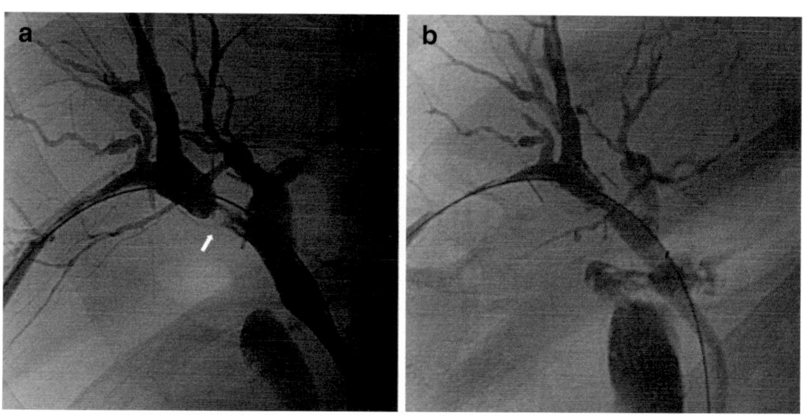

Fig. 21.5 A 54-year-old man with stenosis at the origin of the right hepatic duct after cholecystectomy, without resolution after multiple bilioplasty procedures. (**a**) Cholangiography shows a stenotic bile duct (arrow) and (**b**) resolution of the stenosis after placement of a degradable stent

ties (American Society of Anesthesiologists classification 3 and 4) [10].

Contraindications
An uncorrectable coagulopathy represents an absolute contraindication. Relative contraindications are porcelain gallbladder, which is hard to penetrate, and gallbladder tumor, for the risk of seeding.

Technique
Under imaging guidance (US, CT, or fluoroscopy), an external drainage is positioned in the gallbladder lumen (Fig. 21.6).

Two approaches are possible: transhepatic and transperitoneal (intrahepatic).

The transhepatic approach is generally preferred since it allows a more stable position of the drainage inside the gallbladder lumen. The access route is subcostal between the midaxillary and the midclavicular lines.

The transperitoneal route is used in patients with bleeding disorders or liver diseases.

Two techniques can be used:

- Seldinger: the same technique used to place a biliary drainage.
- Trocar: drainage is assembled over a stiff cannula with a sharp trocar, and it can be placed in a single step into the gallbladder lumen.

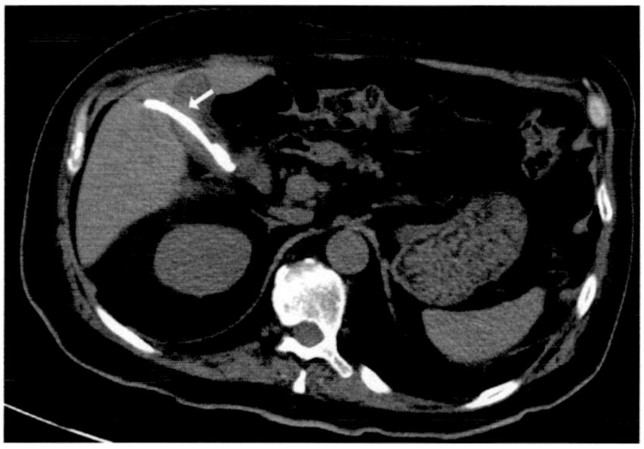

Fig. 21.6 A 66-year-old man with acalculous cholecystitis. A CT image shows transhepatic cholecystostomy in the cholecystic lumen

Complications
Complications are rare. Pneumothorax, bile peritoneum, biloma, bowel perforation, and hemorrhage can happen.

Outcome
Technical success is achieved in nearly 100% of cases. Clinical success is defined by the resolution of sepsis, with a decrease of fever (temperature <37.5 °C) and reduction of blood count below 10,000/mm^3 or by 25% of preprocedural level within 72 hrs. Clinical improvement is achieved in 56–93% of patients.

For acalculous cholecystitis, the drain can be removed at the resolution of the inflammation after a trial period of 48 hours [15].

21.2 Hepatic Procedures

21.2.1 General Considerations

Interventional radiology plays a key role in diagnostic and therapeutic purposes.

Arterial Catheterization Technique
Selective catheterization of the hepatic artery is required to perform liver procedures.

This aim is achieved through catheterization of the common femoral artery punctured under fluoroscopic or US guidance above the femoral head to prevent intra-abdominal bleeding.

After cutaneous anesthesia, a needle is advanced at a 45° angle. A pulsatile flow confirms the access. An atraumatic stiff guidewire is inserted through the needle hub, the needle is removed, and a sheath or catheter can be inserted over the wire [16]. The stiff guidewire is exchanged with a non-stiff hydrophilic guidewire, and this is advanced to the interested arterial vessel.

Venous Catheterization Technique
Central venous catheterization is required for procedures like transjugular intrahepatic portosystemic shunt (TIPS). Usually, the internal jugular vein is accessed. Practical steps do not differ from arterial puncture, and a nonpulsatile blood

flow through the needle hub confirms correct positioning.

Portal Catheterization Technique

Transhepatic portal catheterization is required for procedures like portal stenting or portal embolization. It is performed under fluoroscopic guidance. A thin needle, 22 or 21 gauge, is advanced toward the porta hepatis and slowly withdrawn while injecting contrast until the portal vein is opacified.

Postprocedural Vascular Access Management

When an arterial procedure is performed, manual compression or a closure device can be used to achieve hemostasis.

In manual compression, pressure is applied above and at the puncture site; a near-occlusive pressure is maintained for 2–3 minutes and gradually reduced over 15 minutes.

Different closure devices for different types of arteriotomies can be used; anyway, their use is contraindicated in case of small-caliber or severely diseased arteries.

After the removal of a sheath/catheter/wire from a venous access, digital pressure hemostasis is performed for 2–5 minutes.

21.2.2 Arterial Procedures: Embolization

Transcatheter arterial embolization is a procedure indicated to:

- Exclude an active hemorrhage.
- Treat vascular malformations.
- Devascularize tumors, also before surgical treatment.

Vascular embolization can be obtained with temporary or permanent materials.

Temporary embolization is performed with absorbable gelatin foam and is recommended when a rapid embolization of an arterial hemorrhage is required, especially in the absence of an evident hemorrhage site (e.g., traumatized patients), when a non-selective temporary embolization is needed (e.g., postpartum bleeding or gastrointestinal bleeding), or to occlude a percutaneous transhepatic access; vessel recanalization is unpredictable, occurring within weeks to months [17].

Permanent occluding devices include:

- Coils: determine a mechanical metal occlusion; they assume coiled configuration upon the exiting catheter, and vessel block is obtained with fibers and swelling hydrogel. Various sizes, configurations, and shapes are available. Coils can be considered when the catheter can be advanced to the target vessel. To avoid distal reconstitution of the injured vessels, distal and proximal embolization (so-called sandwich technique) is recommended when possible. This is accomplished by placing coils distal and proximal to the site of vessel injury (Fig. 21.7) [18].
- Particles are micron-sized solids that lodge at the precapillary/capillary level. Particles can be deployed within end arteries when a distal arteriole or organ embolization is desired; they lead to ischemia of the distal tissue/organ. Particles cannot be used in case of vascular shunting or collateral vasculature. They are useful in tumor treatments like transcatheter arterial chemoembolization (TACE), after chemolipiodol administration.
- Plug occluding devices include Amplatzer, a woven nitinol-expandable mesh cylindrical plug. It mechanically occludes target vessels. A precise positioning and a short landing zone are necessary for it to work.
- Liquids can be used for complex embolic targets requiring embolic penetration beyond the catheter tip. They can be injected into the nidus (arteriovenous malformations), used to irreversibly occlude damaged target vessels, or employed in the treatment of neoplasms (e.g., hepatocellular carcinoma (HCC)). Ethanol, Lipiodol, onyx, and N-butyl cyanoacrylate ("glue") are some examples of liquid embolic agents.
- Sclerosing agents: they cause vessel occlusion through thrombosis and fibrosis. Their use is recommended for varicose veins, venous malformations, or pelvic congestion syndrome.

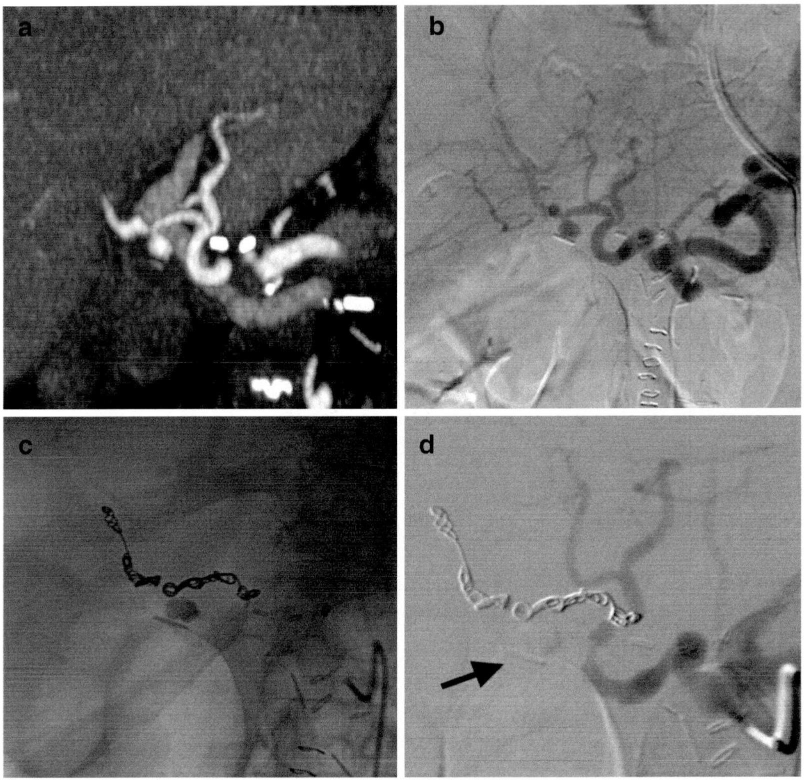

Fig. 21.7 A 63-year-old woman with right hepatic artery pseudoaneurysm after pancreatic surgery. (**a**, **b**) Computed tomography angiography (**a**) depicts the pseudoaneurysm, confirmed by angiography (**b**). (**c**) Bleeding is treated by positioning coils upstream and downstream, to prevent revascularization (sandwich technique). (**d**) The final control shows complete exclusion of the pseudoaneurysm (*arrow*)

- Oncologic agents: drug-eluting beads (DEBs) are bound to chemotherapeutics and delivered to tumors, resulting in high concentrations of the drug. Radioactive particles can be embedded into microspheres for selective internal radiation therapy.

The most feared complications are nontarget embolization, hemorrhage, and excessive tissue ischemia resulting in necrosis. Postembolization syndrome can occur.

21.2.3 Portal Vein Embolization

Portal vein embolization (PVE) consists of the embolization of a portal branch before surgical treatment in patients with primary or metastatic hepatic tumors, to induce hypertrophy of the unembolized liver lobe. It is generally performed on the right portal branch in a diseased right lobe, to induce hypertrophy of the left lobe (Fig. 21.8). The right lobe is usually large enough for a left lobe resection without left portal branch embolization. This strategy increases the future liver remnant (FLR) by 10–46% within 6–8 weeks [19].

Indications

Preoperative PVE is appropriate when the FLR volume is ≤20% of total liver volume (TLV) in patients with normal liver function, ≤30% of TLV in patients with intermediate liver disease, and ≤40% of TLV in patients with well-compensated hepatic fibrosis or cirrhosis [20].

Contraindications

Absolute contraindications are uncorrectable coagulopathy, complete lobar portal vein occlusion, extensive invasion of the portal vein by tumor, or overt clinical portal hypertension.

Relative contraindications are massive ascites (paracentesis is required before the procedure) and biliary dilation within FLR (biliary drainage of FLR before PVE is necessary to promote hypertrophy).

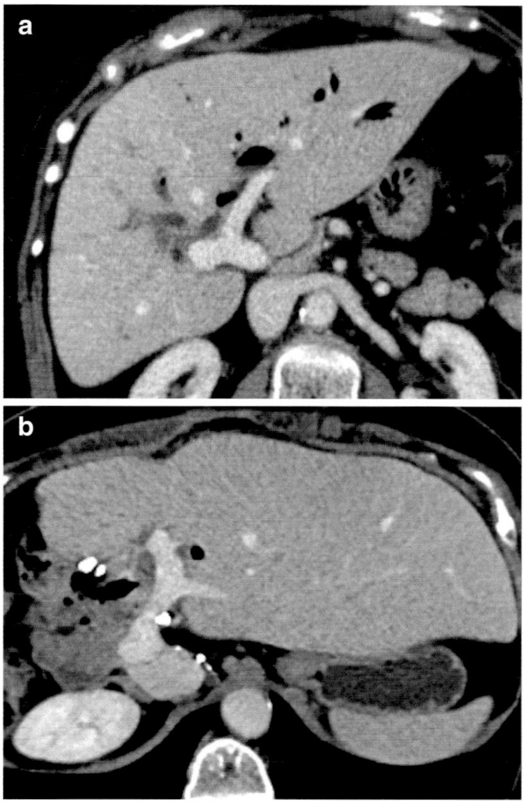

Fig. 21.8 Portal-phase CT performed immediately after right portal branch embolization (**a**) and after right hepatectomy (**b**) show left hepatic lobe hypertrophy obtained thanks to the procedure

Procedure

Ipsilateral or contralateral approaches to the portal vein can be performed. The contralateral approach is easier, but FLR needs to be traversed, with the risk of damaging it. The ipsilateral approach avoids transversing the FLR, but portal branch catheterization is more difficult due to their sharp angle. Once the portal vein is approached, embolic material is delivered until stasis is achieved. Embolic agents described for PVE include n-butyl cyanoacrylate and ethiodized oil, fibrin glue, ethanol, and microparticles (Fig. 21.9) [21].

Complications

The most feared complications are nontarget embolization or thrombosis and hemorrhage. Major periprocedural complications include hemobilia, subcapsular hematoma, infection, and bile leak; minor periprocedural complications include fever and abdominal pain. Transient transaminitis can occur in up to 35% of patients.

21.2.4 Portal Hypertension Treatment Techniques: Transjugular Intrahepatic Portosystemic Shunt and Portal Vein Stenting

Portal hypertension is typically the result of cirrhosis (90% of cases). It is defined as a hepatic venous pressure gradient bigger than 6 mmHg; above 10 mmHg varices may develop, while above 12 mmHg varices may bleed, and other complications can occur like ascites, splenomegaly, thrombocytopenia, and hepatic insufficiency, with hepatic encephalopathy.

TIPS and portal vein stenting are used to treat posthepatic and intrahepatic (TIPS) and prehepatic (portal vein stenting) portal hypertension.

21.2.4.1 Transjugular Intrahepatic Portosystemic Shunt

TIPS is a percutaneously created connection within the liver between the portal and systemic circulations, which diverts portal blood flow into a hepatic vein.

Indications

Indications to perform TIPS include:

- Variceal hemorrhage: TIPS is useful as rescue therapy in patients with active variceal bleeding in case of failure of first-line approaches like endoscopic and pharmacologic treatments. Rates of immediate hemostasis after TIPS range from 90 to 100% [22].
- Portal hypertensive gastropathy, if initial therapy fails and bleeding is severe and refractory.
- Refractory ascites or hepatic hydrothorax not controlled by medical therapy or requiring repeated paracentesis or thoracentesis.
- Budd-Chiari syndrome: hepatic venous outflow tract obstruction not due to cardiac dis-

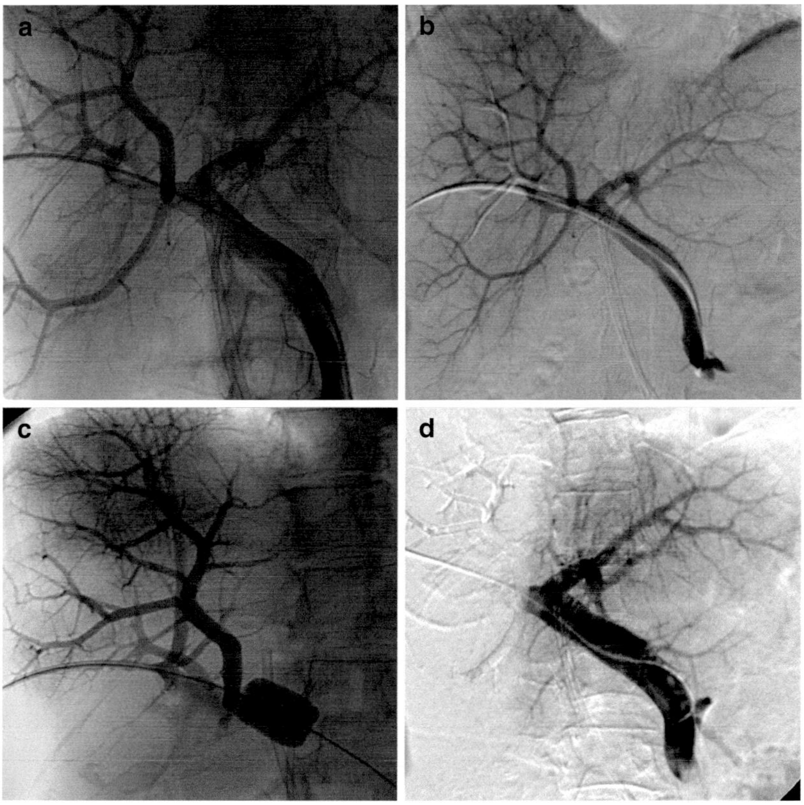

Fig. 21.9 A 68-year-old woman with Klatskin 3a cholangiocarcinoma, candidate to right hepatectomy. Portal embolization was performed to increase FLR. (**a**, **b**) The right portal branch is catheterized. (**c**) An angioplasty balloon is inflated in the right branch to prevent delivery of embolic agent in the left lobe, and then an embolic agent is injected. (**d**) The final control shows complete embolization of the right portal branch and normal vascularization of the left lobe

ease, pericardial disease, or sinusoidal obstruction syndrome (veno-occlusive disease). TIPS placement may be an option:
  - In symptomatic patients with acute or subacute Budd-Chiari syndrome who do not benefit from other treatments.
  - As a temporary measure to treat portal hypertension complications before liver transplantation.
  - In patients with chronic Budd-Chiari syndrome and complications of portal hypertension.

  Anyway, Budd-Chiari is associated with a higher risk of TIPS stenosis or thrombosis than other conditions [23].
- Others: hepatorenal syndrome and sinusoidal obstructive syndrome.

Contraindications

Although there are no absolute contraindications to TIPS creation, several relative contraindications are described:

- Elevated right or left heart pressures.
- Heart failure or severe cardiac valvular insufficiency.
- Rapidly progressive liver failure: elevated model for end-stage liver disease (MELD) score (MELD >24) is associated with a 30-day mortality of 60%.
- Severe hepatic encephalopathy.
- Systemic infection or sepsis (higher risk of TIPS stent colonization).
- Unrelieved biliary obstruction.
- Polycystic liver disease.

- Extensive primary or metastatic hepatic malignancy.
- Severe, uncorrectable coagulopathy [24].

Cross-sectional preprocedural imaging is mandatory to confirm portal vein patency, to evaluate for competing portosystemic shunts, and to demonstrate location/extent of varices and anatomic relationship between portal and hepatic veins.

Procedure

TIPS creation. The right hepatic to right portal vein is the preferred approach. Before proceeding with TIPS creation, free hepatic venous pressure (FHVP) and wedged hepatic vein pressure (WHVP) are usually obtained. WHVP is a measure of hepatic sinusoidal pressure, obtained by occluding the hepatic vein with a balloon. The difference between WHVP and FHVP represents an indirect measure of portal vein pressure. Portal vein access is the most difficult part of the procedure; the optimal intrahepatic portal vein access site is the right portal branch at least 1 cm from the main portal vein bifurcation. Once the portal right branch is accessed with a Colapinto needle, a hydrophilic catheter is exchanged for a calibrated pigtail catheter used to determine the appropriate stent length. Then, an appropriate diameter/length stent is deployed, with a covered portion extending from the portal vein entry site to the hepatic vein/inferior vena cava (IVC) junction and a 2 cm uncovered portion located in the portal vein; the uncovered portion ensures right and left portal branch perfusion. After stent deployment, an angioplasty balloon dilation is performed. Post-TIPS pressure measurements of the portal vein, hepatic vein, and inferior vena cava are obtained, and post-TIPS pressure gradient is determined: if measures are satisfactory, the procedure is completed (Fig. 21.10).

TIPS revision is required in case of stent malfunction, when refractory ascites, stenosis, occlusion, or thrombosis occurs. TIPS is recanalized with percutaneous transluminal angioplasty, or stent placement can be repeated.

TIPS reduction can be performed when an overly effective TIPS causes liver failure or refractory encephalopathy: the goal is to decrease or occlude flow through the shunt.

Outcome

TIPS is a standardized procedure with a high success rate (95%), which guarantees improved control of ascites in 60–85% of cases. However, new or worsened encephalopathy occurs in 25–30% of patients, depending on shunt diameter and degree of portosystemic gradient reduction; often it can be treated medically, but TIPS reduction may be necessary. On the other hand, TIPS stenosis, occlusion, or thrombosis can occur, requiring TIPS revision.

The most fearful periprocedural complication is hemorrhage, which can be intraperitoneal or intraparenchymal. Bile duct injury, acute liver failure or acute increase of cardiac output, central venous, pulmonary wedge pressures which can lead to acute pulmonary edema, and congestive heart failure represent other common complications.

21.2.4.2 Portal Vein Stenting

Prehepatic portal hypertension is determined by noncirrhotic benign or malignant conditions.

The most frequent benign condition is postsurgical adhesive fibrosis, after liver transplant or hepato-biliopancreatic surgery, followed by pancreatitis [25, 26].

Malignant conditions account for mass effect from a surrounding tumor, direct tumor invasion of the pulmonary vein (PV), or PV thrombosis due to a hypercoagulable state in cancer patients [27]. Moreover, the reduced portal blood inflow into the liver parenchyma and the development of portal hypertension limit the options for treating tumors with surgery or transcatheter hepatic arterial chemoembolization [28]. Portal stent placement is indicated to relieve symptoms of portal hypertension and to prevent future adverse events related to untreated PV stenosis.

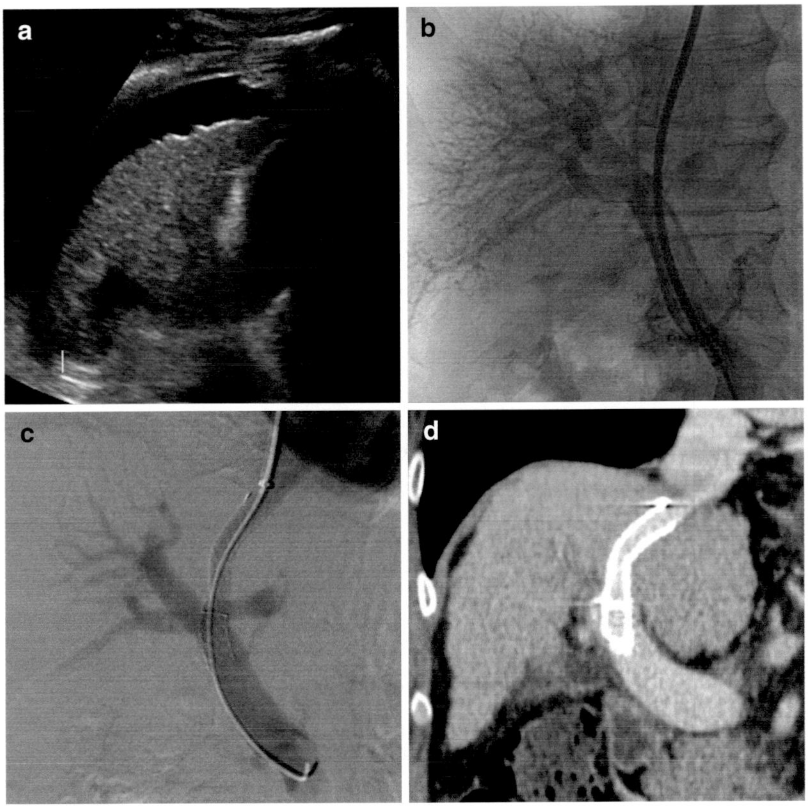

Fig. 21.10 A 60-year-old man with hepatitis C virus-related cirrhosis, refractory ascites, and variceal bleeding. (**a**) US shows a cirrhotic liver surrounded by ascites. (**b**, **c**) TIPS confection is performed between the middle hepatic vein and the right portal branch. (**d**) CT performed 3 months after the procedure demonstrates the metallic stent, patent

Procedure

After diagnostic angiography with confirmation of significant stenosis, stenting is performed using balloon-expandable stents or self-expanding nitinol stents 40–60 mm in length and oversized in diameter by 1–2 mm as compared with the adjacent PV; balloon-expandable stents guarantee a more precise result (Fig. 21.11). In cases of residual stenosis, stents are dilated with balloons at the size of the prestenotic portal segment.

Complications

Major complications include liver abscesses, intraperitoneal bleeding, bile injury, or biliary bleeding [25]. Other mild complications have been reported (fever and abdominal pain).

Outcome

Recent studies described long-term stent patency of 91% in stenosis determined by benign conditions and varying from 64% to 100% for stenosis related to malignant conditions [27].

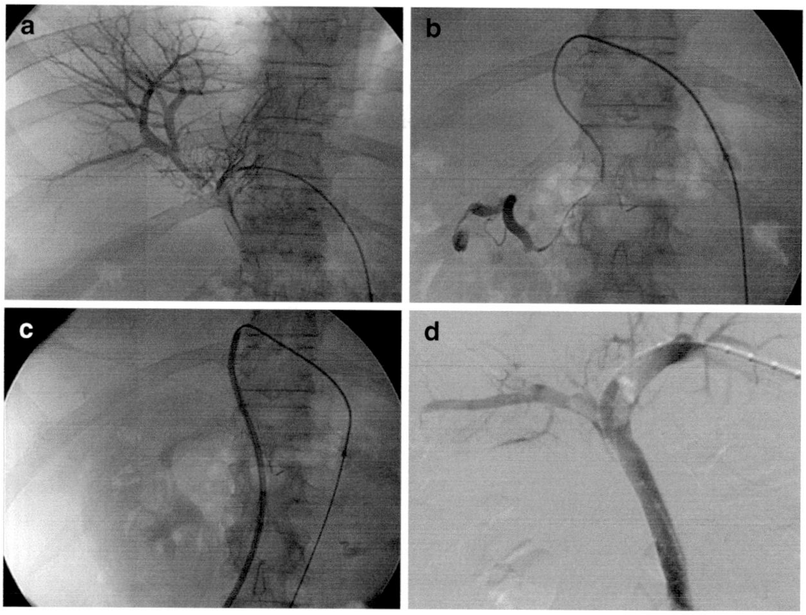

Fig. 21.11 A patient with complete occlusion of the portal vein. (**a**) Left access through S3 was performed. Venography shows complete obstruction of the portal vein. (**b**, **c**) After surpassing the stenosis, angioplasty is performed, and a stent is positioned. At the final control (**d**) portal vein is now patent

21.3 Hepatic and Pancreatic Oncologic Procedures

21.3.1 Hepatic Vascular Procedures: Transcatheter Arterial Chemoembolization

TACE is a transcatheter treatment for hepatic primitive and metastatic tumors by intra-arterial injection of a chemotherapeutic agent with or followed by embolic particles. It takes advantage of the fact that cancers receive blood supply from the hepatic artery, whereas liver parenchyma has a dual supply from the hepatic artery and portal vein. The antitumor effect is due to ischemic necrosis and the prolonged concentration of the chemotherapeutic drug within the tumor.

Two major subtypes of TACE are described:

- Conventional TACE uses Lipiodol as a carrier agent for chemotherapeutic cytotoxic drugs like mitomycin-C, doxorubicin, or cisplatin. Chemolipiodol mixture is injected directly into the hepatic artery via a catheter, and it is preferentially retained within abnormal tumor microvasculature. Chemolipiodol mixture is followed by a particulate embolic agent to produce ischemia and decrease washout of chemotherapeutic from the target.
- Drug-eluting bead transarterial chemoembolization (DEB-TACE) uses beads impregnated with chemotherapeutic agents, such as doxorubicin or irinotecan. Embolic beads have decreased washout into systemic circulation compared with chemolipiodol (less systemic adverse effects) and act as occlusive embolic agents, giving an ischemic effect.

DEB-TACE has been demonstrated not to be superior to conventional TACE in efficacy and safety [29].

Indications

- HCC: Barcelona Clinic Liver Cancer (BCLC) is one of the most used HCC staging classifications, comprehensive of four stages based on the extent of the primary lesion, performance status, vascular invasion, and extrahepatic spread. BCLC system recommends TACE only for nonsurgical patients in intermediate stage B; anyway, indications for TACE are extended, for example, in stage 0, A, or B patients who are waiting for liver transplantation to prevent the tumor from progressing ("bridge to transplant"; Milan/UNOS criteria for liver transplantation: 1 tumor <5 cm or up to 3 tumors <3 cm, no extrahepatic disease, no vascular invasion) (Fig. 21.12) [30].

- Metastatic neuroendocrine tumor (NET): nonsurgical candidates with liver-predominant disease or major symptoms uncontrolled by octreotide are the best candidates [31, 32].

Contraindications

- Liver failure: hyperbilirubinemia >2 mg/dl, Child-Pugh class C liver disease, and liver parenchyma involved by tumor >50%.
- Portal vein thrombosis without the development of portal-portal collateral flow. When portal vein thrombosis occurs, transarterial hepatic radioembolization can be considered (microspheres loaded with a radioactive compound such as yttrium-90 or iodine-131/rhenium-188-labeled Lipiodol) [33].
- Arterioportal or arteriovenous shunting that cannot be safely reduced during the procedure.
- Poor baseline functional status: ECOG Performance Status Scale ≥2.

Preprocedural Assessment

Contrast-enhanced CT or MRI should be performed to assess tumor burden (number and dimension of tumors, liver-confined disease, and liver involvement <50%), vascular anatomy, and portal patency.

Laboratory parameters should be evaluated: renal functionality, bleeding risk (international normalized ratio <1.5, platelet count >50,000/μl), and markers of liver function, liver injury, and cholestasis. Preprocedure prophylactic antibiot-

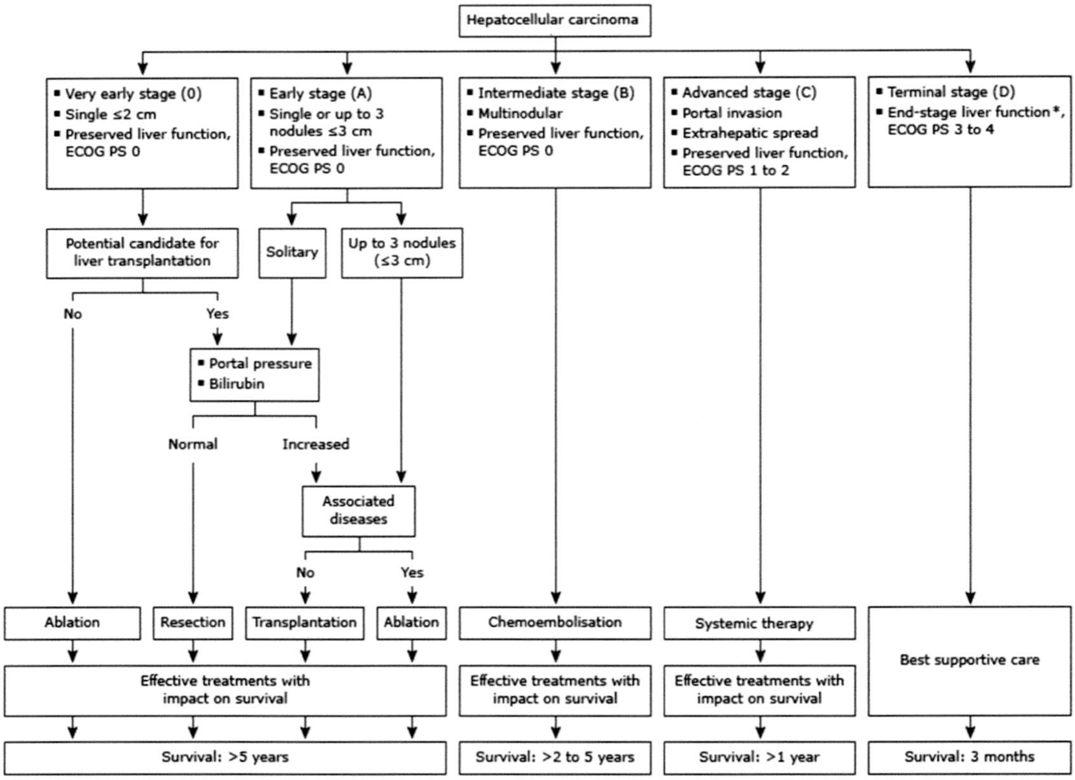

Fig. 21.12 Barcelona Clinic Liver Cancer – Staging System

ics with a broad spectrum should be administered.

Procedure

After the common femoral artery is accessed, a diagnostic angiography of the superior mesenteric artery is mandatory to check for an origin of the right hepatic artery from it (found in up to 30% of the population) [34], and portal vein patency is controlled. The guidewire is advanced through the celiac axis until the lumen of the proper hepatic artery (origins from the celiac axis in 89% of cases). Subselective right and left hepatic angiographies are obtained, as indicated by tumor location. Treatment should be performed from a position as selective as possible; cystic artery and right gastric artery are nontarget arteries. Chemoembolic material is administered into the target vessel under fluoroscopy. The procedural endpoint is blood stasis in all pedicles supplying the tumor and flow preservation in nontargeted arteries (Fig. 21.13).

Postprocedural Complications and Management

Liver failure can occur, due to hepatic insufficiency or hepatic infarction. Other periprocedural complications include access site complications, nontarget embolization, and postembolization syndrome (fever, pain, and nausea). Delayed complications are hepatic abscess onset, chemical cholecystitis, and biliary stricture or necrosis.

Clinical and imaging assessment of the outcome can be planned 4 weeks after the treatment.

21.3.2 Hepatic and Pancreatic Biopsies

A biopsy consists of nonfocal tissue acquisition from an organ, to assess diffuse disease, or targeted tissue acquisition from a lesion, using a large-gauge needle to perform pathologic or microbiological analyses.

Fine-needle aspiration (FNA) requires a smaller-gauge needle, and cytological analyses are usually performed on the acquired sample.

Indications

Indications are to diagnose, stage, or grade diffuse parenchymal diseases, to evaluate lesions of unknown etiology, and assess for pathologic, microbiologic, or cytological analyses; to grade or stage a known malignancy.

Contraindications

Contraindications are uncorrectable bleeding diathesis, lack of safe access, and presence of echinococcal cysts (due to the risk of anaphylaxis).

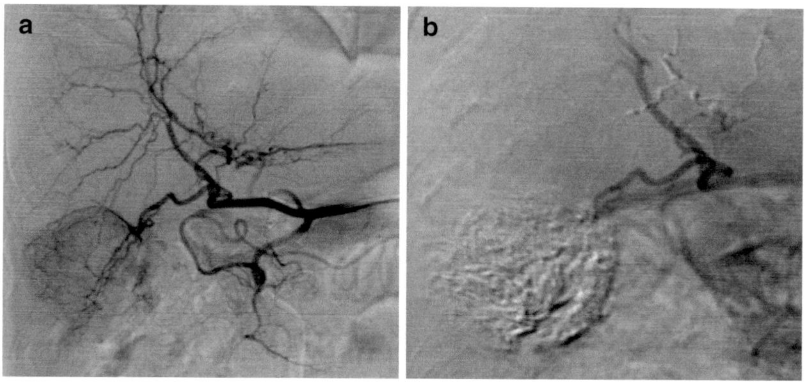

Fig. 21.13 A 68-year-old woman with HCC. (**a**) Angiography performed before the procedure shows staining of the neoplasm located in the right hepatic lobe. (**b**) After chemoembolization, the control shows the disappearance of the tumor staining

Procedure

Preprocedural imaging is reviewed before starting to assess lesion location, surrounding structures, and the best route to the lesion. Biopsies can be performed under US (Fig. 21.14) or CT guidance. US guidance does not use radiations, has lower costs than CT, and provides real-time anatomy and needle position information; however, it is limited by body habitus and by gas and bone; moreover it requires experience and hand-eye coordination. CT guidance guarantees a better resolution of the target but is more expensive and requires longer procedure times and radiation exposure.

Single-needle or coaxial-needle techniques have been described to perform FNAs or biopsies.

The coaxial-needle technique allows to obtain multiple samples, while the coaxial-needle technique is in place, minimizing the number of passes through tissues; moreover, tract embolization is allowed, if bleeding occurs. However, the coaxial-needle technique can be difficult to apply for superficial lesions and has an increased risk of bleeding because the coaxial needle must be large enough to accept the biopsy/FNA device.

Hepatic Procedures While performing nonfocal biopsies, subcostal or subxiphoid accesses are preferred to intercostal access, because they cause less pain and pneumo–/hemothorax risk is reduced. If target lesion biopsy is required, normal hepatic parenchyma should be present along the needle path, to provide a tamponade effect if hemorrhage occurs.

Pancreatic Procedures Pancreatic US-guided biopsies can be performed transabdominally or under endoscopic ultrasound (EUS) guidance. With the transabdominal approach, the US probe gives the chance to displace intestinal bowel loops if they are interposed in the needle tract and allows to avoid the dilated pancreatic duct. The risk of postprocedural pancreatitis is comparable to EUS-guided procedures [35].

Complications

Pain or vasovagal reaction may occur after the procedure. Hemorrhage is the most feared complication.

21.3.3 Percutaneous Ablation of Malignant Lesions

Ablation of malignant lesions can be done by applying thermal or non-thermal local therapies to achieve lesion eradication or reduction under imaging guidance (US or CT).

Indications are to cure liver lesions of 3–5 cm or less, to alleviate symptoms in inoperable tumors, or to control disease progression through debulking.

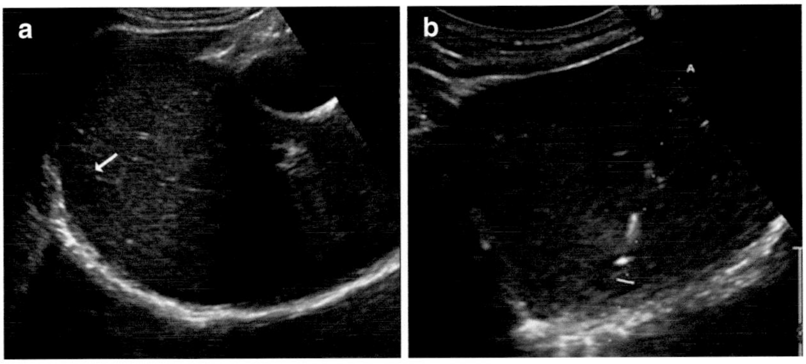

Fig. 21.14 A patient with pancreatic adenocarcinoma and a hepatic lesion. (**a**) At US, the lesion appears hypoechoic to the surrounding hepatic parenchyma (arrow). (**b**) To confirm the nature of the lesion, a US-guided percutaneous biopsy was performed. The image shows the correct placement of the needle, with the tip inside the lesion. Cytology confirmed the metastatic nature of the lesion

21.3.3.1 Thermal Ablations

Thermal ablation of a tumor may occur with extremely high or low temperatures that induce cell membrane injury, apoptosis, and coagulative necrosis.

Heat-ablated lesions can be differentiated into three zones:

- Central zone, near the application tip, which undergoes coagulative necrosis.
- Peripheral zone of sublethal hyperthermia for the cells. Heat reaches this zone from the central zone thanks to heat conduction.
- Surrounding zone of the tissue unaffected by ablation.

Tumor destruction occurs in two phases, through direct and indirect damage.

Direct cellular damage requires a temperature of at least 60 °C to develop rapidly, thanks to protein denaturation. A temperature of 40–45 °C leads to cellular damage only after prolonged exposure (30–60 minutes). Many mechanisms of damage have been proposed, such as membrane destabilization, mitochondrial dysfunction, and inhibition of DNA replication.

Indirect damage is delayed heat damage induced after cessation of thermal ablation. Proposed mechanisms are apoptosis, ischemia, and stimulation of immune response [36].

Complete thermal ablation of a lesion is reached if the entire lesion volume and an external normal parenchymal margin are treated at cytotoxic temperatures.

Subtypes of thermal ablations are radiofrequency ablation (RFA), microwave ablation (MWA), cryoablation, laser ablation, and high-intensity focused ultrasound (HIFU).

Radiofrequency Ablation

This technique is performed by placing one or more radiofrequency electrodes inside the tumor. A high-frequency alternating current generates temperatures between 60 and 70 °C by inducing frictional heating when the tissue ions attempt to follow the changing direction of the current. Frictional heating causes coagulative necrosis of the lesion. Higher temperatures char the tissue immediately surrounding the probe, making the treatment useless because burned tissue increases its impedance and limits electrical conduction to the surrounding areas.

This technique is less effective in inhomogeneous tissues and near vessels larger than 3 mm: the flow of the vessels cools the surrounding area, a phenomenon called the heat-sink effect.

Cell damage also releases many immunogenic substrates, activating inflammatory responses against the tumor [37].

Microwave Ablation

In MWA an antenna is placed inside the tumor to create an intratumoral magnetic field between 900 and 2500 MHz. The oscillating magnetic field forces water molecules to continuously realign (rotating dipoles) and generate heat.

MWA does not rely on electric currents and is not subject to tissue conductivity or impedance: tissues can be heated faster and at higher temperatures than RFA (100–150 °C).

Compared to RFA this technique is less sensitive to heat-sink effects and can better heat larger volumes of the tissue, but it is a weak stimulator of the antitumoral inflammatory response [38].

21.3.3.2 Non-thermal Ablation

Irreversible Electroporation

To perform electroporation a probe is used to generate high voltage electrical pulses that alter the electric potential of cellular membranes, creating nanoscale defects in them and increasing their permeabilization.

Electroporation can be reversible or irreversible. Irreversible Electroporation (IRE) occurs when the magnitude and duration of the electrical pulses overwhelm the capacity of adaptation of the cell, causing its death. At least 80–100 pulses and a voltage amplitude of 3000 V are required.

The non-thermal nature of the technique, if set correctly, does not damage nearby structures (especially blood vessels), allowing the ablation of lesions untreatable with thermal techniques [39].

Hepatic Percutaneous Treatments

RFA and MWA are the most used techniques to treat hepatic primitive and metastatic lesions.

RFA must ablate the lesion with a rim of at least 5–10 mm to address the microscopic, nonvisible spread of neoplastic cells. Generally, a probe covers an area of 5 cm of maximum diameter, allowing the treatment of lesions up to 3 cm. Lesions cannot be treated if near the hepatic dome, liver capsule, heart, and major vascular or biliary structures.

MWA is effective in the treatment of larger lesions (measuring up to 5 cm) and of neoplasms near blood vessels, not being affected by the heat sink effect [40, 41].

Indications

Ablation techniques can be used to treat:

- HCC: indications, according to the BCLC, are patients of 0 and A class noncandidate for liver resections.
- Metastatic disease: ablation is reported in colorectal and NET liver metastasis. There are no clear indications, but it has to be oligometastatic liver disease.

Contraindications

Contraindications are a life expectancy inferior to 6 months, Child-Pugh C cirrhosis, active infection, decompensated liver disease, vascular or bile ducts invasion, extrahepatic spreading of the disease, coagulative alterations, and absence of a percutaneous window.

Follow-Up

Serial follow-up is important:

- Imaging (with the same modality of preprocedure imaging): a successful treatment causes tumor necrosis, with a lack of contrast enhancement of the lesion. It should be performed 1–2 months after the treatment.
- Laboratoristic: blood tumor markers and measurement of liver function.

Complications

Complications can be immediate (hemorrhage) or delayed (biliary strictures, infections, and tumor track seeding). Due to the development of systemic inflammatory response, a post-ablation syndrome can occur from 2 to 10 days after the procedure, with self-limiting fever, myalgia, and fatigue onset.

Outcome

In patients with unresectable early-stage HCC smaller than 3 cm, RFA is the most commonly used technique. Complete necrosis of the lesion is reported in 90% of procedures, with 5-year survival rates of 40–70%. MWA of lesions up to 5 cm presents a similar outcome.

Treatment of metastasis allows a 5-year disease-free survival of 23.9% compared to 39.7% of surgery [41].

Pancreatic Percutaneous Treatments

Indications

Locally advanced pancreatic adenocarcinoma (stage III) that remains stable after chemotherapy can be treated with ablation techniques to control a local, unresectable disease.

RFA is difficult to perform for the risk of damaging structures around and inside the tumor, as the duodenum and vessels. For this reason, it is rarely performed, only in specialized centers and in mass-forming pancreatic neoplasms.

IRE is a new technique, preferred as safer than RFA: being a non-thermal procedure, it can be used to treat neoplasms entailing vessels [42, 43].

Complications

Reported complications range from hemorrhage to thrombosis, pseudoaneurysms, development of abscess and pancreatic fistula, and intestinal burn lesions.

Follow-Up

Follow-up exams after the procedure include:

- Blood tumor markers: carbohydrate antigen 19–9 and carcinoembryonic antigen levels.
- Imaging: CT or MRI performed 1 month after ablation and then every 2 or 3 months [16].

Outcome

For both RFA and IRE, oncologic results are controversial. Many studies have shown no increase in overall survival of patients who underwent these procedures compared to those who did not [42].

References

1. Perez-Johnston R, Deipolyi AR, Covey AM. Percutaneous biliary interventions. Gastroenterol Clin N Am. 2018;47(3):621–41.
2. Tapping CR, Byass OR, Cast JEI. Cytological sampling versus forceps biopsy during percutaneous transhepatic biliary drainage and analysis of factors predicting success. Cardiovasc Intervent Radiol. 2012;35(4):883–9.
3. Ayuso JR, Pagés M, Darnell A. Imaging bile duct tumors: staging. Abdom Imaging. 2013;38(5):1071–81.
4. Brown KT, Covey AM. Management of malignant biliary obstruction. Tech Vasc Interv Radiol. 2008;11(1):43–50.
5. Farges O, Regimbeau JM, Fuks D, Le Treut YP, Cherqui D, Bachellier P, et al. Multicentre European study of preoperative biliary drainage for hilar cholangiocarcinoma. Br J Surg. 2013;100(2):274–83.
6. Kapoor BS, Mauri G, Lorenz JM. Management of biliary strictures: state-of-the-art review. Radiology. 2018;289(3):590–603.
7. Fidelman N. Benign biliary strictures: diagnostic evaluation and approaches to percutaneous treatment. Tech Vasc Interv Radiol. 2015;18(4):210–7.
8. Copelan A, Kapoor BS. Choledocholithiasis: diagnosis and management. Tech Vasc Interv Radiol. 2015;18(4):244–55.
9. Kiriyama S, Kozaka K, Takada T, Strasberg SM, Pitt HA, Gabata T, et al. Tokyo guidelines 2018: diagnostic criteria and severity grading of acute cholangitis. J Hepatobiliary Pancreat Sci. 2018;25(1):17–30.
10. Mayumi T, Okamoto K, Takada T, Strasberg SM, Solomkin JS, Schlossberg D, et al. Tokyo guidelines 2018: management bundles for acute cholangitis and cholecystitis. J Hepatobiliary Pancreat Sci. 2018;25(1):96–100.
11. Koch M, Garden OJ, Padbury R, Rahbari NN, Adam R, Capussotti L, et al. Bile leakage after hepatobiliary and pancreatic surgery: a definition and grading of severity by the International Study Group of Liver Surgery. Surgery. 2011;149(5):680–8.
12. Mansueto G, Gatti FL, Boninsegna E, Conci S, Guglielmi A, Contro A. Biliary leakage after hepatobiliary and pancreatic surgery: a classification system to guide the proper percutaneous treatment. Cardiovasc Intervent Radiol. 2020;43(2):302–10.
13. Mauri G, Michelozzi C, Melchiorre F, Poretti D, Pedicini V, Salvetti M, et al. Benign biliary strictures refractory to standard bilioplasty treated using polydoxanone biodegradable biliary stents: retrospective multicentric data analysis on 107 patients. Eur Radiol. 2016;26(11):4057–63.
14. Wallace MJ. Image-guided interventions in oncology. Surg Oncol Clin N Am. 2014;23(4):937–55.
15. Ginat D, Saad WEA. Cholecystostomy and Transcholecystic biliary access. Tech Vasc Interv Radiol. 2008;11(1):2–13.
16. Brandt CW. Diagnostic imaging. Interventional procedures. 2nd ed. Salt Lake City: Elsevier, Inc.; 2017.
17. Miyayama S, Yamakado K, Anai H, Abo D, Minami T, Takaki H, et al. Guidelines on the use of gelatin sponge particles in embolotherapy. Jpn J Radiol. 2014;32(4):242–50.
18. Lopera JE. Embolization in trauma: principles and techniques. Semin Intervent Radiol. 2010;27(1):14–28.
19. Vennarecci G, Laurenzi A, Santoro R, Colasanti M, Lepiane P, Ettorre GM. The ALPPS procedure: a surgical option for hepatocellular carcinoma with major vascular invasion. World J Surg. 2014;38(6):1498–503.
20. Vauthey JN, Dixon E, Abdalla EK, Helton WS, Pawlik TM, Taouli B, et al. Pretreatment assessment of hepatocellular carcinoma: expert consensus statement. HPB. 2010;12(5):289–99.
21. May BJ, Madoff DC. Portal vein embolization: rationale, technique, and current application. Semin Interv Radiol. 2012;29(2):81–9.
22. Zhu Y, Wang X, Xi X, Li X, Luo X, Yang L. Emergency Transjugular intrahepatic portosystemic shunt: an effective and safe treatment for uncontrolled Variceal bleeding. J Gastrointest Surg. 2019;23(11):2193–200.
23. Bachet JB, Condat B, Hagège H, Plessier A, Consigny Y, Belghiti J, et al. Long-term portosystemic shunt patency as a determinant of outcome in Budd-Chiari syndrome. J Hepatol. 2007;46(1):60–8.
24. Dariushnia SR, Haskal ZJ, Midia M, Martin LG, Gregory Walker T, Kalva SP, et al. Quality improvement guidelines for transjugular intrahepatic portosystemic shunts. J Vasc Interv Radiol. 2016;27(1):1–7.
25. Shan H, Xiao XS, Huang MS, Ouyang Q, Jiang ZB. Portal venous stent placement for treatment of portal hypertension caused by benign main portal vein stenosis. World J Gastroenterol. 2005;11(21):3315–8.
26. Khan A, Kleive D, Aandahl EM, Fosby B, Line PD, Dorenberg E, et al. Portal vein stent placement after hepatobiliary and pancreatic surgery. Langenbeck's Arch Surg. 2020;405(5):657–64.
27. Park JH, Yeo JH, Kim YS, Ahn HK, Sym S, Shin D, et al. Portal vein stent for symptomatic malignant portal vein stenosis: a single-center experience. Curr Probl Cancer. 2020;44(2):100476.
28. Zhou ZQ, Lee JH, Song KB, Hwang JW, Kim SC, Lee YJ, et al. Clinical usefulness of portal venous stent in hepatobiliary pancreatic cancers. ANZ J Surg. 2014;84(5):346–52.
29. Raoul JL, Forner A, Bolondi L, Cheung TT, Kloeckner R, de Baere T. Updated use of TACE for hepatocellular carcinoma treatment: how and when to use it based on clinical evidence. Cancer Treat Rev. 2019;72:28–36.
30. Forner A, Llovet JM, Bruix J. Hepatocellular carcinoma. Lancet. 2012;379(9822):1245–55.
31. Pavel M, Baudin E, Couvelard A, Krenning E, Öberg K, Steinmüller T, et al. ENETS consensus guidelines

for the management of patients with liver and other distant metastases from neuroendocrine neoplasms of foregut, midgut, hindgut, and unknown primary. Neuroendocrinology. 2012;95(2):157–76.
32. De Baere T, Deschamps F, Tselikas L, Ducreux M, Planchard D, Pearson E, et al. GEP-NETs update: interventional radiology: role in the treatment of liver metastases from GEP-NETs. Eur J Endocrinol. 2015;172(4):151–66.
33. Sacco R, Conte C, Tumino E, Parisi G, Giacomelli L, Metrangolo S, et al. Transarterial radioembolization for hepatocellular carcinoma: a review. J Hepatocell Carcinoma. 2016;3:25–9.
34. Favelier S, Germain T, Genson PY, Cercueil JP, Denys A, Krausé D, et al. Anatomy of liver arteries for interventional radiology. Diagn Interv Imaging. 2015;96(6):537–46.
35. Terracciano F, Marra A, Ippolito AM, Bossa F, Sitajolo K, Amoruso A, et al. Transabdominal ultrasound-guided pancreatic biopsy: a neglected but safe, effective and inexpensive procedure that needs to be re-juvinalized. J Ultrasound. 2021;24(2):175–82.
36. Chu KF, Dupuy DE. Thermal ablation of tumours: biological mechanisms and advances in therapy. Nat Rev Cancer. 2014;14(3):199–208.
37. Hong K, Georgiades C. Radiofrequency ablation: mechanism of action and devices. J Vasc Interv Radiol. 2010;21(8S):S179–86.
38. Lubner MG, Brace CL, Hinshaw JL, Lee FT. Microwave tumor ablation: mechanism of action, clinical results, and devices. J Vasc Interv Radiol. 2010;21(S8):S192–203.
39. Geboers B, Scheffer HJ, Graybill PM, Ruarus AH, Nieuwenhuizen S, Puijk RS, et al. High-voltage electrical pulses in oncology: irreversible electroporation, electrochemotherapy, gene electrotransfer, electrofusion, and electroimmunotherapy. Radiology. 2020;295(2):254–72.
40. Decadt B, Siriwardena AK. Radiofrequency ablation of liver tumours: systematic review. Lancet Oncol. 2004;5(9):550–60.
41. Izzo F, Granata V, Grassi R, Fusco R, Palaia R, Delrio P, et al. Radiofrequency ablation and microwave ablation in liver tumors: an update. Oncologist. 2019;24(10):e990–e1005.
42. Paiella S, De Pastena M, Romeo F, D'Onofrio M, Fontana M, Pea A, et al. Ablation treatments in unresectable pancreatic cancer. Minerva Chir. 2019;74(3):263–9.
43. Timmer FEF, Geboers B, Ruarus AH, Schouten EAC, Nieuwenhuizen S, Puijk RS, et al. Irreversible electroporation for locally advanced pancreatic cancer. Tech Vasc Interv Radiol. 2020;23(2):100675.

Correction to: Chronic Pancreatitis: Differentiation from Pancreatic Adenocarcinoma

Cristiana Boldrini, Valerio Di Paola, Luca Russo, Simone Palma, Maria Luisa De Cicco, Silvia De Vizio, Angelica Marra, Silvia Amodeo, Roberta Dattoli, and Riccardo Manfredi

Correction to: Chapter 13 In: B. Sureka (ed.), *Hepato-Pancreatico Biliary Imaging*, https://doi.org/10.1007/978-981-95-1699-5_13

- Corrections needed:
  - Bibliographic Citation 1 must be replaced.
  - Citation 27 must be replaced with a new reference.
  - Citation 28 must also be replaced with a new reference.

- Correct references:
  - **CITATION 1:**
    Schima W, Böhm G, Rösch CS, Klaus A, Függer R, Kopf H. Mass-forming pancreatitis versus pancreatic ductal adenocarcinoma: CT and MR imaging for differentiation. Cancer Imaging. 2020;20(1):52.

  - **CITATION 27:**
    Yadav AK, Sharma R, Kandasamy D, Pradhan RK, Garg PK, Bhalla AS, et al. Perfusion CT–can it resolve the pancreatic carcinoma versus mass forming chronic pancreatitis conundrum? Pancreatology. 2016;16:979–87.

  - **CITATION 28:**
    Zhang TT, Wang L, Liu HH, Zhang CY, Li XM, Lu JP, Wang DB. Differentiation of pancreatic carcinoma and mass-forming focal pancreatitis: qualitative and quantitative assessment by dynamic contrast-enhanced MRI combined with diffusion-weighted imaging. Oncotarget. 2017 Jan 3;8(1):1744–59. https://doi.org/10.18632/oncotarget.12120.

The updated version of this chapter can be found at https://doi.org/10.1007/978-981-95-1699-5_13

© The Author(s), under exclusive license to Springer Nature Singapore Pte Ltd. 2026

B. Sureka (ed.), *Hepato-Pancreatico Biliary Imaging*,
https://doi.org/10.1007/978-981-95-1699-5_22

MIX
Papier aus verantwortungsvollen Quellen
Paper from responsible sources
FSC® C105338

If you have any concerns about our products,
you can contact us on
ProductSafety@springernature.com

In case Publisher is established outside the EU,
the EU authorized representative is:
Springer Nature Customer Service Center GmbH
Europaplatz 3, 69115 Heidelberg, Germany

Printed by Libri Plureos GmbH
in Hamburg, Germany